PRINCIPLES OF VETERINARY THERAPEUTICS

PRINCIPLES OF
VETERINARY THERAPEUTICS

BY
R EINSTEIN
R S JONES
A KNIFTON
G A STARMER

Longman
Scientific &
Technical

Longman Scientific & Technical,
Longman Group UK Limited,
Longman House, Burnt Mill, Harlow,
Essex, CM20 2JE, England
and Associated Companies throughout the world.

First published 1994

ISBN 0 582 02963 5

British Library Cataloguing in Publication Data
A CIP record for this book is available from the British Library

Set in 10/12.5 pt Plantin
Produced by Longman Singapore Publishers (Pte) Ltd.
Printed in Singapore

CONTENTS

Contents

PREFACE

This book is primarily intended for students of veterinary science. However, pharmacology is a rapidly changing discipline and this book will also be of value to practising veterinarians who need access to current texts. The authors' aim is to explain basic pharmacology as a foundation for therapeutic practice. A deliberate decision not to include reference lists at the conclusion of each chapter reflects the opinion of the authors that undergraduate students are unlikely to find these useful.

As with most subjects in the study of veterinary science, pharmacology and therapeutics are complicated by considerable species variation. The problem is compounded in these disciplines because much of the information base for both the fundamental principles of pharmacology and the applied aspects of therapeutics is derived from studies in man. However, it is commonly found that the mechanism of action of drugs is similar in man and animals and in many instances drugs originally developed for use in man have become established in veterinary medicine. The converse, movement of drugs from animal use to use in man, is less common, but not unknown. In this book, where data relating to the actions, effects and uses of a drug have been obtained from human studies, this point is noted but the reader should be aware of the possibility of applying the information to animals and the potential for the use of that drug in animals.

The problem of doses to be used in different species is another which commonly confronts the veterinarian. Various sources often give conflicting information on dose size. The doses in this book were selected after consideration of the manufacturers' data sheets (where applicable) and consultation with colleagues who have recognized expertise in the field of medicine concerned. The reader is also referred to the recent publication of *The Veterinary Formulary* by the Royal Pharmaceutical Society of Great Britain.

The rapidity with which knowledge in pharmacology is growing and the continual evolution of new drugs present problems in the control of medications administered to food animals. Furthermore, at the time of writing, a product licence review was in progress in the United Kingdom. Thus both the availability of drugs and the withdrawal periods for those which are available are constantly changing and an awareness of the status of any medication to be prescribed must remain the responsibility of the veterinarian.

We are particularly grateful to our many colleagues in the Department of Veterinary Preclinical Science and Veterinary Clinical Science at the University of Liverpool who have given freely of their time and advice and also to Dr I. E. Hughes, University of Leeds, Associate Professor E. J. Mylecharane, Dr J. E. Maddison and Ms A. McGregor (University of Sydney) for their comments and suggestions. The help and stimulus of many generations of students are also gratefully acknowledged.

R. EINSTEIN
R. S. JONES
A. KNIFTON
G. A. STARMER
August 1993

CHAPTER 1

INTRODUCTION

Introduction—general principles of pharmacology

What pharmacology is all about

In the broadest sense, a drug is any chemical substance which modifies the function of living tissue. Pharmacology is the study of the properties of drugs and their actions on living tissue. Practical considerations dictate that the main focus of attention is on those drugs which maintain or restore health. The science of pharmacology is closely linked with a number of other biological sciences—physiology, biochemistry, toxicology, microbiology and pathology. Pharmacology can be divided into a number of sub-disciplines. Pharmacodynamics is the study of how drugs work and the effects they produce. In pharmacokinetics the movement of drugs within the body is studied. The rates at which drugs are absorbed, distributed into body compartments, metabolized and excreted are measured or calculated. This forms the basis for the determination of optimal dosage schedules. Clinical pharmacology is the study of the effects of drugs in the clinical situation and includes the kinetics of drugs under clinical conditions.

Therapeutics is the application of the science of pharmacology in the clinical situation. Thus, the practice of therapeutics—the use of drugs in the treatment of disease—is a major part of the work of the veterinarian. A sound knowledge of the science of pharmacology, together with some aspects of toxicology, will provide the best basis for rational therapeutics.

Sources of drugs

The earliest drugs for use in both human and veterinary medicine were derived from plant sources. Later, the extraction of active principles from animals provided useful drugs. With a few notable exceptions, the drugs most commonly used today are synthetic chemical compounds, although plants may still provide the starting material for these syntheses. The use of synthetic drugs allows more stringent quality control and obviates the need for biological standardization of plant or animal extracts. It is interesting to note that some of the older drug mixtures, which contain plant material, are still manufactured. To what extent they are prescribed and used is not known.

Standardization of drugs

The commercial production of pure chemical substances for use as medicines does not usually present insurmountable problems. The majority of drugs in use today are synthesized by drug companies and strict quality control is part of the standard procedure. There are still some drugs which are prepared by isolation of an active principle from a natural source, either animal or plant. In these cases, where it may not be possible to purify the substance completely, standardization is more difficult. The older method of assay in a biological system (bioassay) is still used. In general, bioassay is a sensitive and accurate method for determining the potency of extracted material, which is expressed in terms of the response it elicits in the test system. This can be quantified in terms of arbitrary units, where a unit of activity refers to a standard preparation and is defined in terms of biological response.

Nomenclature

One of the common problems in the early stages of the study of pharmacology is the dauntingly long list of drug names which confronts the student. To further aggravate the trouble, every drug has at least three names, and often many more. The three names which all drugs have are:

1. Chemical name. This is a precise chemical description of the structure of the compound and, as such, may be long and unsuitable for general daily use.
2. Approved (generic, trivial, official or nonproprietary) name. In the very early days of investigation of a new drug it is usually known by a company code number. If some potentially useful biological activity is detected, further experiments are conducted and when the drug is approved for use, an approved name is given to the compound. From that time, regardless of which manufacturer synthesizes the drug, it will retain the same approved name. A number of substances have American approved names which differ from the English names. For example, the approved names of the same analgesic drug are pethidine in the UK and

meperidine in the USA. Where this applies, both names are given in this book. These differences should be borne in mind when consulting American texts.

3. Trade (or brand) name. When a drug is ready for sale the manufacturer will give the product a trade name. This name distinguishes the company's brand of a particular drug from that of any other manufacturer. Where a drug is marketed by a number of different companies, it will have a corresponding number of different trade names. Furthermore, it is not uncommon for a company to include the same drug in a number of different combinations and formulations, hence the possibility of a multiplicity of names.

In this book, as is customary in textbooks, approved names are used throughout. Trade names are usually used when writing prescriptions; commercial interests will ensure that the veterinarian becomes aware of these. Different preparations of the same drug are not necessarily equi-efficient as medicines, but a debate on the merits of brand name vs. generic prescribing is beyond the scope of this book.

References, pharmacopoeias

The *British Pharmacopoeia (Veterinary)* is published every five years. It contains 'Information relating to substances and articles which are or may be used in the practice of veterinary medicine or veterinary surgery'. It consists of monographs describing the preparation of veterinary medicines, except where these are included in the *British Pharmacopoeia* (which is concerned primarily with medicines for human use) and a Formulary, in which the general requirements for dosage forms are laid down. In the Formulary, all monographs are included in full, regardless of listing in the *British Pharmacopoeia*. Thus, those concerned with veterinary medicines have a statement concerning the quality of each product which is expected to be demonstrable at any time during its accepted shelf-life.

Information on actions, uses and doses also appears for many products. This, in contrast to the other sections, is not mandatory. Other areas covered are specifications for immunological products, definitions of reagents, methods of analysis to be used and infra-red spectra for the identification of substances.

The *European Pharmacopoeia* is published by the Council of Europe. Many of its monographs are included in the *British Pharmacopoeia* and the *British Pharmacopoeia (Veterinary)* in an edited format, so as to be consistent with other material.

A veterinary version of the British National Formulary has recently been released. Drug information is structured by body system, disease group and drug type. Special attention is being paid to the use of medicines not licensed for veterinary use, withdrawal periods and withholding times for milk and drug doses for common species.

Legal controls

Before a new drug is approved for veterinary use in the UK, the Veterinary Products Committee carefully examines the data relating to its actions and possible toxicity which must be submitted by the manufacturers. Similar controls are present in other countries. Drugs which are approved for use in humans are also subject to strict control procedures. A more detailed description of the laws relating to the use of medicines is given in Appendix 1.

Prescription writing

A prescription, written by a veterinarian, is required before a drug can be dispensed for animal use. The information which must be included in a veterinary prescription and the conventions of prescription writing are discussed in Appendix 2.

Principles of drug action

Drug–receptor interactions

Although drugs have been in use throughout recorded history, it was only around the turn of the 20th century that the concept of 'receptive substances' (later called receptors) was introduced. Interaction of drugs with receptors is now known to be responsible for the actions of most drugs. Receptors can be any functional macromolecular component of the organism. They are often associated with cell membranes or they may be special sites or enzymes. Interaction between a drug and its receptor depends on the (usually reversible) binding of the drug to the receptor. The bonds formed are most commonly ionic, hydrophobic, van der Waals or hydrogen bonds. Less frequently drugs may bind to their receptors by covalent bonds. For bond formation to occur, the drug and receptor must have complementary structures. The structural requirements for binding may be quite stringent, so that slight changes in the structure of a drug may alter its activity. Such alterations in activity can range from a slight or considerable increase in effectiveness to a reduction in activity which may lead to complete abolition of the original effect, or even antagonism. Thus, the study of 'structure–activity' relationships is of major importance in the rational development of new drugs.

After the binding of a drug to its receptor, a change occurs in the function of the cell. Where the receptor is on the cell membrane, transmembrane signalling strategies enable the interaction between the drug and its receptor to eventually produce a characteristic response in the cell. Some drug–receptor interactions result in an alteration of the membrane permeability by opening or closing ion channels in the cell membrane and thereby altering the electrical potential across the membrane. Drugs which modify the ion channels for Na^+, K^+ and Ca^{2+} have been identified.

Transmembrane signalling may be achieved by the generation of a 'second messenger'. For example, when the hormone adrenaline interacts with its receptors (β-adrenoceptors), a guanosine triphosphate-binding signal transducer protein (G-protein), located on the cytoplasmic side of the cell membrane, is activated. The activated G-protein stimulates the cytoplasmic enzyme adenylate cyclase, which facilitates the conversion of adenosine triphosphate (ATP) to cyclic-adenosine-3',5'-monophosphate (cAMP). cAMP is the 'second messenger'. An increase in its concentration in the cell causes the phosphorylation of proteins, which, in the case of enzymes, results in an alteration of their activity. This is the first step in a chain of reactions which leads to the observed response. In some cells, stimulation of membrane-bound receptors leads to the activation of guanylate cyclase and the generation of cyclic 3',5'-guanosine monophosphate as a second messenger.

Another second messenger system, responsible for the actions of some neurotransmitter substances and hormones, involves the stimulation of phospholipase C. The action of the enzyme generates diacylglycerol and inositol-1,4,5-triphosphate. These second messengers then activate other enzymes, including protein kinases.

As described above, the binding of a drug to a receptor depends on the structure of the drug. Once binding has occurred, a response may be brought about, in which case the drug is called an agonist and is said to have intrinsic activity or efficacy at the receptor. Many commonly used drugs mimic the actions of neurotransmitters or hormones by interacting at the receptors for these substances. Complete agonists are those which elicit the greatest possible response when they interact with their receptors. Those agonists which, even with large doses, can elicit a response which is less than the tissue's maximum response are called partial agonists.

Drugs which have affinity for a receptor, but produce no effect are called antagonists. Although they have no intrinsic activity, they may exert significant effects by inhibiting the action of naturally occurring agonists at that receptor. These drugs are pharmacological antagonists. Antagonism of the effect of a natural mediator (or drug) can also be achieved by a physiological antagonist, i.e. a drug which works at a different site to produce a physiological effect which is opposite to that produced by the agonist. An example of physiological antagonism can be seen in the gut, where noradrenaline (activating α-adrenoceptors) relaxes smooth muscle and thus antagonizes the stimulant effects of acetylcholine (activating muscarinic receptors).

Non-specific drug action

In a relatively small number of cases, drugs can be shown to be effective without strict structure–activity relationships. Examples of such drugs are general anaesthetics, where a variety of chemically diverse substances all produce the same effect. The potency of a general anaesthetic is closely correlated to its oil : water partition coefficient. It is likely that rather than binding to a specific receptor, general anaesthetics have a more diffuse effect on the lipid layer of cell membranes. Other examples where the physicochemical nature of the drug determines the mode of action are the adsorbents (e.g. activated charcoal) and chelating agents (e.g. desfer-rioxamine). These drugs are effective antidotes in that they prevent the absorption of some poisons and metal ions from the gastrointestinal tract by sequestration. Mannitol is another example of a drug which causes an effect which is not due to a drug–receptor interaction. The diuretic effect of this drug depends on the fact that it is not reabsorbed after filtration by the glomerulus. The osmotic pressure of mannitol in the glomerular filtrate results in the retention of water in the nephron thereby causing a diuretic response.

The relationship between drug dose and pharmacological response

The pharmacological response to a drug normally depends on the amount of drug which reaches the site of action which, in turn, is related to dosage or the amount of drug administered by the chosen route. The concentration–response curve, shown in Fig. 1.1a, illustrates the basic relationship between drug concentration and observed response in a tissue which has been mounted in an organ bath. It can be seen from the figure that, in general terms, as the concentration of the drug is increased, the response it elicits increases until a maximum response is attained. The plot is normally hyperbolic. In a whole animal, the concentration of the drug at the site of action is not usually known and the observed response can only be related to the dose administered. Furthermore, in a whole animal, the shape of the curve may be altered if the drug acts at more than one site in the body or

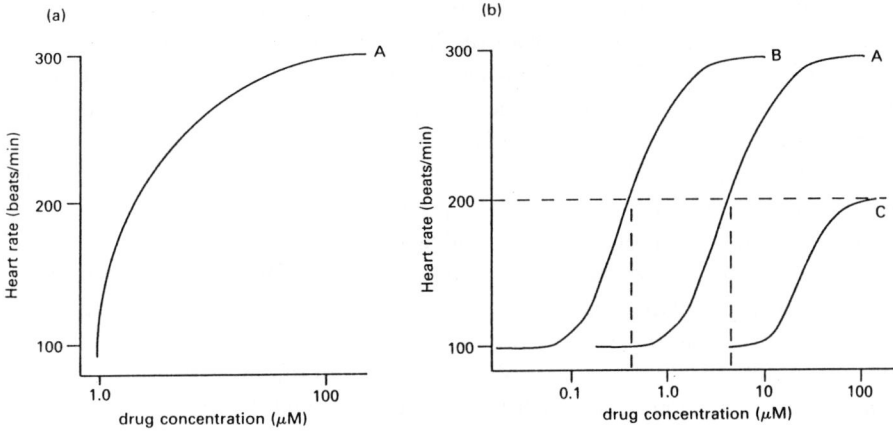

Figure 1.1 (a) Relationship between the concentration of drug A (arithmetic scale) and response in isolated guinea pig atria, mounted in an organ bath. (b) Effect of increasing concentrations of drugs A, B and C on the heart rate of isolated guinea pig atria. Drugs A, B and C all act at the same receptor. Note that the concentration is plotted on a logarithmic scale. The threshold concentration for drug A is 1 μM.

if the response to the drug elicits some reflex reaction which may alter the effect of the drug.

For more convenient mathematical manipulation, the concentration–response curve can be transformed to a log concentration–response curve, as shown in Fig. 1.1b. This transformation results in a sigmoidal curve, in which the central portion of the curve is almost linear. This permits the presentation of a wide range of concentrations on a more compact scale. The log concentration–response curve illustrates a number of important principles of drug action and is used in the calculation of characteristic variables for drugs.

From Fig. 1.1b it can be seen that there is a threshold concentration, below which no response can be observed. Once the threshold concentration is reached, increasing the concentration will result in an increased response until a maximum response is elicited. Further increases in concentration have no additional effect.

The slope of the log concentration–response curve gives some information about the mechanism of action of the drug. If two drugs act at the same receptor, their log concentration–response curves will have similar slopes. In clinical practice, the slope of a log dose–response curve can be used to estimate the expected increase in response from an increase in dose. The steeper the slope of the log dose–response curve, the more difficult is the determination of a suitable dose for that drug because only small changes in dose will produce large changes in response.

The intrinsic activity of a drug, or the maximal effect it is capable of eliciting, can also be inferred from the log concentration–response curve. An example is shown in Fig. 1.1b, where drug A and drug C act on the same receptor. Drug A is capable of increasing the rate of beating of an isolated heart to 300 beats/min, while drug C, regardless of concentration, is only able to increase the rate to 200 beats/min. Drug C has a lower intrinsic activity than drug A and is referred to as a partial agonist.

The potency of a drug can be calculated from the location of its log concentration–response curve along the dose axis. The affinity of the drug for its receptor, which is a function of the structure of the drug, is a major determinant of its potency. It is usual to refer to the potency of one drug relative to that of another. For example, in Fig. 1.1b, the log concentration–response curves for two drugs, A and B, are shown. It can be seen that the linear portions of the curves are parallel, indicating that the drugs act at the same receptor. It is also clear that a 5 μM solution of drug A is required to increase the heart rate to 200 beats/min, while a 0.5 μM solution of drug B will produce the same effect. The relative potency of drug B can be calculated by choosing a mid-range response and dividing the concentration of drug A needed to produce that response by the concentration of drug B which produces the same response. Drug B is thus 10 times as potent as drug A. Clinically, potency is of little concern, as long as it is practicable to administer the drug in doses which elicit the desired effects.

Concentration–response curves for drugs are affected by the presence of antagonists. In the case of competitive antagonists, the log concentration–response curve for an agonist is shifted to the right, the extent of the shift depending on the concentration of antagonist. An example is shown in Fig. 1.2a, where some features of competitive antagonism can be seen. The log concentration–response curves remain parallel in the presence of different concentrations of antagonist and the maximum response to the agonist is not diminished. Thus, competitive antagonism is reversible if sufficient agonist is present to overcome the antagonism. As the name implies, the extent of antagonism depends on competition between agonist and antagonist for the receptor sites. As the concentration of either is increased, so is the likelihood of drug–receptor interaction.

Some antagonists shift the log concentration–response curve of an agonist to the right and also reduce the maximum response which can be attained, as shown in Fig. 1.2b. These may be non-competitive antagonists.

The log concentration–response curves shown in Fig. 1.1b suggest that a given concentration of drug will produce a response of a certain magnitude. In practice, if the same range of concentrations is administered to an isolated tissue several times, the response to each concentration will vary somewhat each time it is given. Such biological variation is found not only within a tissue or a whole animal, but also among individuals of the same species. Thus, if

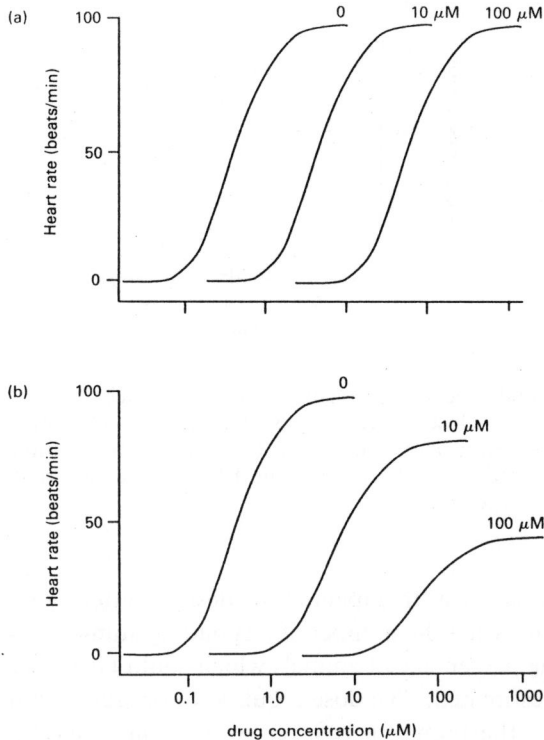

Figure 1.2 (a) Log concentration response curves for a drug A, alone and in the presence of a competitive antagonist at two different concentrations (10 μM and 100 μM). (b) Log concentration–response curves for a drug A alone and in the presence of a non-competitive antagonist at two different concentrations (10 μM and 100 μM).

a test dose of drug is given to a number of animals, the response measured in each animal will not be exactly the same and if the dose is repeated on another occasion, the response in any animal on the second occasion may be different from the one measured initially.

Animal experiments are routinely used in the early stage of testing of a new drug. Where the drug is intended for use in humans, the problem of variation in responses among species complicates the interpretation of the results. In veterinary practice, the problem of species differences is of fundamental clinical significance.

Quantal dose–effect curves (Fig. 1.3) are generated by the administration of increasing doses of a drug to groups of animals and then measuring the number of animals in each dose group which have responded. Again, the fundamental relationship dictates that as the dose is increased, the number or proportion of animals which respond is increased. The critical 'response' can

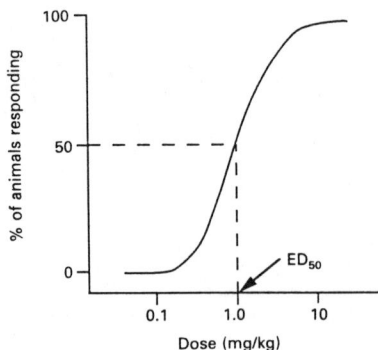

Figure 1.3 Quantal dose–response curve. Groups of mice (10 per group) were dosed with a hypnotic drug. Dose of drug was plotted on the x axis, on a logarithmic scale. In each group the number of mice asleep 60 minutes after dosing was counted and plotted (as a percentage) on the y axis. The ED_{50} is the dose required to produce a response in 50% of the animals.

be defined and can be a 'therapeutic' (or desired) effect, or a sign of toxicity or death. By expressing the number of responding animals as a percentage, the graph allows the percentage of animals which could be expected to respond to any dose to be estimated. The dose required to produce the therapeutic effect in 50 per cent of the animals is referred to as the *median effective dose* (ED_{50}), while the dose required to cause death in 50 per cent of animals is the *median lethal dose* (LD_{50}).

In practice, when drugs are being administered to animals for therapeutic purposes, it is necessary to have an appreciation of the separation of the therapeutic and toxic doses or margin of safety. One measure of this is given by the *therapeutic index*, which is defined as the ratio of the median lethal dose to the median effective dose ($LD_{50} : ED_{50}$). The higher the therapeutic index, the greater is the margin of safety of the drug. Another measure of interest is the ratio of the median toxic dose to the median effective dose ($TD_{50} : ED_{50}$).

The definitions of some other terms used in pharmacology are given below.

Selectivity or *specificity* of drug action refers to the potential of the drug to produce a particular effect at lower doses than those required to produce other effects. The selectivity of two drugs may be compared by measuring the binding affinity of each drug for different receptors or by comparing the ED_{50} values for their different effects *in vivo*. In the clinical situation, selectivity is often assessed by comparing the doses required to produce therapeutic effects with those which produce toxic effects.

Selectivity may be an intrinsic property of the drug or be affected by other factors. For instance, if the drug is applied locally, say to the eye, its potential to produce systemic effects is greatly reduced and its selectivity is thus enhanced.

Tolerance occurs when an animal requires increasing doses to produce the same effect, i.e. repeated administration of a constant dose results in diminishing effects. Cross-tolerance may occur within a group of drugs, so that repeated administration of one member of the group results in the development of tolerance to the other members of the group.

Idiosyncratic reactions are those reactions to a drug which are unexpected or very infrequently observed.

Synergism in response to two drugs occurs when the response to the drugs administered concurrently is greater than the sum of the individual responses which would be expected if the drugs were administered alone. Such interactions between drugs are also referred to as *potentiation*.

As described above, the intensity of the response to a drug is proportional to the concentration of the drug at the site of action, and in a whole animal this is usually proportional to the plasma concentration. The main objective in drug administration is to attain an adequate concentration of the drug at the site of action as quickly as possible and to maintain it for as long as necessary.

The factors which determine the concentration at the site of action are the absorption of the drug from its site of administration, its distribution through the body, its metabolism or biotransformation and its excretion. The quantitative study of the factors which influence the concentration of drug at the site of action as a function of time is called pharmacokinetics (see page 32). In veterinary pharmacology, interspecies variability in the pharmacokinetics of drugs is of major importance.

Drug absorption

Absorption is the process by which drugs enter the body. Knowing the rate of absorption of the drug is important because, in part, it allows inferences to be made about the onset of its action. The extent of absorption is also important, because it determines the magnitude of the response to the drug. Factors which influence absorption include the bioavailability of the drug, the ability of the drug to cross membranes and the route of administration.

The first requirement is that the drug is released from its dosage form and dissolves in the body water. The formulation of the drug (e.g. particle size in the case of griseofulvin and prednisolone) may determine the rate of dissolution of the dose form. The characteristics of the formulation of one manufacturer may differ significantly from those of another; the result is that one product may give higher blood levels than another and the dose forms are said to have different bioavailability. Differences in the bioavailability of two batches of the same drug from the same manufacturer may also occur. Bioavailability may be of major importance where the difference between therapeutic and toxic blood levels is small (e.g. digoxin).

Drug passage across membranes

For a drug to reach its receptor site it must normally cross membrane barriers. Such barriers are present at various levels in the animal, restricting free passage of water and other solutes. Barriers from the external environment include the skin and cornea, the gastrointestinal epithelium and the lung epithelium. Internal barriers include capillaries, various cell barriers, the blood–brain barrier, the renal tubular epithelium, the peritoneum and the placenta.

Reaching the receptor site may be a relatively simple process, as in the application of a drug to the bathing fluid of an isolated organ, or more complex, as in administering a drug to an animal by mouth to produce an action on the heart muscle. In both cases, the movement of the drug across cell membranes is of major importance.

The ability of a drug to cross membranes and to reach its site of action depends largely on its physical properties, including molecular size, molecular shape and solubility in aqueous and lipid phases. Factors such as the ability of the drug to chelate metal ions or surface activity may also exert an influence.

A diagrammatic representation of the structure of a membrane is shown in Fig. 1.4. The phospholipid bilayer is arranged so that the hydrocarbon chains point inwards and so create a hydrophobic phase. At intervals along

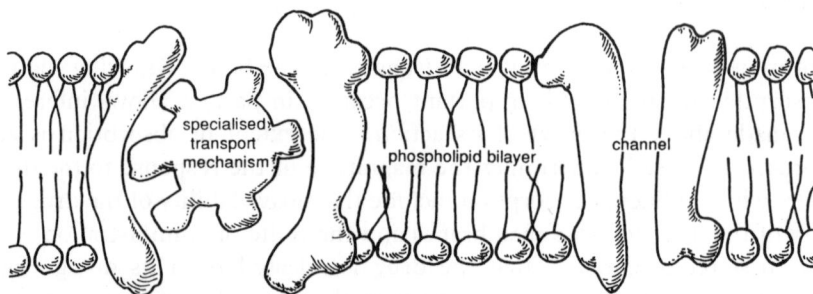

Figure 1.4 Membrane structure showing the arrangement of the phospholipid bilayer, channels within the membrane and specialized transport mechanism.

the membrane there are channels formed by complexes of membrane proteins and lipids. These channels, which are not static and may move about the membrane, allow the transport of ions or molecules with particular characteristics. A number of different transport mechanisms may also occur in cell membranes. These are responsible for the movement of naturally occurring substances or ions across the cell membrane, either with or against a concentration gradient.

The mechanisms by which drugs cross membranes include lipid diffusion, aqueous diffusion and active transport (using specialized carriers or transporters).

Lipid diffusion

Lipid-soluble drugs can move through membranes by passive diffusion, which involves dissolution in the lipid component of the cell membrane and passage down a concentration gradient. The drug enters the cell through one cell membrane barrier, crosses the intracellular compartment and leaves the cell in a similar manner, to enter another extracellular compartment. Drugs which use this method of transport must have high lipid solubility. They must also have aqueous solubility to facilitate transport from the aqueous medium in contact with the lipid membrane layer.

Although the concentration of a lipid-soluble drug at the membrane influences permeation rate, as does the absorptive area, the relative solubility of the drug in lipid and water is usually the most important determinant of its behaviour at cell membranes, i.e. whether it permeates into the membrane or stays in the aqueous phase. This critical factor is termed the oil : water partition coefficient from which the true membrane : buffer partition coefficient can be calculated. In general, the higher the oil : water partition coefficient, the faster the absorption across membranes. This is due to hydrophobic force repelling the drug and pushing it into the membrane.

In the intestine, however, the enormous surface area, which is configured into villi with a hydrophilic microenvironment, becomes the overriding factor. The drug must have some water solubility to gain access to the membrane and there is an optimum value for the oil : water partition coefficient. Above this value, the drug's access to the membrane becomes progressively blocked.

pH and drug ionization

Almost all drugs are either weak acids or weak bases. Thus they exist in aqueous solution in both acid and base forms which have different solubilities in water and lipids based on their charge (polarity). For ionic species, the degree of ionization is important in determining the rate of absorption: the non-ionized form is able to diffuse across membranes but the low lipid solubility of the ionized form will greatly slow its passage.

The Henderson–Hasselbalch equation describes this situation:

for weak bases
$$pH = pK_a + \log \frac{[base]}{[acid]} \qquad [1.1]$$

$$\log \frac{[base]}{[acid]} = pH - pK_a \qquad [1.2]$$

or for weak acids
$$pH = pK_a - \log \frac{[acid]}{[base]} \qquad [1.3]$$

$$\log \frac{[acid]}{[base]} = pK_a - pH \qquad [1.4]$$

K_a is the acid dissociation constant, i.e. the equilibrium constant for the dissociation that yields free hydrogen ions. pK_a is the pH at which 50 per cent dissociation occurs; i.e. $pK_a = pH$ when [base] = [acid].

When [base] = [acid],

$$\log \frac{[base]}{[acid]} = \log 1 = 0 \text{ and } pH = pK_a \qquad [1.5]$$

It is, of course, the degree of ionization at the site in question which determines the extent of absorption (i.e. the pH at the site of absorption and the pK_a of the drug).

Consider a tertiary amine which is a weak base. When uncharged, it can accept a proton (H^+). The pK_a tends to be high (7–11). In the intestine, at high pH, the drug will be un-ionized and will have a high oil : water partition coefficient and can be absorbed readily. In the stomach, at low pH, the drug will be ionized and will have a low oil : water partition coefficient and will thus be poorly absorbed.

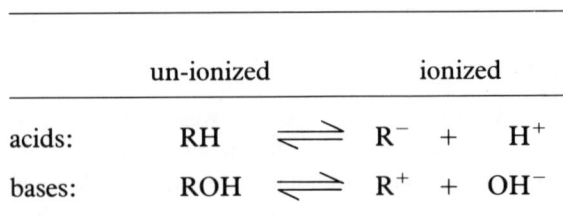

	un-ionized		ionized	
acids:	RH	$\rightleftharpoons$	$R^- +$	H^+
bases:	ROH	$\rightleftharpoons$	$R^+ +$	OH^-

In an acid environment, the surplus of H^+ pushes the equilibrium for acids towards the left and the un-ionized species will be dominant. Thus, in acid conditions, as in the stomach, drugs which are weak acids (e.g. aspirin) are likely to be absorbed. Similarly, absorption of basic drugs will occur more readily in alkaline environments, such as the small intestine. This was illustrated by Tavell in 1940. When strychnine, which is a base, was introduced into the ligated stomach of a cat (pH = 2.0), the drug was not toxic. When sodium bicarbonate was added to raise the pH, the drug was absorbed and the cat died. It should be noted, however, that a great increase in surface area (e.g. small intestine cf. stomach) can swamp the effects of ionization for both charged and uncharged molecules.

Aqueous (passive) diffusion of water-soluble drugs

The movement of small water-soluble drugs across membranes occurs most commonly by a process of passive diffusion. This depends largely on molecular size. The cell membrane channels are about 4–8 nanometres wide and restrict the passage of molecules with relative molecular mass larger than 150–200. Drugs which are highly water-soluble are absorbed mainly by this mechanism (e.g. ascorbic acid; molecular weight = 176). In these cases, the solubility of the drug in the lipid bilayer and the concentration gradient across the membrane determine the rate of transfer of the drug. Small (molecular weight <200), water-soluble molecules (either polar or non-polar) are able to cross epithelial barriers (e.g. gut and lung, which have very tight junctions) in association with water, which moves through the hydrophilic ('aqueous') pores in response to hydrostatic or osmotic differences. The degree of hydration (i.e. association with water molecules) may restrict passage of a compound by effectively increasing its molecular size. This applies especially to pores between endothelial and mesothelial cells of the same tissue (e.g. smooth muscle). Other cell layers (e.g. capillary endothelium) have much larger pores (up to 80 nanometres) which may allow drugs with molecular weights of up to 80 000 to pass. An exception is in the brain capillaries which form an important part of the blood–brain barrier.

Absorption through channels

At intervals along the cell membrane there are channels which are formed by complexes of membrane proteins and lipids. These channels are not static and may move about the membrane. They allow the transport of ions or molecules with particular characteristics.

Facilitated diffusion of drugs

In some cases, relatively selective carrier molecules have been found to facilitate diffusion across membranes. The carrier molecule combines with the drug to produce a readily absorbable complex which then dissociates. No energy appears to be required. Some amino acids (e.g. L-dopa) are absorbed into the brain in this way.

Active transport of drugs

In some tissues or cells specialized transporter proteins are present. Active transport implies an energy-dependent process which moves certain compounds against a concentration gradient, either into or out of the cell. These processes can usually be blocked and/or saturated. Drugs which are substrates for these carriers may be actively transported. For example, iodine is transported into thyroid tissue; catecholamines and 5-hydroxytryptamine are transported into neuronal cells; and weak acids (e.g. penicillin) are actively transported into the renal tubule.

Pinocytosis and phagocytosis of drugs

Drugs with high molecular weights (>1000) are generally absorbed by either pinocytosis or phagocytosis. Drugs which are tightly bound to plasma proteins may also be absorbed in this way (e.g. topical antibacterials such as polymyxin B and bacitracin).

Routes of administration

The usual aim of drug therapy in animals is the entry of the drug into the blood for transport to its ultimate site of action. Exceptions include deliberate avoidance of entry into blood, perhaps to localize the effect (e.g. use of vasoconstrictors with local anaesthetics) or where the drug will not get to its site of action just by entering the blood (e.g. antibiotics in meningitis) and must be given directly into the cerebrospinal fluid.

Drugs are most commonly administered by the oral (or enteral) route or by by a number of parenteral routes (by injection). Sometimes drugs are inhaled, applied directly to the skin or instilled into body cavities.

Topical administration

This implies direct application to the relevant area (e.g. ear, eye, mouth/throat, nose, skin, teat, urethra, vagina, etc.).

Skin

Drugs which are applied to the skin are usually intended for local action but some can be rapidly absorbed, even through intact skin, and these can produce general systemic and toxic effects (e.g. pesticides, corticosteroids). Where a systemic effect is required, absorption can be optimized by the use of an appropriate vehicle. There are many variants (paints, solutions, creams, ointments, powders, etc.) for use in specific circumstances. Differences in drug absorption between species may be due to different skin structures.

Enteral administration

Sublingual

The oral mucosal (sublingual) route is occasionally used in veterinary medicine. It is very effective for a limited number of drugs because absorption is rapid and there is no exposure to gastric acid or biotransformation in the liver before the drug gains access to the general circulation. The limitations of this route are that most drugs are either not absorbed from the buccal mucosa or are too irritant to be held in the mouth.

Oral administration

A variety of dose forms are used including both solids (pills, tablets, capsules) and liquids (suspensions, solutions). With the exception of those required to exert a local effect in the throat or gut, they need to be absorbed from the gastrointestinal tract. The graded pH changes throughout the gastrointestinal tract and the huge mucosal surface with a high blood flow ensure that most drugs are absorbed to some extent.

Since passive diffusion is generally involved in the absorption of drugs after oral administration, those drugs which are lipid soluble are more readily absorbed. A large number of other factors are also involved in determining the rate and extent of absorption of the drug into the general circulation. These include pH, solubility, gastric emptying, intestinal motility, gastric and/or intestinal biotransformation (e.g. penicillin), binding of the drug to the gut contents and bioavailability.

There are many species differences in the rate and extent of absorption of orally administered drugs. For example, carnivores tend to absorb drugs more rapidly than herbivores and the absorption of drugs by ruminants is different from that in monogastric animals. In general, although the ruminal epithelium does have some absorptive capacity, the large volume of the rumen dilutes the drug and delays its absorption. Fermentation by rumen microflora may result in the destruction of some drugs. Oral administration of drugs to ruminants is thus generally limited to those which are required to act in the gastrointestinal tract. Acid in the stomach of many species may destroy the drug (e.g. some penicillins).

Absorption occurs predominantly from the small intestine because of its very large surface area. Thus, gastric emptying time is an important determinant of the rate of absorption of orally administered drugs. The presence of food may delay drug absorption (e.g. phenylbutazone).

Once absorbed from the gastrointestinal tract, drugs in the portal venous blood are exposed to the metabolizing enzymes in the liver. Here, some drugs are extensively destroyed before they reach the general circulation; this is known as the 'first pass effect'. The doses of drugs which are subject to significant first-pass metabolism need to be adjusted accordingly.

Rectal administration

Drugs are occasionally introduced into the rectum in the form of suppositories or enemas. Drugs administered this way are not subject to first-pass metabolism in the liver. This route may be useful when the patient is vomiting or where the drug has a particularly offensive odour or taste.

Parenteral administration

The administration of drugs by injection usually results in a more rapid onset of action than when given by mouth. The problems of drug destruction by gastric acid or first-pass metabolism by the liver are avoided. There are disadvantages, however. There is a need for sterility of equipment and injection site, and discomfort or pain for the patient may occur, especially if repeated injections are required. In veterinary practice, the assistance of someone qualified to administer the injection often increases the cost of treatment.

Intravenous injection

Administration of a drug directly into the circulation overcomes the need for absorption and results in virtually instantaneous effects. This is of major importance in emergency situations and for drugs which may be irritant if injected into muscle or subcutaneous tissue. Except where a rapid onset of effect is required (especially in the induction of general anaesthesia), intravenous injections are usually made slowly with constant patient monitoring. Slow infusions can be used to maintain the plasma concentration at some fixed level. With some drugs, problems with vein irritation may predispose to thrombus formation, which may also be associated with the presence of catheters.

High drug concentrations are rapidly attained by this route and the possibility of adverse reactions is increased. Drugs formulated as suspensions or oily solutions cannot be given by intravenous injection (e.g. procaine penicillin).

Intra-arterial injection
This route is occasionally used to target a drug (e.g. cytotoxics) to a specific tissue.

Subcutaneous injection
Subcutaneous injection is commonly used in animals. There is a relatively constant rate of absorption which depends on the degree of vascularity of the area. In poorly vascularized areas (e.g. the scruff of the neck), absorption may be slow and erratic. Conversely absorption may be quite rapid if the drug is injected over a well-vascularized muscle. Absorption from subcutaneous injections in a patient in shock will be limited by intense peripheral vasoconstriction. This route of administration is only suitable for small volumes of non-irritant drug solutions. Depot preparations which are implanted subcutaneously and slowly dissolve over a period of weeks or months, reduce the need for frequent injections.

Intramuscular injection
Absorption after intramuscular injection also depends on the blood flow to the muscle. In most cases, peak blood levels can be expected within 30 minutes but absorption may be reduced in shocked patients where there is a reduction in the blood flow to muscle. Administration of drugs in aqueous media results in rapid absorption, especially if a deep site is used. The rate of absorption is considerably slower from suspensions or oily solutions. These differences can be used to advantage if a long duration of action is required (such as with depot or slow-release formulations). Intramuscular administration is used for drugs which are too irritant to be given subcutaneously or are only available as suspensions which cannot be given intravenously.

Intraperitoneal injection
The intraperitoneal route can be used for large volumes, and absorption is rapid. It is seldom used in clinical practice, except intra-operatively. It is a common route of administration in experimental procedures. Some of the dose of a drug administered this way is absorbed via the mesenteric vessels and will be subject to metabolism in the liver.

Intrathecal injection
Here the drug is introduced directly into the cerebrospinal fluid, thus by-passing the blood–brain barrier. Drug irritancy may cause a chemically-induced meningitis.

Epidural administration
Local anaesthetics can be given by this route in some animals to produce regional anaesthesia.

Intra-articular injection
Anti-inflammatory drugs (e.g. corticosteroids) are sometimes introduced directly into joints, avoiding the need for high circulating levels. Meticulous attention to aseptic procedures is necessary and there is a need to distinguish infection from a flare-up of the disease.

Inhalation
Administration via the lungs using gases, volatile liquids or nebulized drug solutions is common in general anaesthesia and in the treatment of respiratory disorders. The lungs provide a very large absorptive area with high blood flow. Drugs usually cross the alveolar epithelium by passive diffusion and gain access to the pulmonary circulation and thence to the systemic circulation. In the treatment of bronchoconstriction with salbutamol or corticosteroids (see Chapter 13) very small aerosol doses are locally effective and there are no systemic consequences.

Distribution

After absorption, drugs are distributed within the body. Endrenyi (1989) has stated that 'administering a drug to a patient is analogous to sprinkling salt all over one's plate with the hope that enough will land on the potatoes'. It is necessary to understand the pattern of scatter of a drug to fully appreciate the nature of its effects.

The distribution of drugs to various sites in the body depends on the ability of the drug to pass through membranes, the blood flow to the area and binding of the drug to plasma proteins or extravascular sites. In veterinary pharmacology, the differences in the relative mass of the gastrointestinal tracts of ruminant and non-ruminant species account for some inter-species differences in drug distribution.

Volume of distribution

The volume of distribution of a drug is the volume of body water in which the drug appears to be dissolved. The distribution of some drugs is limited to the plasma, some may also enter the extracellular fluid and others may distribute throughout the total body water. The volume of distribution of an ionized compound which cannot enter cells thus corresponds to the extracellular space and that of a non-polar compound corresponds to the total body water. Knowing the volume of distribution of a drug is important because it gives some indication of the concentration that can be expected in the plasma after a given dose. The calculation of volume of distribution is described later (see page 35).

Sites of drug distribution

Total body water

Ethanol is a commonly used drug which equilibrates with total body water but does not distribute into fat. When administered on a bodyweight basis, higher blood ethanol concentrations are attained by women than by men because females have a lower body water : body fat ratio. This may be of personal forensic significance to the veterinarian.

Extracellular water

The plasma and the interstitial fluid make up the extracellular fluid (ECF). The total volume varies among species and among individuals of the same species. An indication of the volume of extracellular water can be obtained by the administration of an intravenous dose of the carbohydrate, mannitol. Kinetic factors may be operative and distribution of a drug in the ECF may occur long before distribution into cells is complete. This means that there is often an initial phase where plasma drug concentrations are higher than might be expected from the dose.

Blood

A few drugs distribute only into plasma water. Many more enter blood cells and/or become bound to plasma proteins.

Binding of drugs to plasma and serum proteins

Most drugs become ionically bound to plasma proteins to some extent. Binding to albumin is most common but globulins and lipoproteins may also bind drugs. Plasma and serum drug concentrations usually express the total of free and bound drug and can be misleading. When the volume of distribution of a drug is calculated, a distinction must be made between bound and free drug since bound drug cannot attain equilibrium. For many drugs, it is essential to know both the extent and affinity of binding so that dosage can be properly adjusted.

Protein-bound drugs are unable to cross membranes, including capillary walls. The dye, Evans' blue, is so strongly bound to plasma albumin that it is almost entirely retained in the plasma. This fact can be used experimentally in the measurement of plasma volume. In inflammation, capillary permeability increases and bound dye escapes into the interstitial fluid. Colorimetric assay of tissue exudates can be used to monitor inflammatory activity.

Protein-bound drugs are generally unavailable to interact with receptors. Some drugs are more than 99 per cent protein-bound and these need to be given in doses which are sufficient to achieve adequate concentrations at the site of action (as opposed to the plasma), or the expected magnitude of the response is likely to be attenuated. If a drug is extensively bound, it may be necessary to give an initial loading dose to achieve therapeutic levels of free drug for delivery to the site of action.

Drug binding to plasma albumin is reversible and the protein–drug complex can be regarded as a reservoir for free drug. Thus when free drug molecules are metabolized and/or eliminated, protein-bound drug molecules dissociate from their binding sites and are released into the blood.

Protein-bound drugs are not filtered at the glomerulus and protein binding tends to extend the time for elimination of the drug and thus the duration of its effects. Where a drug is subject to proximal tubular secretion (e.g. organic acids, such as penicillin), active removal of free drug into the tubular urine results in an immediate local adjustment of the dissociation equilibrium, enabling more free drug to be available for secretion.

The number of protein-binding sites is not infinite. When all sites are occupied, a minor increase in the dose of a drug may induce a major increase in the free plasma concentration of the drug with possibly toxic consequences. It should also be noted that plasma albumin concentrations are reduced in some disease states (e.g. arthritis) and where there is malnutrition or starvation. In these cases, the dose of drugs which are normally extensively protein-bound may need to be adjusted.

Plasma protein-binding sites are not usually very specific and drugs with similar physicochemical characteristics may compete for available binding sites. The affinity of binding varies considerably among drugs. Thus elevated concentrations of one drug, displaced from binding sites by a second drug, may lead to harmful drug interactions. For example, the non-steroidal anti-inflammatory drugs are usually very strongly protein-bound (>99 per cent for meclofenamic acid). The anticoagulant, warfarin, is less strongly protein-bound and the concomitant administration of conventional doses of warfarin and a non-steroidal anti-inflammatory drug can result in overt warfarin toxicity. Drugs may also compete with endogenous substances (e.g. free fatty acids, bilirubin) for protein-binding sites.

The veterinarian should be aware of the important species differences in the nature and extent of the protein binding of some drugs.

Binding of drugs to other cellular constituents

A therapeutically relevant example of this phenomenon is that of copper taken up and stored in hepatocytes. Animals show no signs of copper toxicity unless some precipitating factor causes the sudden release of large amounts of copper into the circulation.

Body fat
Lipid-soluble drugs tend to accumulate in fat (e.g. chlorinated hydrocarbon insecticides). Since adipose tissue is poorly vascularized, both drug accumulation and release are slow. The storage capacity is great—adipose tissue has been referred to as a 'bottomless pit'—but if fat depots become depleted (e.g. during starvation), stored drugs may be released, causing acute toxicity (e.g. DDT in wild animals).

Tissue binding
Some tissues can be shown to accumulate significant quantities of drugs. Accumulation can occur when the drug is a substrate for an active uptake mechanism. Drugs which are bound at sites other than plasma proteins will have correspondingly reduced plasma levels and appear to have a large volume of distribution, which may greatly exceed the volume of total body water. Examples of drugs which accumulate in tissues include tetracyclines, which are taken up into bone, and iodine, which is stored in the thyroid. Compounds that are tissue-bound are protected from metabolic and excretory processes and thus they tend to have a long half-life in the body. Radioactive strontium (^{90}Sr) is strongly bound to bone and has a half-life in the body of several years.

Other factors affecting drug distribution

The blood–brain barrier

Lipid solubility is the principal determinant of the ability of a drug to cross biological membranes and those which are poorly lipid-soluble have a restricted distribution. The central nervous system presents a special situation for drug distribution. The endothelial cells of the brain capillaries are joined by tight junctions and since there are no intercellular pores, there is little movement of water. The blood–brain barrier thus only allows the entry of lipid-soluble drugs which can cross the endothelial cell membranes. These restrictions are relaxed somewhat when inflammation is present and in this situation the transfer of sufficient amounts of some antibiotics enables effective treatment of meningitis.

The placenta

Lipid-soluble drugs are most likely to cross the placenta. This is particularly important in the early stages of pregnancy, when drugs can interfere with organogenesis. During delivery the neonate can be exposed to the effects of drugs, such as anaesthetics, which are administered to the mother. After delivery the neonate may experience toxic effects from these drugs because it has been removed from the maternal detoxifying capacity and its own metabolic activity is, as yet, undeveloped.

The rumen

The distribution of a drug into the rumen may influence its pharmacokinetics in a number of ways. The drug will be diluted in the ruminal contents, the plasma concentration of the drug will be correspondingly reduced and the rumen may act as a reservoir for drug absorption. Some drugs are metabolized by rumen microflora and others change the rumen microflora.

Redistribution of drugs

Redistribution may be important in the termination of drug action. An example is thiopentone, which is one of the most common injectable anaesthetic induction agents. Thiopentone is highly lipid-soluble and intravenous injection results in a rapidly attained blood–brain equilibrium. The patient is thus quickly and smoothly anaesthetized. After induction of anaesthesia with thiopentone, the patient is usually transferred to an inhalational anaesthetic. The anaesthetic effect of thiopentone is short-lived because it is rapidly redistributed to the muscles and fat, the blood level falls and the drug moves out of the brain into the blood. Thus redistribution of thiopentone is responsible for its short duration of action.

Drug biotransformation

The animal body treats most drugs (correctly) as foreign compounds which should be eliminated. Although a few drugs are excreted unchanged (e.g.

ether), the high lipid-solubility of most drugs (which is responsible for their biological activity) makes them difficult to eliminate. To be efficiently excreted by the kidney, non-polar drugs must be converted to more polar metabolites. The chemical modification of drugs in the body is termed metabolism or biotransformation. Highly water-soluble drugs (e.g. quaternary ammonium compounds) do not require this type of biotransformation. Drugs may be dealt with by more than one metabolic pathway, which may vary according to the dose, the presence of other drugs and a variety of factors which relate to species and to the particular patient. An extreme example is chlorpromazine, which has 10 to 12 major and scores of minor metabolites.

Drug biotransformation is usually a necessary prelude to excretion but biotransformation can also activate drugs. For example, chloral hydrate is metabolized in the liver to trichloroethanol, the active hypnotic agent. Chloral hydrate can thus be regarded as a prodrug. Another example is the anthelmintic, febantel, which is activated to febendazole and oxyfendazole. Biotransformation can sometimes prolong the action of drugs by converting them into metabolites with residual activity (e.g. the minor tranquillizer, diazepam, is metabolized to oxazepam).

The usual outcome of drug biotransformation is a reduction of pharmacological activity. The hepatic enzymes which are most concerned with drug biotransformation are found in the smooth endoplasmic reticulum of hepatocytes. They are referred to as microsomal enzymes because they occur in a particular (microsomal) fraction of liver homogenates.

Drug biotransformation is generally divided into two phases. Phase I reactions (oxidation, reduction, hydrolysis) increase the suitability of the drug for Phase II reactions (conjugation). Phase I reactions do not always alter the biological activity of the drug but Phase II conjugates are usually water-soluble and inactive. An exception is morphine-3-glucuronide, which has recently been found to be a more powerful analgesic than the parent compound. It should also be noted that conjugation reactions can occur outside the liver and that some drugs do not require Phase I biotransformation before conjugation. Furthermore, more than one route of biotransformation may be operative at the same time and one drug may give rise to a number of different metabolites.

Phase I reactions

Oxidation

These reactions are common and are usually carried out by mixed function oxidases (e.g. ethanol is oxidized firstly to acetaldehyde, then to acetate and finally to carbon dioxide and water). Hydroxylation is frequently the first step in an oxidative sequence but the hydroxy derivatives are often very unstable and sometimes highly toxic (e.g. the N-hydroxylation of aromatic amines gives hydroxylamines, which are carcinogenic and cause methaemoglobin formation). Dehydrogenation, oxidative dealkylation (which usually involves removal of an alkyl group from nitrogen or sulphur) and oxidative deamination are other ways in which drug molecules are biotransformed.

The presence of molecular oxygen, nicotinamide adenine dinucleotide phosphate (NADPH) and cytochrome P450 (polysubstrate mono-oxygenase) enzymes is required for oxidative biotransformation reactions. Cytochrome P450 is the name given to a group of haem proteins which bind to carbon monoxide to give products which absorb strongly at 450 nm. About 20 per cent of smooth endoplasmic reticulum protein in the liver is made up of cytochrome P450.

Metabolic oxidation reactions can also occur in the cytoplasm (e.g. alcohol dehydrogenase) and in mitochondria (e.g. monoamine oxidase, which metabolizes adrenaline).

Reduction

Biotransformation by reduction is a less common pathway, but such reactions are important in the metabolism of drugs which contain disulphide, azo or nitro groups (e.g. chloramphenicol—nitro reduced to amino). Under anaerobic conditions, cytochrome P450 can act as a reductase. Reduction reactions also occur when halogen substituents are replaced by hydrogen, double bonds are saturated and aldehydes and ketones are converted to alcohols.

Hydrolysis

Plasma esterases (e.g. pseudocholinesterase) hydrolyse a large number of esters (e.g. acetylcholine) and some amides. A number of transmitter substances and some drugs (e.g. procaine and pethidine) are metabolized in this way. Esterases are also present in most tissues.

Phase II reactions

Phase II biotransformations occur in the cytoplasm and/or the microsomes and usually produce water-soluble and biologically inactive metabolites. These energy-dependent reactions normally result in the formation of metabolites with increased polarity which can be readily excreted by the kidney. They are most likely to occur when the drug or its Phase I metabolite has a hydroxy, carboxyl, amino or thiol substituent. A number of different types of reaction occur.

The most common Phase II reaction is conjugation with glucuronic acid to form a glucuronide. This glucuronylation occurs with many drugs and Phase I metabolites which combine with uridine diphosphoglucuronic acid in the presence of a glucuronyl transferase. The group of enzymes required for glucuronylation may be deficient in some species, strains and individuals (e.g. human neonates cannot glucuronylate the antibiotic chloramphenicol).

The water solubility of some drugs can be increased by acetylation in the presence of an acyl transferase and with acetyl-CoA serving as the donor. Acetylation reactions occur mainly in the liver but also can be carried out in the spleen, lungs and gastrointestinal tract. Acetylation does not always successfully increase water solubility and the acetylated derivatives of the earlier sulphonamides (e.g. sulphathiazole) were prone to crystallize in the renal tubules, causing mechanical damage. Some individuals are poor acetylators and certain drugs are highly toxic to these patients (e.g. isoniazid).

Glycine conjugation is an essentially similar reaction to acetylation; e.g. salicylate is conjugated with glycine to form salicyluric acid. This pathway has a limited capacity and above a certain dose level salicyluric acid is no longer the principal metabolite of aspirin. Thus an increasing proportion of the dose is excreted as salicylate, which is more toxic to the renal tubular epithelium. Conjugation with glutamine can also occur.

Conjugation with sulphate is an important detoxification route for some alcohols and phenols (e.g. paracetamol and some androgens and oestrogens). Erythrocytes are protected against oxidant stress by conjugation reactions with glutathione, which occur in the cytoplasm.

Drug metabolism at sites other than the liver

It should be noted that enzymes in the gastrointestinal tract, lung, kidney and blood can all play a role in biotransformation, to either activate or terminate the action of drugs. In the intestine, conversion of prodrugs to the active molecular species (e.g. pivampicillin to ampicillin) is increasingly being used as a manoeuvre to increase absorption. Hydrolysis of succinylcholine by pseudocholinesterase, with the resultant termination of its effect, occurs in the blood.

Factors affecting metabolism

Species differences

One of the problems facing the veterinarian in the application of pharmacological principles to practice is that of differences in drug metabolism in different species. The usual outcome is a variation in duration of action of the drug. Some of these differences are well documented. For example, pigs lack the ability to provide sulphate for conjugation although they possess the sulphotransferase enzymes required for sulphate conjugation. Cats are deficient in glucuronyl transferase and metabolize drugs like paracetamol and the salicylates poorly. Dogs are unable to acetylate aromatic amino groups (e.g. sulphonamides) and these drugs have a much longer duration of action than might be expected. Ruminants have low levels of plasma pseudocholinesterase and suxamethonium may have an extended effect in these animals compared with that in cats, dogs and horses.

Enzyme induction

Chronic administration of some drugs increases the activity of the liver microsomal enzymes responsible for their metabolism, thus reducing the effect of the drug and making it necessary to increase the dose (e.g. pentobarbitone increases its own hydroxylation). This process is termed enzyme induction and is expressed either as stimulation of enzyme synthesis or inactivation of synthesis inhibition. Such metabolic changes may account for an observed tolerance to the drug.

Induction of metabolizing enzymes by one drug may also increase the metabolism of other drugs. For example, phenobarbitone increases the metabolism of aminopyrine, griseofulvin, dicoumarol, phenytoin and hydrocortisone. A number of environmental contaminants have been shown to produce similar effects. Inhibition of drug-metabolizing enzymes has also been reported.

Other factors

Drugs may compete for a particular metabolic pathway. When two such drugs are given together one is usually metabolized preferentially, leaving abnormally raised levels of the other drug; e.g. when diazepam and cimetidine are co-administered in many species, diazepam levels are increased for this reason.

Diseases, hormonal status, age, nutritional status and other factors may also alter enzyme activity. Neonates and young animals often lack metabolic enzymes, particularly those involved in oxidation and glucuronidation. In elderly animals, there may be reduced liver function and a consequent reduction in the ability to metabolize drugs. Similar considerations apply when liver disease is present. Changes in drug distribution may influence biotransformation (e.g. congestive cardiac failure and renal disease).

Toxic metabolites

With some drugs the action of the parent drug is terminated by metabolism but the metabolites cause toxic reactions. Although this may not occur when the drug doses are low, after administration of high doses, the normal (safe) pathway may be saturated and it is possible for alternative pathways to yield toxic metabolites. For example, the toxic effects on the liver which are produced by high doses of paracetamol are due, in part, to an overload of the glucuronide and sulphate conjugation capacity. In this situation, the normally minor metabolites, hydroxylamines and nitroso compounds, are produced in large amounts and cause glutathione depletion.

Drug excretion

Some drugs are excreted unchanged but the vast majority of drugs undergo biotransformation to more water-soluble metabolites which can be excreted via the kidneys. This is the commonest route for drug excretion. The liver may also be involved when drugs are excreted into the bile (e.g. ampicillin) and some volatile substances can be excreted via the lungs. Saliva often contains low concentrations of drugs and, in a sense, this may also be regarded as a mechanism of excretion, except that saliva is likely to be swallowed and does not contribute significantly to drug clearance. Secretion of drugs into milk may also be of importance in animal husbandry.

Renal excretion

The functional units of the mammalian kidney are the nephrons. Each nephron is made up of a glomerulus, proximal convoluted tubule, loop of Henle, distal convoluted tubule and collecting duct.

Glomerular filtration

Arterial blood passes first to the glomerulus, where some of the plasma water and its contents are filtered out passively along the concentration gradient. The glomerulus has large pores (400–600 nm in diameter) between the cells which allow passive diffusion of molecules with molecular weights of up to about 68 000 (i.e. small proteins). Glomerular filtration rate is measured by the clearance of inulin or creatinine which are freely filtered at the glomerulus and are not reabsorbed from the renal tubule. Glomerular filtration rate can be reduced in disease and this can significantly prolong the stay of a drug in the body. Thus, in patients with impaired renal blood flow or impaired renal function, drug doses may have to be reduced (e.g. gentamicin) according to the creatinine clearance.

Many drugs and drug metabolites gain access to the glomerular ultrafiltrate but plasma proteins do not pass into the tubular urine under normal conditions. It follows that protein-bound drugs will not enter the tubule by glomerular filtration. As indicated earlier, local dissociation of bound drug occurs readily in the glomerulus once the free drug has crossed the membrane.

Tubular reabsorption and tubular secretion

The major function of the kidneys is homeostasis: to conserve water and to separate substances which are required by the body from those which are not. Most of the water in the glomerular filtrate is reabsorbed along the nephron, from proximal tubule to collecting duct. Active and passive absorption mechanisms and active secretion mechanisms operate along the nephron to reabsorb substances which need to be retained and to secrete those which require elimination. Only a small proportion of the glomerular filtrate is voided as urine.

Tubular reabsorption

Non-ionized drug molecules can leave the tubule by passive diffusion as their concentration is increased by the reabsorption of water. Ionized drugs and drug metabolites are not reabsorbed in this way and thus the pH of the tubular urine, which determines the proportion of ionized molecules, is a major determinant of the rate of excretion of acidic and basic drugs and thus the duration of their action. For example, the excretion of salicylic acid, a weak acid, is enhanced in alkaline urine because it will be highly ionized and unable to cross membranes and thus will remain in the nephron to be voided. Acidic urine increases the excretion of basic drugs (e.g. amphetamines).

Manipulation of urinary pH is sometimes used to hasten the removal of a drug in an overdose situation (e.g. alkalinization of the urine in salicylate poisoning). Extending the duration of action of a drug requires a urinary pH change in the opposite direction. Carnivores usually have an acidic urine (pH 5.5–7) whereas the pH of the urine of herbivores is usually much higher (pH 7–8).

Active reabsorption may also occur. Almost the entire glucose content of the tubular urine is actively reabsorbed. Like most active transport mechanisms, this is capacity-limited and if the limit is exceeded, glucose appears in the urine.

Tubular secretion

Tubular secretion occurs by both passive lipid diffusion and active transport pathways. Active transport mechanisms can move drugs and their metabolites into the tubular urine, often in an ionized state. These processes require energy and can move substances against a concentration gradient. Such processes are used for the elimination of both endogenous (e.g. uric acid) and exogenous (e.g. benzylpenicillin) acids. Benzylpenicillin is rapidly excreted and thus it has a very short half-life. This can be extended by giving an inactive competitor for the excretion pathway (e.g. probenecid).

Differences may occur in the ways in which closely related drugs are handled by the kidney. For example, in cattle a high proportion of an ampicillin dose is filtered at the glomerulus whereas cloxacillin is eliminated mainly by tubular secretion.

Non-renal excretion

Liver–biliary excretion

Drugs or their metabolites may be excreted into the bile. This is a two-step process involving transfer from the plasma into the hepatocyte and from the hepatocyte into the biliary system. Drugs are then delivered to the intestine in the bile. Some drug metabolites are reabsorbed from the intestine (see below) and others are eliminated in the faeces. Some Phase II conjugates (especially glucuronides) are broken down in the intestine and the unconjugated drug or drug metabolite is then available for reabsorption.

Dogs, rats and chickens are regarded as being efficient biliary excretors whereas rabbits, guinea pigs and monkeys are poor excretors.

Enterohepatic circulation

Enterohepatic circulation of drugs is said to occur when, after excretion into the bile, the drug is reabsorbed from the gastrointestinal tract. This may be followed by further biliary excretion, and continued reabsorption of the drug may extend its duration of action. The amount of drug excreted and reabsorbed declines with each cycle (e.g. tetracyclines and some steroids). Because of hepatic recycling, ampicillin concentrations often exhibit a slower rise and fall than other penicillins.

Milk

The excretion of drugs into milk may pose hazards for suckling animals, even though the total amount transferred in this way is likely to be low. Since the pH of cow's milk is slightly more acid than that of the plasma, basic drugs which are lipophilic tend to be concentrated in the milk. It is important that the farmer is alerted to the appropriate drug withdrawal periods where milk from treated cattle or goats is to be used for human consumption. A perceived problem is the possible sensitization of the consumer to antibiotics.

Expired air

Pulmonary excretion is the main route of elimination of volatile substances or gases, notably the general anaesthetics. The efficiency of this route depends on the removal of drug in expired air and its replacement by drug-free inspired air. The concentration gradient then favours transport of more drug from the blood to the alveolus.

Saliva

Many drugs are transported into saliva. This could be important in animals (e.g. cows) which produce large volumes of saliva. Most of the saliva output is swallowed and the drug is presumably reabsorbed.

Pharmacokinetics

The concentration–response curves illustrated in Fig. 1.1 can be readily obtained from a simple isolated organ preparation where it can be assumed that the concentration of drug in the organ bath is in equilibrium with the concentration of drug at the receptor site. In a more complex situation, where a drug is administered to an animal in, for example, tablet form, a multitude of variables influence the concentration of drug that is present at the receptors at any time (Fig. 1.5). The ability to estimate the amount of drug available to receptors is necessary for any prediction of the magnitude of the response to that drug or for the interpretation of an observed response in terms of the amount of drug present. The quantitative description of the movement of drugs within the body forms the basis for the sub-discipline of pharmacokinetics.

The aim of pharmacokinetic studies is to provide a detailed analysis of drug levels which might be anticipated in critical target tissues where either therapeutic or toxic effects are expected to be manifested. Thus, mathematical analyses of the processes of absorption, distribution and elimination of drugs are combined to predict or interpret the relationship between blood levels of drugs and time. The assumption that there is a general association between

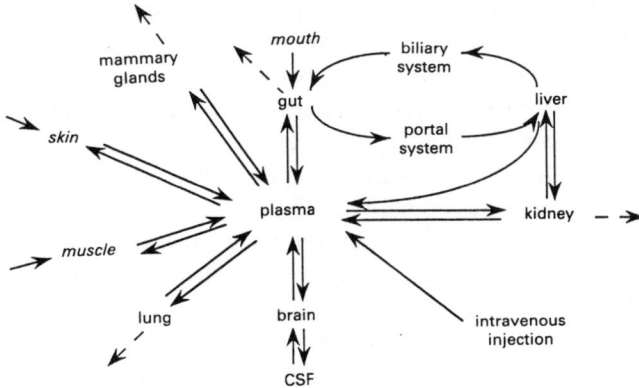

Figure 1.5 Variables determining the concentration of a drug in the plasma and hence at the site of action. Dashed arrows show possible sites of drug loss.

the levels of drug in plasma and those at the receptors (and thus an association between the drug level in plasma and response) is fundamental to most pharmacokinetic studies, but is not always strictly correct.

The commonly observed species differences in the intensity and duration of effect of a number of drugs are most likely to be related to variations in the pharmacokinetics of the drugs among species. Often these arise from differences in the metabolic capacity of the species concerned. Pharmacokinetic data for a drug obtained from studies in animals are not only useful in helping to understand the response to that drug, but may also yield useful principles which could be applied to the prediction of the response to other drugs.

The use of drugs licensed for human use only

Some diseases that occur relatively infrequently in animals may be treatable with drugs approved for human use only. In these cases, the forecast profits from the marketing of the drugs for veterinary applications are insufficient to encourage drug manufacturers to embark on such a marketing programme. Such drugs can be legally obtained by veterinarians for the treatment of animals under their care.

The mechanism of action of drugs in animals is often the same as that in humans, but the kinetics may be very different, leading to significant differences in magnitude and duration of effect. Information about the kinetics in animals of the drugs licensed for human use may be difficult to find or may not be available. The manufacturer may have some relevant information, gleaned during the development of the drug.

Animal size will obviously have an important influence on the dose of drug to be administered. In the case of any one species, calculation of the dose according to bodyweight will usually provide a useful method of adjustment of dose. When extrapolation across species is necessary this simple calculation will not always be adequate. In these cases differences in the metabolism and excretion of the drug in different species may exert a major influence on determination of the required dose. Thus in one of the common laboratory animals, the rat, metabolism and excretion are usually more rapid than in larger animals and man, and relatively more drug per unit bodyweight is required to produce a given effect. The increased metabolic rate is a function of relatively greater size of the liver and also a greater body surface area per unit bodyweight. For this reason it is often more useful to relate dose to body surface area than to bodyweight. It should be noted that there are exceptions to these general rules and even when they do apply, there may be variations in the responses in different species which cannot be predicted on the basis of either bodyweight or surface area.

Absorption

Unless injected intravenously, drugs must be absorbed from the site of administration into the blood to be transported to their sites of action. It is not difficult to appreciate that the rate of absorption will have a significant influence on the amount of drug present at receptor sites at any time after administration and is thus an important pharmacokinetic parameter. Most commonly, absorption of drugs is according to first-order kinetics, i.e. the amount of drug absorbed at any given time depends on the concentration gradient at that time. Once the drug is absorbed, it is rapidly removed and thus, in practice, first-order kinetics usually implies that the rate of absorption is proportional to the amount of drug available for absorption.

There are certain situations when the rate of absorption of a drug is constant and in these cases the absorption is said to follow zero-order kinetics. Examples include the administration of inhalational general anaesthetics, when the drug is continuously supplied in a fixed concentration, and absorption from 'sustained release' formulations in which components of the dose form are designed to disintegrate at different times and thus provide an almost constant supply of drug.

Distribution

The distribution of drugs in the body is a more rapid process than either absorption or elimination. Drugs are distributed into compartments which are defined in terms of the molecules which penetrate them. A compartment can be considered to be a group of tissues or organs for which the rates of uptake and loss of a drug are similar. Since the blood flow to a tissue or organ determines the rate of drug delivery to that site, organs are grouped in compartments according to the proportion of the cardiac output they receive. Thus the central compartment consists of plasma and highly perfused lean tissue, including heart, lung, brain, spinal cord, kidney, liver and glands. Muscle and skin are less well perfused. Areas of considerably lower or negligible perfusion include fat, bone, teeth, ligaments, cartilage and hair and these comprise the peripheral compartment.

A graphical representation of plasma concentration of drug vs. time is shown in Fig. 1.6 and reflects the distribution of the drug into body compartments. Thus, after an intravenous injection of a drug (so that absorption need not be taken into account), the initial decline in plasma level is due to the distribution of drug and the slower decline represents the elimination phase, during which plasma levels fall as the drug is lost from the body.

An important determinant of the plasma level of a drug is the volume of its distribution, which can be calculated from the formula

$$\text{Volume of distribution } V_d = \frac{\text{Total amount of drug in body}}{\text{Concentration of drug in plasma}} \qquad [1.6]$$

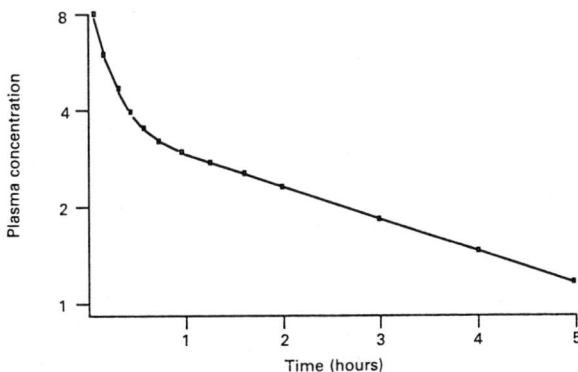

Figure 1.6 Plasma concentrations of a drug after intravenous injection. The concentration declines rapidly initially, as the drug is distributed to body compartments. During the slower elimination phase, the fall in plasma level is due to the loss of drug from the body.

This volume reflects the total space in which that drug is 'diluted' and may be equivalent to any one of the body fluid volumes. However, it should be noted that the V_d gives no indication of the pattern of distribution of the drug. Thus, in the average man (70 kg), a drug which is restricted to the plasma will have a V_d of approximately 3 l, while if it is distributed throughout the total body water (e.g. ethanol), the V_d will be approximately 42 l.

From studies in man and animals, the V_d of many drugs is found to be considerably more than the volume of total body water. In these cases, an apparently enormous V_d is calculated because of the low concentration of drug in the plasma. The small denominator in the equation is a result of drug sequestration in muscle, fat and other storage sites. Age, sex, and the presence of disease can all alter the V_d of drugs and thereby influence the plasma levels of drug.

Elimination

The amount of drug present at the site of action is also influenced by the rate at which it is eliminated from the body. The processes of metabolism and excretion are responsible for elimination, which usually begins as soon as compounds reach the circulation and are transported to the liver and/or kidney. (In some cases, transformation may begin in the gastrointestinal tract, before drug absorption, or in the 'first pass' through the liver.)

For most drugs, metabolism follows first-order kinetics (i.e. the rate of metabolism depends on the amount of drug available). If the enzyme responsible for metabolism of a drug is saturated at the levels of drug attained in the plasma, the metabolism proceeds at a constant rate and thus is a zero-order phenomenon. The two most common examples of drugs for which this occurs are ethanol and aspirin. The rate-limiting step in the hepatic metabolism of ethanol is the conversion of ethanol to acetaldehyde, catalysed by the enzyme alcohol dehydrogenase. This enzyme becomes saturated at blood ethanol concentrations as low as 0.02 g/100 ml. Thus, at blood ethanol concentrations above this, metabolism of ethanol proceeds at a constant rate. Similarly, therapeutic doses of aspirin (especially those in the higher range, used for inflammatory conditions), saturate the drug-metabolizing enzymes and zero-order metabolism occurs.

Excretion of drugs by the kidney usually follows first-order kinetics. The rate constant of elimination (K_{el}) is the sum of the rate constants of metabolism and excretion and thus, for most drugs, elimination also follows first-order kinetics. In Fig. 1.7 plasma concentration of a drug at different times is shown. It is assumed for simplicity that absorption and distribution of the drug are complete. The plasma concentration can be plotted on a linear scale, as in Fig. 1.7a, or on a logarithmic scale, as in Fig. 1.7b. In the latter case, the exponential decline of plasma concentration is transformed to a straight line, the slope of which is equivalent to the rate of elimination. In the example shown, the log plasma concentration declines by 0.5 per hour, i.e. 50 per cent of drug in plasma at any given time will be eliminated in 1 hour.

The data in Fig. 1.7b can also be used to calculate the plasma half-life of the drug, i.e. the time taken for the concentration of drug in the plasma to decline to half of its original value. This is achieved by selecting a particular point on

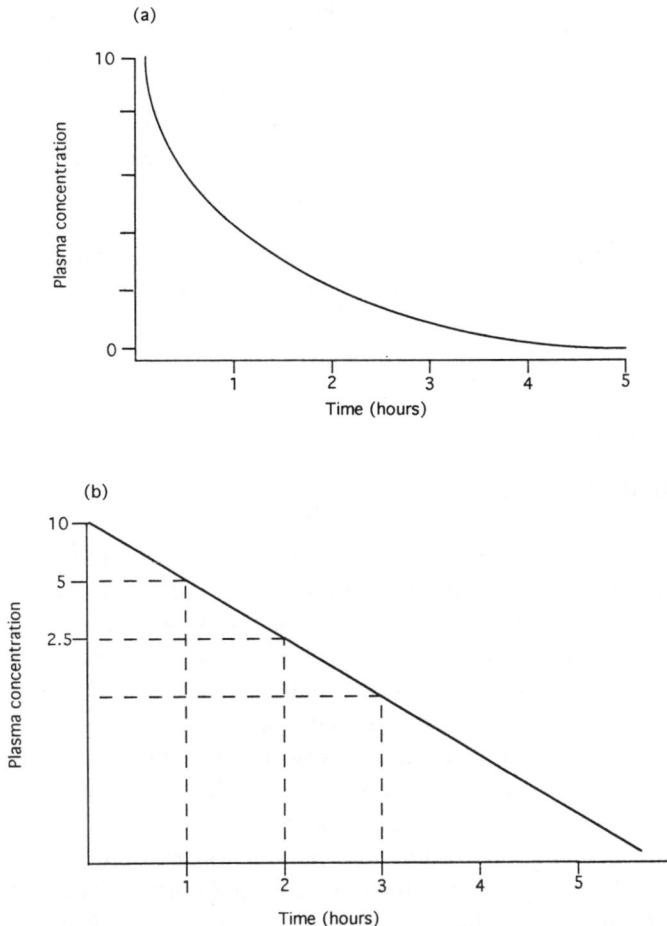

Figure 1.7 Plasma concentration–time curves during the elimination phase of a drug plotted on (a) linear and (b) logarithmic scale. The slope of the line in (b) is equivalent to the elimination rate.

the line, reading the plasma concentration at that time and determining how long it would take for that plasma concentration to be halved. Factors which may increase the half-life of a drug include sequestration into tissues or active tubular reabsorption.

Another approach to quantifying the elimination of a drug is the measurement of its clearance or removal from the body or a specific part of the body. Blood (or plasma) clearance, defined as the volume of blood (or plasma) cleared of the drug in unit time, is often the most convenient to measure. Total body clearance of a drug is determined by its volume of distribution and the rate at which it disappears from the body and is calculated from the formula

$$\text{Clearance} = \text{Volume of distribution} \times \text{Elimination rate constant} \quad [1.7]$$

Drugs may be removed from the body by a number of different organs, including, most commonly, the liver, kidneys and lungs. Total body clearance of a drug is the sum of the clearances by all of the tissues and organs which participate in the elimination of that drug. Plasma clearance, often a good indicator of total body clearance of a drug, may not indicate the real rate at which the drug is being removed from the body. For instance, in cases where plasma clearance measurements suggest rapid clearance, sequestration of the drug at other sites in the body may result in a reduced total body clearance.

Bioavailability and response

The term bioavailability refers to the rate and extent of drug absorption into the circulation after administration. In situations where the drug is administered by intravenous injection, all of the drug enters the circulation. Drugs administered by other routes are absorbed to varying extents, depending on the nature of the drug and the route of administration. For instance, after oral administration, some drugs may be completely absorbed, others may not be absorbed at all and many will be absorbed to some intermediate extent. The proportion of the dose of drug absorbed is clearly an important factor in the determination of the concentration at the site of action.

Measurement of the area under the plasma concentration vs. time curve (AUC) allows an estimate of the fraction of drug absorbed. The factors which determine the area under the curve are the total amount of drug which enters the circulation, volume of distribution and rate of elimination. The calculation of the fraction of drug absorbed after oral administration is based on the Law of Corresponding Areas, which states 'where the dose, volume of distribution and elimination rate constant are equal, the areas under the curves are equal, regardless of the shapes of the curves'.

For example, if a given drug is administered by intravenous injection, its volume of distribution is the same as when it is administered by the oral route. The elimination rate constant is also unaffected by route of administration. Thus, if a particular dose of the drug is administered intravenously on one occasion and by mouth on another, any difference in the area under the curve must be due to different amounts of drug entering the circulation. In the case of intravenous injection, the drug is injected directly into the blood and thus the dose is equal to the amount in circulation. Where the drug is administered orally, absorption may be incomplete, resulting in a reduced area under the curve. Indeed, the ratio of the areas under the curves in these cases is a quantitative measure of the extent of absorption of the drug after oral administration.

i.e.

$$\text{Fraction of oral dose absorbed} = \frac{\text{AUC (oral)}}{\text{AUC (intravenous)}} \qquad [1.8]$$

The bioavailability of a drug also refers to the rate of its entry into the circulation. This is most commonly influenced by the formulation of the drug and variations in bioavailability of drug in preparations from different commercial sources have important implications. An example of plasma concentration vs. time curves achieved after oral administration of a hypothetical drug, available in two different formulations, is shown in Fig. 1.8. The areas under the two curves are equal, so the extent of

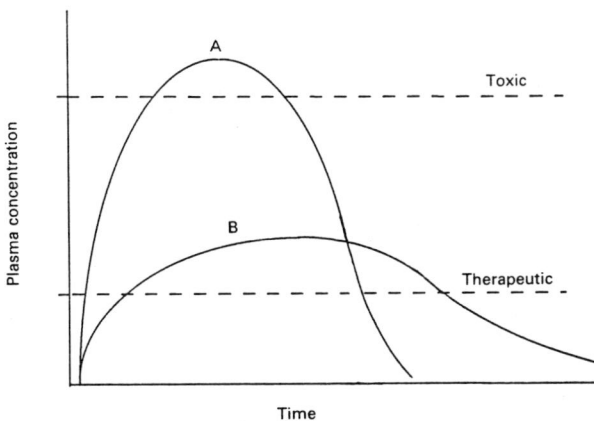

Figure 1.8 Plasma concentration–time curves for two different formulations, A and B, of the same drug. The areas under the two curves are equal.

absorption is the same. The rate of absorption of A is faster than that of B, so that the therapeutic plasma level is achieved more rapidly. However, the rate of absorption of A is so rapid that plasma levels in the toxic range are reached. Furthermore, since the drug is eliminated with first-order kinetics, the high plasma levels result in rapid elimination in the early stages and plasma concentration soon declines below therapeutic levels. Formulation B, in contrast, takes a little longer to achieve therapeutic levels, but there is no overshoot to toxic levels and there is a longer time during which the drug is present at therapeutic levels.

CHAPTER 2

THE AUTONOMIC NERVOUS SYSTEM

Introduction

The autonomic nervous system includes the nerves, ganglia and plexuses which innervate a very wide range of tissues and organs in the body including those of the cardiovascular, respiratory, gastrointestinal and genito-urinary systems. The system is of major importance in homeostatic control and therefore drugs which have the ability to interfere with the normal functioning of the autonomic nervous system have the potential to cause widespread effects in the body. The somatic nerves which innervate the skeletal muscles are not a part of the autonomic nervous system but their function may be altered by drugs which affect autonomic nervous activity. Where this is the case, the relevant pharmacology is included here (for further details of the drugs which affect skeletal muscles see Chapter 7).

Many students of pharmacology find that the study of the autonomic nervous system is a difficult task because of the vast array of drugs which affect the various components of the system and the wide range of actions and side-effects that each of the drugs may have. The task can be made much easier if one tries to understand the normal function of the system and then to learn, in general terms, how each particular drug interacts with it. The actions and many of the side-effects of the drugs can then be logically deduced and only unusual responses need special mention. This chapter is arranged with this approach in mind. First the organization of the autonomic nervous system and the concept of neurotransmission are described. The normal function of the system is then explained and this is followed by a description of the drugs which may affect it. The actions and side-effects of these drugs are explained in terms of how the drug affects autonomic function, and attention is drawn to any peculiar aspects of the drug which do not follow logically from knowledge of its major autonomic action. In this chapter a brief mention will be made of the therapeutic applications of the drugs, but more detail can be found within the sections that deal with the individual systems involved. In most cases cross-references are included in the text.

Organization of the autonomic nervous system

The autonomic control of various body systems involves the transmission of information from the viscera to the central nervous system in afferent (usually non-myelinated) fibres. Reflex responses can be elicited from a number of sites in the central nervous system; the most important involve the spinal cord, medulla oblongata, limbic system, hypothalamus and the cerebral cortex. The subsequent transmission of the impulse to elicit an appropriate response in the periphery is via efferent fibres which emerge in cranial and spinal nerves. These preganglionic nerves synapse, at the ganglia, with postganglionic nerves which then transmit the impulse to the end organ. Thus the impulse crosses at least two synapses before a response is elicited.

Neurotransmission

The mechanism by which a nerve impulse crosses the synapse and either excites a postganglionic nerve or causes a response, has only been well understood for the last 65 years. In the early years of the 20th century experiments with extracts of adrenal glands and drugs isolated from plants, showed that chemical substances could elicit responses which were similar to those produced by stimulation of autonomic nerves. In 1921 Otto Loewi performed experiments in which an isolated frog heart was perfused with physiological solution and the vagus nerve stimulated. The heart rate slowed in response to the stimulation. The perfusing solution was collected and used to perfuse a second isolated heart. Loewi observed that the rate of the second heart slowed as the solution passed through it. Thus it was concluded that a chemical substance or neurotransmitter was released from the vagus of the first heart during the stimulation period and that this substance produced the response in the second heart after being carried to it in the perfusing fluid.

In order to describe the scheme of events involved in the normal functioning of autonomic nerves, the example of blood pressure control can be used. If blood pressure falls, the pressure-sensitive receptors in the carotid sinus and aortic arch detect the fall and transmit the appropriate information, via the afferent autonomic nerves, to the central nervous system. The medulla and hypothalamus are both involved in the integration of the information and in the resultant output, which is transmitted initially via preganglionic sympathetic nerves. The depolarization of these nerves causes the release of a neurotransmitter from the nerve endings, which then interacts with specialized receptor sites on the postganglionic neurones. The consequent depolarization of these nerves leads to the release of neurotransmitter in close proximity to the blood vessels. Interaction of the transmitter with postsynaptic receptors on the blood vessels causes vasoconstriction and an increase in blood pressure. Events similar to these occur continuously, as the autonomic nervous system controls blood pressure, respiration, digestion, temperature, urinary output and most other visceral functions.

Division of the autonomic nervous system

The efferent branch of the autonomic nervous system is divided into two main systems, the sympathetic and parasympathetic nervous systems (Fig. 2.1). This division is made on anatomical and functional grounds.

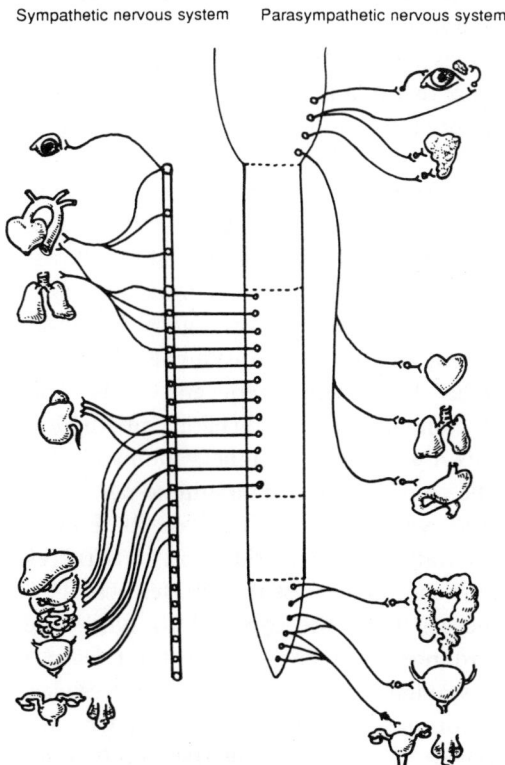

Figure 2.1 Sympathetic and parasympathetic divisions of the autonomic nervous system. For details, see text.

Parasympathetic nervous system—the preganglionic nerves of the parasympathetic nervous system emerge from the spinal cord at the cranial and sacral level. They convey their impulses to the ganglia, which, in this system, are usually in close proximity to the structure being innervated, and which in turn stimulate the short postganglionic nerves. Parasympathetic activity is generally associated with energy conservation.

Sympathetic nervous system—the thoracic and lumbar regions of the spinal cord are the areas from which the sympathetic preganglionic neurones emerge. They are short nerves which synapse with the paravertebral sympathetic ganglia. These lie in a chain on either side of the vertebral column. The ganglia have neural connections with each other. There are some sympathetic ganglia, e.g. in the abdomen, pelvis, bladder and rectum, which are not part of the chain. Because of the location of the ganglia, postganglionic sympathetic nerves are generally longer than those in the parasympathetic nervous system.

The adrenal medulla is an important component of the sympathetic nervous system. Anatomically, histologically and functionally it behaves as a sympathetic ganglion. On being stimulated by the transmitter released from the preganglionic nerve which innervates it, the adrenal gland responds by releasing chemical messengers into the circulation. Activity in sympathetic nerves and the adrenal medulla is usually associated with energy expenditure, particularly in times of stress, and the system is often referred to as the 'fight or flight' system.

The innervation of the major systems of the body by autonomic nerves is shown in Fig. 2.1. It can be seen that most of the viscera are innervated by both parasympathetic and sympathetic nerves. This allows for the adjustment of the activity of these organs by alterations in the activity of either component of the autonomic nervous system. Most organs are under the predominant control of either sympathetic or parasympathetic systems; for instance, although the heart has both sympathetic and parasympathetic innervation, heart rate is usually controlled by vagal (parasympathetic) activity. Note that blood vessels receive only sympathetic innervation and therefore arterial blood pressure is under the control of the sympathetic nervous system.

Drugs may produce wide-ranging effects on the body by interfering with normal processes of transmitter function and it is therefore appropriate to consider the different components of transmitter activity (Fig. 2.2).

All autonomic nerves have the capacity to synthesize their transmitter substance. The substance must be available for release when required and this is ensured by storage of the transmitter in vesicles in the autonomic nerves. There is a complex mechanism, triggered by the depolarization of the nerve, which results in the release of transmitter into the synaptic cleft. Having crossed the synapse, the transmitter is able to combine with receptors to initiate a response. Receptors on the nerve terminals, called presynaptic

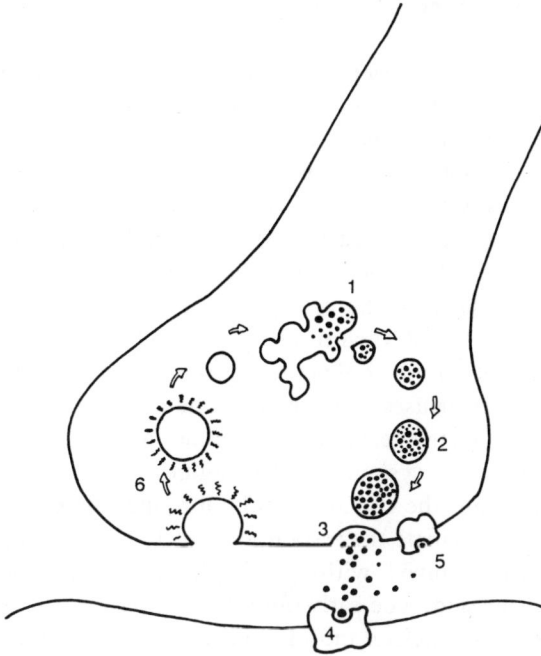

Figure 2.2 Mechanisms exist in autonomic nerves for (1) synthesis, (2) storage and (3) release of transmitter when the nerve is depolarized. The transmitter interacts with postsynaptic receptors (4) to produce a response. Interaction with presynaptic receptors (5) may be important in control of transmitter release. The vesicle is re-formed (6) after transmitter release.

receptors, are thought to be involved in the control of transmitter release and may also be stimulated. A most important feature of the system involves the mechanism for the termination of transmitter activity. It is necessary, for efficient function, that the transmitter be destroyed or removed rapidly. This ensures that the autonomic nervous system has the ability to influence function on a moment-to-moment basis.

Parasympathetic nervous system

The neurotransmitter in the parasympathetic nervous system, both at the ganglia and postganglionically, is acetylcholine. This chemical, initially named 'vagusstoff' by Loewi, is also the transmitter in motor nerves and therefore some of the drugs which affect acetylcholine influence not only autonomic function but also the function of skeletal muscle.

Cholinergic nerves have a carrier system which is responsible for the uptake of choline from the extracellular fluid into the nerve. This step appears to be the rate-limiting one in the biosynthesis of the transmitter. The synthesis of acetylcholine from choline and acetyl coenzyme A (CoA) is catalysed by the enzyme choline acetyltransferase. The enzyme is widespread throughout nervous tissue, with high concentrations in peripheral cholinergic nerves.

Acetylcholine is stored in vesicles within the nerve terminals, with some also being free in the cytoplasm of the cell. There is a continuous, spontaneous background release of small quantities of acetylcholine from cholinergic nerves. On depolarization of the nerve terminal there is an increase in intracellular Ca^{2+} which causes the acetylcholine-containing vesicles to fuse with specialized areas on the terminal membrane, and this is followed by a greatly increased release of vesicular acetylcholine. This effect is dependent on the influx of Ca^{2+} into the cell and can be inhibited by excess Mg^{2+}.

The receptors which mediate the responses to acetylcholine vary, depending on whether they are involved with ganglionic, postganglionic or skeletal neuromuscular transmission. The early observation by Dale, that the responses of autonomic ganglia and skeletal muscle to acetylcholine could be mimicked by the application of nicotine to these receptor sites, led to the classification of these as nicotinic receptors. The receptors at postganglionic autonomic sites were termed muscarinic receptors because, when stimulated by the alkaloid muscarine, the responses were similar to those produced by parasympathetic stimulation. Although this classification is still valid, the results from later extensive investigations by many other scientists have revealed differences within the classes of muscarinic and nicotinic receptors.

The earliest differences described were the differences in the nicotinic receptors at the ganglia and those at the skeletal neuromuscular junction. The discovery that some drugs (e.g. tubocurarine) could antagonize the effects of acetylcholine at the receptors in skeletal muscle much more effectively than those at autonomic ganglia, and that other drugs (e.g. hexamethonium) had selectivity for ganglionic sites, indicated that the nicotinic receptors at these locations were likely to have some structural differences. This contention was supported by the discovery of drugs capable of selective stimulation of one or other of the nicotinic receptor types. Thus nicotinic receptors are either ganglionic or are involved with transmission at the skeletal neuromuscular junction.

More recently differences within the class of muscarinic receptors have been demonstrated. Initially the different potency of an antagonist at anatomically distinct receptor sites formed the basis for the conclusion that two types of muscarinic receptors exist. The original observations, that the muscarinic receptors in autonomic ganglia, oxyntic cells of the stomach and in some areas of the central nervous system are similar to each other and different to most of those in smooth muscles, have been convincingly confirmed. These receptors were named M_1 receptors. Since then, at least five different subtypes of muscarinic receptor (M_2, M_3 etc.) have been postulated. This subdivision is relatively recent and there is no general agreement about which of the muscarinic receptors (other than M_1) belong in each group.

The distinction between different subtypes of both nicotinic and muscarinic receptors was initially described in terms of the anatomical location of the subtypes. While the generalizations based on these early observations still hold true, it should be noted that accurate receptor identification depends on determining the affinity of the receptor for selective agonists or antagonists. This can be done by receptor binding experiments *in vitro*, or by observation of responses of the receptors to the selective agents *in vivo*. Results from such experiments indicate that although one subtype may be the predominant receptor at any given site, it is quite possible that a minority of the receptors of the other subtype(s) coexist at that site.

The role of the parasympathetic nervous system in the homeostatic control of various body functions is summarized in Table 2.1, where it can be seen

Table 2.1 Responses to stimulation of muscarinic receptors

Effector	Response
Eye	
Iris, sphincter muscle	Contraction—miosis
Ciliary muscle	Contraction—focus for near vision
Salivary glands	Secretion
Lacrimal glands	Secretion
Heart	
SA node	Reduced heart rate
AV node	Reduced conduction velocity
Blood vessels	Vasodilation (most of doubtful physiological significance)
Lungs	
Smooth muscle	Contraction—bronchoconstriction
Glands	Secretion
Gastrointestinal tract	
Smooth muscle	Increased motility and tone—peristalsis
Sphincters	Relaxation
Glands	Secretion
Gall-bladder	Contraction
Bladder	
Detrusor muscle	Contraction
Sphincter	Relaxation
Exocrine glands	Secretion

that the system has widespread effects throughout the body. It is important in the control of the amount of light entering the eye and its focusing for near vision. Stimulation of parasympathetic nerves generally leads to an increase in the output of secretions from glands, whether these be tears, gastric acid or the secretions from the nasopharyngeal and bronchial glands. As mentioned previously, this system is associated with periods of energy conservation and this is reflected in the muscarinic responses of slowed heart rate and slowed atrioventricular (AV) conduction in the heart. The gastrointestinal response to parasympathetic stimulation also demonstrates the principle of energy conservation, i.e. the increase in peristalsis and in the secretions from salivary and other glands enables the efficient digestion of food and extraction of the energy from it. Presynaptic cholinergic receptors have been shown to occur on parasympathetic and sympathetic nerves. These receptors are believed to be involved in the modulation of transmitter output. Once acetylcholine has been released from nerve terminals and has had its effect on the postsynaptic receptors, it is appropriate that it is rapidly removed from the synapse. In the normal functioning of the autonomic nervous system the most efficient maintenance of homeostasis depends on the ability of the system to respond quickly to changes in the environment. An important feature of this is that the responses are short-lived and thus an efficient mechanism for the removal of transmitter is required. In the case of the parasympathetic system, acetylcholine is rapidly degraded in the synapse by the enzyme acetylcholinesterase. Choline and acetic acid are liberated by the reaction and the choline is then available for uptake into the nerve to be used in the synthesis of acetylcholine. The enzyme, which occurs in neurones, at autonomic neuro-effector junctions and at motor end-plates, is largely responsible for the termination of the effects of acetylcholine. There is another enzyme (serum cholinesterase or pseudo-cholinesterase), which occurs in plasma and at some other sites, that is also capable of hydrolysing acetylcholine. This enzyme can hydrolyse other esters and it is involved in the metabolism of drugs, such as the muscle relaxant suxamethonium and the local anaesthetic procaine.

Bearing in mind the normal processes involved in the biosynthesis, storage and release of acetylcholine, its actions at muscarinic receptors and the mechanism responsible for its inactivation, the actions of drugs which interfere with these processes and the responses to these drugs can be explained.

Although drugs which inhibit the uptake of choline into cholinergic nerves are known (e.g. hemicholinium) and there are some substances capable of inhibiting the actions of choline acetyltransferase, none of these exerts any clinically useful effect. Various toxins are known to have effects on the release of acetylcholine. Clostridium botulinum, an anaerobic bacterium, produces a highly potent toxin which exerts its effect by inhibiting the release of acetylcholine from cholinergic nerves. The inhibition of transmitter release from the phrenic nerve to the diaphragm results in death from respiratory failure. Drugs also may influence the actions of acetylcholine by combining with its receptors and either mimicking or blocking its actions. Cholinergic agonists which stimulate muscarinic receptors are called parasympathomimetic agents; those which are antagonists at muscarinic receptors are called para-sympatholytics.

Parasympathomimetic drugs

Besides acetylcholine itself, there are a number of naturally occurring alkaloids which stimulate muscarinic receptors. These include arecoline, muscarine and pilocarpine. Arecoline is the active principle of the betel nut, chewed for its euphoric effect and as a digestive aid by the people of the East Indies. The nut is the seed of *Areca catechu*. Arecoline also has some activity at nicotinic receptors. Muscarine (Fig. 2.3) has been isolated from the poisonous mushroom, *Amanita muscaria*. Because its action is limited almost exclusively to stimulation of muscarinic receptors, it has played an important role in the study of the receptors of the autonomic nervous system. Pilocarpine is found in the leaves of the tree, *Pilocarpus jaborandi*, and is a potent muscarinic agonist with only weak nicotinic effects. The actions of all of these compounds are due to their ability to stimulate muscarinic receptors and can be easily predicted from an appreciation of the contents of Table 2.1.

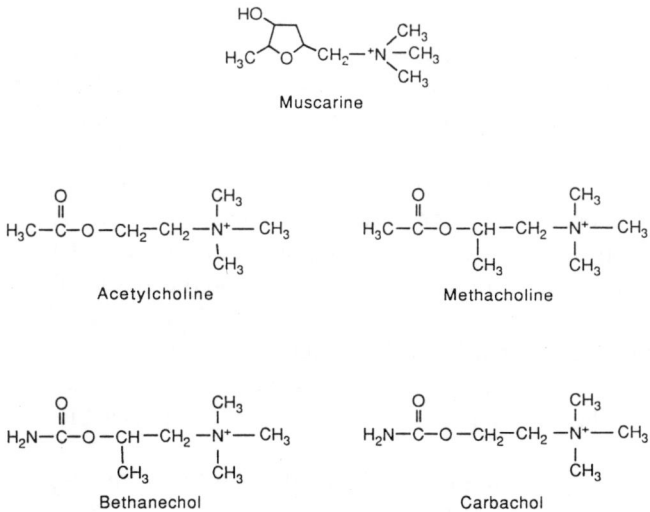

Figure 2.3 Structural formulae of muscarinic agonists.

Acetylcholine is of little use in clinical practice since it has a very short duration of action and it is not selective for muscarinic receptors. A number of parasympathomimetic agents have been synthesized, the main aim being to produce a selective muscarinic agonist with more persistent activity. Relatively slight chemical modifications of the acetylcholine molecule (Fig. 2.3) have resulted in synthetic parasympathomimetic agents with significantly increased selectivity and prolonged duration of action.

Methacholine (Fig. 2.3) is a more selective muscarinic agonist than acetylcholine, with only slight nicotinic activity. It is also less susceptible to the actions of acetylcholinesterase and hence has a longer duration of action than the transmitter. Bethanechol (Fig. 2.3) has virtually no nicotinic activity and is even more resistant to acetylcholinesterase than methacholine. It is therefore a more selective and longer-lasting agonist than methacholine. Carbachol (Fig. 2.3) is also resistant to hydrolysis and therefore has a long duration of action, but it has considerable nicotinic activity.

Like those of the naturally occurring alkaloids, the main actions of the synthetic muscarinic agents can be predicted from Table 2.1. Some qualitative differences have been observed. Methacholine has the most pronounced effect on the cardiovascular system, producing vasodilation and either a direct depression of heart rate or a reflex rise in heart rate, depending on dose and route of administration. Carbachol and bethanechol are more effective stimulants of the smooth muscle of the gastrointestinal and urinary tracts.

Therapeutic uses of parasympathomimetics

With the exception of pilocarpine, the alkaloids are not widely used clinically. Where muscarinic activity is required, it is more common to use one of the synthetic parasympathomimetic agents. The side-effects of the drugs in this group are those which arise from stimulation of muscarinic receptors in organs other than the target organ and include excessive salivation, cardiac slowing and bronchoconstriction.

Pilocarpine is used in the treatment of glaucoma, by the local application of a solution of pilocarpine nitrate. The stimulation of the muscarinic receptors in the ciliary muscle of the lens and the sphincter muscle of the iris results in spasm of accommodation and constriction of the pupil. There is a pull on the scleral spur opening the trabecular meshwork, an increase of the drainage angle and increased aqueous outflow through the open angle and trabecular meshwork. Pilocarpine is often the drug of choice when therapy is initiated as other, more potent drugs may cause pupillary block and worsen the glaucoma.

When tear secretion is inadequate in the syndrome of 'dry eye' in dogs (keratoconjunctivitis sicca, KCS), pilocarpine is also used, either topically applied or administered by mouth, often in conjunction with one of the artificial tear preparations used in human ophthalmology (p. 326). Such therapy requires constant nursing care, and more recently a surgical approach has been used. The parotid duct is transposed to suture the papilla into the conjunctival sac. There are many reports of the successful use of this technique.

Carbachol has been used as a stimulant of the gastrointestinal tract, but bethanechol, which is more specific for the gastrointestinal tract, may be a better choice. Care should always be taken to ensure that no obstructions exist before the use of such stimulants. Poor bladder function, particularly in small animals, is another indication for bethanechol, after ensuring that there is no obstruction to urination.

Feline dysautonomia was first described in 1982 and similar dysautonomias have been reported in the horse (grass sickness), dog and man. The pathogenesis is unknown, but pre- and postganglionic neurones of the sympathetic and parasympathetic systems undergo degeneration, leading to variable clinical signs. Typically, in the cat, there is inappetence, dehydration, dry oral and nasal mucosae, dilated pupils with third eyelid protrusion, reduced lacrimation, oesophageal dysfunction, urinary retention or incontinence, and constipation. The prognosis is poor (about 50 per cent respond satisfactorily to therapy) and several months of treatment may be required. In addition to fluid therapy, parasympathomimetic drugs are used, with variable benefit, to promote salivation and lacrimation and to aid gut and bladder function. Bethanechol is used, but absorption may be irregular. Pilocarpine or physostigmine, administered as eye drops, are absorbed and produce systemic effects. They should not be used more than twice daily nor in combination. Enemas (e.g. Micralax) and laxatives such as liquid paraffin or danthron (Dorbanex Forte suspension, 2–5 ml daily) are often necessary in addition to parasympathomimetics. Cats which respond to initial treatment may suffer episodes of recurrent constipation, which can be satisfactorily managed with danthron.

Doses

Glaucoma
   pilocarpine 1.0–2.0 per cent, applied topically, 3–4 times daily.

KCS
   pilocarpine 0.25–0.5 per cent, applied topically several times daily, as
      required. 1 per cent ophthalmic preparation, administered p.o., 1
      drop per 5 kg twice daily in food, increase by 1 drop every third day,
      until signs of excessive lacrimation.

Poor bladder function
   bethanechol   dogs   5–25 mg t.i.d.
                   cats   2–5 mg b.i.d.

Feline dysautonomia

bethanechol   2.5 mg p.o., b.i.d.
pilocarpine   1 per cent, 1–2 drops to the eye, b.i.d. ⎫ 5–20 min
physostigmine 0.5 per cent, 1–2 drops to the eye, b.i.d. ⎭ before feeding

Antimuscarinic drugs

Drugs which antagonize the actions of acetylcholine at muscarinic receptors are sometimes referred to as atropinic, since atropine is regarded as the prototype drug of this class. All of the drugs in this group have a mode of action similar to that of atropine, i.e. they act as competitive antagonists at the muscarinic receptor. The action of the drugs at any site can be predicted from the knowledge of the effects of acetylcholine at that site, and, more particularly, from an understanding of the involvement of the parasympathetic nervous system in the function of the tissue or organ in question.

Atropine (dl-hyoscyamine) (Fig. 2.4) is the active principle of *Atropa belladonna*, also known as deadly nightshade. It is a very potent, selective muscarinic antagonist, having little effect at other sites until large doses are used. It is a relatively non-selective antagonist at muscarinic receptors.

Blockade of normal muscarinic function by atropine is most readily observed in glands, where there is inhibition of salivation, lacrimal secretions and sweating. (Although the sweat glands are under sympathetic control, the transmitter is acetylcholine.) As the dose of atropine is increased, effects on the eye become apparent and there is dilation of the pupil and paralysis of accommodation, with the lens fixed for far vision. A rise in intraocular pressure may occur in animals predisposed to narrow angle glaucoma (see page 323). The effects of atropine on heart rate are variable. A fall in heart rate may occur in response to low doses. This is believed to be a centrally

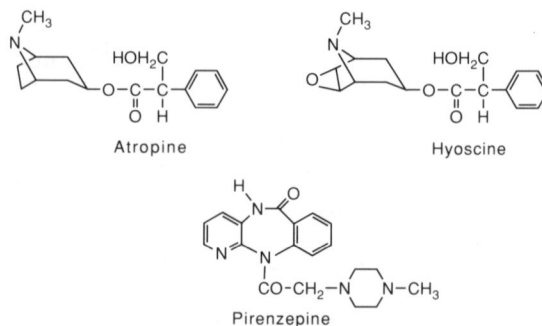

Figure 2.4 Structural formulae of muscarinic antagonists.

mediated response since it does not occur with parasympatholytics which do not penetrate the central nervous system. When the dose is increased, heart rate increases due to blockade of cardiac muscarinic receptors. Atropine relaxes the muscles of the bladder. With relatively large doses the tone and motility of the gastrointestinal tract are reduced, but even at these doses effects on gastric acid secretion may not be significant. Atropine is effective after oral or parenteral administration or after local application to the eye.

Most of the side-effects of atropine are due to the fact that it blocks muscarinic sites throughout the body and when, for example, blockade of receptors in the lungs is required, then the effects of blockade of all other receptors are 'side-effects'. Many of the toxic effects of atropine are due to excessive muscarinic receptor blockade. There is a weak and rapid pulse. Temperature increases due to inhibition of the sweat gland activity. In the central nervous system, toxic doses of atropine produce stimulation and animals may become excited, but this is followed by depression when the toxicity becomes more marked. (It is of interest to note that rabbits can tolerate high doses of atropine, or ingest large amounts of deadly nightshade because they have an enzyme capable of metabolizing atropine.)

Hyoscine (scopolamine) (Fig. 2.4) is isolated from *Hyoscyamus niger* (henbane) and has muscarinic antagonist activity similar to that of atropine. The peripheral effects of hyoscine are qualitatively similar to those of atropine. At doses which cause similar inhibition of salivation, it is less effective than atropine as a vagolytic. Although hyoscine generally produces depression of the central nervous system in man, responses in animals are variable and, in some, it may produce considerable excitement.

Hyoscine-N-butyl bromide is a quaternized form of hyoscine and as such will not cross the blood–brain barrier. Drugs of this type appear to have selectivity for the muscarinic receptors in the gut.

Glycopyrronium is a synthetic quaternary ammonium compound which is more effective as an inhibitor of gastric acid secretion and as an antisialogogue than atropine. The tachycardia is usually less than that caused by atropine.

Hyoscine methobromide and hyoscine methonitrate, like the other quaternary amines, lack central nervous activity and are poorly absorbed from the gastrointestinal tract.

Propantheline has antispasmodic activity with fewer side-effects than other parasympatholytics.

Homatropine, eucatropine and tropicamide are antimuscarinic agents with durations of action considerably shorter than that of atropine. The effects of homatropine are no longer evident after 24 hours. Eucatropine, which dilates the pupil but does not induce cycloplegia, is effective for up to 1 hour.

Pirenzepine (Fig. 2.4) is a relatively new antimuscarinic agent, which appears to be a selective antagonist of the muscarinic receptors involved in the secretion of gastric acid (M_1 receptors).

Therapeutic applications of antimuscarinic drugs

Atropine is used in pre-operative medication, where it reduces salivary secretions and secretions in the respiratory tract, which allows improved gaseous exchange. It also protects the heart from excessive vagal activity during surgical procedures and thereby prevents marked slowing of heart rate. However, it is now accepted that it is probably best to treat bradycardia by the specific injection of atropine when it is required. Glycopyrronium is a useful alternative antimuscarinic for pre-operative medication.

Atropine or glycopyrronium are also used in combination with neostigmine or edrophonium, in the reversal of neuromuscular blockade (see page 166). Some bradyarrhythmias, where excessive vagal activity may be involved, respond to atropine. Ocular examination, without natural reflex responses to light, can be performed after local application of antimuscarinics. Since the effects of atropine can last for 3–4 days, in these cases it is more suitable to use one of the drugs with a shorter duration of action; tropicamide (duration of action 6–12 hours) is the drug of choice. Other antimuscarinics used in ophthalmology include homatropine and cyclopentolate. Great care must be taken in patients with glaucoma since any antimuscarinic agent can increase intraocular pressure and precipitate an attack.

In treatment of poisoning by anticholinesterases, atropine is most effective at preventing the signs which are due to excessive muscarinic activity (see below).

The antispasmodic effects of antimuscarinic drugs can be clinically useful in treatment of muscle spasm in the gastrointestinal or urinary tracts. Propantheline produces muscle relaxation with relatively few side-effects. Hyoscine methobromide and hyoscine-N-butyl bromide are also used as gastrointestinal antispasmodics.

In the treatment of calf scours the addition of an antimuscarinic agent to the antibiotic medication slows the transit of the antibiotic through the gastrointestinal tract and enhances its effectiveness. Pirenzepine is the only M_1 selective muscarinic antagonist available for general use. It is effective at reducing acid output from the oxyntic cells of the stomach. (For further comment on the use of antimuscarinics in gastrointestinal disorders, see page 269.)

Doses

atropine

horse, cattle	30–60 μg/kg s.c.
pig	20–40 μg/kg s.c.
sheep	80–160 μg/kg s.c.
dog, cat	30–100 μg/kg s.c.
	(44 μg/kg is most commonly used).

Ocular
atropine	1 per cent solution
homatropine	1–2 per cent solution
eucatropine	2–10 per cent solution

For use in pre-anaesthetic medication or in combination with neostigmine for reversal of neuromuscular blockade.

glycopyrronium
horse	1–3 μg/kg i.v.
dog	2–8 μg/kg i.m. or i.v.

hyoscine-N-butyl bromide
horse	80–120 mg i.v.
cattle	80–100 mg i.v. or i.m.
calf, pig	20–40 mg i.v. or i.m.
piglet	4–8 mg i.v. or i.m.
dog	4–10 mg i.v. or i.m.

Drugs which block metabolism of acetylcholine

A variety of drugs which inhibit the action of acetylcholinesterase are available. They are of interest for their therapeutic applications and toxicological importance, since many of them are used as pesticides and are involved in cases of poisoning. It is not difficult to predict the responses to drugs which have anticholinesterase activity. Most of their actions are due to the build-up of acetylcholine released from parasympathetic nerves and therefore are very similar to the effects of the muscarinic agonists.

Reversible anticholinesterases produce their effects by reversibly combining with the active site of the enzyme. After a period of time the drug is either metabolized by the enzyme or diffuses away; in either case the enzyme is then able to continue with the metabolism of acetylcholine in the normal way. The structures of neostigmine, physostigmine and edrophonium, three of the reversible anticholinesterases, are shown in Fig. 2.5.

Some of the agents commonly used as pesticides are organophosphorus derivatives (Fig. 2.5). The interaction between these drugs and acetylcholinesterase involves the formation of a covalent bond between the phosphorus atom of the drug and the active site of the enzyme. This type of bond is most unusual in pharmacological drug–receptor interactions and, unless there is some early, specific intervention, an irreversible inhibition occurs.

Physostigmine (eserine) is a naturally occurring alkaloid, isolated from the calabar bean, with reversible anticholinesterase activity. A number of unpleasant side-effects limit its general clinical use and the synthetic substance neostigmine is more commonly used.

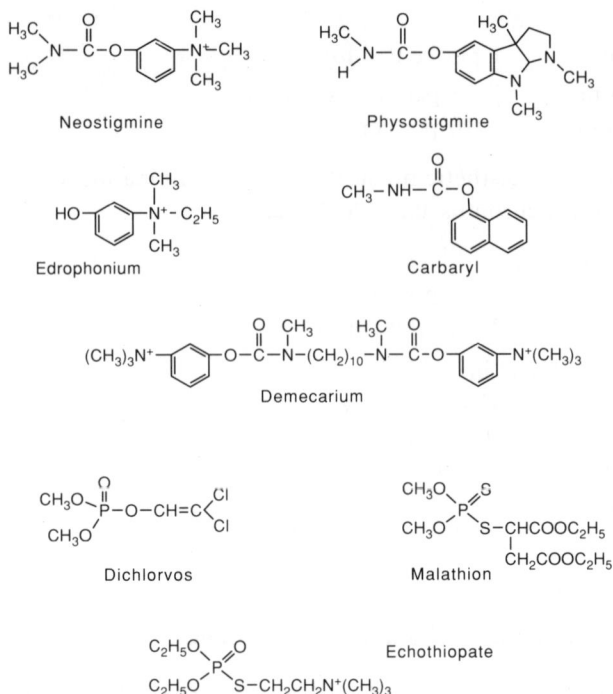

Figure 2.5 Structural formulae of anticholinesterases.

Neostigmine combines with the active site of acetylcholinesterase and is very slowly hydrolysed. During the prolonged period required for the hydrolysis of the drug, the active site of the enzyme is unavailable for the metabolism of acetylcholine. Thus the levels of transmitter increase and its effects are more pronounced. Pyridostigmine is closely related to neostigmine and has a similar mode of action. Demecarium consists of two neostigmine molecules connected by a series of ten methylene groups (Fig. 2.5). It is more potent and has a longer duration of action than neostigmine. Edrophonium is a quaternary alcohol which combines with acetylcholinesterase but is not a substrate for hydrolysis. Its duration of action is much less than that of carbamates such as neostigmine and physostigmine as it simply diffuses away from the active site of the enzyme after a short period of time.

Side-effects of anticholinesterases are similar to those of the directly acting muscarinic agonists because they are due mainly to the increased levels of transmitter which can accumulate in the absence of normal metabolism.

The irreversible anticholinesterases or organophosphorus insecticides are mainly of toxicological significance as domestic animals are likely to come into contact with them when they are used in the home or on the farm. Those commonly used as ectoparasiticides include dichlorvos (Fig. 2.5) and coumaphos. Carbaryl is the most commonly used carbamate-based agricultural and garden insecticide. Its actions are similar to those of the organophosphorus group, but less persistent.

Some of these insecticides are thiophosphates, which need to be converted to phosphates to become active. These are generally less toxic in mammals because the conversion occurs much less rapidly than in insects. The drugs are also readily inactivated by mammalian metabolism. Thus a degree of selective toxicity is present. It should be stressed, however, that although there may be a difference in the reaction of insects and mammals, these compounds are all extremely potent poisons and great care, for both man and animals, should be taken in their handling, use and disposal.

The 'irreversible' nature of the action of these drugs arises from the formation of a particularly stable bond between the enzyme and inhibitor. In the early stages of the interaction it is possible to cleave the bond between the hydroxy-serine residue at the active site of the enzyme and the phosphorus atom of the inhibitor. After an 'ageing' period, the enzyme is permanently phosphorylated and no regeneration of active enzyme is possible.

Most of the commonly used drugs are very lipid soluble and are readily absorbed after oral ingestion, inhalation of sprays or on contact with skin. Early signs of acute poisoning with anticholinesterases vary, depending on the route of ingestion of the poison. In each case, the effect seen is due to high concentrations of acetylcholine at the site of contact, i.e. vomiting and diarrhoea if via the oral route, bronchoconstriction and copious bronchial secretions if inhaled, and local vasodilation, sweating and muscle twitching if via skin. Because of the rapid distribution of the compounds, after a short while signs of poisoning occur in all systems. The heart rate is slow because of enhanced vagal action at the S–A node. Marked ocular effects, miosis and ciliary spasm are obvious. Besides the autonomic effects of high levels of acetylcholine, there is also an effect at the skeletal neuromuscular junction. Initially the increased levels of transmitter cause muscle twitching, but as the toxicity progresses a depolarizing blockade of the nicotinic receptors occurs and the skeletal muscle becomes paralysed.

The drugs easily cross the blood–brain barrier and cause restlessness, confusion and ataxia. In severe cases, convulsions followed by coma may occur. In the absence of treatment, central respiratory paralysis, combined with peripheral respiratory distress due to bronchoconstriction, increased secretions and skeletal muscular weakness, will eventually kill the animal. Chronic exposure is sometimes associated with the development of a neuropathy characterized by demyelination and axonal degeneration. The inhibition of an enzyme other than acetylcholinesterase is thought to be involved.

Exposure to lower doses of drug may not be fatal, and with repeated or prolonged exposure animals develop tolerance to the effects of the anticholinesterases. This may be due to desensitization of the cholinergic receptors or increased production of enzyme.

Effective treatment of poisoning by the organophosphorus anticholinesterases begins with removal of any unabsorbed poison if local skin contact has been involved. This requires thorough washing of the affected area, taking care not to contaminate personnel involved in treatment of the poisoned animal. Muscarinic responses to the excessive acetylcholine can be effectively treated with atropine; large doses should be used (1 mg/kg) and the animal observed to ensure that more atropine is administered if required. General supportive therapy, with anticonvulsants, artificial ventilation or other measures as required, should be instituted as appropriate.

Cholinesterase reactivators, such as pralidoxime (up to 10 mg/kg, repeated after 1 hour, if required) and obidoxime (up to 10 mg/kg), are able to cleave the covalent bond formed between the drug and enzyme and regenerate the activity of the enzyme. They are only effective if administered soon after poisoning, i.e. before ageing of the enzyme–inhibitor complex. Both pralidoxime and obidoxime are charged molecules and thus do not cross the blood–brain barrier. They appear to have most beneficial effects at the skeletal neuromuscular junction.

Therapeutic uses of anticholinesterases

The drugs are used in the treatment of glaucoma, where the local application of the drug to the eye allows the accumulation of high levels of acetylcholine, which then contracts the sphincter muscle of the iris and the ciliary muscle and thus facilitates drainage of the aqueous humour. The elevated intraocular pressure is reduced. The irreversible anticholinesterases dyflos (di-isopropylfluorophosphonate) or echothiopate (Fig. 2.5) are also used.

Neostigmine is used in general anaesthesia to reverse the effects of muscle relaxants (see page 166) and also in the treatment of myasthenia gravis, which has been reported in dogs and, less commonly, in cats. The presenting signs are due to defective neuromuscular transmission. There is evidence that, as in humans, some cases may arise from the development of antibodies against the acetylcholine receptors on skeletal muscle. Neuromuscular junctions anywhere in the body may be affected but typically there is marked muscular weakness on exercise, difficulty in swallowing, facial paresis and ptosis. The beneficial effect of neostigmine (or pyridostigmine) is thought to be due to the increased levels of acetylcholine at the motor endplate, strengthening contraction of the skeletal muscle. When using anticholinesterases in the treatment of myasthenia gravis, dosage is adjusted according to response and it must be appreciated that excess anticholinesterase causes prolonged muscle depolarization, which clinically resembles myasthenia gravis itself. In some cases, therapy can be discontinued after a few weeks without relapse.

The response to an intravenous injection of edrophonium (1–2 mg) is a useful diagnostic aid. About 1 minute after injection, paresis should disappear and the animal should eat, drink and walk normally for about 15 minutes, whilst the effect of the drug persists.

Doses

Glaucoma
   echothiophate or demecarium
      Initially 1 drop of 0.25 per cent solution daily, then adjusted
      according to response.

Reversal of muscle relaxation
   neostigmine
      horse, cow, pig, sheep   0.05 mg/kg i.v.
      cat, dog   0.1   mg/kg i.v.

Myasthenia gravis
   steroid therapy plus
   neostigmine 0.5 mg/kg p.o. t.i.d.
   or pyridostigmine 2 mg/kg p.o. t.i.d.

Sympathetic nervous system

As in the parasympathetic nervous system, acetylcholine is the transmitter at sympathetic ganglia. The postganglionic nerves release noradrenaline (nor-epinephrine) as their transmitter substance. Although adrenaline (epinephrine) itself is not a neurotransmitter, the nerves are usually referred to as 'adrenergic'. Adrenaline is more correctly described as a hormone, which is released from the adrenal medulla during periods of sympathetic activity and whose effects reinforce those of the neuronally released noradrenaline. As mentioned earlier, the adrenal medulla behaves like a sympathetic ganglion, but in response to stimulation instead of exciting a postganglionic nerve, it releases its catecholamine content—a mixture of adrenaline and noradrenaline. The naturally occurring substances adrenaline and noradrenaline, their precursor dopamine and the synthetic drug, isoprenaline (isoproterenol), are sometimes called catecholamines. This term refers to the benzene ring with two adjacent hydroxyl groups, the 'catechol' nucleus which is common to all their structures (see Fig. 2.7).

The synthesis of noradrenaline, as it occurs in adrenergic nerves, is shown in Fig. 2.6. The rate-limiting step in this pathway is the conversion of tyrosine to dihydroxyphenylalanine (DOPA), catalysed by the enzyme tyrosine hydroxylase. There is a mechanism which is responsible for the uptake of dopamine into intracellular storage vesicles. The final steps in the biosynthesis of noradrenaline take place within the vesicles, where the transmitter is stored in combination with ATP and the protein, chromogranin. In the adrenal medulla the enzyme phenylethanolamine N-methyltransferase catalyses the formation of adrenaline by the transfer of a methyl group to the nitrogen atom of noradrenaline (Fig 2.6). This enzyme does not occur in neuronal tissue. Adrenaline is stored in the chromaffin cells of the adrenal medulla.

Release of noradrenaline from sympathetic nerve terminals occurs when the nerve is depolarized (Fig. 2.8). As in the case of cholinergic nerves, the process depends on the presence of Ca^{2+} and involves the release of vesicular contents of noradrenaline after fusion of the vesicles with the membrane of the nerve terminal. In the adrenal medulla, acetylcholine, released from preganglionic nerves, acts on nicotinic receptors and the resultant depolarization causes adrenaline release in a similar manner.

A number of different receptors appear to be responsible for the responses to noradrenaline. The classification of adrenergic receptor types by Ahlquist in 1948 was initially based on the responses of different tissues to agents which stimulated adrenergic receptors (or adrenoceptors). After studies of the effects of these compounds on isolated cardiac muscle, lung tissue and

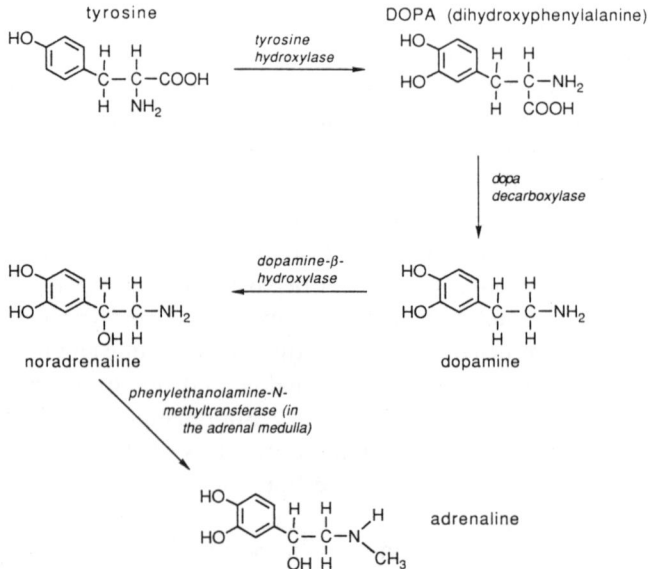

Figure 2.6 Biosynthetic pathway for noradrenaline and adrenaline.

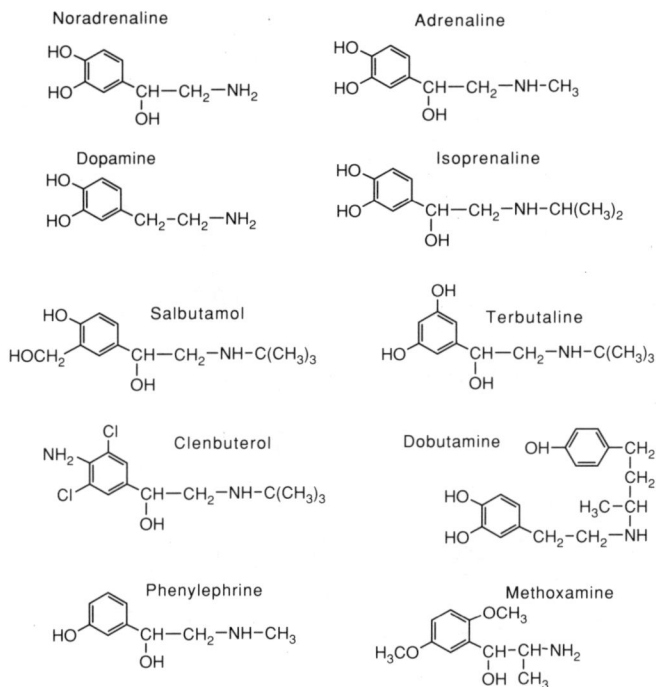

Figure 2.7 Structural formulae of sympathomimetic amines.

strips containing vascular smooth muscle, he found that the order of potency was as follows:

vascular smooth muscle: noradrenaline > adrenaline >>> isoprenaline
cardiac muscle: isoprenaline > adrenaline > noradrenaline
bronchial smooth muscle: isoprenaline > adrenaline >>> noradrenaline

Ahlquist named receptors which did not respond to isoprenaline (like those in vascular smooth muscle) α-adrenoceptors, and those where isoprenaline was the most potent agonist (like those in heart and lung) β-adrenoceptors. He was unable, at that time, to differentiate between the β-adrenoceptors in the heart and lung. With the availability of many more agonists, and particularly with the development of antagonists at these receptors, Lands and his colleagues introduced the terminology of β_1- and β_2-adrenoceptors in 1967. According to the findings from their experiments, Lands classified receptors such as those in the heart, where isoprenaline was the most potent agonist and where noradrenaline was quite a potent agonist, as β_1-adrenoceptors. The receptors where isoprenaline was the most potent agonist, but noradrenaline had little or no activity, like those in the lung, were classified as β_2-adrenoceptors.

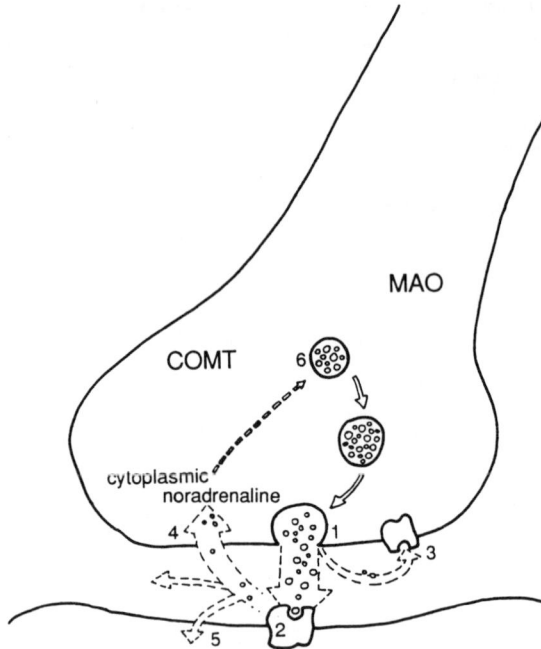

Figure 2.8 Diagrammatic representation of the sympathetic nerve terminal. (1) Noradrenaline is released when the nerve is depolarized. The transmitter crosses the synapse and (2) stimulates postsynaptic receptors. (3) Stimulation of presynaptic receptors reduces further transmitter output. Transmitter action is terminated by (4) Uptake$_1$, into the nerve terminal, and (5) Uptake$_2$, into other cells. Some transmitter may be carried away from the synapse in the blood. Noradrenaline in the cytoplasm can be taken back into vesicles (6) or is metabolized by intracellular catechol-*O*-methyltransferase (COMT) or monoamine oxidase (MAO).

In more recent years differences in α-adrenoceptors have also been recognized. The early work of Ahlquist measured responses of postsynaptic receptors, i.e. those which mediated the responses of the end organ to transmitter released from the nerves which innervated it. More recent work has demonstrated the existence of presynaptic receptors, i.e. those on the nerve terminal itself (Fig. 2.8). Stimulation of these receptors by noradrenaline results in an inhibition of further transmitter output. The receptors fit the broad classification of α-adrenoceptor but they differ from the classic α-adrenoceptors studied by Ahlquist. With the discovery of selective agonists and antagonists, it has now become possible to distinguish between subtypes of α-adrenoceptors and, following the terminology which was used for β-adrenoceptors, they have been named α_1- and α_2-adrenoceptors.

The effects of noradrenaline at α- and β-adrenoceptors are summarized in Table 2.2. It is considered acceptable to generalize about the populations of

Table 2.2 Responses to stimulation of adrenergic receptors

Effector	Response and receptor type
Eye	
Iris, radial muscle	Contraction—mydriasis α_1
Ciliary muscle	Relaxation β
Eyelid	Opening of the palpebral fissure α_1
	Contraction of the nictitating membrane α_1
Salivary glands	Secretions—viscous α_1, β
Heart	
S–A node	Increased heart rate β_1
Muscle	Increased force of contraction, increased conduction velocity β_1
A–V node	Increased conduction velocity β_1
Blood vessels	
Visceral, skin, mucosa	Vasoconstriction α_1
Skeletal muscle	Vasodilation β_2
Lungs	
Smooth muscle	Bronchodilation β_2
Gastrointestinal tract	
Smooth muscle	Relaxation α_1, β_1, β_2
Sphincters	Contraction α_1
Liver	Glycogenolysis α, β
Fat	Triglyceride release α, β
Kidney	Renin release β_1
Bladder	
Detrusor muscle	Relaxation β
Sphincter	Contraction α
Uterus	Relaxation in dioestrus β_2
	Contraction in oestrus α
Spleen	Contraction of capsule α
Skin	Contraction of piloerector muscles α
Skeletal muscle	Tremor β_2
Adrenergic nerve terminals	Reduced transmitter release α_2

receptors in specific organs or tissues, although it has been clearly shown that there are many instances where mixed receptor populations exist. For example, in the case of different types of α-adrenoceptors as described above, it is generally found that postsynaptic α-adrenoceptors are of the α_1 type and presynaptic receptors are α_2-adrenoceptors. There have been many experiments, however, in which α_1-adrenoceptors have been demonstrated in presynaptic locations and α_2-adrenoceptors in postsynaptic locations. Thus Table 2.2 shows the predominant receptor type for each action of transmitter and represents the one of greater pharmacological importance.

Since periods of activity in the sympathetic nervous system tend to involve the whole body in its effort to handle stress, the adrenal medulla is usually stimulated at these times and the response to neuronally released noradrenaline is compounded by the response to circulating adrenaline. The neurotransmitter and the hormone combine to help the animal in 'fight or flight' and most of the responses can be predicted if the physiological needs or general appearance of an animal in this situation are considered.

The eyes actually 'widen with fright' because of the effect of noradrenaline on the muscles of the eyelids and because the pupil is dilated. In the cardiovascular system a number of different responses combine to shunt blood to the skeletal muscle to provide the increased energy needed to 'fly' or fight. This is efficiently achieved by the constriction of blood vessels which supply areas which are not of immediate importance for the present emergency, so blood flow to the viscera, skin and glands is reduced to a minimum. Stimulation of the β_2-adrenoceptors in the blood vessels which supply the skeletal muscles ensures these vessels are dilated and blood flow through them can increase. The cardiac stimulation, both rate and force of contraction, increases cardiac output, thus ensuring a good supply to the skeletal muscles and vital organs. Improved oxygenation of the blood is achieved by dilation of the bronchioles, and increased supplies of energy for the working muscles are ensured by the breakdown of glycogen and fat.

An interesting response in animals (which also occurs to some extent in man) is the contraction of the pilomotor muscles, which causes the hair to rise and may alert the opponent or make the animal appear more daunting. Sweat secretion is increased; the nerves involved are anatomically and functionally sympathetic, but in this case the transmitter released is acetylcholine.

Stimulation of the α-adrenoceptors of the splenic capsule causes contraction which results in a discharge of blood into the circulation. This effect could be of significance for the protection of an animal under conditions of stress, such as those associated with severe blood loss or hypoxia, when stimulation of the sympathetic nervous system is known to occur.

Both α- and β-adrenoceptors are found in the uterus; the number of each is species-specific and also dependent on the prevailing hormonal tone. In general, increased progesterone levels are associated with an increase in the number of uterine β-adrenoceptors.

The interaction of noradrenaline and adrenaline with β-adrenoceptors results in the stimulation of a membrane-bound enzyme, adenylate cyclase. The enzyme catalyses the conversion of ATP to adenosine 3′,5′-monophosphate (cyclic AMP), which then phosphorylates intracellular proteins. The final response depends on the cell type and the nature of the proteins which are phosphorylated. Rapid dephosphorylation of the proteins occurs when the receptor occupation ceases and any cyclic AMP remaining is broken down by phosphodiesterase.

A number of mechanisms exist to ensure the rapid inactivation of noradrenaline. The majority, 80 – 90 per cent, is taken back into the nerve terminal by an active mechanism called $Uptake_1$ (Fig. 2.8). This system has a high affinity for noradrenaline, which is returned to the interior of the cell where it can then, by a different mechanism, be taken up into the storage vesicles. The process called $Uptake_2$ has a higher affinity for adrenaline and is responsible for the uptake of catecholamines into non-neuronal tissue. There are also two enzymes capable of metabolizing noradrenaline and adrenaline. Monoamine oxidase (MAO) is found mainly in the mitochondria and will oxidatively deaminate noradrenaline that enters the cell or is released intraneuronally. Catechol-O-methyltransferase (COMT), a cytoplasmic enzyme, methylates catecholamines at the 3-hydroxyl position, producing inactive metabolites. The enzyme is distributed widely and is responsible for the rapid inactivation of circulating adrenaline and noradrenaline.

A considerable number of drugs interfere with the normal function of the sympathetic nervous system. Compounds which affect the synthesis, storage or release of noradrenaline, those which either mimic or inhibit its actions at adrenergic receptors, and those which inhibit its uptake all have the capacity to produce widespread effects in the body. Many of these drugs are important in human medicine; some of them are also important in veterinary practice.

The biosynthesis of noradrenaline is inhibited by drugs which inhibit tyrosine hydroxylase, the rate-limiting enzyme in the pathway. The drugs which have the capacity to do this (e.g. α-methyltyrosine) have no clinical application in human or veterinary medicine. Other substances (e.g. α-methyldopa) also interfere with noradrenaline synthesis, by substituting for the normal substrate, DOPA, and resulting in the formation of α-methylnoradrenaline. The actions of this 'false transmitter' in the periphery and, probably more importantly in the central nervous system, account for its antihypertensive effect in man, but there is no veterinary use for α-methyldopa.

Storage of noradrenaline can also be affected by drugs. Reserpine, an alkaloid from the shrub Rauwolfia serpentina, interferes with the normal function of the transmitter storage vesicles in the sympathetic nerves. The transmitter is therefore metabolized by the intraneuronal MAO and stores of noradrenaline are depleted. Reserpine was widely used in the past, as an antihypertensive and as a tranquillizer, but newer drugs have largely replaced it. It still has a place in experimental pharmacology, in the investigation of the importance of catecholamine stores in any response, although in some species it can produce unpredictable and harmful central effects.

Adrenergic neurone blockers are drugs which inhibit the release of noradrenaline from sympathetic nerves. These compounds are all substrates for Uptake$_1$ and, once inside the nerve, prevent further release of transmitter. Guanethidine, the prototype of this class, like reserpine, is no longer commonly used as an antihypertensive because of the many side-effects which result from the inhibition of sympathetic function. Bretylium is another adrenergic neurone blocker which finds some use as an anti-arrhythmic agent (see page 230).

All of the drugs which inhibit the normal processes of synthesis, storage and release of noradrenaline have similar actions. These can be predicted from the information in Table 2.2. The most obvious effects are in the cardiovascular system, where the sympathetic nervous system plays a dominant role in control of blood pressure. In the absence of sympathetic tone to blood vessels there is generalized vasodilation and a fall in blood pressure. Reflex adjustments of blood pressure are also inhibited, leading to orthostatic hypotension. In the gastrointestinal tract, the unopposed parasympathetic tone results in increased motility, with diarrhoea being a common problem. Besides the disturbance of normal control, the animals affected by these drugs do not have the ability to respond appropriately to stressful situations. Modern therapy relies on more selective drugs, reducing the need to obtund the whole sympathetic nervous system in order to deal with one, relatively small aspect of it.

Sympathomimetic drugs

Drugs which mimic the actions of noradrenaline may act either by direct combination with adrenoceptors or by inducing the release of noradrenaline. The latter method requires that the drug is taken up into the nerve (by Uptake$_1$) before inducing the release of noradrenaline from the nerve. Most of the drugs which do this also have the ability to interact directly with adrenergic receptors, i.e. they have a mixed action.

Adrenaline, despite its relatively short duration of action, is an important drug. It has the ability to stimulate α-, β_1- and β_2-adrenoceptors. The pressor response to adrenaline is less than that to noradrenaline because the vasoconstrictor effects of adrenaline (mediated via α-adrenoceptors) are counteracted, to some extent, by its vasodilator effects (mediated via β_2-adrenoceptors). Its actions are rapidly terminated by Uptake$_2$ and metabolism by MAO and COMT. Its clinically useful actions include cardiac stimulation, vasoconstriction and bronchodilation (see below).

Most commercially available preparations of adrenaline contain antioxidants because adrenaline is easily oxidized in the presence of heat or light. The oxidation product, adrenochrome, is coloured pink and any batch of adrenaline solution which is discoloured in this way (or which is brown, indicating further oxidation) must not be used.

Noradrenaline has little clinical application. Because it has little or no β_2-adrenoceptor stimulant activity, the pressor response to noradrenaline is more marked than that after adrenaline. This results in stimulation of the baroreceptors which respond by slowing heart rate. The final response observed in an animal depends on the combined effect of direct stimulation of cardiac β_1-adrenoceptors and reflex slowing.

Dopamine, the natural precursor of noradrenaline (Fig. 2.6), is an agonist at α- and β-adrenoceptors and also at dopamine receptors. The latter are found in the renal artery where stimulation by dopamine results in an increase in renal blood flow. Dopamine is an important transmitter in the central nervous system, but in the periphery it is probably of significance only in the kidney. It has been used in humans in the management of acute heart failure but the veterinary clinical use of dopamine is limited.

Isoprenaline (Fig. 2.7), one of the synthetic catecholamines used in the initial classification of β-adrenoceptors, is a directly acting, non-selective agonist, i.e. it stimulates both β_1- and β_2-adrenoceptors. Its cardiac stimulant action, via the β_1-adrenoceptors, results in an increase in heart rate and force of contraction while the stimulation of β_2-adrenoceptors in blood vessels tends to reduce blood pressure. Since there is no α-adrenoceptor stimulation to counteract the vasodilation, even though the heart is beating more forcefully, mean blood pressure falls and the baroreceptor response to this further increases heart rate.

The most widely used β_2-adrenoceptor stimulants are salbutamol, terbutaline and, especially for veterinary use, clenbuterol (Fig. 2.7). These drugs all have similar effects, causing effective bronchodilation by stimulation of the β_2-adrenoceptors in the bronchial muscle, with little or no effect at cardiac β_1-adrenoceptors. The separation of cardiac and bronchial activity is increased when the drugs are administered by inhalation, since there is then direct delivery of the drug to the site of action and the need for high circulating levels is reduced.

β_2-Adrenoceptor agonists also relax the myometrium and clenbuterol is a potent agonist at this site, with a prolonged duration of action. Isoxuprine, which has some β-adrenoceptor stimulant activity, has also been used to relax uterine muscle. A common side-effect of administration of β_2-adrenoceptor stimulants is tremor in skeletal muscle.

The problems of tachycardia and arrhythmias associated with the use of adrenaline as a cardiac stimulant led to the design of a series of experiments to find a substance which would retain the inotropic effects of adrenaline but have reduced chronotropic and arrhythmogenic activity. Dobutamine, a synthetic catecholamine with a structure, as its name implies, similar to that of dopamine (Fig. 2.7), was found to fulfil the criteria most satisfactorily.

Selective α_1-adrenoceptor agonists, such as phenylephrine and methoxamine (Fig. 2.7), cause an increase in blood pressure which elicits the baroreceptor reflex response and thereby reduces heart rate. They may be useful in situations where vasoconstriction is required without direct cardiac effects, e.g. during anaesthesia to increase blood pressure. However, great care must be taken when animals are anaesthetized by halogenated hydrocarbon anaesthetics, since many of these sensitize the heart to the arrhythmogenic actions of adrenoceptor agonists. Local application of drugs of this nature may be useful in decongesting nasal mucous membranes and reducing nasal discharge.

All of the α-adrenoceptor agonists described above stimulate α_1-adrenoceptors. α_2-Adrenoceptor agonists are used in veterinary medicine, but their actions are a result of interaction with α_2-adrenoceptors in the central nervous system. Drugs in this class include xylazine and detomidine, which are used as sedatives (see page 126-7), and clonidine, which is used as an antihypertensive in man. Clonidine has no veterinary application.

The sympathomimetic effects of the drugs described above are exerted largely through direct stimulation of either α- or β-adrenoceptors and in some cases partly by the liberation of noradrenaline. The only substance which is purely indirect in its action is tyramine, a naturally occurring amine, found in a variety of foods for human consumption (e.g. cheese, red wine, yeast or beef extracts) and in a number of plants, with the possibility of high levels in silage. As an indirectly acting amine, tyramine is a substrate for Uptake$_1$ and displaces noradrenaline from the nerves. Normally, after oral ingestion, tyramine is metabolized in the gut by MAO. Therefore no sympathomimetic effect occurs, unless animals have been treated with drugs which inhibit the actions of MAO (see page 72).

Therapeutic uses of sympathomimetic amines

Adrenaline is most effective in the treatment of anaphylactic shock, where it increases both heart rate and force of contraction, increases blood pressure by its cardiac stimulant and vasoconstrictor actions, and helps to alleviate the bronchoconstriction associated with the release of mediators of the allergic response. It is administered intramuscularly or intravenously and is often so rapidly effective that the signs of anaphylaxis may abate while the injection is being given.

The cardiac stimulant action of adrenaline is also useful in the management of acute cardiac arrest, after the heartbeat has been restored by some physical means (electric shock, external cardiac massage). Intravenous injection is necessary in these cases, for rapid onset of effect. Adrenaline may also be used to restore the heartbeat in the asystolic heart. Intracardiac injections are required, but these should be avoided if the chest is closed since fibrillation may be induced or exacerbated and damage to the coronary vessels or conducting system is possible. In weakly fibrillating hearts, administration of adrenaline may produce coarse fibrillation, which can then be electrically (usually) or chemically defibrillated.

There are some disadvantages associated with the use of adrenaline as a cardiac stimulant. The interaction with cardiac β_1-adrenoceptors results in an increase in the force of contraction, but also in heart rate. In situations where the heart muscle is in failure, the increase in inotropy is required, but the tachycardia represents an increased burden for the heart. At the higher heart rate there is usually an increase in oxygen demand, and the increased work performed is less efficient in terms of oxygen usage. Furthermore, with higher doses of adrenaline, or when the heart is sensitized by the presence of halogenated hydrocarbon general anaesthetics, cardiac arrhythmias can occur. The use of dobutamine in the emergency treatment of heart failure (see page 218) overcomes some of the problems encountered with adrenaline.

Solutions of local anaesthetic may contain added adrenaline, where its vasoconstrictor activity reduces local blood flow, slowing the rate of removal of the local anaesthetic from the site of injection and hence prolonging its duration of action (see page 175). Adrenaline is also useful as a vasoconstrictor in the temporary control of bleeding from small blood vessels and capillaries, but the possibility of reactive vasodilation and secondary bleeding as the reaction wears off must be considered. Application directly at the site of bleeding by swabs soaked in adrenaline will clear an operative field if required. Care must be taken with high doses as the resultant ischaemia may lead to local necrosis and delayed healing, and also in the presence of hydrocarbon anaesthetics, when the heart may be sensitized to the arrhythmogenic actions of adrenaline.

Isoprenaline is used as a cardiac stimulant in emergencies. Because of the nature of such conditions, the drug must be administered by intravenous injection, although it is effective after subcutaneous injection or inhalation. The latter route of administration was used formerly when the β_2-adrenoceptor stimulant activity of isoprenaline was used to induce bronchodilation. Because of the lack of selectivity of the drug, stimulation of the cardiac β_1-adrenoceptors increased heart rate and this tachycardia was an undesirable side-effect. With the development of more selective β_2-adrenoceptor agonists (salbutamol, terbutaline and clenbuterol), isoprenaline is no longer used as a bronchodilator (see Chapter 13).

The use of β_2-adrenoceptor agonists to relax uterine muscle is increasing. The therapeutic use of these drugs is described on page 313.

Isoxuprine, although chemically similar to the β-adrenoceptor agonists, induces a vasodilator response which is not completely antagonized by β-adrenoceptor antagonists. It is used in the management of navicular disease (see page 205) to improve the blood supply to the navicular bone. It must not be used in pregnant animals or after arterial haemorrhage.

Phenylephrine is used as a decongestant and as a mydriatic, to permit examination of the fundus.

Doses

Drugs with catecholamine-based structures are less effective after oral administration because they are destroyed by MAO in the gut.

adrenaline
cattle, horse   4–8 μg/kg i.m. or s.c.
                2–4 μg/kg slow i.v.
dog, cat   0.5–10 μg/kg s.c., i.m. or slow i.v.

isoprenaline
dog   10 ng/kg/min i.v.

isoxuprine
horse   60–90 mg/100 kg b.i.d. for 21 days followed by
               90–120 mg/100 kg twice daily for 14 days, then
               reduced over a further 3 week period.
Doses should be administered p.o., 30 min before feeding. Treatment is repeated intermittently, as indicated by clinical response.

phenylephrine
Pressor effects   dog   0.088 mg/kg i.v., approx. double this s.c. or i.m.
Decongestant   0.125 per cent solution applied topically.

Sympatholytic drugs

In general, these are antagonists at either α- or β-adrenoceptors. Only one, labetalol, blocks both types of adrenergic receptor.

Early α-adrenoceptor antagonists (phenoxybenzamine, phentolamine) were unselective in their ability to block α_1- and α_2-adrenoceptors. Clinical applications were limited and they have been largely replaced by the selective α_1-adrenoceptor antagonist, prazosin (Fig. 2.9). The most important action of prazosin is the blockade of α_1-adrenoceptors in the smooth muscle of blood vessels. The stimulation of these receptors by noradrenaline is responsible for maintenance of vascular tone, and in the presence of prazosin there is a reduction in resistance in both arteries and veins. Since prazosin is a selective α_1-adrenoceptor antagonist, it has no effect at the α_2-adrenoceptors located on the nerve terminals and therefore does not alter the control of transmitter release.

The response of any physiological system to a β-adrenoceptor antagonist depends on the degree of sympathetic tone present in that system at the time. Thus, in an animal at rest, where there is little background sympathetic tone,

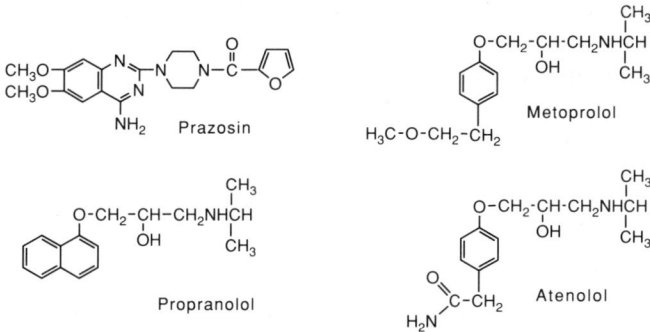

Figure 2.9 Structural formulae of adrenoceptor antagonists.

the administration of a β-adrenoceptor antagonist has little effect on the heart rate, force of contraction or blood pressure. The drugs do, however, reduce the cardiovascular response to exercise or stress. One of the oldest and the most extensively studied drugs of the group is propranolol (Fig. 2.9), which is a non-selective, competitive antagonist at β-adrenoceptors.

The main problems associated with the use of β-adrenoceptor antagonists like propranolol occur in animals with compromised cardiovascular or respiratory systems. In heart failure the sympathetic nervous system contributes significant cardiac stimulant tone and the administration of a drug (e.g. to control a tachyarrhythmia) which antagonizes this effect may exacerbate the failure. Similarly, in animals with compromised pulmonary function, there is an increased risk of bronchospasm when a β_2-adrenoceptor antagonist is administered. The use of selective β_1-adrenoceptor antagonists reduces the risk, but it should be remembered that these drugs are only selective, and there is the possibility that some β_2-adrenoceptor blockade may occur and the likelihood of this increases with increasing doses. Examples of β_1-selective antagonists are atenolol and metoprolol (Fig. 2.9).

Therapeutic uses of adrenoceptor antagonists

The most common use of prazosin is in the treatment of hypertension in man, but its use in the management of cardiac failure is increasing (see page 219).

β-Adrenoceptor antagonists are very widely used in human clinical medicine, in angina, hypertension, cardiac arrhythmias and migraine. In veterinary practice their use is limited to the treatment of cardiac arrhythmias in dogs (see page 229) and occasionally in the management of heart failure (see page 222).

β-Adrenoceptor inhibition in the eye reduces the formation of aqueous humour and local application of antagonists is beneficial in the treatment of glaucoma. Timolol is the drug of choice. Each application provides relief for 12 hours, with little or no effect on pupil size. There is some risk of systemic absorption through the conjunctiva or nasal mucosa.

Doses

Adrenoceptor antagonists: see Chapters 10 and 16.

Drugs which inhibit noradrenaline removal

Uptake$_1$ is inhibited by drugs which are known as tricyclic antidepressants (imipramine, amitriptyline, desipramine). As their name implies, they are used in the treatment of depression in man, but they have no therapeutic application in veterinary medicine.

The action of monoamine oxidase is inhibited by another group of drugs, which are also used in the treatment of depression and have antihypertensive activity in man. It should be noted that although these applications are not relevant to veterinary clinical practice, both monoamine oxidase inhibitors and tricyclic antidepressants are considerably more toxic in dogs than in man and instances of fatal and near fatal poisoning after accidental ingestion of these drugs have been reported.

Some drugs which are used for other applications may, as a side-effect, inhibit the activity of MAO. An example of this is furazolidone, used as a chemotherapeutic agent, which is metabolized into a compound with MAO inhibitory activity. High levels of tyramine can occur in some plants and silage and, in animals treated with furazolidone, such ingested tyramine would no longer be destroyed in the gut. Thus it may enter the circulation, be taken up into sympathetic nerve terminals and cause release of noradrenaline. The most serious consequence of this sequence of events is the development of a hypertensive crisis.

Ganglionic transmission

Acetylcholine is the transmitter at both sympathetic and parasympathetic ganglia. Thus it is released from the preganglionic nerves and, after crossing the synapse, it stimulates receptors on the postganglionic nerves. These receptors were originally classified as nicotinic, although it is now known that a number of different types of receptors, including muscarinic receptors, also occur on postganglionic nerves.

The response to nicotine is complex and results from the combination of the effects of initial stimulation of sympathetic and parasympathetic ganglia and sites in the central nervous system, followed by depression at these sites. The adrenal medulla and carotid and aortic chemoreceptors are also stimulated by nicotine. The sum of these effects results in increased blood pressure and heart rate and respiratory stimulation. The drug is a potent toxin and salivation, vomiting and muscle fasciculation follow with slightly higher doses. If the dose is increased further, the depressant effects of nicotine become obvious, with death from central respiratory failure and weakness of the skeletal muscles required for breathing.

Drugs which antagonize the effects of nicotine at autonomic ganglia are called ganglion-blocking drugs. The side-effects of these drugs are numerous, as the normal function of the entire autonomic nervous system is inhibited by their action. With the development of more selective antagonists at adrenergic and cholinergic receptor sites, ganglion-blocking agents are no longer used.

CHAPTER 3

HORMONES AND AUTACOIDS

Hormones are the natural secretions of endocrine glands. They are transported to distant sites in the body where they interact with receptors to produce characteristic responses. Aspects of the endocrine system relating to the anti-inflammatory actions of hormones of the adrenal cortex and to reproduction are discussed in Chapters 8 and 15 respectively. This chapter describes the therapy of disorders of the pancreas, thyroid, pituitary and adrenal glands and the clinical applications of the anabolic steroids.

Other naturally occurring substances exert their effects in the immediate area of their release. These substances are called 'autacoids', a term derived from Greek, meaning self-remedy. The substances include histamine, serotonin (5-hydroxytryptamine or 5-HT), prostaglandins, leukotrienes (see Chapter 8) and the endogenous polypeptides. They are very potent substances and many appear to be involved in physiological and pathological processes. The actions of histamine and serotonin and some of their antagonists are described in this chapter. Although there is no therapeutic application for these autacoids, their antagonists are used in human and veterinary medicine.

Hormones

The pancreas

Insulin is a polypeptide hormone (molecular weight approx. 6000), released from the pancreas. It consists of two amino acid chains, linked by two disulphide bridges. The amino acid sequence of insulin shows some species variation, although the specific activities of most mammalian insulins are similar. Glucagon, also released from the pancreas, is a smaller (molecular weight about 3500), single chain polypeptide. There appears to be no difference in the amino acid sequence of glucagon molecules from different species.

The islets of Langerhans consist of α cells (about 25% of the islet cells), which produce glucagon, and β cells (about 60% of islet cells), which produce insulin. The remaining cells secrete somatostatin and pancreatic polypeptide. The actions of insulin are related to the storage of fuels, including glucose, amino acids and fatty acids. The presence of these and gastrointestinal hormones associated with digestion stimulate release of insulin. The islet cells are innervated by both sympathetic and parasympathetic nerves. Stimulation of the sympathetic nervous system, associated with stress and energy expenditure, inhibits the release of insulin via α-adrenoceptor stimulation. Conversely, acetylcholine, released from parasympathetic nerves stimulates muscarinic receptors on the islets and thereby induces insulin release.

Insulin binds to cell membrane receptors and increases the intracellular uptake of glucose, amino acids, fatty acids and K^+. Within the cells, glucose metabolism, protein synthesis and deposition of fat and glycogen are all enhanced. These anabolic actions of insulin are increased by its actions to inhibit glycogenolysis, gluconeogenesis and lipolysis.

In general terms, the actions of glucagon are antagonistic to those of insulin; it is a hormone of fuel utilization. The food products, hormones and neurotransmitters which control the release of insulin also control the release of glucagon. Usually the effect on glucagon secretion is opposite to the effect on insulin secretion. For example, a rise in blood glucose leads to an increase in insulin release and a reduction in the release of glucagon.

The opposing effects of glucagon and insulin in healthy animals maintain the blood glucose concentrations within normal limits. These actions are not confined to carbohydrate metabolism; the pancreatic hormones have a complex and incompletely understood role in regulating intermediary metabolism. Besides the metabolic effects, glucagon is also a potent stimulant of rate and force of cardiac contraction.

Insulin and glucagon are readily inactivated in the liver and kidney. Thus the half-life of both of these hormones is of the order of 5 minutes.

Disorders of the pancreas

Diabetes mellitus
The most common endocrine disorder of the pancreas causes diabetes mellitus, characterized by an absolute or relative lack of pancreatic insulin, resulting in

glucose intolerance. This is relatively common in dogs and cats and may be due to deficient insulin production by the pancreatic islets of Langerhans (primary diabetes), or to antagonism of insulin by other hormones (secondary diabetes). Progestogens, thyroid hormone and glucocorticoids all antagonize insulin so that long-term therapy with these hormones may induce secondary diabetes mellitus. This action of progestogens results from the release of pituitary growth hormone which causes peripheral insulin resistance.

Lack of insulin causes hyperglycaemia with consequent glycosuria, osmotic diuresis (polyuria) and polydipsia. The appetite may be normal or increased, although there is commonly weight loss due to tissue catabolism. The deficiency of insulin causes lipolysis but fat metabolism is incomplete, with a consequent increase in plasma free fatty acids and formation of ketones. The excretion of acetone in the breath accounts for the characteristic smell associated with diabetic patients.

The drugs available for treatment of diabetic animals are insulin or those which, after oral administration, produce a hypoglycaemic response. Insulin is obtained commercially from the pancreas of cattle and pigs. Administration by injection is necessary to avoid denaturation in the gastrointestinal tract.

Table 3.1 Insulin preparations

Preparation	Peak activity (hours)	Duration of action (hours)
Soluble insulin	0.5–6	1–10
Isophane insulin	8–12	12–24
Protamine zinc insulin	5–14	24–36

Subcutaneous injections are the most common route of administration but, under certain circumstances, intravenous administration is necessary. A variety of preparations of insulin are available and are listed in Table 3.1. They are designed to provide formulations with different rates of onset of action and duration of action. These times may vary between species; the figures shown in Table 3.1 relate to dogs and are usually lower in cats, which metabolize insulin more rapidly. Soluble (regular or crystalline) insulin is the only formulation suitable for intravenous administration, although it can also be given by other parenteral routes. It has a rapid, short-lived action and is used in hospitalized animals, particularly for treatment of diabetic ketoacidosis. Isophane insulin (insulin zinc suspension) is a modified preparation of protamine zinc insulin, with an intermediate duration of action. It is commonly used for initiating therapy in cases of uncomplicated diabetes. Some patients may require twice daily administration. Protamine zinc insulin is a long-acting preparation, suitable for a single daily injection. It is a combination of insulin, zinc chloride and protamine, which provides depot therapy by delaying the absorption of insulin from the subcutaneous injection site.

The sulphonylureas (including tolbutamide and chlorpropamide), one of the groups of oral hypoglycaemic drugs, are believed to act, at least initially, by stimulating the secretory activity of the β-cells of the islets of Langerhans. They induce hypoglycaemia in normal, but not pancreatectomized, experimental animals. An action to lower blood glucagon concentration and/or an increased binding of insulin to tissue receptors may also be involved. These latter actions may also contribute to the hypoglycaemic actions of the biguanides (e.g. metformin), which do not depend on stimulation of insulin release. In general, oral hypoglycaemic drugs have proved to be of little value in veterinary therapeutics, probably because the diabetes is often too severe and the patients are already insulin dependent when first presented. Metformin (250–500 mg b.i.d.) has been used in dogs with mild glucose intolerance associated with obesity.

Treatment of pancreatic disorders

Uncomplicated diabetes mellitus

Most cases of diabetes mellitus present as uncomplicated insulin-dependent diabetics. A glucose tolerance test may be necessary when, after urine analysis and measurement of fasting blood glucose levels, the diagnosis is uncertain.

The need for daily injections of insulin, regular monitoring of urinary glucose levels and careful attention to diet and exercise must be discussed at the outset with the owner to determine whether treatment is feasible. Since diabetes may be precipitated by long-term administration of glucocorticoids or progestogens, this should be corrected where possible. Entire bitches should be spayed when blood glucose has been stabilized. If the cause of secondary diabetes can be removed before the islet cells become exhausted, the condition may be reversible. For example, there are reports of megestrol acetate-induced diabetes mellitus in cats when this progestogen was used to treat dermatoses. Drug withdrawal and insulin therapy have generally effected resolution of the diabetes over periods ranging from 10 days to 8 months. Occasionally cats have required insulin indefinitely.

Dietary therapy in conjunction with insulin facilitates glycaemic control and reduces daily insulin requirements. The calorie intake should be adjusted to correct obesity and maintain an ideal body weight. There is merit in feeding high fibre, and suitable proprietary foods are available for dogs and cats.

Stabilization on insulin should be carried out with the animal hospitalized, since daily (at least) monitoring of blood and urine glucose concentrations is necessary. The objective is to achieve and maintain a normal blood glucose concentration (3–5 mmol/l) at the time of peak insulin activity (see Table 3.1), or a minimal glucosuria in the pre-dosage morning sample. Therapy should be initiated with an intermediate-acting insulin preparation, given subcutaneously once daily.

Starting dose: cat 1 unit; dog <10 kg 2 units; dog >10 kg 4 units

Dosage routine

1. A morning sample of urine is collected and tested for glucose and ketones (e.g. Keto-Diastix). A glucose concentration of 5–12.5 mmol/l is ideal and in these cases the dose of insulin should be the same as on the previous day. If there is no detectable glucose, the dose of insulin is reduced by up to 2 units, because the overnight blood glucose concentration could be very low. A glucosuria of 50–100 mmol/l indicates an increase of up to 2 units on the previous day's dose.
2. After testing the urine, one-third of the daily food allowance is given, followed immediately by the pre-determined dose of insulin. The purpose of the small morning feed is to prevent an insulin-induced hypoglycaemia. If the food is refused, only half of the dose of insulin should be given that day.
3. The remainder of the daily feed should be given 8 hours after insulin injection. Ideally, blood glucose concentration will then peak at a time when insulin is increasing tissue uptake of glucose at a maximal rate, although it will be apparent from Table 3.1 that there is considerable individual variation in response to insulin.
4. The animal can be discharged when the insulin requirement has been approximately the same for several consecutive days and the owner appraised of all aspects of management.

Acute hypoglycaemia
This is the most common crisis in a diabetic patient, with signs varying from muscle twitching and lethargy to convulsions and coma. It is usually caused by insulin overdosage, particularly if the animal has not eaten, or has had excessive exercise. The condition is corrected with oral glucose syrup (smeared on the tongue if unconscious) or a feed containing glucose powder. In an acute emergency, i.v. glucose (1 ml/kg, 50 per cent solution) can be administered.

Destabilization problems
In addition to acute hypoglycaemia, which requires emergency treatment, a patient may exhibit clinical signs of diabetes or hypoglycaemia or persistent morning glucosuria after being stabilized on insulin and discharged. The

owner's comprehension and compliance must initially be investigated since most cases of instability are due to irregular feeding or exercise and improper administration of insulin, and thus are easily resolved.

If instability persists after eliminating compliance causes, the animal should be hospitalized and blood glucose concentrations measured at intervals of 4 hours over a 24-hour period. Differential diagnosis of the cause of the instability can be made on the basis of the assays.

Insulin-induced hyperglycaemia

This is caused, paradoxically, by overdosing with insulin. There is an initial sudden hypoglycaemia which stimulates the release of adrenaline, noradrenaline and glucagon. The combined effect of these is a rebound hyperglycaemia (>16 mmol/l). The excessive degree of morning glucosuria prompts the owner to increase the insulin dose still further. In these cases, the insulin dose should be halved and the animal restabilized.

Rapid exogenous insulin metabolism

This occurs in some animals which, therefore, become hyperglycaemic between injections. The blood glucose concentration becomes normal after insulin injection, but within 18 hours exceeds 11 mmol/l. The treatment of these animals should be changed to the longer-acting protamine zinc insulin.

Insulin resistance

Insulin resistance is the likely cause of destabilization when the insulin requirement increases and is confirmed by consistently high blood glucose concentrations (>16 mmol/l) throughout the 24-hour period. The antagonism may be due to other hormones or to the development of antibodies against exogenous insulin. Porcine insulin is probably less antigenic than bovine insulin in dogs.

Diabetic ketoacidosis

Patients presenting with decompensated ketoacidosis are less common than those with uncomplicated diabetes. They present with depression, tachypnoea, vomiting, dehydration and eventually coma. Intensive therapy is required to correct the fluid deficit, acid–base balance and elevated blood concentrations of glucose and ketones.

The fluid deficit is commonly 10–20 per cent of bodyweight and intravenous Compound Sodium Lactate Injection is the preferred replacement solution. Blood glucose concentrations usually exceed 20 mmol/l and are reduced initially with soluble insulin, the only form which can be administered intravenously. It may be given by drip (1 unit/kg/h) or, at the same dosage, as intravenous boluses, repeated every 2 hours until the blood glucose concentration is reduced by 50 per cent. The animal is then treated as an uncomplicated case. Oral potassium supplementation for a few days is advisable. Serum potassium concentration may be low in ketoacidosis and this is exacerbated by insulin, which stimulates uptake of potassium into tissues.

Hyperinsulinism

Rarely, islet cell tumours of the pancreas in ageing dogs, especially boxers, cause indiscriminate overproduction of insulin with consequent profound hypoglycaemia. The initial signs of trembling and weakness progress, over a period of weeks, to incoordination, ataxia, muscle twitching, generalized seizures and episodes of fainting. Diagnosis is made on the basis of persistently low blood glucose concentration and radioimmunoassay of blood insulin concentration (>50 μU/ml).

Surgical removal of the tumour has been recorded but it is often small and difficult to locate. Several approaches to medical treatment, in addition to feeding frequent small meals and intravenous administration of 50 per cent dextrose solution to effect, have been described.

Diazoxide is a non-diuretic thiazide, which causes a transitory hyperglycaemia by various mechanisms. It exerts an α-adrenoceptor agonist-like action on islet beta cells, which decreases insulin secretion. It also stimulates the release of endogenous catecholamines.

Dose

5–30 mg/kg p.o. b.i.d.

Streptozocin is an antitumour drug which has a fairly selective action against islet cells. It is used in man to treat insulin-secreting tumours. Its clinical use in the dog is under investigation.

The thyroid

Iodide is absorbed from the gut and actively transported from the circulation to be concentrated in the thyroid gland. Here it is oxidized to iodine and coupled to tyrosine, forming mono-iodotyrosine and di-iodotyrosine. Oxidative coupling of these iodinated intermediates results in the formation of the active hormones L-thyroxine (T_4) and L-tri-iodothyronine (T_3) (Fig. 3.1), which are stored in the thyroid in combination with thyroglobulin. The activity of the thyroid gland is controlled by thyroid-stimulating hormone (TSH; thyrotrophin) from the anterior pituitary. The release of TSH is stimulated by thyroid insufficiency and depressed by excessive thyroid hor-

Thyroxine (T$_4$)

3,5,3'-Tri-iodothyronine (T$_3$)

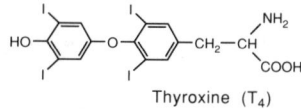

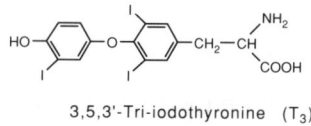

Figure 3.1   Structure of thyroid hormones.

mone output. The actions of TSH include stimulation of the synthesis of thyroid hormones and hydrolysis of thyroglobulin with consequent release of T$_3$ and T$_4$.

The thyroid gland also secretes the hormone calcitonin, in response to hypercalcaemia. Calcitonin opposes the action of parathyroid hormone and it may have a function in the rapid control of hypercalcaemia.

Actions of thyroid hormones

Thyroid hormones are important in the control of metabolic rate in all tissues. Under their influence, increased metabolic rate is associated with an increased glycogenolysis, peripheral glucose utilization and mobilization of fat. Some of these actions appear to involve β-adrenoceptors. In conjunction with other hormones, they are necessary for normal differentiation, development and function of nervous, reproductive and skeletal tissues. The growth phase of hair is activated and thyroid deficiency commonly causes characteristic changes in the skin and coat. The characteristic signs of congenital thyroid hypoplasia (cretinism) illustrate quite dramatically the important role of thyroid hormones in normal development.

Thyroid preparations

Thyroid extract is comparatively unrefined, poorly stable and has been superseded by synthetic L-thyroxine or liothyronine (L-tri-iodothyronine). Both are well absorbed after oral administration (T$_3$ almost completely). T$_3$ has a more rapid onset of action and a shorter duration of action than T$_4$ (24 hours and 7 days respectively) and is also more potent.

Antithyroid drugs

The thionamides, mainly propylthiouracil and methimazole (Fig. 3.2), are used to inhibit thyroid hormone synthesis. This is achieved by inhibition of

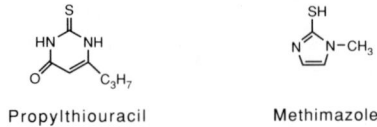

Propylthiouracil   Methimazole

Figure 3.2   Structure of antithyroid thionamides.

the incorporation of iodine into tyrosyl residues and the coupling of these to form thyroid hormones. The drugs may take some weeks to be effective, while the existing stores of thyroid hormones are depleted.

Hyperthyroidism

Hyperthyroidism has been described in dogs and, more frequently, in cats. In cats, there is usually hyperplasia of the gland but in dogs it is often due to thyroid neoplasia, which may be malignant. The enlarged thyroid (goitre) is usually palpable. The excessive output of thyroid hormones increases metabolic rate and leads to weight loss, polyphagia, muscle weakness, restlessness, polyuria, heat intolerance, tachycardia and tachyarrhythmias.

Partial thyroidectomy (carefully preserving the parathyroids) is the treatment of choice but is futile after tumour metastasis. Prognosis after surgery in cats is good. The β-adrenoceptor antagonist propranolol is useful for controlling tachyarrhythmias pre-operatively.

Alternatively, antithyroid drugs such as propylthiouracil (50 mg/kg t.i.d.) may be used if the condition is not associated with malignancy, but levels of T_3 and T_4 need to be monitored during stabilization and at intervals thereafter.

Hypothyroidism

Hypothyroidism, with a decreased concentration of T_3 and T_4 in the circulation, appears to be more common than hyperthyroidism in domesticated animals. It may arise from a deficiency of iodine, malfunction of the thyroid gland itself (primary hypothyroidism), or be due to deficient output of TSH from the pituitary gland (secondary hypothyroidism).

Iodine deficiency can occur in any species, but is rare in dogs and, indeed, is difficult to produce experimentally. The diagnosis is confirmed by a low protein-bound iodine level in the plasma (<2.4 µg/100 ml). In ruminants, it may be due to deficient iodine intake or to deficient absorption due to a high calcium intake or a high brassica diet. Hypotrichosis in pigs ('hairless pigs') is usually an inherited condition, but is sometimes the result of an iodine deficiency.

Affected cattle have enlarged thyroid glands with reduced libido in bulls and irregular oestrus in cows. Calves from affected dams are either born weak or dead or are aborted; thyroid hyperplasia is found at post-mortem examination. The signs are similar in ewes and often more marked in goats.

The treatment of iodine deficiency is to increase the iodine level in the feed, usually by salt licks with added iodide. Affected ewes late in gestation may be dosed with potassium iodide.

In dogs primary and secondary hypothyroidism are most common in middle-aged individuals of the larger breeds. Most cases (90 per cent) are due to thyroid hypoplasia or lymphocytic thyroiditis and others (secondary hypothyroidism) to TSH deficiency. Clinical signs usually develop insidiously over several months. There is commonly a history of lethargy, weight gain without polyphagia and intolerance to cold. Affected animals have bilateral thinning of the coat with thickening and hyperpigmentation of the skin and usually seborrhoea. Oestrous cycles are irregular and there is a lack of libido in dogs. Diagnosis is based on clinical signs and laboratory evaluation, usually radioimmunoassay, of T_3 and T_4.

Treatment of primary or secondary hypothyroidism is by administration of a thyroid replacement, usually for the remainder of the patient's life. An increase in physical activity is usual within 2 weeks of beginning treatment with either L-thyroxine or liothyronine, but improvement in the condition of the skin and coat may not be obvious for several weeks.

Doses

thyroxine   20–40 μg/kg p.o. daily, in divided doses. If there is
                 no satisfactory response after 2–3 weeks, the dose may
                 be increased each week by 50 μg. The dose should be
                 reduced immediately if signs of overdosage (restlessness,
                 polydipsia) appear.

liothyronine   2–3 μg/kg p.o. 3 times daily. The initial dose is adjusted
                 according to the response, until the minimum effective
                 dose is established.

The pituitary

The pituitary is composed of two major parts, with different embryological derivations—the anterior pituitary or adenohypophysis, and the posterior pituitary or neurohypophysis (Fig. 3.3). Two, chemically similar peptide hormones, oxytocin and antidiuretic hormone (ADH, vasopressin), are synthesized in the hypothalamus and are transported via neurosecretory fibres to storage sites in the posterior pituitary, from which they are released as required.

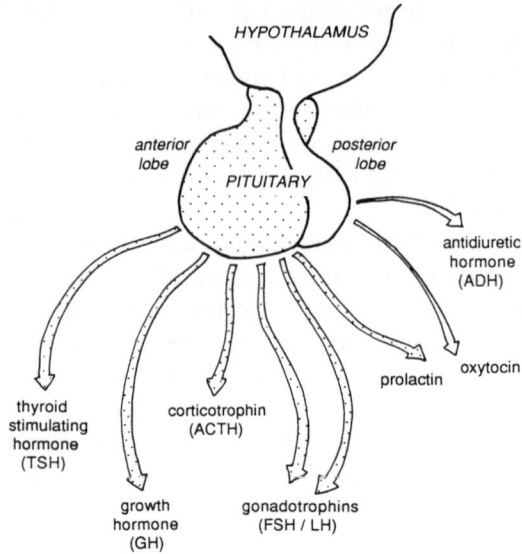

Figure 3.3 Release of hormones from the pituitary. Antidiuretic hormone and oxytocin are released from the posterior pituitary. The anterior pituitary releases thyroid-stimulating hormone, growth hormone, corticotrophin, prolactin and the gonadotrophins.

The mammalian anterior pituitary produces trophic hormones (thyroid-stimulating hormone, corticotrophin and two gonadotrophins) which stimulate other endocrine glands to release their hormones. The other anterior pituitary hormones, for example, somatotrophin (growth hormone) and prolactin (lactogenic hormone) have direct actions. The release of each of the adenohypophyseal hormones is controlled by specific releasing hormones which are secreted by the hypothalamus and reach the pituitary gland via the hypophyseal portal venous system. Most of the pituitary hormones are described in other chapters in their appropriate context, such as reproductive function; antidiuretic hormone and growth hormone are discussed in this section.

Antidiuretic hormone (ADH, vasopressin)

Antidiuretic hormone is a nonapeptide, released from the pituitary in response to an increased plasma osmolarity (detected by hypothalamic osmoreceptors) or to a decreased blood volume (detected by baroreceptors in the thoracic veins). Ethanol inhibits release of the hormone with a consequent (and well-attested) diuresis.

The hormone acts on cell membrane receptors (V_2) in the distal convoluted tubule and collecting duct, which activate adenylate cyclase. Consequent formation of cyclic AMP leads, via an incompletely understood series of responses, to an increase in the permeability of the luminal cell surface to water and thereby an increased water reabsorption. In very large doses, ADH has a direct contractile action on the smooth muscle of blood vessels (at V_1 receptors). Its action on coronary blood vessels precludes the use of ADH at such high doses.

ADH must be administered parenterally since it is rapidly degraded by enzymes in the gastrointestinal tract. Even after injection or nasal insufflation, the presence of peptidases in the liver, kidneys and tissues ensures a short duration of action. Synthetic analogues of ADH are available. Desmopressin (1-deamino-8-D-arginine vasopressin) is a more potent antidiuretic and has reduced pressor activity. It is more resistant to degradation by peptidases and thus has a longer duration of action. It is administered intranasally, either as drops or via an atomizer.

Diabetes insipidus

Diabetes insipidus is the syndrome arising from the failure of the distal renal tubules to concentrate urine; it occurs occasionally in the dog and cat. It may be due to the failure of ADH synthesis or release (central diabetes insipidus) associated with trauma, neoplasia or inflammation, or to failure of the kidneys to respond to the hormone (nephrogenic diabetes insipidus) because of renal necrosis or fibrosis. The typical signs are a sudden onset of severe polyuria, often with nocturia, and a compensatory severe polydipsia, usually in an otherwise apparently well animal. The daily intake of water often exceeds 100 ml/kg bodyweight and the daily urine output usually exceeds 90 ml/kg.

Diagnosis is confirmed by the low specific gravity of the urine (<1.010), which the animal fails to concentrate when water is restricted. Administration of ADH usually produces a marked improvement in cases of central diabetes insipidus. Failure to concentrate the urine after administration of ADH indicates nephrogenic diabetes insipidus.

Treatment

ADH is ineffective in cases of nephrogenic diabetes, but is the most effective treatment for central diabetes. Injection of Vasopressin B.P. (Pitressin) has been used, but the effect lasts for only a few hours. A longer duration of affect is achieved with use of desmopressin.

The thiazide diuretics (see Chapter 12) paradoxically reduce polyuria in diabetes insipidus. Salt intake must be restricted and the thiazides then cause an excessive reabsorption of sodium chloride and water in the proximal renal tubules. This reduces the volume delivered to the distal tubules, with a consequent reduction in the volume of free water that can be formed. Thiazides are less effective than ADH in central diabetes insipidus, but are invaluable in patients with nephrogenic diabetes insipidus. Because they can be administered orally, they are a convenient alternative to ADH therapy.

An alternative agent to ADH or thiazide diuretics is chlorpropamide. This oral hypoglycaemic drug, although rarely effective in animals as a substitute for insulin (see above), is sometimes more effective than hydrochlorothiazide in the treatment of diabetes insipidus. It appears to act by potentiating the renal response to ADH and, like the thiazides, promoting reabsorption of sodium chloride and water. Since it also stimulates insulin secretion, owners should be warned of signs of hypoglycaemia.

Doses

vasopressin	2 units i.m. or s.c., adjusted according to the response
desmopressin	5 μg i.m. daily, adjusted according to the response
hydrochlorothiazide	2–4 mg/kg twice daily, p.o.
chlorpropamide	
dog	10–40 mg/kg p.o. once daily
cat	50 mg p.o. per day.

Growth hormone

Growth hormone (GH), also known as somatotrophin (STH), is a complex protein hormone with a molecular weight of approximately 22 000 for most species. There are species differences in the sequence of amino acids (191 in humans) and varying degrees of species specificity in response to GH when it is administered in experimental studies or clinically. For example, humans respond only to primate GH and in domesticated animals, refractoriness and other adverse effects develop with the use of heterologous hormone.

The output of GH is controlled by a balance between growth-hormone releasing hormone (GHRH) and growth-hormone-release inhibitory hormone (GHRIH; somatostatin), which are produced from the hypothalamus. Various factors influence the output of GH, possibly by modifying the secretion or activity of the hypothalamic regulating hormones. Plasma levels of GH are increased during sleep and by hypoglycaemia, exercise, stress and α-adrenoceptor agonists. Conversely, hyperglycaemia, glucocorticoids and β-adrenoceptor agonists inhibit GH output.

Effects of GH

GH is produced throughout life and affects virtually every tissue and organ in the body. During pre-puberty it stimulates growth and subsequently remains one of the important regulating factors, in conjunction with other hormones, of the metabolism of carbohydrates, proteins and fats. GH mobilizes adipose tissue and increases fatty acid oxidation. Protein metabolism is markedly influenced by GH, which promotes nitrogen retention, increases transport of amino acids into tissues and accelerates their incorporation into protein. GH also affects lactation, and utilization of this property is currently a controversial matter (see 'Bovine somatotrophin' below).

Peptides released mainly from the liver, but also from kidney and muscle, in response to GH, appear to mediate many of the responses described above; these are called somatomedins. Somatomedins also regulate GH output by a negative feedback mechanism. As with GH itself, somatomedins are species specific and can be distinguished immunologically.

Being a protein, GH must be administered parenterally. The plasma half-life of GH is only about 20 minutes but the somatomedins which it induces have a half-life of several hours. This is probably due to the binding of somatomedins to larger plasma proteins.

Disordered GH production

Adult acromegaly due to an excess of GH has been described in dogs. The condition is occasionally caused by pituitary hyperplasia but more commonly by excess progestogens during metoestrus in middle-aged bitches or when administered to control oestrus. The signs are polydipsia, polyuria, panting, abdominal enlargement and thickened skin. GH levels in the plasma are measured by radioimmunoassay to confirm the diagnosis. The treatment is to withdraw any progestogen therapy and then carry out ovariohysterectomy.

Pituitary dwarfism is due to deficient GH production in early life with a consequent deficiency of somatomedins and stunted growth. The disorder most commonly affects German Shepherd dogs, where it is inherited as an autosomal recessive condition, usually affecting only a single dog in the litter. In contrast to congenital hypothyroidism (cretinism), the pituitary dwarf is normal in proportions and throughout life retains the dimensions of a puppy with a characteristically soft coat. Diagnosis is confirmed by radioimmunoassay of plasma GH levels.

Treatment is not normally attempted, since affected animals are usually well accepted by owners. There are reports of successful treatment using bovine GH (bovine somatotrophin, BST) administered subcutaneously (10 IU) on alternate days for 1 month. Treatment of human hypopituitary dwarfs has produced striking effects in some cases, by inducing normally proportioned growth.

Bovine somatotrophin (BST)

It has been known for many years that administration of BST to lactating cows increases milk production. During World War II, heroic attempts were made to utilize this for economic purposes. However, pituitaries from about 20 cows were required to extract sufficient BST to provide a single daily dose for one cow! In 1982, pure BST was produced, like human somatotrophin, by recombinant-DNA techniques and trials are currently in progress to assess its usefulness as a management tool in dairy farming. It is not yet available commercially.

Lactating cows, treated with BST, produce more milk. Although they eat more food to adjust their metabolism to the increased output, there is a significant increase in the milk-to-feed ratio and feed utilization is increased by about 10 per cent. The use of BST in this way, if it is eventually permitted to be commercially available, may seem paradoxical since the supply of milk in the European Community (EC) and the USA currently exceeds demand. (A system of milk quotas is in operation in the EC.) However, the use of BST enables the same amount of milk to be produced from fewer cows, which is an argument for its strategic use. Studies to date indicate increases in milk yield of about 12 per cent under normal farm management conditions.

Trials are currently in progress to assess the safety of administration of BST for several lactation periods in cows. For example, the potential effects on the incidence of mastitis, metabolic diseases and on reproductive performance, including subsequent development of the calf, must be determined. With reference to consumer safety, it is known that BST occurs naturally in cows' milk at a concentration generally less than 2 parts per billion; there appears to be no evidence for an increase in cows treated experimentally with BST. It is assumed that BST, being a protein, would be completely degraded in the digestive tract and indeed by pasteurization. These consumer safety aspects, together with potential effects on the composition and quality of milk from treated cows, are also being evaluated.

At the time of writing, the European Commission has delayed a decision on the commercial use of BST in the EC to assess the results of ongoing studies on consumer safety, animal welfare, economics and consumer opinion on the acceptability of milk from treated cows.

The adrenal glands

Two different types of corticosteroid hormone are secreted by the adrenal glands:

1. Mineralocorticoid, i.e. aldosterone, which is involved in the control of Na^+ and water excretion. The secretion of aldosterone is controlled by the renin-angiotensin-aldosterone system; the actions of aldosterone and drugs which inhibit these actions are described in Chapter 12.
2. Glucocorticoid, i.e. hydrocortisone (cortisol) and corticosterone. These have important effects on metabolism and anti-inflammatory activity.

Glucocorticoid secretion is controlled by the hypothalamus-pituitary-adrenal axis (Fig. 3.4). Corticotrophin-releasing factor (CRF) is secreted by the hypothalamus and stimulates the release of adrenocorticotrophic hormone (ACTH, corticotrophin) from the anterior pituitary. Release of the glucocorticoids from the zona fasciculata of the cortex is induced by the actions of ACTH on the adrenal glands.

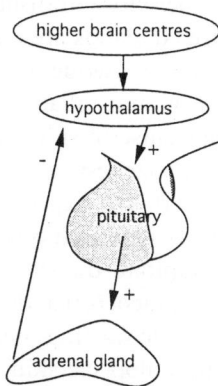

Figure 3.4 The hypothalamic-pituitary-adrenal axis controls the release of hormones from the adrenal cortex. Stimulation (+) of hormone release is by the hypothalamus via the pituitary. A negative feedback mechanism exists whereby high blood levels of hormone inhibit further hypothalamic-induced stimulation.

Blood levels of the glucocorticoids are controlled by three factors:
(a) Stress—release of CRF, ACTH and glucocorticoids is stimulated by stressful situations, including excitement, injury and pyrexia.
(b) Circadian rhythm—in the horse, sheep, pig and dog, plasma hydrocortisone levels are highest in the morning. In the cat, the peak occurs in the evening.
(c) Glucocorticoids (whether endogenous or synthetic) exert a negative feedback effect on the hypothalamus and pituitary, suppressing the release of CRF and ACTH.

Pharmacological actions of glucocorticoids

Glucocorticoids are potent anti-inflammatory agents and are widely used in the management of a variety of inflammatory reactions. Details of these actions are described in Chapter 8. Some of the actions of the glucocorticoids which account for the observed anti-inflammatory activity are also involved in the mediation of the immunosuppressive activity of these agents. The release of neutrophils from bone marrow and reduction of their entry into inflammatory sites; the direction of eosinophils out of the peripheral circulation and away from inflammatory sites; monocytopenia; and an inhibition of the entry of lymphocytes into inflamed tissue all contribute to the immunosuppressive response. Furthermore, there is a reduction in T-cell proliferation (due to inhibition of production of interleukin$_2$) and a suppression of the production of some types of antibodies in some species.

The glucocorticoids influence a wide range of metabolic processes. In healthy animals, these are important in the control and maintenance of normal function. Signs of hypo-activity (Addison's disease) or hyperactivity (Cushing's syndrome) of the adrenal glands are due to inadequate or excessive levels of the hormones and the consequent disturbance of metabolism. Where glucocorticoids are used as anti-inflammatory drugs, their influence on metabolic activity may be the cause of side-effects.

Glucocorticoids increase gluconeogenesis and decrease the peripheral utilization of glucose. In ruminants, this is expressed in increased blood sugar levels. In other species, the excess blood glucose is stored as liver glycogen. Corticosteroid therapy may precipitate diabetes mellitus in incipient cases. Protein catabolism is increased by glucocorticoids. This may lead to atrophy of the lymphatic tissues, skeletal muscle wasting, defective tissue repair, stunted growth in young animals and thin, alopecic skin. Concurrent hypercalcaemia may cause calcinosis cutis. Subcutaneous injections of depot corticosteroids are contraindicated, particularly in dogs, because of these effects on skin. In bone, catabolism of the protein matrix and calcium loss lead to the development of osteoporosis.

Increased metabolism of fat and its redistribution to the lumbar area, liver and omentum occur with corticosteroids. Excessive levels of glucocorticoids also lead to polydipsia and polyuria. These effects are probably due to inhibition of the release or actions of antidiuretic hormone and adaptation usually occurs after a few days' therapy.

In the gastrointestinal tract, the glucocorticoids inhibit the renewal of surface epithelial cells, thus predisposing to ulceration. This becomes of clinical significance when the hormones are used concurrently with ulcerogenic drugs (e.g. aspirin) or in dogs undergoing surgery for intervertebral disc protrusion, which also predisposes to gut ulceration.

Suppression of the hypothalamic-pituitary-adrenal (HPA) axis is an important factor when glucocorticoids are used systemically. The enhanced anti-inflammatory potency of the synthetic agents is accompanied by a proportional increase in the ability to suppress the HPA axis. A single dose of a synthetic glucocorticoid will suppress endogenous hydrocortisone secretion, but with a short course of therapy (days) the patient will be protected from untoward effects by the exogenous steroid. After cessation of long-term therapy, however, the HPA axis may be suppressed for weeks and this can lead to complications if the animal is stressed. For example, a single i.m. injection of a 'depot' formulation of prednisolone acetate in cattle lasts about 2 weeks and may suppress the HPA axis for about 5 weeks. In dogs, withdrawal of glucocorticoids after 4 months' therapy can precipitate an Addisonian crisis, even though (due to protracted therapy) patients may show signs of adrenal hyperactivity. Thus local application of corticosteroids should be practised where possible and depot preparations used only where absolutely necessary. Where systemic administration is required, problems of HPA axis suppression may be reduced by gradually reducing the dose, to allow endogenous hormone secretion to be re-established. Alternate-day therapy is less suppressive and should be considered where therapy for long periods is indicated. Using this technique, a drug like methylprednisolone, which will depress the HPA axis for less than 36 hours, is administered on alternate days. This allows the HPA axis to function normally on the non-dose days, while the anti-inflammatory activity of the drug persists. Minimal disruption occurs if the daily dose is administered at the time when endogenous hormone levels are highest and ACTH is naturally suppressed (in the morning for dogs and in the evening for cats).

Synthetic glucocorticoids

Corticosteroids are mainly used for their anti-inflammatory and immuno-suppressive actions. It would be ideal to manipulate the structure of hydro-cortisone to enhance these effects and eliminate the mineralocorticoid actions, metabolic effects and potentially dangerous suppression of the HPA axis. It has proved possible to separate mineralocorticoid and glucocorticoid actions (Table 3.2) but not, at present, to isolate the others. The potency (compared to hydrocortisone) with respect to metabolic and anti-inflammatory actions and HPA axis suppression, increases in parallel in the synthetic glucocorticoids.

Table 3.2 Potency (with respect to hydrocortisone) and half-life of corticosteroids

Drug	Glucocorticoid potency	Mineralocorticoid potency	biological half-life (h)★
Hydrocortisone	1	1	8–12
Cortisone	0.8	0.8	8–12
Prednisolone	5	0.8	12–36
Prednisone	4	0.8	12–36
Methylprednisolone	5	Negligible	12–36
Triamcinolone	5	Negligible	12–36
Dexamethasone	30	Negligible	36–54
Betamethasone	25	Negligible	36–54
Flumethasone	100	Negligible	36–54
Desoxycorticosterone	Negligible	50	8–12
Fludrocortisone	15	100	8–12

★Refers to free steroid, the duration of action depends on the ester used.

Preparations for injection, oral administration and local application are available. The injectable formulations have varying degrees of water solubility, which determine the speed of absorption after intramuscular injection. Highly soluble esters are suitable for intravenous administration or are rapidly absorbed after intramuscular injection (methylprednisolone as the sodium succinate, betamethasone as the sodium phosphate, dexamethasone as the sodium phosphate). Less soluble esters have an intermediate duration of action (dexamethasone trioxan undecanoate, methylprednisolone acetate, dexamethasone phenylpropionate and dexamethasone acetate), while the insoluble preparations are only very slowly absorbed and are active for a number of weeks (triamcinolone acetonide). Some formulations combine a mixture of a soluble ester, for rapid initial effect, with an insoluble ester for sustained action.

Glucocorticoids are often administered as tablets to small animals. These usually contain acetates, which are readily hydrolysed to the free base in the gut, or free steroids (prednisolone, betamethasone, dexamethasone, flumethasone).

Various glucocorticoid esters are formulated as creams or ointments for local skin application or as drops for eyes and ears. An antibacterial, such as neomycin, is often incorporated.

Therapeutic uses of glucocorticoids

Replacement therapy
Primary adrenocortical insufficiency (Addison's disease) occurs in dogs, but is not common. The output of both mineralocorticoids and glucocorticoids is reduced in these patients. Vomiting, weakness and collapse with shock due to hypovolaemia through failure of renal regulation occur in acute insufficiency. Rapid therapy is required to treat patients in shock and includes intravenous saline (0.9 per cent), one of the soluble glucocorticoid preparations (see above) i.v. and daily dosing with desoxycorticosterone acetate (1–3 mg/day, i.m.) until the crisis is controlled.

Signs in animals with a chronic disorder include lethargy, inappetence and weight loss. Therapy in these animals (and for maintenance after acute failure) requires a preparation with combined mineralocorticoid and glucocorticoid activity, such as fludrocortisone acetate (0.1–0.5 mg daily). The dose should be adjusted to maintain K^+ levels which, along with Na^+ levels, should be regularly checked. Animals should have added Na^+ in the diet, with free access to water.

Secondary adrenocortical insufficiency, arising from inadequate ACTH secretion, can be due to pituitary disease or iatrogenic suppression of the HPA axis. Glucocorticoid levels are depressed, but aldosterone secretion is not affected. Short-acting glucocorticoids (hydrocortisone or prednisolone), to produce physiological levels of hormones in the circulation should be used to minimize HPA axis suppression. The normal output of hydrocortisone in dogs is 1 mg/kg/day. This dose of hydrocortisone tablets or 0.1–0.2 mg/kg prednisolone should be used. The doses should be administered in the morning in dogs and in the evening in cats, to mimic the circadian rhythm. Increased doses will be required during stress, particularly before surgery.

Glucocorticoids are used with cytotoxic drugs such as cyclophosphamide to treat lymphoma and leukaemia in dogs and cats (see page 529), to induce parturition or abortion in ruminants and as an adjunct to fluid therapy in shock (see page 242). The metabolic actions of the glucocorticoids are utilized in the management of bovine ketosis. A single injection is often effective in raising blood glucose levels, reducing blood ketones and reducing milk production. A combination of soluble and longer-acting esters is usually used. These agents are less effective in the treatment of pregnancy toxaemia in sheep; they probably work when they are successful in inducing abortion.

As well as their use in the treatment of inflammatory reactions, corticosteroids are also first-line therapy in autoimmune diseases, where circulating antibodies are directed against the host's own tissues, e.g. pemphigus, haemolytic anaemia and systemic lupus erythematosus. Treatment requires high doses of prednisolone (2–5 mg/kg daily, in divided doses, followed by alternate-day therapy, if the condition responds).

Treatment of Cushing's syndrome (hyperadrenocorticism)

Hyperadrenocorticism in dogs is not uncommon; the most common signs include polydipsia, polyuria, polyphagia, abdominal distension, skin changes and lethargy. Diagnosis of this syndrome can be confirmed by the measurement of plasma hydrocortisone levels. At least 80–85 per cent of cases of Cushing's syndrome are thought to be due to pituitary tumours. In the relatively few cases where adrenal tumours are the cause, surgical adrenalectomy is recommended. The adrenocorticolytic drug mitotane is effective in patients with pituitary tumours. The drug is cytotoxic (see page 539) and care should be taken by personnel handling it.

Alternative drug therapies, which have not yet been widely used, include those agents which inhibit the synthesis of corticosteroids and those which inhibit the secretion of ACTH. Ketoconazole, an antifungal agent, has been shown to lower serum hydrocortisone levels and this action may be of use in Cushingoid dogs. Metyrapone, aminoglutethimide and trilostane are other drugs which inhibit adrenal steroid synthesis and have potential therapeutic applications. The dopamine antagonist bromocriptine and the 5-HT antagonist cyproheptadine may, by inhibiting the release of ACTH from the pituitary, be effective in the management of Cushing's syndrome.

Anabolic steroids

Several hormones have anabolic (tissue-building) properties, e.g. insulin, growth hormone, oestrogens (via release of growth hormone and insulin), progestogens (via release of growth hormone) and androgens. Conventionally, however, the term anabolic steroids is used to describe derivatives of testosterone in which the androgenic activity (on the reproductive system) has been reduced (but not eliminated) relative to the tissue-building activity.

Actions of anabolic steroids

When administered to mammals, the anabolic steroids induce an accelerated growth of the musculoskeletal system. Experimental studies in rodents and ruminants have shown that, unlike the anabolic response to oestrogens and progestogens, this is a direct action of the hormones and does not depend on the release of other hormones such as insulin or growth hormone.

There is a continuous turnover of amino acids between the amino acid pool and muscle tissue; growth and regeneration after tissue injury or wasting requires a net anabolism between opposing anabolic and catabolic activity. Experimental studies indicate that the effect of the anabolic steroids is to decrease the rate of protein catabolism, thereby inducing a net anabolism. The hormones stimulate appetite, but adequate intake of dietary protein is obligatory for their anabolic action.

The anabolic steroids also act on the renal tubules and increase retention of Ca^{2+}, PO_4^{3-}, K^+ and Na^+. The increased Ca^{2+} retention and anabolic effect on the protein bone matrix enhances bone growth if the epiphyseal plates are not closed. Excessive dosing in early life can hasten closure of the plates and prevent further growth of long bones.

Clinical applications

Anabolic steroids are sometimes used to aid convalescence after specific therapy for infectious diseases, such as parvovirus or endoparasitism, which may cause marked weight loss. In aged animals there is anecdotal evidence for improvement in muscle tone and renal function and, postoperatively, enhanced tissue regeneration.

Anabolic steroids have been used as long-term therapy in cases of osteoporosis, where they increase Ca^{2+} retention and decrease bone resorption. After fracture repair, particularly in aged animals, they enhance the formation of bone matrix, promote Ca^{2+} retention and stimulate the synthesis of chondroitin sulphate in connective tissue. They are thus useful in cases of delayed fracture healing. There are reports that anabolic steroids increase tendon strength in young horses and hasten recovery from tendon injuries.

The drugs are contraindicated in animals with androgenic-dependent tumours. In addition, excessive dosing may induce masculinizing side-effects and, in growing animals, premature ossification of the epiphyses.

The use of anabolic steroids for fattening food animals is now prohibited in the EC (see 'Hormone growth promoters' below).

Available preparations and doses

Many anabolic steroids are available for use in human and veterinary medicine but only a selection of those with veterinary product licences will be described here. Structural modifications of testosterone are designed to increase the ratio of anabolic : androgenic activity and to improve the pharmacokinetic profile.

One such modification is the removal of the 19-methyl group of testosterone to form nandrolone (19-nor-testosterone) (Fig. 3.5). This reduces the androgenic activity of the molecule and, by adding different side-chains at carbon-17, different esters with prolonged durations of action are produced.

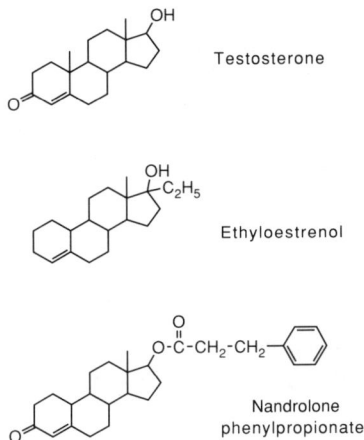

Figure 3.5 Some of the anabolic steroids in veterinary use.

Doses

nandrolone laurate
    dog and cat   1 mg/kg s.c. or i.m.
    repeat at intervals of 3 weeks if necessary.

nandrolone phenylpropionate
    dog   up to 50 mg s.c. or i.m.

    cat   up to 25 mg s.c. or i.m.
    repeat at 7–10-day intervals if required.

nandrolone decanoate,
    dog, cat   1–3 mg/kg weekly

Trenbolone acetate also lacks the 19-methyl group and has additional double bonds in the molecule. This product was formerly licensed for the treatment of pregnancy toxaemia in sheep, but under current legislation (see below) this is prohibited.

    dog, cat   2–5 mg i.m. twice weekly
                       or 4–10 mg weekly i.m.

Boldenone undecenoate is an anabolic steroid of therapeutic interest. The manufacturer's current data sheet refers to its use not only in dogs and cats, but in horses not intended for human consumption. Clearly, there are differences in interpretation of the legislation relating to the use of the hormones.

    dog, cat   2.5 mg/kg s.c. or i.m. every 2–4 weeks

    horse   25 mg per 45 kg i.m. every 2–4 weeks
    (not intended for human consumption)

    geldings   half the above dose, at twice the frequency, to avoid
                       masculinizing side-effects.

Ethyloestrenol differs from the anabolic steroids described above in that the structural modifications render it effective by oral administration. Modifications of this type, with alkyl groups attached in the α position at C-17 (Fig. 3.5), show some hepatotoxic effects in humans. However, several hundred times the normal dose of ethyloestrenol is necessary experimentally to produce signs of cholestatic hepatitis in dogs. When liver function is already impaired, close supervision during treatment is prudent.

    dog, cat   approx. 0.05 mg/kg daily,
                     normally for 10–14 days.

Hormone growth promoters

The steroid sex hormones—oestrogens, progestogens, androgens—and their synthetic analogues such as the stilbenes (oestrogenic) and anabolic steroids (see above) have been used to increase the growth rate of farm animals. Their efficacy in increasing protein deposition, with a consequent accelerated growth rate, is well documented. There is also increased feed conversion efficiency and production of a leaner carcass. The products were implanted subcutaneously as pellets in the ear and any remaining at slaughter was discarded when the carcass was dressed.

However, the use of hormones as growth promoters in food animals is now banned in the EC following public concern about consumer safety. The demonstration of high levels of residues of diethylstilboestrol (DES) in veal-based baby foods in Italy led, in 1980, to a national ban on the sale of such foods. The residues were apparently due to illicit administration of DES in oil intramuscularly to veal calves. Subsequent publicity relating to the risk of cancer in humans associated with DES was rapidly followed by an effective consumer boycott of the purchase of veal in continental Europe. An EC Directive was produced (which was to be implemented by national legislation) to prohibit the use of stilbenes in farm animals. The UK legislation (1982) prohibits the sale or supply of stilbenes (benzoestrol, dienoestrol, hexoestrol, stilboestrol and its salts and esters) for use in veterinary medicines and the relevant veterinary product licences have been withdrawn. The Regulations also specifically prohibit the use of all stilbenes in farm animals.

Before the ban on stilbenes, the use of other hormone growth promoters in the EC was also under review. A vociferous consumer lobby wanted to prohibit the use of all hormones in food animals following the stilbenes affair. Against this had to be weighed the value of hormones in veterinary therapeutics (see Chapter 15) and scientific evidence that the proper use of hormone growth promoter implants was not only of economic value, but presented no danger to the consumer.

For example, in countries such as Germany, where most beef is produced from intact males, the meat would contain up to 10 times more natural hormones than in artificially treated animals. Implantation in the ear prevented the intake of significant amounts of hormone by the consumer. Further, growth-promoting hormones, with the exception of the stilbenes, are rapidly metabolized and excreted by the enterohepatic system.

However, EC Directives were introduced to prohibit the use of hormones for growth promotion. In the UK the Directives are enacted by Regulations (1988), the relevant sections of which are reproduced below, unadorned. The definitions contained in the legislation should be noted. The prohibition applies to all domesticated animals except dogs and cats: the definition may imply food animals, but does not say so. Synthetic anabolic steroids are growth promoters because they have some sex hormone activity. Therapeutic treatment is defined in a very restrictive manner in the Regulations.

(1) Subject to paragraph (2) below, no person shall administer, or knowingly cause or permit to be administered, to animals, by any means whatsoever, any hormone growth promoters.

(2) The prohibition in paragraph (1) above does not apply to the administration—

   (a) by a veterinary surgeon or a veterinary practitioner—

      (i) for therapeutic treatment in the form of an injection of oestradiol-17-β, progesterone or testosterone or those derivatives of these substances which readily yield the parent compound on hydrolysis after absorption at the site of application; or

      (ii) for the termination of unwanted gestation or the improvement of fertility; or

   (b) by, or under the direct responsibility of, a veterinary surgeon or veterinary practitioner for the synchronisation of oestrus or the preparation of donors or recipients for the implantation of embryos.

In these Regulations—

"animals" means domestic animals of the bovine species, swine, sheep, goats, solipeds and poultry, and wild animals of these species and wild ruminants which have been raised on a holding;

"hormone growth promoters" means any substance which has an oestrogenic, androgenic or gestagenic action;

"injection" does not include implantation;

"therapeutic treatment" means the treatment of a fertility problem diagnosed by a veterinary surgeon or a veterinary practitioner in an animal not intended for fattening.

(From: The Medicines (Hormone Growth Promoters) (Prohibition of Use) Regulations 1988 (SI 1988 No. 705). H.M.S.O.)

Autacoids

Histamine

Histamine is an imidazole derivative; its structure is shown in Fig. 3.6. It is synthesized *in vivo* by the action of the enzyme histidine decarboxylase on the amino acid histidine. In the periphery, histamine is found in the mucosal layer of the stomach and is stored in basophils or in mast cells in a bound,

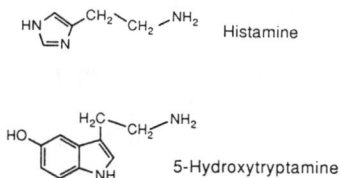

Figure 3.6 Structure of histamine and 5-hydroxytryptamine.

inactive form. It is also present in the brain, where storage sites which are not associated with mast cells have been demonstrated. Many venoms and stings contain histamine, although other active substances are present and may be more significant in determining the toxicity of the venom or sting. Histamine appears to be important in a number of physiological and/or pathological processes, including acute allergic and inflammatory reactions, gastric acid secretion and central nervous system neurotransmission.

Release of histamine can be triggered by a variety of different factors. Some drugs and/or their vehicles, notably tubocurarine, polymyxin, morphine and cremophor EL, induce the release of histamine, which may be responsible for some of the observed side-effects of these drugs. Although damage to mast cells results in degranulation and histamine release, drug-induced release of this type does not involve injury to mast cells.

Histamine release also occurs in certain immune mechanisms. When sensitized mast cells or basophils, with IgE antibodies attached to their surface membrane, are exposed to the appropriate antigen, the cell degranulates and releases histamine. Mast cells are found in high concentrations at potential sites of injury, including the mouth, nose, feet, internal body surface and in blood vessels, particularly at bifurcations. IgG- or IgM-mediated immune responses also release histamine, although it should be noted that a wide variety of other mediators are also released in these immunological responses.

Actions of histamine

The responses to histamine are mediated via three distinct receptor subtypes: H_1-, H_2- and H_3-receptors.

In the cardiovascular system, histamine is a potent vasodilator. Both H_1- and H_2-receptors are thought to be involved in this response. The hypotensive effect of histamine initiates a baroreceptor reflex response and heart rate increases. The direct inotropic effect of histamine on cardiac muscle is mediated via H_2-receptors. The relaxation of vascular smooth muscle in response to histamine is accompanied by an increase in capillary permeability. It appears that separation of endothelial cells allows the leakage of fluid and relatively large molecules, including other mediators of inflammation, into the perivascular tissue.

Histamine-induced stimulation of H_1-receptors on sensory nerve endings is associated with pain and itching. The release of histamine is an important component of the reaction to both plant and insect stings.

The effects of histamine on vascular receptors and those on sensory nerve endings combine to produce the characteristic response in the skin, referred to as the 'triple response', i.e. local reddening, wheal and flare (Fig. 3.7). The reddening is due to vasodilation of small blood vessels. Increased capillary permeability and the associated leakage of fluid into the perivascular tissues is responsible for the wheal. Histamine-induced stimulation of sensory nerve endings initiates impulses in other branches of the affected axons which cause vasodilation, or the flare.

Smooth muscle in both the gastrointestinal tract and the respiratory system contracts in response to histamine. These responses are mediated via H_1-receptors. Uterine smooth muscle is also sensitive to the contractile effects of histamine. There is considerable variation in susceptibility of different species to the smooth muscle effects of histamine. Guinea pigs are the most sensitive species; dogs are more sensitive than horses. Interestingly, histamine induces tracheal relaxation in cats and sheep.

Stimulation of H_2-receptors on the parietal cells induces secretion of gastric acid and also stimulates production of gastrin and intrinsic factor. The more recently identified H_3 receptors appear to be located mainly at presynaptic sites on nerves and may have a role in the modulation of transmitter release.

Histamine agonists

A number of synthetic compounds that stimulate histamine receptors are available. Some of these have considerable selectivity for receptor sub-types. These agents have no therapeutic applications in veterinary medicine and are most commonly used in experimental studies involving histaminergic mechanisms. In contrast, drugs which antagonize the effects of histamine have a number of important therapeutic applications.

Antihistamines

The response to histamine can be antagonized either by drugs which are competitive antagonists at the histamine receptors or by those which work at some other receptor site and have opposing physiological effects. The latter are referred to as physiological antagonists. In practice, adrenaline is most commonly used to counteract the effects of massive release of histamine associated with severe allergic reactions and anaphylactic shock.

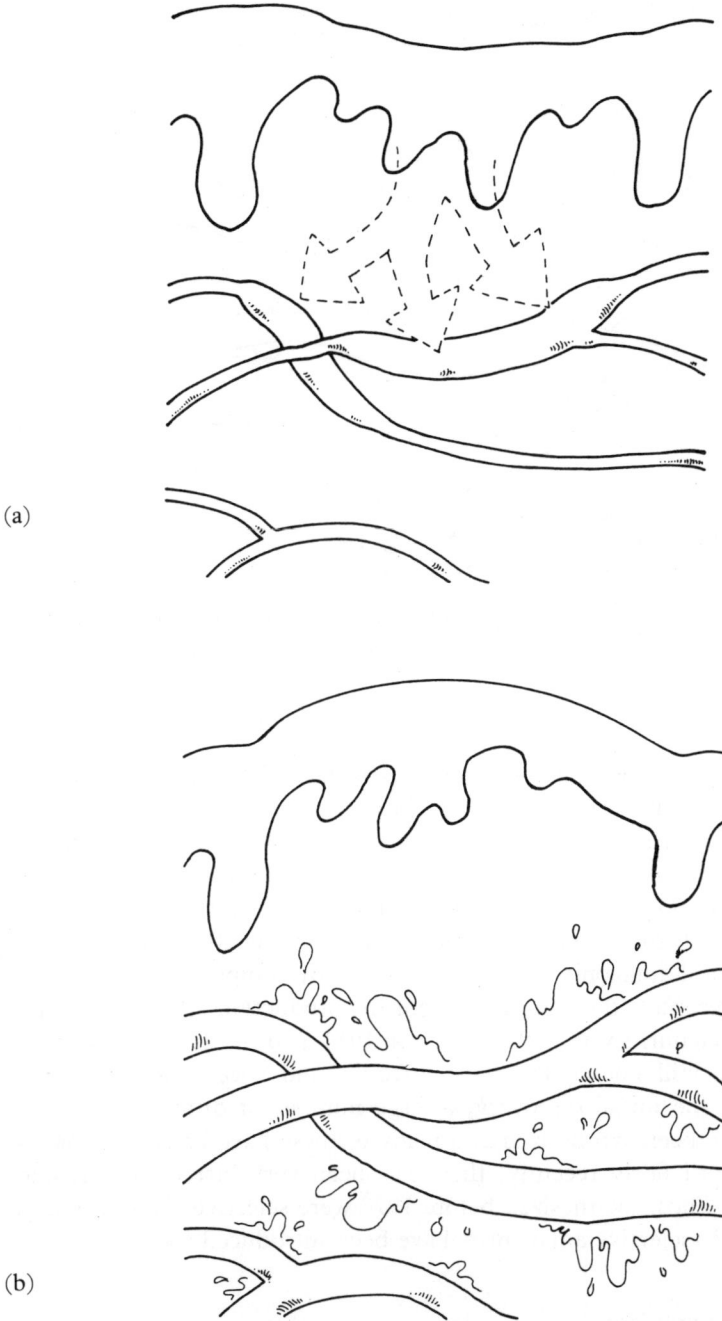

Figure 3.7 The triple response to histamine. (a) Local release of histamine causes vasodilation and the characteristic reddening. (b) The capillaries become more permeable and fluid leaks into the tissue, causing a wheal.

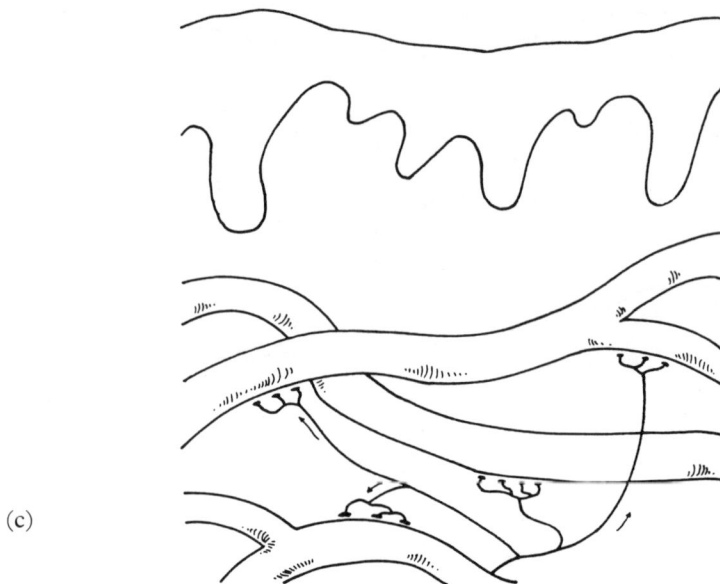

(c)

Figure 3.7   (c) The flare is associated with histamine-induced stimulation of sensory nerve endings and the consequent impulses in axonal branches, which cause vasodilation.

In these reactions, the signs and symptoms associated with histamine release include profound vasodilation, resulting in a marked fall in blood pressure, bronchoconstriction and oedema of the tongue and glottis. Adrenaline does not affect the interactions of histamine at its receptor sites, but its vasoconstrictor activity (at α-adrenoceptors) and bronchodilator activity (at β-adrenoceptors) physiologically antagonize the potentially life-threatening effects of histamine.

Pharmacological antagonists exert their effects by competitive inhibition at the histamine receptor; they do not prevent the production of histamine. The first of these antagonists was in clinical use in 1944, and the drug, mepyramine (pyrilamine), is still one of the most effective and specific antagonists in its class. Since the initial discovery, a large number of different histamine antagonists have been synthesized and many of these have been available for clinical use. Until fairly recently, there has been very little real difference between them. Those synthesized before 1970 were selective H_1-antagonists; both H_1- and H_2-selective antagonists have been introduced since then.

H_1-receptor antagonists

The general structure of H_1-receptor antagonists is shown in Fig. 3.8. The drugs can be classified into a number of chemical subgroups and an example of the drugs in each of these is also shown in Fig. 3.8. The action common to these drugs is antagonism of H_1-receptor-mediated responses, but many of them have a range of effects at clinical doses. Other actions include α-adrenoceptor antagonism, 5-HT antagonism, antimuscarinic and local anaesthetic effects. Thus, when used as antihistamines, they may have a number of side-effects which may or may not be related to these actions.

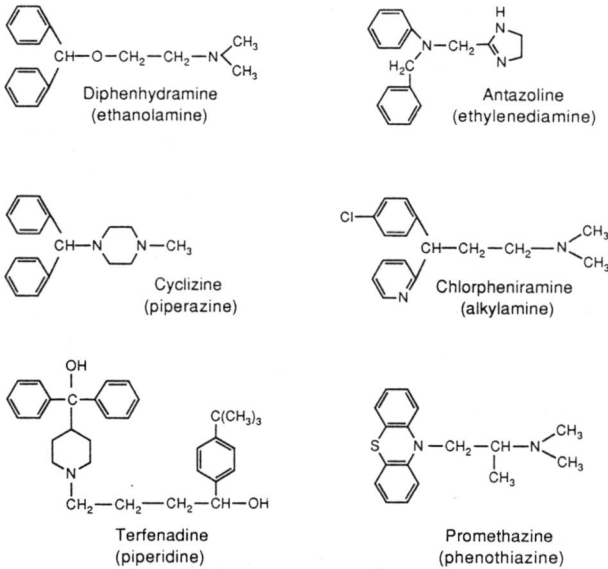

Figure 3.8 Histamine H_1-receptor antagonists.

Sedation is the most common side-effect of the antihistamines. The intensity of this reaction varies with different drugs in the group and also between individuals. Some human patients are particularly sensitive and will find that a particular antihistamine is an effective hypnotic, while others may not be affected at all by the same drug. In some cases, a degree of tolerance to the sedative effect of antihistamines develops over time. Terfenadine and mequitazine are two of the newer antihistamines which do not easily cross the blood–brain barrier and are thus significantly less sedative than some of the older drugs.

The side-effects of urinary retention, blurred vision and dry mouth are all associated with the anticholinergic activity of antihistamines. A useful 'side-effect' of the antihistamines is their ability to reduce nausea and vomiting and to prevent motion sickness. They are less effective once sickness is present. If administered over a long period, anorexia, vomiting, and constipation or diarrhoea may occur.

The local anaesthetic effect of the antihistamines can be useful when these drugs are used topically as antipruritic agents.

All of the antihistamines are effective after oral administration. Most of them are lipid soluble and are widely distributed throughout the body, including the central nervous system.

Uses

The most common use of antihistamines is the alleviation of signs of allergic reactions, including skin allergies and oedema and for histamine-mediated phenomena including pruritus, urticaria, dermatitis, gut oedema in pigs, pulmonary emphysema in horses and cattle and reactions to insect stings. The drugs are most effective if administered prior to the allergic challenge and cannot be expected to reverse the effects of histamine already at receptor sites. It should also be remembered that allergy and inflammation involve a large number of mediators and the antihistamines cannot be expected to suppress the responses to all of these.

The most potent antiemetics are diphenhydramine and promethazine, but both of these have considerable sedative effects. Drugs in the piperazine group are also effective in the prevention of motion sickness and may be preferable because their sedative effects are less marked.

H₂-receptor antagonists

The first antihistamine which was selective for H_2-receptors was discovered in 1972. Those currently available are cimetidine and ranitidine (Fig. 3.9). The newer drugs in this class, famotidine and nizatidine may soon be available for veterinary use.

Blockade of H_2-receptors reduces the secretion of gastric acid by histamine, gastrin and muscarinic agonists. The drugs are capable of reducing acid secretion by more than 90 per cent without any effect on gastrointestinal muscle function.

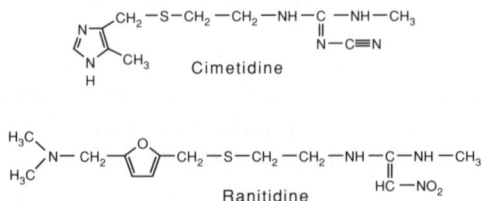

Figure 3.9 Histamine H_2-receptor antagonists.

Uses

Since peptic duodenal ulcers affect 10 per cent of adults in the Western world, H_2-receptor antagonists are widely used to promote healing and prevent ulcer recurrence. They are also used to relieve symptoms and promote healing of gastric ulcers.

Their use in veterinary medicine is not widespread, but they may be beneficial in gastric ulceration and in conditions producing hypersecretion of acid, such as the Zollinger–Ellison syndrome. Here they may be used as a primary treatment or in preparation for surgery for removal of the gastrin-secreting tumour. H_2-receptor antagonists may also be beneficial in controlling haemorrhagic gastritis induced by uraemia and for the treatment of ulcers in foals.

Inhibition of autacoid release

The actions of histamine can also be reduced by drugs which reduce degranulation of the mast cells that results from immunological triggering of antigen–IgE interactions. The only 'release inhibitor' available is sodium cromoglycate (cromolyn sodium). The drug does not reduce the response to histamine or other mediators which have been released; thus it is useful only as a prophylactic. It is used in horses for treatment of allergic respiratory disease. The only effective means of delivery is by aerosol directly to the lungs; a face mask is required.

Serotonin or 5-hydroxytryptamine (5-HT)

5-HT (Fig. 3.6) is found in both plant and animal tissue and in venoms and stings. In animals, it occurs in platelets, in mucosal chromaffin cells of the intestine (the major source of 5-HT), in the pineal gland (where it is the precursor of melatonin) and in the central nervous system. It has a variety of effects, most of which show considerable species variation. The 5-HT receptors which mediate the responses to this autacoid have been shown to be of at least four different subtypes. These are named 5-HT_1-, 5-HT_2-, 5-HT_3- and 5-HT_4-receptors. In addition, both 5-HT_1- and 5-HT_2-receptors appear to be heterogeneous and have been further divided into subtypes.

The cardiovascular response to 5-HT is complex and variable. It can produce either vasodilation or vasoconstriction, depending on the vascular bed and species involved. Most other smooth muscle contracts in response to 5-HT. Pain and itch sensory nerve endings are stimulated by 5-HT and this effect contributes to the response to stings.

As in the case of histamine, there are no therapeutic applications for 5-HT, but a recently-discovered selective 5-HT_1- receptor agonist, sumatriptan, has been found to be effective in migraine.

Antagonists at the 5-HT receptor include lysergic acid diethylamide, cyproheptadine (which also blocks histamine receptors) and ketanserin. Ketanserin is a relatively selective 5-HT_2-receptor antagonist. The 5-HT receptor antagonists are being investigated for the treatment of hypertension and, in cancer patients, the reduction of nausea and vomiting associated with chemotherapy. To date they have no applications in veterinary medicine.

CHAPTER 4

MINERALS AND VITAMINS

In order to remain healthy and to maintain optimum productivity, all animals require adequate levels of a diverse group of both inorganic minerals and organic micronutrients (vitamins). These substances are necessary for normal body functions, and signs of deficiency appear in animals with inadequate intake or synthesis. Prophylaxis or therapy for deficiency states aims to provide sufficient quantities of these micronutrients for normal function to be maintained. Supplementation of vitamin or mineral intake may be particularly important in animals with reduced food intake and during periods of additional stress, including pregnancy and lactation and in disease. Signs which indicate inadequate vitamin or mineral intake can usually be quite easily treated with supplements, followed by careful attention by the owner to the animal's diet. A wide variety of commercial vitamin preparations are available.

Calcium, phosphorus and magnesium

Calcium is the major cation of hydroxyapatite, the basic component of bone, where it is present with phosphorus in the ratio Ca : P of 2 : 1. It is also a vital element in the excitation-contraction coupling in smooth, skeletal and cardiac muscle, in transmission of neural impulses and in release of neurotransmitters. Magnesium ions are also important in transmitter release, where their actions tend to oppose those of calcium ions. Thus, the balance between the levels of these two minerals is essential for the maintenance of normal neuromuscular transmission.

The major site of storage of magnesium in the body is in bone, where it is vital for normal metabolism. Magnesium is also an important cofactor in a number of metabolic pathways. Most of the phosphorus in the body (80 per cent) exists in combination with calcium in bones and teeth. It is an important element in the transfer of energy, through the formation of high-energy phosphates (adenosine triphosphate).

Parathyroid hormone, calcitonin and vitamin D are all involved in the maintenance of normal levels of calcium and phosphorus. The rate at which these minerals are absorbed from the gastrointestinal tract is dependent on the body's requirements and is controlled by vitamin D. Vitamin D also increases the reabsorption of calcium from the renal tubules.

The amount of calcium absorbed from dietary sources is influenced by the level of phytic acid and its salts in the feed. Calcium (and also magnesium) bind to the phosphate radicals of phytic acid, forming insoluble and unavailable complexes. Thus where grain, which contains high levels of phytic acid, is a major constituent of the diet, calcium absorption may be limited.

The calcium and phosphorus requirements of growing animals are greater than those of adults. Growing animals deposit calcium and phosphorus in bone when blood levels are sufficiently high. The requirements of lactating animals are higher than those of growing animals.

Metabolic disorders and mineral deficiencies

Milk fever (parturient paresis)

Milk fever is associated with an imbalance between the intake and output of calcium. It is usually associated with the movement of minerals into the colostrum and milk near the time of parturition. The animals are unable to mobilize bone calcium or to increase intestinal and renal absorption of calcium. It is associated with calving in cattle, and occurs, less commonly, in late pregnancy or during lactation in sheep and goats. There is a possibility that a defect in vitamin D function is involved. Milk fever is more common in older cows and in some breeds of cattle (especially Jerseys).

The disease is characterized by severe hypocalcaemia, with blood calcium levels below 1.5 mmol/l, compared to the normal levels of 2.2–2.6 mmol/l. Hypophosphataemia and hypomagnesaemia may also occur.

Treatment
Administration of calcium is effective in reversing the signs. A rapid increase of plasma levels follows the intravenous injection of the mineral, and muscle twitching, defecation, urination and eructation may occur. The total amount

of calcium injected is considerably less than that excreted into the milk and is only a small fraction of the readily exchangeable calcium in the body. However, even the brief restoration of plasma calcium levels appears to restore normal gut function, improve the appetite and re-establish normal homeostatic mechanisms for the control of calcium movements. If the hypocalcaemia is still evident after 24 hours, further doses of calcium may be required.

Calcium borogluconate is the treatment of choice. Although calcium gluconate is also effective, the inclusion of boron increases the solubility and stability of the solution. There is no evidence to suggest that addition of magnesium and phosphorus to the solution is of advantage, except in cases of hypomagnesaemia (<0.85 mmol/l) and hypophosphataemia (<1.35 mmol/l).

Since high-calcium diets during pregnancy are reported to increase the incidence of milk fever, the use of a low calcium/high phosphorus diet in the period before calving has been advocated as a preventative measure. Animals on this diet have high levels of parathyroid hormone and increased absorption of dietary calcium. Prophylactic administration of vitamin D for up to a week prepartum has been reported to reduce the incidence of the disease.

Dose

calcium borogluconate
cow	50–400 ml of 40 per cent solution i.v.
sheep	15–50 ml of 40 per cent solution i.v.
goat	15–50 ml of 40 per cent solution i.v.

Puerperal tetany

In the bitch (and less commonly in the cat) puerperal tetany occurs near the time of peak lactation, approximately 1–3 weeks postpartum. The observed neuromuscular tetany is thought to be due to an altered sensitivity of motor nerve fibres associated with a loss of stabilizing membrane-bound calcium. This condition can be complicated by hypoglycaemia.

Treatment with calcium gluconate (approximately 1 ml/kg of 10 per cent solution), administered by *slow* intravenous injection is effective within 15 minutes. Removal of the puppies from the bitch (and weaning, if possible) prevents further calcium depletion.

Transit tetany

In horses transit tetany is produced by the stress of transportation. Long periods of fluid therapy can also produce a diaphragmatic flutter which is synchronous with the heartbeat. Animals are treated with calcium boro-gluconate, administered i.v. to effect.

Rickets

Rickets occurs in growing animals where there is a deficiency of calcium and/or vitamin D. In these cases, calcium hydrogen phosphate, calcium lactate or calcium hydrogen lactate may be used in conjunction with vitamin D.

Hypophosphataemia

Hypophosphataemia can occur in cows, in the presence or absence of hypocalcaemia. This is treated by intravenous administration of phosphorus-containing solutions, followed by oral supplementation.

Hypomagnesaemia (grass tetany)

Grass is a relatively poor source of magnesium and cattle grazed on grass pastures are more likely than most other animals to suffer from magnesium deficiency. Hypomagnesaemia commonly occurs in lactating cows, which have a fairly high daily loss of magnesium and are thus particularly susceptible to sudden reductions of magnesium intake. Cold, wet and windy conditions appear to increase the risk of development of hypomagnesaemia.

Treatment of hypomagnesaemia, in the absence of other metabolic disorders, is by injection of magnesium sulphate (25 per cent) or magnesium dextrose solutions. Intravenous administration should be at a very slow rate, with careful cardiac monitoring. Serum magnesium levels will be raised for 3–6 hours after i.v. dosing. Administration of an additional dose by subcutaneous injection will maintain serum levels of magnesium for 24 hours. If hypocalcaemia is also present, injection of calcium borogluconate with magnesium or combined calcium, phosphorus, magnesium solution is appropriate.

Prevention of grass tetany requires the addition of magnesium to the diet. A variety of methods, including application of magnesium-containing fertilizers to the soil, spraying foliage with magnesium oxide and oral supplementation with magnesium, have been effective.

Cobalt

Vitamin B_{12} is synthesized in the forestomach of ruminants. It is essential for cell division and thus for generation of new red blood cells. The vitamin contains 4 per cent cobalt, and ruminants, unlike other animals which receive preformed vitamin B_{12} in their diets, require a dietary source of elemental cobalt. Deficiency of cobalt results in reduced blood volume and oxygen-carrying capacity. Other signs of cobalt deficiency include anorexia and weight loss. In severe cases, wasting and emaciation may occur and affected animals may die. Deficiency of this trace element is a common cause of anaemia in cattle grazing where soils contain less than 2 ppm of cobalt. These occur in specific areas of Australia, New Zealand, Africa, USA and the UK.

Treatment of deficiencies

The aim is to provide an adequate intake of cobalt. This may be achieved by dressings of cobalt sulphate or chloride for the pasture, where 0.5 kg of cobalt sulphate/hectare provides adequate levels for 3–4 years. Where the pasture is inaccessible, the addition of cobalt salts to feed or oral dosing may be used. Cobalt-containing bullets for oral administration provide a source of slow-release cobalt, but the formation of an insoluble coating of calcium phosphate decreases the rate of release of the mineral after a few weeks. A more recent preparation releases cobalt from a slowly dissolving glass.

Toxicity

There is a considerable margin of safety and cobalt toxicity is extremely unlikely to occur in ruminants.

Dose

Daily dose for prophylaxis:
cattle	25 mg
calf	10 mg
sheep	5 mg
lamb	2.5 mg

Treatment doses:
cattle	500 mg
calf	200 mg
sheep	100 mg
lamb	50 mg

Copper

Copper is an essential component of a number of enzymes and a required cofactor for the actions of others. It is also important for the absorption and utilization of iron. Following intestinal absorption, copper is stored in a small protein molecule, metallothionein, which also binds zinc and cadmium. High levels of dietary molybdenum and sulphate result in the formation of insoluble copper thiomolybdate complexes and thereby reduce copper absorption. Thus in high-molybdenum soils, dietary requirements of copper are higher.

Signs of deficiency in sheep include change in wool growth and hypochromic anaemia. Demyelination of nerves in the brain and spinal cord may occur in lambs, causing swayback. In cattle, excess molybdenum often results in reduced copper absorption and consequent deficiency syndrome. Anaemia is common; other signs vary. Before instituting copper supplementation, animals should have their copper status checked by laboratory testing.

Treatment of deficiencies

Administration of copper to pregnant ewes reduces the incidence of congenital swayback in lambs. Copper may be administered in a variety of ways. Dressing of pastures in areas known to be deficient in copper has proved effective. The problem is common in Australia and New Zealand, where farmers determine the amount of copper required for each area. Addition of copper to feed or the provision of mineral licks are also effective. Copper sulphate is used for pastures, as a feed additive and for licks. Copper oxide needles in gelatin capsules may be administered orally. The copper in this formulation is slowly released over a number of weeks.

Parenteral administration of copper has proved successful. Copper heptonate, edetate and methionate can be administered subcutaneously or intramuscularly. Complexed formulations of copper (e.g. copper diethylamine oxyquinoline sulphonate) are also suitable for subcutaneous injection. Reactions at the site of injection may occur after parenteral administration of copper salts.

Toxicity

Toxic reactions to acute, excessive copper intake are rare. They include salivation, severe colic and purging, which may cause circulatory collapse. The passage of green faeces (due to the presence of a copper-chlorophyll complex) is a useful diagnostic feature.

Chronic administration of copper results in the accumulation of excessive amounts in the liver. The condition is asymptomatic until a precipitating factor (e.g. physical effort, fasting) causes release of large amounts into the bloodstream and consequent haemolysis. Death may follow within 1–4 days. The veterinarian and farmer should be aware of all sources of copper; examples include food additives for growth promotion; copper presented as licks or used in anthelmintics; and copper-contaminated pasture after spraying copper-containing fungicides on fruit trees. Oral and parenteral supplementation should not be used together.

The dose for sheep needs to be carefully controlled since they, especially lambs, are particularly susceptible to poisoning. Other ruminants are also sensitive, but less so. Pigs, in contrast, are relatively resistant to the toxic effects of copper but the practice of adding copper to pig meal may be dangerous because of the difficulty in achieving uniform mixing.

Copper chelating compounds may be of benefit in the treatment of acute toxicity. Calcium EDTA and penicillamine are used. Chronic toxicity is managed by the administration of ammonium molybdenate and sodium sulphate. Further accumulation of copper is prevented and liver stores are slowly depleted.

Doses

copper (as calcium copperedetate)
    cattle   100–200 mg s.c.
copper (as methionine complex)
    cattle   40–120 mg i.m.
    sheep   40 mg s.c. or i.m.
    lamb   10 mg s.c. or i.m.
copper (as heptonate)
    sheep   25 mg i.m.
copper (as cuproxoline)
    cattle   12–60 mg s.c.
    sheep   6–12 mg s.c.

Vitamins

Vitamin A

Vitamin A occurs as vitamin A_1 (retinol) (Fig. 4.1) and vitamin A_2 (3-dehydroretinol); both are formed from various fat-soluble carotenes, which serve as provitamins. The major source of vitamin A for food animals is β-carotene. The carotenoids occur in green vegetables, carrots, hay and dairy products. Enzymic conversion of these to vitamin A occurs in the liver and gastrointestinal tract. Fish liver oils are also a rich source of the vitamin.

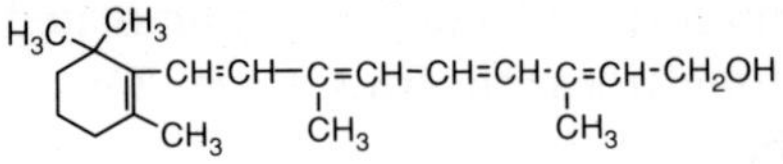

Vitamin A_1 (retinol)

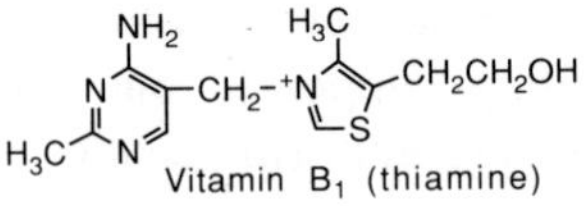

Vitamin B_1 (thiamine)

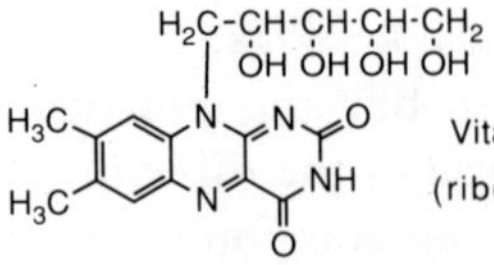

Vitamin B_2 (riboflavine)

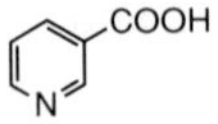

Vitamin B_3 (niacin)

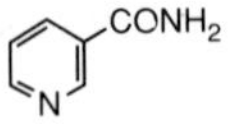

Nicotinamide

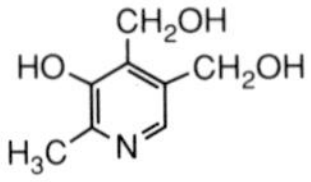

Vitamin B_6 (pyridoxine)

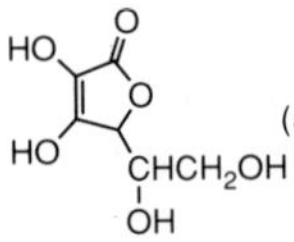

Vitamin C (ascorbic acid)

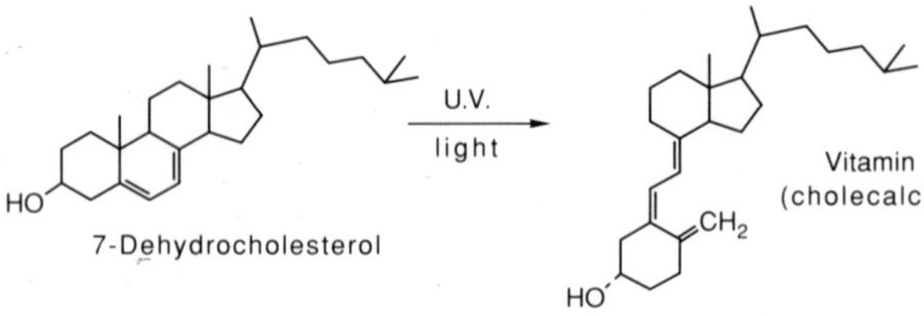

7-Dehydrocholesterol

Vitamin D_3 (cholecalciferol)

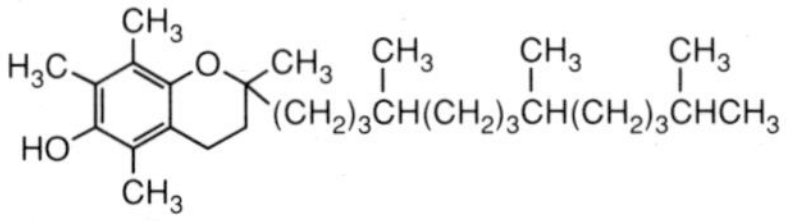

Vitamin E (α-tocopherol)

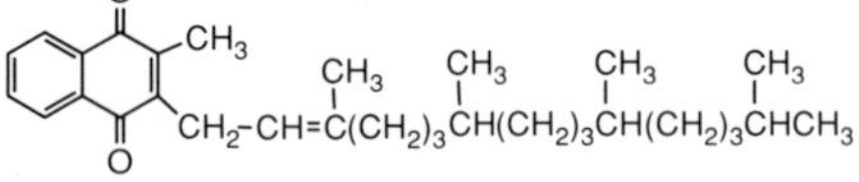

Vitamin K_1

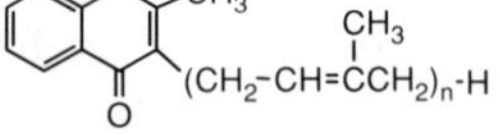

Vitamin K_2 ($n = 1\text{-}13$)

Figure 4.1 Vitamins.

Commercial preparations contain vitamin A_1, derived from saltwater fish, usually cod or halibut. Vitamin A is stored in the liver, which can hold enough to maintain animals through seasonal periods of low vitamin intake. Normal function of epithelial tissue of the retina, skin and respiratory mucosa depends on adequate levels of vitamin A. It is required for the formation of mucus-secreting cells, which synthesize glycoproteins, and for the formation of rhodopsin, which is necessary for activation of visual neural pathways. Vitamin A also has an important role in reproduction, where it is required for spermatogenesis and maintenance of pregnancy.

Supplementation is especially important during pregnancy, lactation and in the neonate. In some disease states the requirement for vitamin A is increased. In cats with upper respiratory tract infection, the stores of vitamin A are depleted and supplementation is required for restoration and maintenance of healthy respiratory epithelia.

Night blindness, due to retinal abnormalities, is an early sign of vitamin A deficiency. Hyperkeratinization of the skin and mucus-secreting epithelia, dryness of the conjunctiva followed by hyperkeratinization, bone deformities, retarded growth and disorders of reproduction may all occur.

Vitamin A deficiency is treated by single, large doses of either synthetic vitamin A or fish oils. The vitamin will be stored in the liver and provide supplementation over a period of several months.

Cats fed on diets which are excessively rich in vitamin A, e.g. those containing a high liver content, may suffer hypervitaminosis A. Spondylitis results from the production of extra bone, especially in the cervical region but also in the leg joints. General depression and anorexia may occur.

Vitamin B group

The B vitamins consist of a number of different, water-soluble substances which are necessary for the normal metabolism of protein, carbohydrate and fats. The maintenance of adequate levels is particularly important during and after infections. In ruminants, these vitamins are synthesized by rumen microflora and deficiencies may become evident when rumen function is abnormal.

Vitamin B_1 (thiamine) (Fig. 4.1) occurs in many cereals and meats. The requirement for thiamine in ruminants is usually met by synthesis in the rumen. Non-ruminants rely on a combination of bacterial synthesis in the digestive tract and ingested thiamine. Deficiency of thiamine is uncommon and when it occurs, ingestion of thiamine antagonists is the most likely cause. Pet animals fed on diets containing only cooked meat may also become deficient in thiamine. Signs of deficiency include neuromuscular incoordination and tremors. Convulsions follow and animals may die of cardiac failure.

Vitamin B_2 (riboflavin) (Fig. 4.1) occurs in milk, meat, cereals, vegetables, fruit and fish, and plays a vital role in a number of enzyme systems. Dietary intake of vitamin B_2 is often marginal and supplements are required.

Nicotinamide, the active form of niacin (vitamin B_3) (Fig. 4.1), is found in meat, cereals, vegetables, fish and milk. It is a component of nicotinamide adenine dinucleotide (NAD) and the phosphate (NADP) which are both necessary for normal metabolic pathways.

Deficiency in dogs causes the characteristic syndrome called black tongue, including erythema, dermatitis, diarrhoea and CNS disturbances. Such deficiencies are unlikely if dogs are fed a normal standard diet. The syndrome responds to supplementation with niacin and nicotinamide.

Vitamin B_6 (pyridoxine) (Fig. 4.1) is a common component of natural feeds and plays an important role in amino acid metabolism. Spontaneous deficiencies are rare.

Vitamin B_{12} (cyanocobalamin) occurs in meat and eggs but since it needs to be synthesized by microorganisms in animal tissue it is not found in vegetable matter. Thus, diets for non-ruminants must contain synthetic vitamin B_{12}, unless some animal protein sources are included. The vitamin contains cobalt and ruminants must have adequate dietary cobalt intake (see above). The liver stores vitamin B_{12} but stores can become depleted if there is an increased rate of tissue breakdown or reduced absorption (which may be associated with alteration in gut flora). Deficiency causes anaemia and reduced wool production, muscle growth or milk production.

Vitamin C

Vitamin C (ascorbic acid) (Fig. 4.1) is synthesized *in vivo* in pigs, sheep, beef cattle and poultry. A deficiency syndrome, hypertrophic osteodystrophy, with pain and swelling in the limbs, has been recognized in dogs. Cats with upper respiratory tract infections may respond well to doses of up to 1 g (i.v.) daily.

Vitamin D

Vitamin D is formed from provitamins, found in both plants and animals. In plants, the provitamin ergosterol is converted by ultraviolet radiation to vitamin D_2 (calciferol). Thus the vitamin D content of plants can be increased by irradiation. In animals, vitamin D_3 (cholecalciferol) is formed by the action of ultraviolet rays on the provitamin, 7-dehydrocholesterol (Fig. 4.1).

Vitamin D is an important regulator of Ca^{2+} homeostasis. It stimulates the synthesis of the calcium-binding protein needed for the transport of Ca^{2+} from the intestinal lumen into the cell. It acts together with parathormone to mobilize Ca^{2+} and PO_4^{3-} from the bone and thus maintain required blood levels of Ca^{2+}. It is also required for renal tubular reabsorption of Ca^{2+} and PO_4^{3-}.

Large seasonal variations in vitamin D levels have been observed in sheep. Low concentrations occur in winter, and this may be exacerbated by the demands of pregnancy. Inadequate mineralization of the bone is associated with vitamin D deficiency and in growing animals this may lead to the development of rickets. In mature animals, demineralization of the bone leads to fractures.

Treatment of vitamin D deficiency is effective; fish meals and irradiated yeast provide useful additional dietary sources of vitamin D. Calcium and phosphorus supplements may also be required. Vitamin D is useful as a preventative measure in cows known to be subject to parturient paresis. Its benefit in these animals is thought to be due to increased absorption of Ca^{2+}.

Vitamin E

Vitamin E consists of a group of tocopherols, of which D-α-tocopherol is the main active compound. Green plants and whole grain cereals are a rich source of this highly fat-soluble vitamin. The antioxidant properties of vitamin E prolong the life of polyunsaturated fatty acids and thereby help maintain the integrity of the cell membrane. Its function is similar to that of a selenium-containing enzyme and it is thus able to protect animals against selenium deficiency (and vice versa). Such deficiencies affect the function of both cardiac and skeletal muscles.

Horses, sheep and cattle in New Zealand and Australia and beef cattle in the UK suffer selenium/vitamin E deficiencies which lead to either acute or chronic nutritional myopathies. Subclinical growth deficits, inappetence and in extreme cases, death, may occur.

Since vitamin E is inactivated by heat, light and oxygen, cats fed on canned foods which contain excessive amounts of fat may develop a deficiency known as pansteatitis (yellow fat disease). The syndrome responds to therapy with vitamin E and glucocorticoids but may be fatal if left untreated.

The most common product used in diet supplementation is α-tocopherol acetate, which is often given in combination with selenium.

Vitamin K

Vitamin K is a fat-soluble vitamin with a variety of forms (Fig. 4.1); it is found in both plant and animal materials. Since it is an essential component of the blood clotting process, deficiencies lead to impaired clotting ability, and in extreme cases to fatal haemorrhage. Microbial synthesis in the rumen and the non-ruminant digestive tract ensure adequate levels are normally available in all species, except poultry. Vitamin K levels may be reduced in situations where absorption is impaired, including diarrhoea or alteration of gut microflora due to use of broad-spectrum antibiotics. The ingestion of antimetabolites (e.g. dicoumarol in sweet clover) reduces the activity of vitamin K. This reduced activity is put to therapeutic use with the oral anticoagulants (see page 204).

Deficiency of vitamin K in poultry leads to increased clotting time and, in more serious cases, haemorrhage. These can be treated by parenteral administration of the vitamin. Prophylaxis requires the maintenance of adequate dietary intake by supplementation with naturally occurring or synthetic vitamin K preparations. Vitamin K preparations are also used in the treatment of warfarin overdose (see page 204).

CHAPTER 5

DRUGS USED FOR PREMEDICATION AND RESTRAINT

Drugs used in premedication for general anaesthesia include analgesics, anticholinergics and those used to reduce stress. The latter group of drugs serves a variety of different purposes. They calm the patient and reduce the stress associated with induction of anaesthesia. This allows a smoother induction of, and recovery from, anaesthesia. In the presence of these drugs, it is usual for the dose of anaesthetic induction agent to be reduced and this reduces the chance of adverse side-effects and toxicity. Catecholamine levels, which are elevated in stressed animals, are lower in those which have been premedicated and thus the risk of cardiac arrhythmias is also reduced.

A wide variety of drugs which exert their primary effects on the central nervous system (CNS) are available. They are useful in the sedation of nervous animals prior to the use of general anaesthetics or, when used in selected combinations, allow relatively simple operative procedures to be performed. Those which calm or sedate patients are called sedatives or anxiolytics. In higher doses, most of the sedatives are hypnotics, i.e. they induce drowsiness and facilitate the onset of sleep. As the response depends on the dose of drug administered, most of the drugs in this category are referred to as sedative-hypnotics. The majority of these drugs, when administered in sufficiently high doses, are capable of inducing general anaesthesia.

The other commonly used CNS depressants in veterinary practice are the neuroleptics. Their main use in human clinical practice is in the management of psychotic patients. The calming properties of this group of drugs are different from those of the sedative-hypnotics and they are not capable of inducing general anaesthesia, irrespective of dose. They are, however, particularly useful in combination with potent analgesic drugs for production of the state of neuroleptanalgesia.

The vagolytic actions of premedicant agents protect the heart from brady-cardia and also help to dry the airways by reduction of secretions in most species, except ruminants. The two main agents which are in clinical use are atropine and glycopyrronium (see page 54).

The use of an analgesic component of premedication is particularly. important in animals which are in pain or are likely to suffer pain. Alleviation of pain is often more effective in the sedation of the patient than use of a sedative on its own. The drugs which are commonly used are the narcotic analgesics (Chapter 8).

Hypnotics and sedatives

Barbiturates

The barbituric acid derivatives are probably the oldest of the drugs used to depress the CNS. The structure of barbituric acid and its commonly used derivatives is shown in Fig. 5.1. Differences in chemical structure within the group account for differences in potency and pharmacokinetics but the basic feature of CNS depression is common to all members of the group. The speed of onset of action of the drugs is greatly influenced by their lipid solubility and thus the ease with which they cross the blood–brain barrier. Thiopentone sodium, the most lipid soluble of the group, has the fastest onset of action and is thus extremely useful in the induction of general anaesthesia.

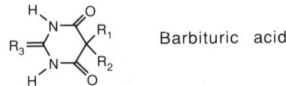

Barbituric acid

Barbiturate	R_1	R_2	R_3
thiopentone	ethyl	1-methylbutyl	S
phenobarbitone	ethyl	phenyl	O
pentobarbitone	ethyl	1-methylbutyl	O

Figure 5.1 Barbiturates used in veterinary practice.

The duration of action of individual barbiturates is determined by redistribution of the drug and by the rates of its metabolism and excretion. Redistribution is the most important factor which influences the duration of action of thiopentone. Thus the general anaesthetic effect lasts for only a short time because the thiopentone is rapidly redistributed from the brain to highly perfused tissues and more slowly to poorly perfused adipose tissue. The medium-acting barbiturates are dependent on hepatic metabolism for the termination of their activity. Drugs which interfere with liver enzymes may either prolong or reduce the duration of action of barbiturates. Chloramphenicol, by the inhibition of liver microsomal enzymes, greatly increases the duration of effect of the medium-acting barbiturates. Phenobarbitone, or other drugs which have the ability to induce hepatic enzymes, reduces the duration of action of the barbiturates. Phenobarbitone is one of the longer-acting barbiturates whose duration of action is influenced, at least in part, by the rate of renal excretion.

The CNS depressant action of barbiturates is thought to involve the inhibitory neurotransmitter, γ-aminobutyric acid (GABA). The response to GABA, following binding to its postsynaptic receptor sites, is the activation of chloride channels, which increases the permeability of the cell to Cl^- (Fig. 5.2). In the presence of the barbiturates, the affinity of GABA for its receptor sites is increased. Furthermore, a high concentration of the barbiturates may directly activate the chloride channels.

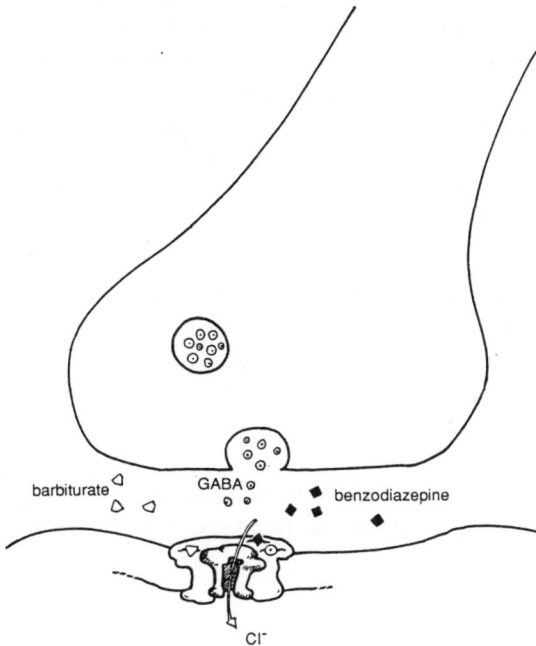

Figure 5.2 Binding sites for benzodiazepines and barbiturates are believed to be associated with Cl^- channels which are activated by the transmitter GABA.

The degree of CNS depression induced by the barbiturates varies from sedation to deep anaesthesia, depending on the dose and the particular drug. A dose-dependent depression of the respiratory centre also occurs. The doses used for sedation or hypnosis do not markedly disturb respiratory reflexes. When anaesthetic doses are administered, depression of respiration becomes detectable. Similarly, in sedative or hypnotic doses, barbiturates have little or no effect on the cardiovascular system. In fact, clinically significant depression of cardiovascular function does not occur until toxic doses are administered. The barbiturates are poor analgesics and may even accentuate the response to pain. Phenobarbitone has a special application in the treatment of convulsions (see below).

Barbiturates are well absorbed after oral administration although the rate of absorption does vary within the group. They are metabolized by the microsomal enzymes in the liver and are also potent inducers of microsomal enzyme activity. They are, therefore, capable of influencing the rate of hepatic metabolism of many other drugs.

In recent years, the use of barbiturates in humans has declined in favour of the benzodiazepines and other, newer drugs. The main factors involved in the change in prescribing habits are the abuse potential of the barbiturates and the fact that they were not uncommonly associated with intended or accidental drug overdoses. In many cases toxicity was increased by alcohol abuse and/or the use of other CNS depressant drugs. In veterinary practice, these problems are less applicable and the barbiturates are still quite widely used. The most commonly used member of the group is phenobarbitone, both as a sedative-hypnotic and as an anticonvulsant. Pentobarbitone is widely used as a general anaesthetic in laboratory animals.

Dose

phenobarbitone (for sedation)

    dog   2–8 mg/kg p.o. 2 or 3 times daily

    cat   0.5–3 mg/kg p.o. 2 or 3 times daily

pentobarbitone

    dog, cat   20–40 mg/kg i.v.

               depending on degree of sedation/anaesthesia required, premedication and rate of administration.

Benzodiazepines

The benzodiazepines were introduced into clinical medicine in the 1960s and, predominantly because of their very low inherent toxicity, they have largely replaced the barbiturates in human medicine. They have anxiolytic and sedative properties which are thought to be due to actions on the limbic system of the brain and particularly on the hippocampus and the amygdala.

Benzodiazepines, by their ability to modulate the coupling mechanism between GABA receptors and their associated chloride channels, enhance GABAergic transmission (Fig. 5.2). The binding site for the benzodiazepines is distinct from that for the barbiturates and, in contrast to the barbiturates, benzodiazepines are unable to directly affect the chloride channel or to induce a state of general anaesthesia, even at high doses.

There are at least 12 drugs in this group and they all induce similar responses although the magnitude and duration of action may vary in different species. They are relatively free from undesirable side-effects and have a wide therapeutic ratio when compared to the butyrophenone and phenothiazine tranquillizers (see below). Those in current use include brotizolam, chlordiazepoxide, diazepam, flunitrazepam and midazolam but only diazepam appears to have been widely used in veterinary anaesthesia. It is commonly used in combination with drugs such as ketamine or with the opioids, for anaesthesia rather than sedation.

Diazepam

Diazepam (Fig. 5.3) is insoluble in water and the injectable solution contains a number of organic solvents. It is not chemically compatible with a number of commonly used drugs and it is not advisable to mix it in a syringe with other drugs. Diazepam has sedative, anxiolytic, muscle relaxant and anticonvulsant properties. There are considerable species differences in sensitivity to the muscle relaxant and sedative effects. Diazepam potentiates most common anaesthetic agents. Unlike the neuroleptic agents, it has no antiemetic action. It produces minimal cardiovascular or respiratory depression and has a wide safety margin. The use of diazepam in the treatment of convulsions is described below.

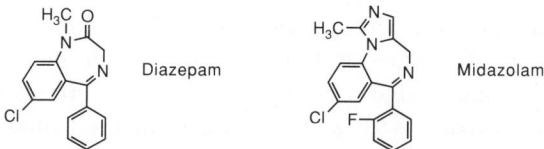

Figure 5.3 Benzodiazepines used in veterinary practice.

The main clinical uses of diazepam are taming of wild or intractable animals, sedation, skeletal muscle relaxation and as an anticonvulsant. The taming effect is useful in the prevention of fighting during the grouping of animals, e.g. during transport of pigs and in zoos. It has been used as pre-operative medication in horses and dogs. In the latter case it may be combined with morphine for prolonged sedation. The undesirable effects of ketamine in the cat and dog may be reduced by premedication with diazepam.

Diazepam is effective after oral dosing but in veterinary practice is more commonly administered by injection. Absorption from intramuscular injection sites is unreliable. The risk of thrombophlebitis after intravenous injection can be minimized by the use of an emulsion formulation.

Dose

All species, up to 1 mg/kg (to a maximum of 10 mg in the dog).

Midazolam

Midazolam (Fig. 5.3) is a water-soluble compound which produces effects similar to those of diazepam. The solution is compatible with other drugs, such as the opioids, in the syringe. The limited data available indicate that the duration of action of midazolam may be slightly shorter than that of diazepam.

Dose

Small animals, up to 0.5 mg/kg for sole use. Lower doses are required when midazolam is used in combination with other drugs.

Zolazepam

This is a diazepam analogue with activity very similar to that of the parent compound. It has been developed specifically for use in combination with tiletamine, a dissociative anaesthetic agent. This combination has been used in a variety of species and produces effective general anaesthesia, muscle relaxation and analgesia with minimum side effects (see page 156). It produces tachycardia, with a slight rise in arterial blood pressure and cardiac output. There is also an initial stimulation of respiration, followed by a mild depression.

Dose

dog	5–10 mg/kg i.v. or 7–25 mg/kg s.c.
cat	5–7.5 mg/kg i.v. or 10–15 mg/kg s.c.
	depending on depth and duration of anaesthesia required.

Chloral hydrate

Chloral hydrate is one of the oldest CNS depressants known in veterinary medicine. It is an effective hypnotic and may induce general anaesthesia if sufficiently large doses are administered. Generally the administration of large doses will produce undesirable side-effects and other, more potent general anaesthetics are preferred.

Rapid metabolism of chloral hydrate by reduction to trichloroethanol occurs (Fig. 5.4) and it is the metabolite that is thought to be the active principle. Trichloroethanol is eventually conjugated with glucuronic acid prior to urinary excretion.

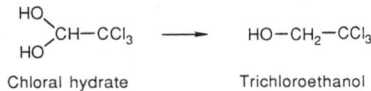

$$\underset{\text{Chloral hydrate}}{\overset{\text{HO}}{\underset{\text{HO}}{>}}CH-CCl_3} \longrightarrow \underset{\text{Trichloroethanol}}{HO-CH_2-CCl_3}$$

Figure 5.4 Metabolism of chloral hydrate to trichloroethanol.

Chloral hydrate is used mainly for sedation in large animals, more usually in cattle but occasionally in horses. In therapeutic doses it does not significantly depress the cardiovascular or respiratory systems. It can be administered orally or by the intravenous route. The irritant nature of chloral hydrate may cause gastric irritation when the drug is administered orally. Similarly, care must be taken to avoid extravascular injection. The onset of action after oral administration may take up to 30 minutes.

Dose

Sedation in the horse
  3–3.5 g/50 kg orally by stomach tube, 5 g/50 kg i.v.

Anaesthesia in the horse
  5–7 g/50 kg i.v.

Sedation in cattle
  cow   30–60 g p.o.
  bull   up to 200 g p.o.

Anaesthesia in cattle
  5–7 g/50 kg i.v.

α-Adrenoceptor agonists

α-Adrenoceptors of the peripheral and central nervous systems are classified as α_1- and α_2-adrenoceptors, according to the actions of specific agonists and antagonists. Stimulation of central presynaptic α_2-adrenoceptors inhibits the release of noradrenaline, leading to a decrease in cortical neuronal activity. This action is responsible for the sedative actions of α_2-adrenoceptor agonists such as xylazine. Stimulation of central α_2-adrenoceptors in cardiovascular control centres results in bradycardia and hypotension; clonidine, a selective α_2-adrenoceptor agonist, is used as an antihypertensive in man.

Xylazine

Xylazine (Fig. 5.5), through its stimulant actions at α_2-adrenoceptors, produces dose-dependent sedation, analgesia and muscular relaxation. It does not cause excitement either on induction of or recovery from anaesthesia. There is considerable species variation in sensitivity to xylazine, with ruminants being most sensitive and pigs the least. Dogs, cats and horses have similar, intermediate sensitivities.

Xylazine   Detomidine

Figure 5.5 α_2-Adrenoceptor agonists used as sedatives.

Xylazine has a variety of effects on the cardiovascular system. In many species an initial increase in blood pressure is followed by a longer period of hypotension. The heart rate decreases and atrio-ventricular blocks of varying degrees are evident. Premedication with atropine reduces these effects. Cardiac output and respiratory frequency decrease and usually the $PaCO_2$ rises and the PaO_2 falls after xylazine administration. It has also been shown to produce hyperglycaemia and hypoinsulinaemia, which is probably due to an α_2-adrenoceptor-mediated inhibition of insulin release. Cats and dogs are likely to vomit after the administration of the drug. Hypothermia is a common feature of xylazine sedation. The drug should not be administered to animals in the latter stages of pregnancy, except at parturition.

Dose

cattle	5–30 mg/100 kg i.m.
horse	0.25–1.1 mg/kg slowly i.v.
	0.5–3 mg/kg i.m.
cat	up to 3 mg/kg i.m.
dog	1–3 mg/kg i.m.

Detomidine

Detomidine (Fig. 5.5) is an α_2-adrenoceptor agonist, with weak α-adrenoceptor affinity. It is a potent sedative and analgesic which has been used widely in horses and to a lesser extent in cattle. The sedation produced by detomidine can be improved by administration in combination with opioids. The combination of choice is butorphanol (0.05–0.1 mg/kg) with detomidine (10 μg/kg). Detomidine has been used successfully as a premedicant alone and in combination with other drugs.

The main side-effects of detomidine are the result of peripheral adrenergic stimulation. Doses as low as 20 μg/kg produce severe hypertension and bradycardia. There are disturbances in cardiac rhythm and both sino-atrial and atrio-ventricular block have been reported. Bradycardia and heart block are maximal at doses of 20 μg/kg and can be prevented by prior administration of atropine. Higher doses produce marked and prolonged hypertension.

The respiratory effects of detomidine are variable but it is usual to observe a slight increase in respiratory rate which does not appear to be of significance. Other consequences of peripheral adrenergic stimulation include ataxia, swaying, sweating, piloerection and increased frequency of micturition. It should not be used in conjunction with sympathomimetic amines and should not be administered to animals in the last month of pregnancy. Trimethoprim/sulphadiazine combination preparations should not be administered to horses sedated with detomidine because potentially fatal cardiac arrhythmias have been reported to occur with this drug combination.

Dose

horse	10–80 μg/kg i.v. or i.m.
cattle	20–80 μg/kg i.v. or i.m.
	according to degree of sedation required.

Medetomidine

Medetomidine is a highly selective α_2-adrenoceptor agonist sedative and analgesic which has been developed specifically for use in dogs and cats. It has been used in combination with a wide variety of other sedative and anaesthetic agents in both species. It produces marked bradycardia and hypothermia; hence efforts should be made to conserve body heat. It also induces vomiting in about 8 per cent of dogs. The specific α_2-adrenoceptor antagonist, atipamezole, has been recommended for the reversal of the CNS effects of medetomidine and it produces a rapid return to consciousness and awareness. Medetomidine should not be used in pregnant animals or in conjunction with sympathomimetic amines.

Dose

dog   10–80 μg/kg i.v. or i.m.
cat   50–150 μg/kg i.m.
         according to degree of sedation required.

Neuroleptics

Drugs in this group are also referred to as ataractics or major tranquillizers. The two major chemical groups used in veterinary practice are the butyrophenones and the phenothiazines. They are used in low doses to produce a calming effect and at somewhat higher doses to produce sedation. Administration of doses above the recommended therapeutic dose is unlikely to induce a greater sedative effect.

Phenothiazines

The phenothiazine (Fig. 5.6) derivatives have a variety of actions. They usually produce sedation in most species, although excitement has been produced in some (e.g. horse) by some drugs in the group (e.g. chlorpromazine). The phenothiazines include chlorpromazine (usually considered the prototype drug), promazine, acepromazine (the most widely used in veterinary medicine), prochlorperazine, perphenazine and triflupromazine.

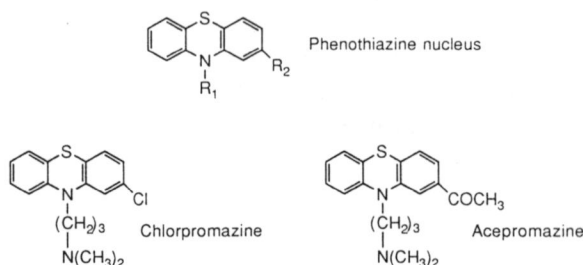

Figure 5.6 Phenothiazine nucleus and some of the derivatives in clinical use.

The main pharmacological action of all the drugs in the group is essentially similar. Differences in potency, kinetics and spectrum of actions account for the differences observed with the clinical use of these drugs. The actions of the phenothiazines are due to blockade of central dopamine receptors. In addition the drugs interact with a number of other receptors both in the brain and peripherally. Thus they have a wide variety of other actions which vary in degree from drug to drug within the group. For example, chlorpromazine has a good sedative action and potent adrenoceptor antagonist activity but is a weak antihistamine. In contrast, promethazine has some sedative action, weak adrenoceptor antagonist activity and is a potent antihistamine. Phenothiazines potentiate most of the common anaesthetic agents and lower the metabolic rate. They are also antiemetic, antipyretic and produce hypotension and hypothermia. The drug which has been the most extensively studied is chlorpromazine.

Chlorpromazine

Chlorpromazine (Fig. 5.6) is a CNS depressant which has its main action on the reticular formation and the hypothalamus with little effect on the cerebral cortex and the spinal cord. It is generally accepted that it potentiates the action of hypnotics, analgesics and anaesthetics.

It has a marked antiemetic action which can be utilized to advantage in anaesthesia and in the treatment of motion sickness. This effect is mediated by blockade of dopamine receptors in the chemoreceptor trigger zone in the medulla. The body's temperature controlling mechanism is also depressed and hence shivering is prevented by chlorpromazine. The drug may also be useful in the treatment of heat-stroke or in the production of hypothermia.

The α-adrenoceptor antagonist action of chlorpromazine accounts for its main effects on the cardiovascular system. Thus it produces peripheral vasodilation, a reduction in peripheral resistance and hypotension. The heart rate is increased and the cardiac output remains unaltered. The vasodilator effect may be useful in maintaining the blood supply to vital areas during shock, although it is more effective in the prevention of shock rather than its treatment. The use of chlorpromazine to treat shock may lead to an extreme fall in blood pressure and death; hence it is important to institute adequate fluid therapy if it is to be used for this purpose. The vasodilator effect may also potentiate the hypotensive effects of local anaesthetics administered epidurally and the phenothiazines should not be used for premedication when this anaesthetic technique is employed.

Chlorpromazine has minimal effects on the respiratory system apart from a suppression of the secretions of the bronchial tree. Whilst it potentiates the actions of muscle relaxants, it has no neuromuscular blocking properties of its own. However, it is said to produce muscular weakness and smooth muscle tone is depressed due to its spasmolytic action. Intestinal spasm and peristalsis are reduced, which may lead to constipation.

The mild antihistamine action of chlorpromazine, together with its sedative properties, may be useful in the treatment of certain skin diseases. Skin rashes in people handling the drug have been reported and therefore adequate precautions should be taken.

The metabolism of chlorpromazine is relatively complex and the number of metabolites produced varies from species to species. The rate of metabolism is variable, even within a species. The main metabolite is chlorpromazine sulphoxide.

The use of chlorpromazine in horses is not normally recommended since excitement and muscular incoordination may occur, although it may occasionally be used in the treatment of tetanus. In cattle, all of the phenothiazine derivatives, including chlorpromazine, tend to prolong the recovery period after general anaesthesia. This may lead to alimentary, respiratory and locomotor problems, thus the drug is not recommended for premedication in cattle. It may, however, be used for sedation which can be combined with local or regional anaesthesia. The drug is useful for premedication or sedation in pigs. It may be administered by intravenous injection into an ear vein or intramuscularly, but the latter is not as predictable. It is also used for premedication and sedation in dogs, cats and sheep.

Dose

horse	0.5–1.0 mg/kg i.m. (occasional use – tetanus)
cattle	0.25–1 mg/kg i.m.
pig	up to 2 mg/kg i.v.
sheep	up to 2 mg/kg i.m. or i.v.
dog and cat	0.5–2 mg/kg i.v.
	1–5 mg/kg i.m.
	up to 5 mg/kg p.o.

Acepromazine

Acepromazine (Fig. 5.6) is used extensively throughout the world as a sedative and premedicant in animals. It is the most widely used phenothiazine derivative in veterinary practice in the UK. The actions of acepromazine are similar to those of chlorpromazine, but it is a more potent drug.

Since acepromazine produces very few aberrant reactions in horses, it is the phenothiazine derivative of choice in this species. Intravenous injection of acepromazine in horses should be performed extremely slowly and halted immediately any untoward signs are observed. It is considered inadvisable to administer acepromazine to breeding stallions as paralysis of the erector penis muscle has been reported following the use of this drug.

In cats and dogs acepromazine can be administered by intramuscular or intravenous routes and orally. It is useful for the prevention of travel sickness in small animals. When used as a premedicant, the dose of anaesthetic required is considerably reduced.

The full effect of acepromazine may not be manifest for up to 1 hour after intramuscular administration and at least 30 minutes should be allowed after dosing before the induction of general anaesthesia. When the drug is administered by intravenous injection, general anaesthesia should not be induced for at least 10 minutes.

Dose

horse, cattle, sheep and pig	0.05–0.1 mg/kg i.m. or slow i.v.
cat and dog	0.05–0.25 mg/kg i.m. or slow i.v.
	1–3 mg/kg p.o.

Butyrophenones

The mechanism of action of the butyrophenones is similar to that of the phenothiazines, i.e. they block dopamine receptors in the CNS. Although they have a higher therapeutic ratio than the phenothiazines, they are more likely to produce extrapyramidal signs of rigidity, tremor and catalepsy. The butyrophenones decrease the dose of anaesthetic induction agents and potentiate both anaesthetics and narcotic analgesics. The respiratory and cardiovascular effects of this group of drugs are minimal, but some hypotension may be produced by α-adrenoceptor blockade.

Azaperone

Azaperone (Fig. 5.7) is a butyrophenone specifically developed for use in pigs, although it has been used in horses and in zoo animals. It produces reliable, dose-dependent sedation following intramuscular or intravenous administration. It is recommended for use as a specific premedicant with metomidate to produce general anaesthesia in pigs. In addition, it has been used to suppress aggression. It is particularly effective in reducing fighting when pigs from different sources are mixed, usually at the weaner stage, and in the reduction of aggression in sows towards their piglets. Azaperone produces a slight hypotension and tends to stimulate respiration in the pig.

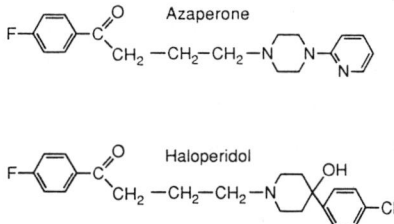

Figure 5.7 Butyrophenone neuroleptics.

Dose

| pig | 1–4 mg/kg i.m., 10 mg/kg i.p. |
| horse | 0.5–1 mg/kg i.v. |

Droperidol

Droperidol is one of the most potent antiemetic drugs available. When administered by intravenous injection, it produces a moderate fall in blood pressure, which is of short duration. This effect does not occur after oral or intramuscular administration. Defecation commonly occurs during the onset of action of the drug. There is no depression of respiration. Droperidol has been used in both pigs and dogs, either alone or in combination with fentanyl to produce neuroleptanalgesia (see below).

Dose

| pig | 0.1–0.4 mg/kg i.m. |
| dog | 2–8 mg/kg (see below for neuroleptanalgesic dose). |

Fluanisone

Fluanisone has similar properties to droperidol. It is used mainly in combination with fentanyl as a neuroleptanalgesic combination in dogs, guinea pigs and rabbits. It has potent antiemetic properties and potentiates the analgesic effects of fentanyl. Fluanisone may also reduce the respiratory and cardiovascular depression produced by fentanyl.

Dose see page 135.

Haloperidol

Haloperidol has similar properties to droperidol but a somewhat longer duration of action.

Thioxanthenes

These are triple ring heterocyclic compounds and their pharmacology is similar to that of the phenothiazines. The only one in the group to have been used in animals is chlorprothixene.

Dose

| pig | 1–2 mg/kg i.v. |
| dog | 2–4 mg/kg i.v. or i.m. |

Drugs used to reduce secretions

The main purpose of including antimuscarinic agents in premedication is to reduce the volume of secretions in the respiratory tract. Because these drugs exert their effect by the blockade of muscarinic receptors, they have the added effect of preventing vagally mediated bradycardia. They should therefore be used during eye surgery when initiation of the oculocardiac reflex may result in marked bradycardia. Similar considerations apply to any surgical procedure during which the vagus may be accidentally stimulated. The drugs most commonly used are atropine and glycopyrronium. The pharmacology of these is described in Chapter 2. The following discussion relates specifically to the use of these drugs in premedication.

Antimuscarinics are rarely used in ruminants because they produce a sticky, thick saliva which is more likely to block the airways than the saliva produced under normal conditions. However, the use of a drying agent is considered most necessary in the cat because the small trachea may be readily blocked, even with relatively small quantities of saliva. Pigs are also quite sensitive in this regard. In dogs, the use of a drying agent is generally a matter for the individual veterinarian to decide. It may be necessary where the breed or the individual patient produces copious quantities of saliva. Horses seldom require a drying agent.

Neuroleptanalgesia

For the performance of diagnostic and relatively minor operative procedures it may be desirable to avoid the use of general anaesthetics. Where possible, it is safer and easier if the operation can be performed using local anaesthetics and/or strong analgesics. However, the administration of analgesics is often associated with a number of undesirable side-effects such as nausea, vomiting and respiratory depression. These effects are particularly marked with the more potent analgesics, such as etorphine and fentanyl. In order to reduce these undesirable effects, a second drug may be administered. The drugs which are used are the neuroleptics, and their usefulness in these combinations is due to their antiemetic activity and to the fact that they have marked sedative actions. Whilst a number of drug combinations have been used, only three or four are available for general veterinary use.

Etorphine and acepromazine

This combination has been produced for use in large animals. Each millilitre of solution contains 2.45 mg etorphine and 10 mg acepromazine. Etorphine is a semisynthetic opioid, with a potency between 1000 and 10 000 times that of morphine. Because of the remarkable potency, only very small quantities of drug are required, even for very large animals. Thus the drug, administered by dart, has been successfully used on its own and in combination with neuroleptics in the capture of wild animals.

In horses, a marked rise in pulse rate occurs after administration of the combination of etorphine and acepromazine, but in other animals pulse rate is likely to fall. Increased blood pressure has been observed in most species. Muscle tremors and spasm, particularly in horses, are also a feature of etorphine/acepromazine neuroleptanalgesia.

Extreme care is essential in the handling of etorphine due to its potentially lethal effects in man. Rubber gloves should be worn while handling the drug but if these should be damaged and the skin surface broken, to even a minor degree, then the area should be washed and medical help summoned immediately. A reversing agent such as naloxone (0.8-1.2 mg) should be injected every few minutes until all symptoms have abated. In the absence of naloxone, diprenorphine may be used. In animals, the effects of the etorphine component are reversed by the administration of diprenorphine at a dose rate approximately equivalent to the etorphine dose.

Dose

horse, cattle, pig	1 ml of the etorphine/acepromazine combination per 100 kg i.m. or i.v., and for reversal a similar volume of diprenorphine.
sheep	0.5 ml of the etorphine/acepromazine combination per 100 kg i.m. or i.v.

Etorphine and methotrimeprazine

This combination has been produced for use in small animals and its use is normally restricted to dogs. Each ml contains 0.074 mg etorphine and 18 mg methotrimeprazine. The corresponding diprenorphine antidote solution contains 0.272 mg/ml. Administration of the drug combination may cause sudden reaction of the animal to noise and may produce depression of respiration, cyanosis and bradycardia. Hence great care must be taken in its use and considerable attention must be paid to the physiological condition of the patient. In older animals, in which major organ function may be impaired, the duration of action may be prolonged.

Dose

1 ml/10 kg and, for reversal, a similar volume of diprenorphine.

Fentanyl and droperidol

The analgesic, fentanyl, is 100 times as potent as morphine and, in combination with droperidol, it has been used extensively in dogs in the USA and Europe. Each millilitre contains 0.4 mg fentanyl and 20 mg droperidol. The neuroleptanalgesic combination is not available in the UK.

Bradycardia and respiratory depression, both associated with the fentanyl component, occur quite commonly. The bradycardia can be offset by the previous administration of atropine. The respiratory depression can be reversed with nalorphine or naloxone.

Dose

dog   1 ml of the drug combination per 10–20 kg i.v.
            1 ml of the drug combination per 5–10 kg i.m.

Fentanyl and fluanisone

This combination consists of 0.315 mg fentanyl and 10 mg fluanisone per ml. The mixture has been used for sedation and neuroleptanalgesia in dogs, guinea pigs and rabbits. Bradycardia is likely to occur and can be reversed with atropine. There may be hypersensitivity to sound and an absolutely quiet environment is essential. Respiratory depression is likely following this drug combination and its use should be avoided in animals with respiratory disease. Renal or hepatic dysfunction are also contraindications. If general anaesthesia is to be induced or maintained with conventional agents, extreme care is necessary as the anaesthetic drugs will be potentiated by the neuroleptic combination. Fentanyl is liable to provoke defecation in a high percentage of dogs. The actions of fentanyl can be reversed with nalorphine or naloxone but the sedative effect of fluanisone persists.

Dose

dog, rabbit, guinea pig   0.5 ml/kg i.m.
                                    (reduced by up to one half in old or debilitated animals).

Drugs used in the treatment of epilepsy

Dogs are far more likely to suffer from epilepsy than other species and, in practice, anticonvulsant treatment is normally limited to the cat and dog. A large number of different drugs have been used in the treatment of epilepsy in man. There are, however, only three drugs—phenobarbitone, primidone and phenytoin—which are widely used in veterinary medicine for seizure control.

Before any treatment is commenced it is essential to have a correct diagnosis and to ensure that the fits are truly epileptic and not due to other causes, such as cardiac conditions. It is also necessary to ensure that the epilepsy is not caused by a condition which may require treatment in its own right. It is also prudent to consider whether there is any risk to the animal or owner if the condition is left untreated.

The object of treatment is to suppress fits by maintaining an effective concentration of the drug in plasma, and hence in the brain, at all times. The frequency of dosing is determined by the plasma half-life of the drug. Treatment is begun with a low dose and this is increased until the fits are controlled or signs of overdosage are seen. Initially control should be attempted with a single drug. The main reason for this is to avoid drug interactions. Liver microsomal enzymes may be induced and one drug may increase the metabolism of the other.

Once a treatment regimen has been established it should be maintained until there is freedom from fits for a 2-year period. If it is necessary or desirable to withdraw treatment, this should be done slowly as sudden changes may precipitate convulsions. Any change from one treatment to another should be carried out gradually over a period of several weeks in order to avoid complications.

Phenobarbitone

Phenobarbitone (Fig. 5.8) specifically depresses the motor cortex and this accounts for its anticonvulsant action. The mechanism of action may involve an interaction with a subgroup of GABA receptors. It is the drug of choice in veterinary practice because it has a wide spectrum of anticonvulsant activity and is effective in all types of epileptic seizures occurring in cats and dogs. It may also be used i.v. (or i.m.) in the control of status epilepticus in the cat. Although it has a sedative action in man, this may not be evident with anticonvulsant doses used in cats and dogs. Higher doses induce ataxia and other signs of sedation. Some patients may become irritable and restless.

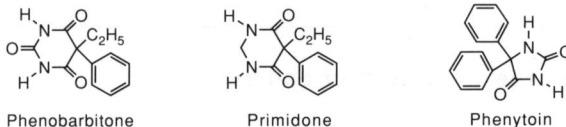

Phenobarbitone   Primidone   Phenytoin

Figure 5.8 Drugs used as anticonvulsants.

Absorption of phenobarbitone after oral administration may be variable, which is one reason why dosage needs to be adjusted for each individual animal. The most reliable way to determine an appropriate dose regime is to monitor plasma phenobarbitone levels. Effective plasma concentrations lie in the range 20–40 μg/ml and dosing should be adjusted accordingly. Phenobarbitone is one of the most potent inducers of microsomal enzymes in the liver. This influences its own metabolism and that of other drugs. The majority of the drug is excreted in the urine, but part is broken down in the liver.

Dose

dog, cat   Initial dose 1–2 mg/kg/day p.o. in one or two doses.
This may be increased to up to 20 mg/kg/day if necessary.

Primidone

Primidone is similar in structure to phenobarbitone although it is not a barbiturate (Fig. 5.8). It is metabolized to two main products, phenobarbitone and phenylethylmalonamide, both of which have anticonvulsant activity. The major side-effect associated with its use is ataxia coupled with sedation and occasionally polydipsia may be seen. Tolerance to these effects may develop with time. It is less satisfactory for use in cats, where increased toxicity may occur. Primidone is also a potent inducer of liver microsomal enzymes.

Primidone has been used in the control of excitement in sows (1 g, twice daily) and to control convulsions in foals suffering from the neonatal maladjustment syndrome (25 mg/kg).

Dose

It is essential to start with low doses in dogs and cats and increase doses gradually every two or three days, until the required effect is produced or the maximum tolerated dose has been given. Monitoring plasma levels is the most reliable method of dose adjustment.

dog, cat   Initial dose 20 mg/kg/day, in 2 or 3 divided doses.
Dose is increased to up to 50 mg/kg/day.

Phenytoin sodium

Phenytoin (Fig. 5.8) produces its anti-epileptic effect by the depression of motor areas of the cortex. It has a number of different actions on neurotransmitters, ionic movements and membrane potentials, which may contribute to its anticonvulsant activity. Potentiation of the inhibitory effects of GABA is thought to be involved. Similar effects on ion conductance also occur in peripheral nerves and the heart and hence it has anti-arrhythmic properties.

Phenytoin is less effective as a general anticonvulsant compared to phenobarbitone, e.g. in the treatment of poisoning. Furthermore, the pharmacokinetics of phenytoin in the dog are such that the achievement of therapeutic plasma levels is difficult. It may be effective in combination with phenobarbitone or primidone, if these are not successful alone in the control of seizures.

Absorption of phenytoin from the intestine is slow and it is highly bound to plasma proteins. There is a considerable delay in the establishment of a steady-state concentration in the body. Several days of oral administration of phenytoin are required in dogs before control of convulsions occurs. The drug is metabolized in the liver. Feline deficiency of glucuronyl transferase leads to an extremely long duration of action in the cat and phenytoin is not recommended in this species.

Minor side-effects such as nausea can occur but usually subside with continued use. A number of allergic reactions have been reported in humans but are not well documented in the dog. The treatment for overdose is non-specific, supportive and symptomatic and includes the administration of oxygen and ventilatory support.

Dose

The optimal dose for each dog must be individually determined.

An initial dose of 10 mg/kg (in divided doses), gradually increased or decreased to maintain control of the epilepsy. Up to 100 mg/kg daily may be necessary for seizure control.

Diazepam

The anticonvulsant efficacy of diazepam in the dog may be limited by its irregular absorption from the gastrointestinal tract and its short half-life. It is used, however, in the management of status epilepticus in the dog and may also be useful for various epileptic seizures in cats.

Dose

Status epilepticus

dog, cat   10 mg boluses, administered i.v.
at 2–4-minute intervals. Up to 3–5 doses may be administered. If this is not effective, pentobarbitone, 3–15 mg/kg i.v. is recommended.

Sodium valproate

Sodium valproate inhibits the metabolism of GABA, but this may only happen at relatively high concentrations and may not be the most important factor in its anticonvulsant effect. It is widely used in the management of human epilepsy but has not yet been fully evaluated in dogs, and opinions of its place in veterinary medicine differ.

Medroxyprogesterone acetate

This potent progesterone (see page 308) has been recommended for the treatment of epilepsy in the dog, but there is little evidence for clinical efficacy.

CHAPTER 6

GENERAL ANAESTHETICS

General anaesthesia is the loss of sensation associated with a state of unconsciousness deliberately induced by drugs. Thus general anaesthetics allow the veterinarian to perform surgical procedures without the patient feeling pain and in the absence of interference from responses to pain. Furthermore, many of the general anaesthetics also improve operating conditions by their ability to produce muscle relaxation.

General anaesthetic agents have been in clinical use for more than 140 years. Until fairly recently, all of the drugs which were capable of inducing a state of anaesthesia were central nervous system depressants. Many of the newer agents, however, appear to have a different mechanism of anaesthetic action.

The basic pharmacological principle of the dose–response relationship applies to the depressant general anaesthetics. In this case, the degree of depression of the central nervous system is related to the concentration of the drug in that system. Low doses of central nervous depressant general anaesthetics induce sedation only, but as the dose is increased, sleep and then unconsciousness occur. Further increases in dose cause coma and death. The levels of anaesthesia are described as four stages.

Stage 1   Fear, struggling, analgesia, breath holding can occur.

Stage 2   Delirium. This response is thought to be due to the depression of inhibitory centres in the brain and includes struggling, increased muscle tone, defecation and urination.

Stages 1 and 2 constitute the induction phase and should be passed through as rapidly as possible.

Stage 3   Surgical anaesthesia.

Plane 1   Light   ⎫   Signs associated with these levels vary
Plane 2   Moderate ⎬   between species. For details, a specialist
Plane 3   Deep   ⎭   text should be consulted.
Plane 4   Failure of circulation and respiration, paralysis of the thoracic muscles.

Most veterinary surgery is conducted under light to moderate surgical anaesthesia.

Stage 4   Coma and death.

The general anaesthetic agents are administered either by inhalation or by injection (most commonly intravenous). Injected anaesthetics reach the central nervous system rapidly and the dose injected determines the magnitude of the response. Since the brain receives a large proportion of the cardiac output, and since the drugs which are used are highly lipid soluble, a high concentration of drug in the brain is rapidly achieved. Thus induction of anaesthesia with an agent which can be injected intravenously is more rapid than with inhalational anaesthetics. Stage I and II are effectively by-passed and excessive struggling and associated excitement are avoided. However, the disadvantages associated with this method of induction must also be considered. The anaesthetist has less control over the depth of anaesthesia produced with intravenous anaesthetics, although, in practice, experienced anaesthetists are unlikely to administer the drugs in overdose. The intravenous anaesthetics are not ideal drugs for prolonged surgical procedures; details of the problems associated with individual drugs can be found later in this chapter. In practice, therefore, most of the intravenous agents are used to ensure smooth induction, after which the animal is transferred to one of the inhalational anaesthetics.

The inhalational agents are gases or volatile liquids. As the patient inspires, the anaesthetic agent reaches the alveoli, then dissolves in the blood in the pulmonary vasculature and is transported to the brain (and other tissues). The partial pressure of the anaesthetic in the inhaled gas determines its partial pressure in the alveoli. The rate at which the gas leaves the alveoli and enters the circulation depends on the difference between the partial pressure of the anaesthetic in the alveoli and that in the blood.

Because the anaesthetics are more fat soluble than water soluble, a greater amount is dissolved in highly lipid tissue like the brain. The high rate of blood flow to the brain also ensures that a considerable portion of the total inhaled drug is delivered there. In the induction stages, absorption of the anaesthetic into the brain (and other tissues) continues until its partial pressure in the tissues is equal to its partial pressure in the inspired air. Thus, the depth of anaesthesia in the steady state will depend on the partial pressure of the gas in the inspired air. Blood flow through the lungs and to the brain will also affect the depth of anaesthesia, as will the efficiency of respiration.

With agents which are highly soluble in the blood, the alveolar partial pressure of the gas falls quickly with the rapid uptake into pulmonary blood. Since arterial blood and brain tensions equilibrate with alveolar tension, the more soluble drugs give slow induction but reach higher concentrations in the brain. Conversely, when a drug has a low tissue solubility, rapid induction is achieved as alveolar tension rises quickly and the drug is present in lower concentrations in the brain.

The rate of onset of anaesthesia may also be influenced by the phenomenon known as the 'concentration effect', whereby higher concentrations of anaesthetic in the inspired air result in a greater rate of increase of partial pressure in the alveoli. There is thus more rapid saturation of the brain and a faster onset of anaesthesia.

The concept of minimal alveolar anaesthetic concentration (MAC) was introduced in 1965 to enable the comparison of relative potencies of anaesthetics. The MAC is defined as the alveolar concentration of an anaesthetic that prevents muscular movement in response to a painful stimulus in 50 per cent of the test subjects. In animals, the stimulus is usually tail clamping. Because the dose–response relationships for anaesthetics are steep, increasing the dose to 1.1 or 1.5 times the MAC ensures satisfactory anaesthesia in most animals. Furthermore, the variability of MAC within a species is small and even between species is remarkably low.

When sufficient time for equilibration is allowed, the partial pressure in the brain is the same as that in blood, which in turn equals the alveolar partial pressure of the anaesthetic. This can be measured and fairly accurately expresses the anaesthetic state. With the MAC defined as 1.0, the state of anaesthesia can be expressed as the ratio of the alveolar concentration to the MAC.

The use of a mixture of inhalational anaesthetic gases is sometimes appropriate. One of the most common combinations is halothane, oxygen and nitrous oxide. When such mixtures are employed the 'second gas effect' influences the rate of uptake of the anaesthetic agent, e.g. the addition of nitrous oxide to a halothane–oxygen mixture. With this combination, there is a large gradient between the tension of nitrous oxide in the inspired gas and the arterial blood in the early stages of induction. Thus, large volumes of gas are taken up and this rapid removal of nitrous oxide increases the tension of the second gases, halothane and oxygen, and augments alveolar ventilation. The higher tension of the second gas results in a steeper tension gradient and a facilitated passage into the blood.

At the termination of the procedure, no further anaesthetic is added to the inspired air. The concentration gradient then causes the diffusion of drug from the blood to the alveolar air, in which it is exhaled. In this way, the blood is cleared and drug in the tissues diffuses into the blood and will eventually be exhaled. Drugs which are very soluble will be present in higher amounts in tissue stores and thus will take longer to be eliminated from the body. Thus the fastest recovery times occur with the most insoluble drugs. The animal begins to recover consciousness when the brain level of anaesthetic falls, although there may still be considerable quantities of drug in the body. A variable amount of the anaesthetic agents (particularly those which are more soluble) may be metabolized. As the animal recovers consciousness, it ascends the stages of anaesthesia in reverse order.

Mechanism of action of general anaesthetics

Most of the current theories of the mechanism of action of the general anaesthetics are based on the original observations by Overton and Myer in the early years of the 20th century of the close relationship between the lipid solubility of the anaesthetics and their potency. This consistent finding has led to the suggestion that the site of action of the general anaesthetics is in the lipid matrix of membranes or in the hydrophobic areas of membrane-bound proteins. The anaesthetics, acting at these sites, are believed to interfere with normal ionic fluxes across membranes and thus influence their excitability. Thus, unlike most of the other drugs in current use, there are no specific receptor sites for general anaesthetics.

Inhalational anaesthetic agents

Halothane

Halothane (Fig. 6.1) is a colourless, volatile liquid at room temperature. It is decomposed by light and hence it is stored in amber bottles, stabilized

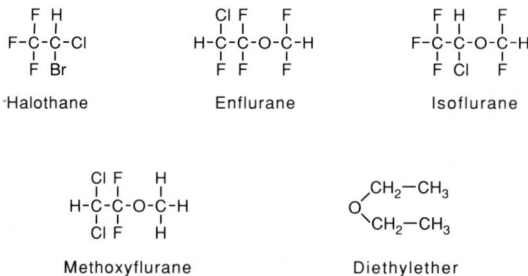

Figure 6.1 Inhalational anaesthetic agents.

by the addition of 0.01 per cent thymol. At clinical concentrations, it is non-explosive, non-flammable and does not react with soda lime.

Halothane is fairly soluble in blood (Table 6.1) and arterial concentrations equilibrate more quickly than with ether, but more slowly than with nitrous oxide. It produces only moderate muscle relaxation, which is usually adequate for the majority of surgical procedures in animals. Halothane is not irritant to respiratory mucosa and it reduces the formation of secretions. However, respiratory depression occurs and hence respiration should be carefully monitored during halothane anaesthesia. It also elicits dose-dependent hypotension, both by ganglion blockade and by direct depression of the myocardium. Since the dose of halothane can be reduced when it is administered with nitrous oxide, hypotension and depression of respiration are correspondingly reduced. In the presence of halothane, cardiac muscle is sensitized to the arrhythmogenic effects of β-adrenoceptor agonists.

Table 6.1 Properties of inhalational anaesthetics

Drug	Boiling point (°C)	Blood/gas partition coeff.	MAC (species) (% v/v)	
Halothane	50.2	2.3	0.9	dog
			1.19	cat
			0.9	horse
Enflurane	56.5	1.78	2.2	dog
			2.37	cat
			2.1	horse
Isoflurane	48.5	1.4	1.5	dog
			1.61	cat
			1.31	horse
Methoxyflurane	104.8	12.0	0.23	dog
Diethyl ether	34.6	12.1	3.04	dog
Trichloroethylene	86.7	9.15	0.6	rat
Nitrous oxide	−88.5	0.47	188.0	dog
Cyclopropane	−32.8	0.46	17.5	dog

Metabolism of up to 20 per cent of a dose of halothane occurs in the liver and in some species it induces liver enzymes. It can produce massive hepatic necrosis in humans but this condition does not appear to be documented in animals. In some species halothane relaxes the uterus and this may lead to postpartum haemorrhage. Furthermore, since halothane crosses the placenta, it may lead to depression of the foetus; its use in obstetric anaesthesia must be carefully considered.

The often fatal condition of malignant hyperpyrexia can be triggered during halothane anaesthesia, either in the presence or absence of suxamethonium. Although this is a relatively rare event, it is well documented in man and pigs and has been reported in a number of other species.

Halothane is probably one of the most widely used anaesthetic agents and can be used to induce and maintain anaesthesia in most species. It is administered by either semi-closed or closed circuit, vaporized with oxygen or oxygen and nitrous oxide. On economic grounds, its use in the larger species is limited to closed-circuit administration and under these circumstances care must be taken, in the use of nitrous oxide, to prevent hypoxia. Halothane should, due to its potency, be administered from an accurately calibrated and temperature-compensated vaporizer. On safety grounds and for ease of resuscitation, administration by endotracheal intubation is preferred to the use of face-masks.

Anaesthesia with halothane should not be deepened in an attempt to increase muscle relaxation because excessive cardiovascular depression can occur with increased doses. It is better practice to administer muscle relaxant drugs (see Chapter 7) and to note that halothane potentiates the actions of the non-depolarizing (competitive) relaxants.

Halothane increases oxygen consumption and this may lead to hypoxia during recovery when the animal is breathing air. The cardiac depressant effect of halothane limits its usefulness for patients with compromised cardiac function.

Dose

Induction	2–4 per cent in oxygen
Maintenance	0.5–2 per cent

Enflurane

Enflurane (Fig. 6.1) is a completely stable and colourless liquid at room temperature. It is non-explosive and non-flammable and does not react with soda lime. It is an extremely potent anaesthetic agent and, due to its relative insolubility, is rapid in onset and termination of effect. An accurately calibrated, temperature-compensated vaporizer is essential. The use of enflurane has been reported in a number of species. It produces good muscular relaxation and also potentiates the actions of the non-depolarizing muscle relaxants. It produces dose-dependent depression of respiration and also depresses the cardiovascular system and renal function. Reports have occurred of the production of convulsions under enflurane anaesthesia in dogs, particularly in the presence of hypocapnia. Potentiation of the arrhythmogenic effects of adrenaline may also occur, but to a lesser extent than with halothane.

Dose

Induction	2–4.5 per cent
Maintenance	0.5–3 per cent

Isoflurane

Isoflurane (Fig. 6.1) is a structural isomer of enflurane. The vapour pressure of isoflurane is similar to that of halothane and hence the vaporizers for these agents are interchangeable. This practice, however, is not to be recommended as it carries the risk of misidentification. Although it resembles enflurane in its physical properties, isoflurane is less soluble in blood and hence induction of and recovery from anaesthesia occur relatively rapidly. Furthermore, it does not have the convulsant properties of enflurane. Isoflurane is a marked respiratory depressant but, in clinical concentrations, it does not depress myocardial function and cardiac output is maintained. The potentiation of the effects of non-depolarizing muscle relaxants is greater with isoflurane than with most of the other inhalational anaesthetic agents. It appears to have little hepatic or renal toxicity, which may be due to the fact that only 0.2 per cent of the drug is metabolized in the liver.

Dose

Induction	2–4 per cent
Maintenance	1–2 per cent

Methoxyflurane

Methoxyflurane (Fig. 6.1) is a clear colourless liquid with a heavy, fruity odour. Prolonged exposure to light will produce a brown colour (due to oxidation of the antioxidant) which is of no significance. Under normal working conditions it is non-explosive and non-flammable. It does not react with soda lime and can be administered in a similar manner to most other volatile agents. It has a relatively high boiling point (105°C) and thus it is not possible to vaporize high concentrations under normal working conditions and this is responsible for the safety of the drug.

Although methoxyflurane is a potent anaesthetic, its high solubility means that induction and recovery from anaesthesia are relatively slow. It is best administered after adequate premedication and barbiturate induction. The slow recovery makes it an undesirable agent to use in large animals. Good analgesia accompanies anaesthesia with methoxyflurane and persists into the postoperative period. Muscle relaxation is also good, especially with deep anaesthesia. Methoxyflurane has similar actions to halothane on both circulatory and respiratory systems and may sensitize the myocardium to the arrhythmogenic effects of adrenaline.

The high fat solubility of methoxyflurane is associated with considerable drug retention and metabolism (up to 50 per cent). The fluoride ions liberated by its metabolism render the distal renal tubule unresponsive to antidiuretic hormone and are thought to be responsible for a high incidence of renal failure in some species. The metabolism of methoxyflurane is thought to vary between species, which may explain the variation in renal toxicity. It is not hepatotoxic.

Dose

Induction	not recommended due to the high solubility of methoxyflurane
Maintenance	0.25–1.5 per cent

Diethyl ether (ether)

Diethyl ether (Fig. 6.1) is a highly inflammable agent which also forms explosive mixtures with air, nitrous oxide and oxygen. It is decomposed by air, heat and light; hence it should be stored in an opaque, sealed container in a cool, dark place.

The high solubility of ether results in slow onset of action. The cardiovascular system is extremely stable during ether anaesthesia and it is not until deep planes are reached that depressive effects occur. Even at this stage, there is no sensitization of the heart to catecholamines. Respiration is stimulated during light ether anaesthesia but is progressively depressed as deeper planes are reached.

Ether is irritant to mucous membranes, increasing oral and respiratory secretions, and it can cause laryngeal spasm in cats and primates. An anticholinergic agent administered as part of the premedication will prevent the increase in secretions. Muscular relaxation is better under ether anaesthesia than with any other volatile agent and thus it is not usually necessary to use muscle relaxants. The effects of non-depolarizing agents are potentiated by ether. Blood sugar rises during ether anaesthesia and renal and hepatic function is depressed. These return to normal within 24 hours.

Because of its low potency, the use of ether is limited to small domestic animals. In these patients it is one of the least toxic and one of the safest anaesthetic agents available. Administration with either oxygen or nitrous oxide and oxygen in a semi-closed circuit is the technique of choice.

Nitrous oxide

Nitrous oxide is a colourless gas which is heavier than air. It is neither flammable nor explosive but will support combustion. It is a powerful

147

analgesic but a weak anaesthetic. It is used mainly as an adjunct to potentiate other agents such as ether and halothane, and rarely as a sole agent in animals. Because of its low potency it must be administered in high concentrations which produce high partial pressures. In practice it should be delivered with oxygen and the oxygen percentage should never be less than 30. Rapid saturation of the tissues occurs because the drug is poorly soluble. Cardiac and respiratory depression are not clinical problems with nitrous oxide. It does not induce any significant muscle relaxation.

At the end of the surgical procedure, when the nitrous oxide is removed from the inhaled air, the insoluble nitrous oxide rapidly leaves the tissues and enters the lungs. Nitrous oxide may form 10 per cent or more of the volume of the expired gas, and partial pressure of oxygen in the lungs may be lowered to a dangerous level by the outward diffusion of nitrous oxide into the alveoli. This diffusion hypoxia is of particular significance in elderly animals or those with compromised respiratory or cardiovascular function. The risk of diffusion hypoxia is reduced by the administration of higher concentrations of oxygen for at least 10 minutes before the patient is allowed to breathe air.

Nitrous oxide will diffuse into any gas-filled cavity in the body and the cavity will expand. Hence it should be used with caution in ruminants, where abdominal and intestinal distension occur, or when a condition such as pneumothorax is present.

Cyclopropane

Cyclopropane is a colourless gas with a pungent odour. It is highly flammable and is explosive in air or oxygen. These properties and its cost limit its use to closed circuits.

Induction of and recovery from anaesthesia with cyclopropane are rapid because of its low solubility. Significant muscle relaxation accompanies anaesthesia. Cyclopropane is a powerful respiratory depressant. In contrast to nitrous oxide, high concentrations of oxygen can be used with cyclopropane. Blood pressure tends to be maintained during cyclopropane anaesthesia until deep levels of anaesthesia are reached. This may be due, in some measure, to the drug's respiratory depressant effect and the retention of carbon dioxide.

When the administration of cyclopropane is terminated, the rapid decrease in carbon dioxide tension in the blood may lead to 'cyclopropane shock'. A fall in circulating catecholamines may contribute to this. Cardiac arrhythmias are common under cyclopropane anaesthesia. It has little effect on hepatic or renal function.

In view of its cost, its inflammable and explosive properties and possible complications, the use of cyclopropane is relatively limited but it still has its advocates for general anaesthesia in ruminants.

Dose

Induction	20–25 per cent
Maintenance	10–20 per cent

Injectable anaesthetic agents

Intravenous administration of injectable anaesthetic agents ensures rapid induction of anaesthesia. Delivery of anaesthetic quantities of the drug to the brain occurs with extreme rapidity due to the combined effects of the high rate of blood flow to the brain and the high lipid solubility of the drugs, which facilitates their passage across the blood–brain barrier with ease. It should be noted that the doses shown for the agents below apply to healthy animals in a good nutritional state. These doses must be adjusted for animals that are very young, aged, debilitated or in a poor nutritional state. Similar care should be taken with animals with electrolyte or acid–base imbalance and those which are diseased, particularly with renal or hepatic involvement. Details of appropriate premedication are given in Chapter 5.

Thiopentone (thiopental) sodium

Thiopentone is a derivative of barbituric acid (a description of the general pharmacology of the barbiturates can be found on page 120). The sodium salt is soluble in water. It is supplied with anhydrous sodium carbonate to prevent the formation and precipitation of free acid on exposure to carbon dioxide. A 5 per cent solution has a pH of 10.8; hence it is extremely irritant and extreme care is essential to ensure that it is not injected extravascularly. Intra-arterial injection can lead to spasm of the artery and gangrene of the area supplied by that vessel. Thiopentone is more lipid soluble than other barbiturates and thus enters the CNS more rapidly. High lipid solubility and high blood flow to the brain combine to ensure rapid onset of action. Following intravenous injection of an anaesthetic dose, consciousness is lost within 30 seconds and general anaesthesia lasts for 5–10 minutes in most species, although full recovery will take much longer. The short duration of anaesthesia is due to the rapid fall of the brain concentration of the drug and distribution into tissues which are less vascular than the brain. In the early stages, most of the drug is transported to muscle. Initially, relatively little drug enters the body fat but some 30 minutes after administration the concentration in adipose tissue begins to rise.

The metabolism of thiopentone occurs at only 10–15 per cent per hour in most species. Metabolism is by side-chain oxidation, mainly by the microsomal enzymes of the liver but also to a small extent in the kidneys and in muscle. The metabolites are excreted by the kidneys and alimentary tract.

Poor muscular relaxation and poor analgesia accompany thiopentone anaesthesia. It depresses the myocardium and cardiac output decreases as plasma concentrations rise. Blood pressure may fall transiently after rapid intravenous injection of thiopentone. This is due to high concentrations of the drug acting on the vasomotor centre. Cardiac arrhythmias are not directly produced by thiopentone but may occur where there is a rise in carbon dioxide tension or hypoxia associated with anaesthesia.

The respiratory system is depressed by thiopentone and short periods of apnoea are common. This is most likely immediately after the rapid injection of thiopentone and is due to the presence of a high concentration in the brain. Reduced sensitivity to CO_2 and direct depression of the brainstem respiratory centres are responsible for the depression of respiration. In the event of cessation of respiration, artificial ventilation must be instituted and maintained until the animal is able to breathe without assistance. Respiratory depression occurs at plasma concentrations lower than those required for cardiac depression. Unless a very considerable overdose has been administered, depression of the cardiovascular system is unlikely to cause clinical problems in healthy animals. The drug produces an increased tendency to laryngospasm in some species and bronchospasm may also be seen.

If large doses or incremental doses of thiopentone are administered, saturation of tissue stores may occur. Under these circumstances the drug remains in brain and blood at relatively high levels and termination of anaesthesia depends on metabolism of the drug. Since this is slow, anaesthesia is prolonged. Prolonged (and occasionally fatal) effects may also occur in hypovolaemia, where the redistribution of drug from brain to other tissues is particularly slow.

Thiopentone crosses the placental barrier and depresses foetal respiration. The neonatal liver is incapable of metabolizing the drug and prolonged respiratory depression may endanger life.

Thiopentone is used as an induction agent in a large number of species. This is achieved by the relatively rapid administration of a single dose of the drug by the 'bolus injection' method. Premedication with one of the phenothiazine tranquillizers such as acepromazine and/or pethidine is recommended in most species. This practice reduces the dose of thiopentone required, produces a co-operative patient for intravenous injection and ensures a quiet recovery. (In order to reduce the risk of regurgitation and decrease the recovery time premedication of ruminants is not often advocated.)

Dose

horse	10 mg/kg or 1 g/90 kg following premedication with acepromazine (0.05–0.1 mg/kg).
	5.5 mg/kg or 1 g/180 kg following premedication with (a) xylazine 1.1 mg/kg i.v. or (b) chloral hydrate up to 100 mg/kg i.v. or (c) guaicol glycerol ether (up to 100 mg/kg) followed by acepromazine (0.05–0.1 mg/kg).
cattle	10 mg/kg or 1 g/90 kg unpremedicated.
sheep and goat	7.5–20 mg/kg i.v.
pig	5–10 mg/kg following premedication.

Note: Care must be exercised with barbiturate dosage in the pig as the response can be variable.

dog and cat	A 2.5 per cent solution is normally used but 1.25 per cent solution may be used in cats and small dogs. A dose of 25 mg/kg is computed and drawn up into a syringe. 7.5–12.5 mg/kg rapid i.v., following premedication with either a tranquillizer and/or an analgesic drug. Increments of a further 2.5 mg/kg can be given to effect.

Note: Thiopentone is rarely used in sight hounds such as the greyhound because recovery may be delayed.

Thiamylal sodium

Thiamylal (Fig. 6.2) is similar in chemical structure to thiopentone. It is 1.25 to 1.5 times more potent than thiopentone and is less likely to be accumulated after large or incremental doses. It has been suggested that thiamylal produces more salivation than thiopentone in both the dog and cat, so that premedication with atropine or glycopyrronium is essential. It is used extensively in the USA but rarely in Europe. Where it is available, it is usually much more expensive than the equivalent dose of thiopentone. It is used in a similar manner to thiopentone; the dose is reduced because of its potency.

Dose

dog and cat	18–23 mg/kg i.v.
pig	18 mg/kg by slow i.v. injection

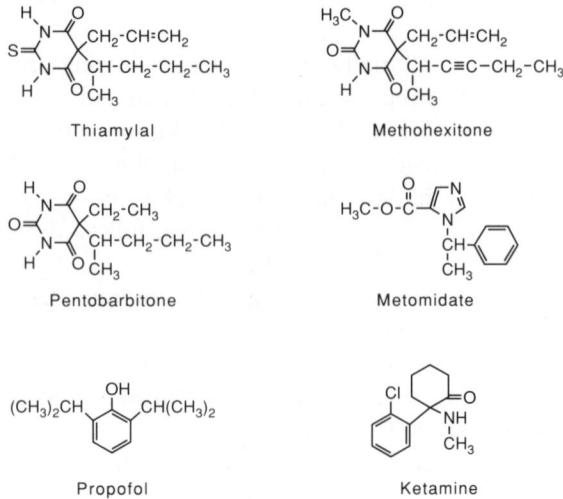

Figure 6.2 Injectable anaesthetic agents.

Methohexitone (methohexital) sodium

Methohexitone (Fig.6.2) is approximately 2.5 times more potent than thiopentone. Recovery of consciousness is more rapid than after thiopentone administration because methohexitone is more rapidly metabolized. It is less irritant to the tissues than thiopentone if accidental extravascular injection occurs.

It is not anticonvulsant, and muscle tremors and even convulsions can occur during induction and recovery from methohexitone anaesthesia. These can be reduced by the judicious use of premedication, rapid intravenous injection and by allowing the animals to recover in quiet and darkened surroundings. Because recovery from methohexitone is more rapid than that from thiopentone, it is a more suitable agent for use in sight hounds.

Dose

dog and cat up to 10 mg/kg after premedication. Half of the dose is injected initially and the rest to effect.

horse 5.5 mg/kg (1 g/180 kg) i.v. after premedication with acepromazine (0.05–0.1 mg/kg).

12.75 mg/kg (1 g/360 kg) after premedication with (a) xylazine 1.1 mg/kg or (b) chloral hydrate up to 100 mg/kg or (c) acepromazine (0.05–0.1 mg/kg) and guaicol glycerol ether up to 100 mg/kg.

cattle   The response is unpredictable but a total dose of
                          up to 2.5 g may be given to adult cattle by slow i.v.
                          injection.
calves   1 mg/kg
sheep and goat   4 mg/kg. A lower dose is recommended if
                          premedication is used.
pig   10–12 mg/kg following premedication.

Pentobarbitone (pentobarbital) sodium

Pentobarbitone (Fig. 6.2) is classified as a medium-acting barbiturate. As
with all members of this group, pentobarbitone depresses respiration and the
cardiovascular system in direct relation to dosage. It is metabolized in the
liver, oxidation is one of the most common mechanisms, and the metabolites
are excreted by the kidneys.

Administration of pentobarbitone is best achieved by slow intravenous
injection of small incremental doses, with adequate time between each dose
and proper assessment of its effect after each dose. Its onset of action is
relatively slow (up to 30 minutes to reach full effect) and Stage I and II of
anaesthesia are more obvious. The recovery period from general anaesthesia
can be as long as 24 hours and adequate supportive therapy, in the form of
heat and fluids, is essential during this time. Excitement during recovery may
be a problem and should be minimized by the maintenance of quiet, warm,
darkened surroundings and adequate premedication.

Although the extensive use of pentobarbitone in routine veterinary anaesthesia
has now been superseded by a number of superior drugs and techniques, it
still has some important applications. It is probably the most widely used
anaesthetic agent in laboratory animals where prolonged, stable anaesthesia
can be achieved without the need for expensive anaesthetic equipment. In
animals which cannot be restrained for intravenous injection, pentobarbitone,
which can be administered by intraperitoneal injection, may be used. It
is also used to control convulsions produced by such agents as strychnine
and, administered in overdose, it is the main drug used for euthanasia in
cats and dogs. In these cases, rapid injection of the drug ensures a high
concentration reaches the brain and produces fatal respiratory and cardiac
depression. Pentobarbitone is a useful drug for the induction of anaesthesia in
sheep and goats. It has a shorter duration of action in these species, probably
due to a more rapid metabolism.

Dose

cat, dog and laboratory animals   up to 30 mg/kg i.v.
     Note: as for thiopentone, excess anaesthetic should be drawn into

syringe, half the computed dose injected relatively rapidly and the remainder 'to effect'. Euthanasia can be achieved by the rapid administration of 70 mg/kg i.v.

pig	up to 30 mg/kg i.v. by intratesticular injection for castration.
sheep and goat	30 mg/kg i.v. for induction in unpremedicated animals.

Metomidate hydrochloride

Metomidate is an imidazole derivative (Fig. 6.2) which was initially introduced for use in pigs but has also been used in birds and horses. The white powder is soluble in water; once dissolved, the solution should be stored in the refrigerator. Metomidate produces good muscle relaxation but has no analgesic properties. It has very little depressant action on the cardiovascular system. It tends to reduce respiratory rate but this is offset by an increase in tidal volume. In pigs, metomidate is usually administered after azaperone premedication.

Dose

pig	under 45 kg	10 mg/kg i.o.	} after azaperone
	over 45 kg	4 mg/kg i.v.	} 2 mg/kg i.m.
birds	10–15 mg/kg i.m.		

Propofol

Propofol (Fig. 6.2) is virtually insoluble in water at room temperature. It is available as a free-flowing oil in water emulsion which contains 10 mg/ml of the active drug. It has anaesthetic properties similar to those of thiopentone in that it is a rapidly acting agent which produces anaesthesia of relatively short duration and is without excitatory side-effects. Its use is compatible with that of all the commonly used premedicants, inhalational anaesthetics and neuromuscular blocking agents. Anaesthesia has been maintained in a number of species by the use of intermittent injection and by infusion of propofol. Cardiovascular and respiratory depression are similar to that seen after thiopentone and Saffan (see page 156). It appears to have little effect on general metabolism, gastrointestinal or renal function.

Dose

dog	premedicated	4 mg/kg i.v. for induction
		0.4 mg/kg/min for maintenance
	unpremedicated	6 mg/kg i.v. for induction.

cat   premedicated   6 mg/kg i.v. for induction.
           unpremedicated 8 mg/kg i.v. for induction.

Dissociative anaesthesia

Dissociative anaesthesia is a state of sedation, catatonia, amnesia and marked analgesia. The name describes the feeling of dissociation from the environment which follows the administration of such anaesthetic agents to humans. Ketamine was the first of these to be used clinically.

Ketamine

The most striking difference between ketamine (Fig. 6.2) and the older injectable anaesthetics is that it can be administered by intramuscular, intravenous or subcutaneous routes and can even be sprayed into the mouth of fractious small animals for oral administration. It produces a state of dissociative anaesthesia and a loss of consciousness with intense analgesia. It is metabolized in the liver and excreted by the kidneys.

Ketamine has a wide margin of safety. Pharyngeal and laryngeal reflexes are normal or only slightly depressed during ketamine anaesthesia. There is little depression of either cardiac or respiratory function. A rise in blood pressure and a slight rise in heart rate may occur, but cardiac output remains unchanged. The respiratory rate may be slightly stimulated but tidal volume may be decreased. In some species, notably the domestic cat, apneustic respiration has been observed. Muscular relaxation is poor and increased muscle rigidity is seen in some species. The problems of muscle rigidity and apneustic respiration can be overcome with suitable premedication. Xylazine appears to be the premedicant of choice in cats, ruminants and horses. In dogs and pigs, acepromazine, diazepam and xylazine have been used. Ketamine stimulates salivation, but this effect can be overcome by the use of anticholinergic premedication.

Ketamine has been used in a wide variety of non-domesticated animals. It is the drug of choice in primates, with the possible exception of squirrel monkeys and marmosets, and has been widely used in zoo species, reptiles and birds.

Dose

The lower doses are useful for short, relatively painless procedures while the higher doses allow more painful surgical operations to be performed.
cat   11–33 mg/kg i.m., i.v. or s.c.
                       22 mg/kg i.m. after premedication with

	xylazine (1.1 mg/kg i.m.) and atropine (0.04 mg/kg i.m.).
horse and donkey	2.2 mg/kg i.v. after premedication with xylazine (1.1 mg/kg i.v.).
pig	2–5 mg/kg i.v. or 12–15 mg/kg i.m. after premedication with xylazine (1.1 mg/kg).
calf, sheep and goat	10 mg/kg i.m. after premedication with xylazine (0.2 mg/kg i.m.) and atropine (0.2 mg/kg i.m.).
non-human primates	10–25 mg/kg i.m.
birds	small species 50 mg/kg i.m. large species 20–40 mg/kg i.m.
snakes and reptiles	up to 50 mg/kg i.m.

Tiletamine hydrochloride

Tiletamine is a dissociative anaesthetic which is more potent than ketamine. It is administered by intravenous or intramuscular injection, although the latter route appears to cause pain. When administered alone, tiletamine produces analgesia and cataleptoid anaesthesia which may be accompanied by convulsive seizures and clonic muscular reactions in some animals, particularly in cats. When the drug is combined with the diazepam analogue, zolazepam (as Telazol), the convulsive and muscular effects may be reduced and better muscle relaxation may be achieved. Salivation is a regular feature of this drug combination and can be controlled by an anticholinergic agent. In dogs tiletamine induces a persistent tachycardia and in cats it produces slight hypotension. Respiratory rate increases and tidal volume is reduced after administration of tiletamine.

Dose

dog	2–13 mg/kg Telazol
cat	2–15 mg/kg Telazol

Steroid anaesthesia

Saffan

Saffan is a combined preparation of the steroids alphaxalone and alphadolone, in the ratio 3 : 1. Alphaxalone is virtually insoluble in water and is dissolved in Cremophor EL. Alphadolone increases the solubility of alphaxalone in Cremophor EL. Saffan has a rapid onset of action, and redistribution and metabolism ensure a short duration of action. The drug can be administered by intravenous or intramuscular injection.

Anaesthesia with the steroid combination is associated with good muscle relaxation. Dose-dependent respiratory depression occurs. Saffan produces hypotension, which is not dose-related, and is accompanied by tachycardia. It should not be used in dogs, because the solubilizing agent causes release of histamine in this species. Use in combination with barbiturates is also contraindicated. Oedema and hyperaemia of the paws occurs in a varying percentage of cats which receive Saffan and the incidence appears to have a regional distribution.

Dose

cat	9 mg/kg i.v. lasts about 10 min. Anaesthesia may be maintained by the administration of supplementary doses or by inhalational agents.
	9–18 mg/kg by deep i.m. into the quadriceps mass. Higher doses may be used for more major procedures.
non-human primates	6–9 mg/kg i.v. for induction
	12 mg/kg i.m. for sedation
	12–18 mg/kg i.m. for anaesthesia

CHAPTER 7

SKELETAL MUSCLE RELAXANTS

Drugs which interfere with skeletal neuromuscular transmission can be divided into two distinct groups. The first, and by far the most important clinically, are the neuromuscular blocking agents, which have a peripheral action and are used to produce blockade during surgery under general anaesthesia. The effects of these peripherally acting drugs have been known for a number of centuries. Early in the 16th century stories of the use of the arrow poison 'ourari' began to reach Europe from South America. It was, however, not until the 1840s that Claude Bernard conducted his classic experiments on the pharmacology of curare. Some 100 years later the drug was introduced into medical anaesthetic practice. Drugs in this group have no effect on the central nervous system; their main effect is to interfere with neuromuscular transmission at the end-plate.

Drugs in the second group are used to reduce spasticity or as adjuncts to the induction of general anaesthesia and are referred to as 'centrally acting muscle relaxants'. However, as one of the members of this group, dantrolene, has no central effects, it may be something of a misnomer.

Neuromuscular blocking agents with peripheral actions

The mechanism of neuromuscular transmission at the skeletal neuromuscular junction is similar to that at autonomic neuroeffector junctions. When the nerve terminal is depolarized, an influx of Ca^{2+} triggers the exocytotic release of acetylcholine. The transmitter diffuses across the synaptic cleft to the nicotinic cholinergic receptors on the motor end-plate. The transmitter–receptor interaction is extremely brief; acetylcholine is bound to its receptors for an average of approximately 2 msec. The interaction increases the permeability of the membrane in the end-plate region to small cations, mainly to Na^+ and K^+ and to a lesser extent to Ca^{2+}. Because the extracellular concentration of Na^+ is greater than that inside the cell, Na^+ moves into the cell and the postsynaptic membrane is depolarized. This change in voltage is the end-plate potential.

The quantity of acetylcholine released from the nerve terminal determines the magnitude of the end-plate potential. If the release is sufficiently large for the end-plate potential to reach the threshold for excitation, depolarization of the muscle membrane occurs and the impulse is propagated along the muscle fibre. Excitation-contraction coupling follows and the muscle contracts. Acetylcholine is readily hydrolysed as it dissociates from the receptor sites. Acetylcholinesterase, bound to the basement membrane of the nerve terminal, is responsible for the rapid inactivation of transmitter and consequent brief duration of action.

Peripheral neuromuscular blocking drugs may exert their action in one of two ways. Competitive antagonists at the nicotinic receptor site, like tubocurarine, prevent acetylcholine reaching the receptor sites and thus induce paralysis. Transmission at nicotinic receptor sites can also be blocked by excessive amounts of depolarizing agonists, like suxamethonium. These drugs induce a period of sustained depolarization of the muscle membrane during which the muscle does not respond to further depolarizing stimuli.

The use of muscle relaxants enables lighter levels of anaesthesia to be employed, with adequate relaxation of the abdominal and thoracic muscles, including the diaphragm. This is important during intermittent positive-pressure ventilation, which is mandatory when these drugs are employed in an anaesthetic regime. They also produce relaxation of laryngeal muscles and are used, in some species, to facilitate endotracheal intubation. In animals which have received a muscle relaxant, respiration should always be controlled until the drug has been metabolized, excreted or antagonized. In view of the humane considerations, drugs of this type should never be administered to animals which are likely to be conscious.

Non-depolarizing muscle relaxants

These are also known as competitive muscle relaxants. Tubocurarine is the prototype and the group includes a number of newer, synthetic drugs such as alcuronium, atracurium, gallamine, pancuronium and vecuronium. These drugs have no effect on the release of acetylcholine but rather produce neuromuscular blockade by direct competition with acetylcholine at the receptor sites at the neuromuscular junction. In addition to the competitive antagonist action, some of the response to higher doses of the drugs in this group may be due to blockade of ion channels in the end-plate.

Paralysis of skeletal muscle rapidly follows the intravenous administration of the competitive muscle relaxants. The small, rapidly moving muscles, like those in the face, eyes and digits are the first to respond. The larger muscles of the trunk, neck and limbs are paralysed next. The diaphragm is the last muscle to be affected. As the patient recovers, muscle tone is regained in the reverse order.

All of the competitive neuromuscular blocking agents used in current clinical practice are quaternary ammonium compounds and bear considerable structural similarities to acetylcholine (Fig. 7.1). The high degree of ionization of drugs in this class inhibits their passage across membranes. Despite their charge, there is no practical problem with absorption since the drugs are administered by intravenous injection to the anaesthetized patient.

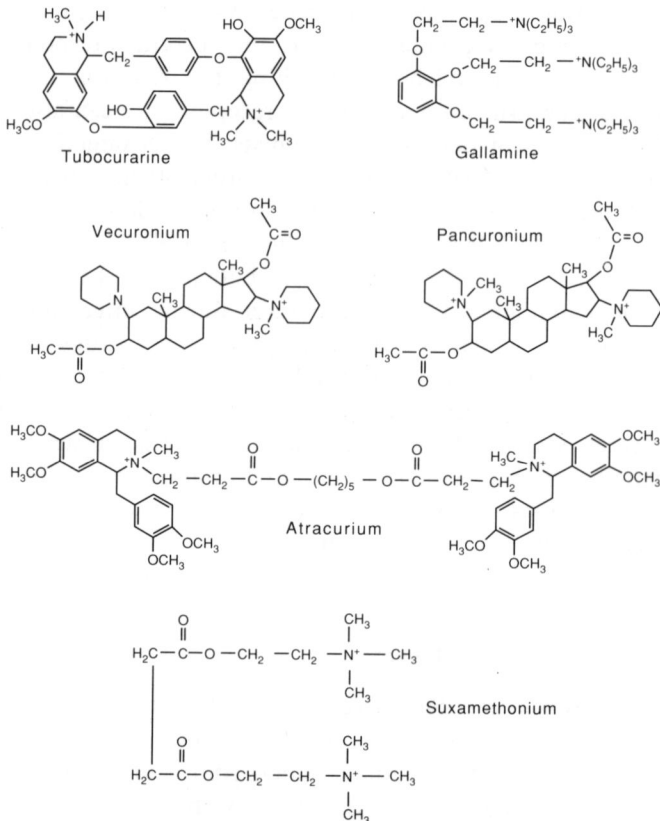

Figure 7.1 Neuromuscular blocking agents with peripheral actions.

Inhalational anaesthetic agents potentiate the neuromuscular blockade produced by the non-depolarizing drugs in a dose-dependent manner. This interaction depends on a number of factors, including the stabilizing action of the anaesthetic on the post-junctional membrane, depression of the central nervous system and changes in blood flow to muscle which increase the proportion of the drug reaching the neuromuscular junction. With regard to potentiation of neuromuscular blockade, the potency of different anaesthetics varies. Isoflurane and enflurane are the most potent, followed by halothane and lastly nitrous oxide.

A number of antibiotics enhance the neuromuscular blockade produced by the non-depolarizing relaxants. Aminoglycoside antibiotics seem to produce the greatest effect, by a combination of reduced acetylcholine release and stabilization of the post-junctional membrane. The actions of both depolarizing and non-depolarizing blockers are also potentiated by local anaesthetics which, if given in sufficiently high doses, can induce neuromuscular blockade themselves. Furthermore, calcium channel antagonists and some other anti-arrhythmic drugs enhance non-depolarizing neuromuscular blocking agents.

Although the use of non-depolarizing muscle relaxants should, in general, be avoided in animals with muscle disease, they have been used, in reduced dosage, in dogs suffering from myasthenia gravis, with adequate monitoring of neuromuscular transmission. They may also be used occasionally to facilitate long-term pulmonary ventilation during intensive therapy. However, in this situation, adequate monitoring of neuromuscular transmission is essential.

Tubocurarine

This agent is regarded historically as the typical non-depolarizing muscle relaxant and is the standard by which the others are compared. The most troublesome side-effect of tubocurarine is hypotension, which is due in part to ganglion blockade and also to the release of histamine from mast cells. Loss of skeletal muscle tone and the consequent reduction in venous return exacerbates the hypotensive effect. The release of histamine is particularly evident in cats and dogs and totally precludes its use in these species. With the availability of newer drugs with few side-effects, it is now rarely used in anaesthesia in other species.

Tubocurarine is not metabolized to any significant extent in animals. About 50 per cent of an injected dose is excreted unchanged in the urine. The exact fate of the remainder is unknown, but biliary excretion is thought to be significant. The relatively short duration of action, about 30 minutes, is probably due to redistribution of the drug. Its use should be avoided in animals with hepatic or renal disease.

Dose (by intravenous injection)

The currently available preparation contains 10 mg/ml.

Species	Initial dose mg/kg	Duration of action minutes	Dosage increments mg/kg
horse	0.3	60	0.05
cattle	0.06	30	0.01
sheep	0.04	30	0.01
pig	0.4	30	0.08

Cat and dog contraindicated, although doses of up to 0.4 mg/kg have been used to produce relaxation for about 30 minutes.

Gallamine triethiodide

This was the first synthetic non-depolarizing muscle relaxant. It induces considerably less release of histamine than tubocurarine. Its vagal blocking action results in increased heart rate and thus use of gallamine should be avoided in situations where tachycardia is considered to be dangerous. The drug is not metabolized and is excreted totally unchanged in the urine. Hence it should not be administered to animals suffering from renal disease. Furthermore, where renal clearance rates are low, the duration of action of gallamine is considerably prolonged.

Dose (by intravenous injection)

Species	Initial dose mg/kg	Duration of action minutes	Dosage increments mg/kg
horse	1	20–25	0.2
cattle	0.5	30–40	0.1
calf	0.4	up to 240	
sheep and lamb	0.4	>120	
pig	1	30	0.2
dog	1	30	0.2
cat	1	15–20	0.2

Alcuronium chloride

Alcuronium chloride is a synthetic derivative of the alkaloid toxiferine, which is obtained from calabash curare. It is a non-depolarizing muscle relaxant of relatively long duration. It does not have any significant histamine-liberating or ganglion-blocking effects in domestic animals. It should not be used in animals with renal disease as it is excreted mainly via the kidney.

Dose (by intravenous injection)

Species	Initial dose mg/kg	Duration of action minutes	Dosage increments mg/kg
horse	0.05	60	0.01
dog	0.1	70	0.02

Pancuronium bromide

This is an amino steroid which is free from hormonal activity. It causes a moderate increase in heart rate and a slight rise in cardiac output. It has little effect on systemic vascular resistance. It is metabolized to some extent in the liver but the major route of excretion is via the kidney. Hence it should be used with extreme caution, or avoided in the presence of hepatic or renal disease.

Dose (by intravenous injection)

Species	Initial dose mg/kg	Duration of action minutes	Dosage increments mg/kg
horse	0.06	40	0.01
cattle	0.04	40	0.008
sheep and goat	0.025	45	0.005
pig	0.1	30	0.02
dog	0.06	30	0.01

Atracurium besylate

This agent induces less histamine release than tubocurarine, but more than most of the other synthetic non-depolarizing muscle relaxants. It has a unique method of metabolism which involves the Hoffmann elimination reaction. Although stable when stored at acid pH, it undergoes spontaneous degeneration in plasma which results in the breakdown of the quaternary group. The drug is also metabolized by ester hydrolysis which is independent of hepatic and renal mechanisms. Hence atracurium is the relaxant of choice in the presence of liver or kidney disease. The major metabolites of atracurium do not have muscle relaxant activity. However, one of them, laudanosine, is only slowly metabolised by the liver and blood levels may rise with prolonged administration of the parent compound. Alkaline solutions, including thiopentone, inactivate atracurium. Hence normal saline should be used as a diluent.

Dose (by intravenous injection)

Species	Initial dose mg/kg	Duration of action minutes	Dosage increments mg/kg*
horse	0.15	30	0.06
sheep	0.5	30	0.2
dog and cat	0.5	40	0.2

*at approx. 20 min intervals

Vecuronium bromide

Vecuronium bromide is a steroid muscle relaxant with a structure very similar to that of pancuronium. It has a medium duration of action. It does not release histamine or influence autonomic ganglia and has no adverse effects on the cardiovascular system. About 15 per cent of the drug is eliminated by the kidney, the rest is probably eliminated into the bile, either as unmetabolized drug or as the 3-hydroxy metabolite of vecuronium. Thus, although not totally contraindicated, its use in patients with renal or hepatic disease should be carefully assessed.

Dose (by intravenous injection)

Species	Initial dose mg/kg	Duration of action minutes	Dosage increments mg/kg
horse	0.1	30	0.02
sheep	0.04	15	0.01
dog and cat	0.1	25	0.02

Depolarizing muscle relaxants

Suxamethonium (succinylcholine) chloride (Fig. 7.1) is the only commonly available and clinically used drug in this group. It consists of two acetylcholine molecules, linked by their acetyl groups. It acts by mimicking the action of acetylcholine at the skeletal neuromuscular junction. Because disengagement from the receptor site is slower than that for acetylcholine, the depolarization persists and the membrane is unresponsive to further impulses. This is termed depolarization or phase I blockade. Since the excitation-contraction coupling necessary to maintain muscle tension requires repolarization and repetitive firing, a flaccid paralysis is produced. Rapid, complete and predictable paralysis follows intravenous injection and recovery is spontaneous as the drug diffuses away from the motor end-plate and is metabolized in the plasma. Paralysis is usually preceded by muscle fasciculation, associated with the initial depolarization, and there may be a transient rise in plasma potassium.

The drug is metabolized by pseudocholinesterase. Prolonged muscle paralysis has occurred in human patients with atypical plasma pseudocholinesterase but this condition does not appear to have been described in animals. However, care is necessary in animals which have received organophosphorus-containing compounds up to 1 month before administration of suxamethonium. These compounds, present in flea collars, some eye drops and anthelmintics, inhibit cholinesterase and thus prolong the duration of action of suxamethonium.

Prolonged paralysis may also occur in dual (or phase II) blockade, which occurs on continued exposure to the drug, after at least three doses. It is associated with the development of a neuromuscular blockade with characteristics of non-depolarizing blockade, following the primary, depolarizing one. In these cases, artificial ventilation should be continued until muscle function is restored. Dual blockade can be diagnosed with a suitable nerve stimulator and/or by administration of a small dose of a short-acting anticholinesterase such as edrophonium. If there is an improvement, i.e. reversal of the non-depolarizing blockade, a full dose of edrophonium or neostigmine may be administered.

The rapid onset and relatively short duration of action make the drug a useful agent for endotracheal intubation. This aspect of its use is of particular importance in pigs, non-human primates and cats. Repeated injections may be given for longer procedures and it is occasionally administered by infusion. Suxamethonium is contraindicated in severe liver disease. The clinical applications of suxamethonium are limited because, unlike the non-depolarizing muscle relaxants (see below), its action cannot be reversed.

Dose (by intravenous injection)

Species	Dose mg/kg	Duration of action minutes
horse	0.1	up to 5
cattle and sheep	0.02	6–8
pig	2	2–3
dog	0.3	25
cat	1.5	5
non-human primates	1	up to 5

Reversal of skeletal muscle relaxation

Since the non-depolarizing muscle relaxants exert their effects, at least in part, by competitive inhibition of acetylcholine at nicotinic receptors at the neuromuscular junction, increasing the local concentration of acetylcholine diminishes the extent of the muscle relaxation. Thus the effects of these drugs are reversed by administration of anticholinesterases. Increases in the local concentration of acetylcholine enhance the effect of depolarizing muscle relaxants and thus the duration of action of suxamethonium can be increased by up to 100 per cent by the administration of anticholinesterases.

Before the administration of any anticholinesterase to reverse neuromuscular blockade, an antimuscarinic drug such as atropine or glycopyrronium should be injected. This is necessary to prevent excessive salivation, bradycardia and other muscarinic responses to accumulated acetylcholine. If the initial dose of anticholinesterase does not produce adequate reversal of the neuromuscular blockade and a repeat dose is required, then the dose of atropine or glycopyrronium should also be repeated.

Dose

atropine
    small animals   30–100 μg/kg s.c.
    large animals   20–60 μg/kg s.c.
                           (see also page 54)

glycopyrronium
    all species   0.1 mg/kg

Edrophonium has a relatively short duration of action and is used mainly to diagnose the presence of dual blockade produced by repeated doses of suxamethonium. Neostigmine is the specific drug for the reversal of non-depolarizing neuromuscular blockade. It acts within 2 minutes of injection and has a duration of action of at least 30 minutes. It is also used in the reversal of dual blockade produced by repeated doses of suxamethonium.

Doses

All i.v., following pretreatment with atropine or glycopyrronium.

edrophonium
    Reversal of neuromuscular blockade   0.5–1.0 mg/kg
        repeat after 5 minutes if reversal is inadequate
    Diagnosis of dual blockade   0.5 mg/kg.

neostigmine methylsulphate
    large animals   0.05 mg/kg
    small animals   0.1 mg/kg
        repeat after 5 minutes if reversal is inadequate.

Centrally acting muscle relaxants

Mephenesin inhibits polysynaptic excitation of motor neurones in the spinal cord and thereby induces muscular paralysis, without loss of consciousness. Originally developed in 1943, its use in anaesthesia has now been abandoned.

Guaiacol glycerol ether (GGE) is a mephenesin-like compound which inhibits polysynaptic spinal reflexes and is currently used as an adjunct to the induction of anaesthesia in horses and cattle. It is also commonly used as a decongestant and antitussive. The drug has little effect on respiration but there may be an increase in rate of ventilation accompanied by a decrease in tidal volume. It produces a moderate degree of hypotension in healthy animals. Solutions of drug at concentrations greater than 15 per cent may produce haemolysis. GGE is excreted in the urine following hepatic conversion to a glucuronide.

In practice, a 10 per cent solution (in water or 5 per cent dextrose) is administered to effect, i.e. the animal becomes ataxic. At this stage, a bolus dose of thiopentone or other intravenous anaesthetic agent can be administered to produce recumbency. The dose of thiopentone recommended (1 g/180 kg) is half the normal dose. In some centres the barbiturate (2–3 g) is mixed with the GGE prior to administration.

Dose

horse and cattle   75–110 mg/kg i.v.

Spasmolytic drugs

Spasticity is associated with hyperexcitability of tonic stretch reflexes, exaggerated tendon jerks and flexor muscle spasms. These signs may be accompanied by muscle weakness. Phenobarbitone and mephenesin have been used in the treatment of spasticity in the past but they lack specific spasmolytic action and any benefit was probably related to general sedation.

Baclofen is a chlorophenyl derivative of GABA (Fig. 7.2). It is an orally effective agonist at GABA receptors and as such may exert its effect by the presynaptic inhibition of the release of excitatory transmitters. Baclofen has been used in the treatment of spasticity in humans but there is little information available on its use in animals.

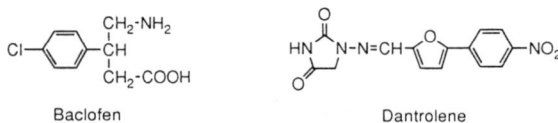

Baclofen   Dantrolene

Figure 7.2 Spasmolytic drugs.

Dantrolene (Fig. 7.2), unlike diazepam and baclofen, exerts its spasmolytic effect by a direct action on the excitation-contraction coupling in skeletal muscle. The relaxant effect is associated with inhibition of the release of calcium from the sarcoplasmic reticulum. Neuromuscular transmission is not affected. Dantrolene has been used specifically in the treatment of malignant hyperthermia. This relatively rare reaction to anaesthetic agents, such as halothane, in combination with neuromuscular blocking agents, such as suxamethonium, has been described in a number of species.

Dose
by i.v. injection

horse	up to 2 mg/kg
pig	up to 5 mg/kg
dog	up to 2 mg/kg

CHAPTER 8

PAIN AND INFLAMMATION

Introduction

The presence of pain in animals is, by necessity, inferred from their reactions. This is in distinct contrast to the situation in humans, who are capable of describing and even anticipating pain. It is, however, a reasonable assumption that pain will exist in animals where it would normally be experienced in humans.

It is well known that surgery involving the eye and its surrounding structures can be distressing to animals. They will often attempt to rub and scratch the area if adequate pain relief is not provided. This is particularly important in view of the relatively intricate nature of some ophthalmic surgery, as major damage can be done by the patient, particularly during the anaesthetic recovery period. Surgery of the ear region is especially painful and, in the absence of adequate analgesia, animals will often shake their heads. This may well initiate a vicious cycle of pain and discomfort, accompanied by repeated head shaking. The trauma associated with orthopaedic surgery of the limbs in all species is extremely painful and therefore adequate postoperative analgesia is essential for these patients. The behaviour of the majority of small animals with conditions requiring spinal surgery suggests these are most painful, and hence analgesia is necessary in both pre- and postoperative periods.

Thoracic surgery, carried out mainly in cats and dogs, does not appear to be extremely painful in animals, provided a lateral approach is adopted. Individual animals may exhibit severe pain, particularly in the immediate postoperative period and more so when chest drains, which are poorly tolerated by most animals, are utilized. Analgesic drugs may be administered with sedative agents if required. Intra-abdominal manipulations in most species of domestic animal appear to be relatively pain free. This is typified by surgery in the ruminant, which is carried out in the standing animal, under local or regional anaesthesia. However, surgery involving the upper abdomen and the perianal area, including the rectum, is known to be painful and hence adequate analgesia is essential.

In order to establish the presence and the extent of pain in animals it is necessary to use one's clinical experience and judgement to interpret the animal's reactions. The common signs of pain in animals are mainly related to the autonomic nervous system and include such features as changes in the diameter of the pupils, alterations in pulse and respiratory rates, panting, sweating and piloerection and vomiting. Other signs of pain include audible and visual indicators such as moaning and other abnormal noises, and changes in posture. There may also be interference with the normal function of organs or systems, such as lameness and unwillingness or inability to eat, defecate or urinate.

Physiology of pain

Perception of pain involves the initial physiological perception of the painful stimulus, known as nociception, which is followed by the conscious or emotional reaction to the pain. Tissue damage *per se* or substances released by damaged tissue are thought to stimulate nociceptive nerve endings, widely distributed throughout the body. The endogenous compounds which may be released include prostaglandins, histamine, 5-hydroxytryptamine, kinins and enzymes (see below). The receptors are non-encapsulated endings of unmyelinated or small, myelinated A fibres which run to the spinal cord via the dorsal root. They synapse in the substantia gelatinosa in the dorsal horn and impulses are transmitted to the ascending lateral spinothalamic tract. The tract forms synapses with thalamic nuclei which then project to the cerebral cortex. The major transmitter of pain impulses in the spinal cord is substance P. The conscious experience of pain involves a complex interaction of cerebral pathways, and relatively little information regarding the nature of this process in domestic animals is available.

The inflammatory process

Inflammation is the body's response to insult or injury. Provided the injury is not sufficient to destroy the structure and vitality of the tissue, the reaction consists of a succession of events which are designed to prevent further injury by localizing and destroying the harmful agent. The stimulus to inflammation may be a living organism or its toxin, a chemical (either introduced or endogenous) or physical trauma. The classic features of inflammation are pain, swelling, redness, heat and loss of function.

Alteration of blood flow to the affected area occurs early in the inflammatory response. Release of vasoactive substances from mast cells increases local blood flow and is responsible for the observed redness. An increase in vascular permeability follows the contraction of capillary endothelial cells. Fluid and proteins escape from the circulation and this inflammatory exudate causes swelling and pain, due to pressure on nerve endings. The exudate also helps to dilute any noxious substances present. Leucocytes move into the area of inflammation and release enzymes, oxygen radicals and mediators to deal with the inflammatory stimulus. Release of kinins and eicosanoids (see below) potentiates the nociceptive response. Phagocytes eventually remove the debris associated with the inflammatory reaction, then repair and regeneration begin.

Mediators of inflammation

Eicosanoids are substances which are derived from a 20-carbon eicosa-tetraenoic acid, arachidonic acid, which is a component of the phospholipids of cell membranes. The eicosanoids are not stored in the body but are synthesized when required. In the case of inflammation, the inflammatory stimulus activates the enzyme phospholipase A_2, which results in the release of arachidonic acid. Two different pathways of arachidonic acid metabolism are possible (see Fig. 8.1). One of the pathways may predominate, depending on the cell involved.

The cyclooxygenase pathway
Conversion of arachidonic acid to the unstable cyclic hydroxy endoperoxide, prostaglandin G_2 (PGG_2), is catalysed by the enzyme cyclooxygenase. (Prostaglandins are described by a letter, which indicates the functional groups attached to the cyclopentane ring, and a number, which indicates the degree of saturation of the aliphatic side-chains.) PGG_2 is converted, by the action of a peroxidase, to PGH_2. A variety of different enzymes catalyse the metabolism of PGH_2 to prostaglandins, prostacyclin or thromboxanes (see Fig. 8.1). As with most endogenously produced active substances, the prostaglandins are rapidly metabolized and excreted. Prostacyclin (PGI_2) is produced mainly by vascular endothelial and smooth muscle cells. It spontaneously hydrolyses to an inactive derivative (half-life approx. 3 minutes). Thromboxane A_2 (TXA_2), released from aggregating platelets, also spontaneously breaks down to the inactive TXB_2.

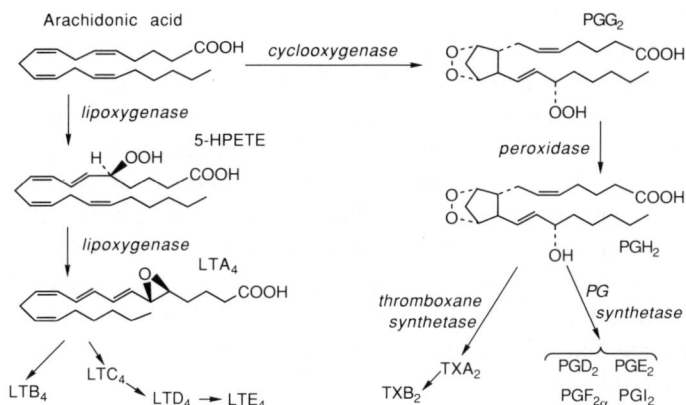

Figure 8.1 Arachidonic acid may be metabolized by the cyclooxygenase or lipoxygenase pathways. The action of cyclooxygenase results in the formation of PGG_2, which is converted, by a peroxidase, to the intermediate PGH_2. Depending on the cell type and the presence of particular enzymes, PGH_2 is then converted to other prostaglandins or to thromboxane A_2. The lipoxygenase pathway results in the formation of the leukotrienes LTA_4–LTE_4, via 5-HPETE.

Eicosanoids bind to cell surface receptors and are capable of eliciting reactions in a wide variety of tissues. These actions are thought to be of major significance in the response to noxious stimuli:

1. Cardiovascular system: PGE_2 and PGI_2 are vasodilators and are responsible for the redness observed in inflammation. $PGF_{2\alpha}$ and TXA_2 are vasoconstrictors. Platelet aggregation is induced by TXA_2 and inhibited by PGI_2.
2. Gastrointestinal tract: muscle in the gastrointestinal tract is contracted by PGI_2 and $PGF_{2\alpha}$. Prostaglandins are associated with the production of gastric and intestinal mucus and stimulate turnover and repair of gastrointestinal epithelial cells.
3. Respiratory tract: the response may be species specific but, in general, PGE_1, PGE_2 and PGI_2 are bronchodilators, while $PGF_{2\alpha}$ and TXA_2 are bronchoconstrictors.
4. Reproduction: prostaglandins play an important role in female reproductive physiology and may also be important for fertility in males.
5. Fever: PGE_1 and PGE_2 increase body temperature, and fever is thought to be mediated by the local release of prostaglandins from the hypothalamus.
6. Inflammation: PGE_2 and PGI_2 have a number of actions which are consistent with the inflammatory response. They induce vasodilation, increased capillary permeability and hyperalgesia. They also enhance the nociceptive response to bradykinin and histamine.

The lipoxygenase pathway

Activation of lipoxygenase in pulmonary tissue, platelets and leucocytes results in the conversion of arachidonic acid to 5-hydroxyperoxyeicosatetraenoic acid (5-HPETE). 5-HPETE is the precursor of leukotriene A (LTA_4), which is then metabolized to LTB_4 or, by a series of reactions, to LTC_4, LTD_4 and LTE_4 (see Fig. 8.1). Less is known about the products of the lipoxygenase pathway than about the prostaglandins and thromboxanes, but they also appear to be important in allergic and inflammatory reactions. LTB_4 is a potent chemo-attractant for neutrophils. It increases leucocyte adherence, degranulation and free radical formation. LTC_4, LTD_4 and LTE_4 all induce bronchoconstriction, mucus secretion and increase microvascular permeability and plasma exudation.

Treatment of pain

The removal or reduction in intensity of the existing cause is an extremely important aspect of the treatment of pain, where this is applicable. This includes the removal of penetrating foreign bodies, the immobilization of a fracture or the reduction of the inflammatory reaction.

The perception of pain can be modified in a number of ways which do not involve the administration of drugs. One of these is the stimulation of local circuits in the spinal cord. This inhibits or reduces transmission of impulses up the main pathways and is typified by the reduction of the pain response from a particular area by gentle rubbing. Higher centres in the brain can also influence pain perception. Activation of the descending inhibitory pathways from the midbrain inhibits ascending transmission of nociceptive stimuli. Cortical activity can also influence the perception of pain. One of the mechanisms which may be involved here is the local release of endogenous opioids.

There are several sites of action of drugs which are used in the management of pain. Local anaesthetics block conduction in nerve fibres and thereby prevent the perception of pain. Inhibition of the transmission of pain impulses at various levels in the central nervous system is responsible for the analgesic effects of most drugs used to alleviate severe pain. Drugs which interfere with the production of the local mediators of nociception are most commonly used to treat inflammation and mild to moderate pain.

The purpose of the inflammatory reaction is to prevent further injury and, most commonly, successful healing follows the acute reaction. In some circumstances, however, the reaction may be inappropriate to the healing process or may be of such intensity that further tissue damage is likely. In these cases treatment with anti-inflammatory drugs is indicated. Drugs used in the treatment of inflammation may act by inhibition of the release of mediators of the inflammatory process or by alteration of the response of cells to an inflammatory stimulus.

Local anaesthetics

Drugs which are used to produce a reversible blockade of conduction of the nerve impulse are called local anaesthetics. In general, susceptibility of nerves to the effect of local anaesthetics varies with size. Smaller nerves are more readily affected, which may explain the variation in the effect of the drugs on different senses. Pain sensation is abolished first, followed by cold, heat, touch and finally deep pressure.

The action of local anaesthetics is due to interference with the movement of Na^+ across the cell membrane (Fig. 8.2). These agents appear to bind to receptor sites on sodium channels and so prevent the changes in Na^+ permeability associated with membrane depolarization. Thus conduction in nerves is blocked. The drugs are weak bases and may exist as cations or in the uncharged form. They are able to penetrate cell membranes in the uncharged state and thus to enter nerve cells. It is the cationic form which is thought to be the active form at the receptor site.

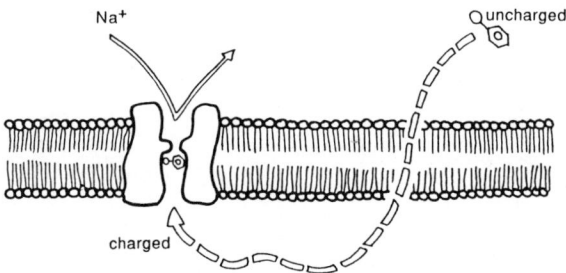

Figure 8.2 Local anaesthetics penetrate cell membranes in the uncharged state. Once in the cationic form, they exert their effects by interfering with the movement of Na^+ across the cell membrane.

If it is considered desirable to prolong the duration of action of a local anaesthetic agent, a vasoconstrictor may be added. This also confers the advantage of reducing the rate of systemic absorption of the local anaesthetic thus reducing the chance of systemic toxicity. Vasoconstriction may be achieved by addition of adrenaline in concentrations which vary from 1 in 50 000 to 1 in 500 000. When local anaesthetics are to be used in the presence of inhalational general anaesthetic agents (e.g. halothane) which sensitize the heart to the action of adrenaline, then local anaesthetic solutions with adrenaline added are best avoided in favour of the plain solution. Felypressin, a synthetic analogue of vasopressin, may also be added to local anaesthetics to produce vasoconstriction.

Toxic effects of local anaesthetics may occur if absorption from the site of injection is rapid and sufficient plasma levels are reached. The chances of this occurring depend on the rate of absorption of the drug and the rate of its metabolism in the liver. Since the rate of absorption from a subcutaneous site is slow, drugs administered by such injections are unlikely to cause toxic effects. Aspiration, to ensure that the needle used to administer local anaesthetics is not in a vein, will avoid toxicity associated with accidental intravenous injection. Signs of toxicity are due to stimulation of the central nervous system, causing restlessness, which may proceed to convulsions. The convulsions are best controlled by the induction of general anaesthesia with a barbiturate such as pentobarbitone or by intravenous diazepam. The convulsions often proceed to depression of the central nervous system and, occasionally, to cardiac failure. This situation is treated by ventilation with an oxygen-enriched atmosphere and such measures for cardiac resuscitation as are considered appropriate.

A large number of compounds may be used to produce local anaesthesia in veterinary medicine. In practice, however, only a few of these are in regular use and only these drugs will be described. Their formulae are shown in Fig. 8.3.

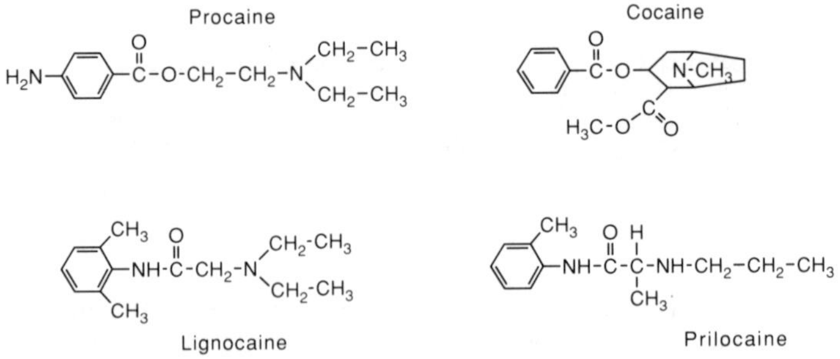

Figure 8.3   Local anaesthetics.

Cocaine

Cocaine is the oldest known local anaesthetic. It is an alkaloid, found in the leaves of a South American shrub, *Erythroxylon coca*. It was widely used as a local anaesthetic for ophthalmic applications and as a central nervous system stimulant. The central effects of cocaine led to its abuse and the drug is now controlled (in the UK) by the Misuse of Drugs Act. Furthermore, although effective in the eye, the inhibition of the blink reflex removes the eye's natural defence mechanism and damage from the undetected presence of foreign bodies may result. It has also been found that repeated application of cocaine to the eye may cause corneal ulceration. Cocaine is toxic when administered parenterally. For these reasons it has largely been superseded by less toxic synthetic compounds.

Procaine

Procaine was the first synthetic compound to replace cocaine and is still in common use. It is a vasodilator and is rapidly absorbed following parenteral injection. Therefore it is best used in combination with a vasoconstrictor. It is ineffective when applied to mucous membranes. It is rapidly metabolized in both liver and plasma. Solutions of up to 4 per cent may be used for local infiltration analgesia and 1–2.5 per cent solutions for epidural analgesia.

Lignocaine

Lignocaine (lidocaine) is one of the most widely used local anaesthetic agents. It is more potent and has a more rapid onset and a longer duration of action than procaine. Lignocaine produces surface anaesthesia when applied to mucous membranes. It is rapidly metabolized in the liver. Solutions of 1 per cent may be used for local infiltration and solutions up to 2 per cent for regional analgesia. Drowsiness and sedation are the first signs of systemic absorption of significant quantities of lignocaine.

Prilocaine

Prilocaine has a similar structure to lignocaine (Fig. 8.3) but has a longer onset and duration of local anaesthetic effect. Like lignocaine, it may induce drowsiness, although its central effects are generally less marked than those of lignocaine. Ortho-toluidine, which can cause methaemoglobinaemia (especially in the cat), is formed as a metabolite of prilocaine.

Proparacaine

Proparacaine is a local anaesthetic solution which is recommended solely for ophthalmic use. It produces very little irritation in the eye when the recommended 0.5 per cent solution is used. It does not produce pupillary dilation.

Techniques for inducing local anaesthesia

A number of techniques are employed for the production of local anaesthesia.

Surface anaesthesia

A 2 per cent solution of lignocaine in a water-miscible viscous base is effective on application to the mucous membranes of the mouth, pharynx, glans penis, vulva and urethra. For procedures in the nose and pharynx, a spray of 10 per cent lignocaine may be used. This preparation is also satisfactory for spraying the vocal cords of cats, pigs and primates to facilitate endotracheal intubation. Aqueous solutions of local anaesthetics do not penetrate the intact dermis.

Surface anaesthesia may also be used for the relief of pain in joints and synovial sheaths. Intra-articular injection of local anaesthetics has been used in the diagnosis of lameness. The majority of joints and tendon sheaths can be injected but an accurate knowledge of the anatomy is essential.

Infiltration anaesthesia

In order to anaesthetize an area of skin for incision it is necessary to inject intradermally in the first instance. The nerve endings are anaesthetized by their direct exposure to the drug. The onset of analgesia is rapid and then subcutaneous injections can be commenced. Reinsertion of the needle for further infiltration, if a long incision is necessary, is carried out through an already insensitive area. Lignocaine, at a concentration of 0.5 per cent, is probably the drug of choice due to its superior spreading powers.

A ring block may be used to anaesthetize a digit or teat. Here it is essential to avoid the use of vasoconstrictors as they may produce ischaemic necrosis of the structure.

A field block may also be used in veterinary anaesthesia to desensitize an area for incision. The technique involves enclosure of the whole of the area within walls of anaesthesia. A variation of this technique has been employed in the flank of cattle as an L-block.

Regional anaesthesia

This technique involves the injection of the local anaesthetic in close proximity to a nerve trunk which then blocks conduction in the sensory nerves to the area which it innervates. Thus no local anaesthetic solution is present at the site of surgery. A large number of techniques are employed to elicit regional anaesthesia in veterinary practice and their discussion is beyond the scope of this book.

Intravenous regional anaesthesia

Using this technique, an intravenous injection of a local anaesthetic is administered into a limb, following the application of a tourniquet proximal to the site of injection. Analgesia persists as long as the tourniquet is in position and sensation returns within a few minutes of the removal of the tourniquet. Basal sedation may or may not be employed. In practice, an injection of 1 per cent plain lignocaine is made into a convenient superficial vein; the total dose should not exceed 5 mg/kg. The technique is limited to the limbs and has been used successfully in cattle, dogs and some other species.

Analgesia of fractures

Local anaesthetic solution can be injected into the haematoma at the site of fracture in order to reduce the pain associated with that fracture. Plain lignocaine (0.5 per cent) is used; up to 5 ml may be injected in small animals and up to 25 ml in large animals.

Opioid analgesics

Although the effects of opioid analgesics have been known for many hundreds of years, the concept of opioid receptors only became widely accepted in the 1960s. During the following years, endogenous ligands for these receptors were identified. It has now been shown that three groups of peptides possessing morphine-like activity occur naturally in the brain—the enkephalins, the endorphins and the dynorphins. Each group of peptides is derived from a genetically distinct precursor polypeptide.

The availability of selective agonists and antagonists at opioid receptors led to the proposal that separate subclasses of opioid receptors exist at different sites. There is evidence to indicate that the various actions of opioid agonists result from interactions with one or more of the receptor subclasses. Thus, both μ and κ receptors are associated with analgesia, dysphoria is mediated via interaction with σ receptors and changes in affective behaviour are due to effects on δ receptors. Results from experimental studies to date indicate that each of the three classes of endogenous opioid peptides binds with some degree of selectivity to one or two of the subclasses of opioid receptor. Thus, enkephalins have selective activity at δ receptors, dynorphins at κ receptors and β-endorphin is equally potent at δ and μ receptors.

The effects of the endogenous opioid peptides are widespread throughout the body. They may influence temperature, respiration, endocrine secretion, the function of the gastrointestinal tract, pain perception and general behaviour. For example, β-endorphin is a potent, long-lasting analgesic when injected into the cerebrospinal fluid. It is likely that the release of endogenous opioids under conditions of severe stress or pain is important in the natural reactions to such circumstances. It is probable that these compounds produce their effects by modulation of the release of other transmitters. In particular, the analgesic response may be due to inhibition of the release of transmitters (such as substance P) from terminals of nerves relaying nociceptive stimuli. In addition to the alteration of the sensation of pain, the opioids act at other centres in the central nervous system and modify the emotional reaction to pain.

The opioid analgesics are those derived from the opium poppy and the related synthetic analgesic substances which act via opioid receptors. The structures of some of those used in veterinary medicine are shown in Fig. 8.4. They are usually used for cases of severe pain. They have selective depressant and excitatory actions on the central nervous system. Amongst the depressant actions are analgesia, sedation, respiratory depression, cough suppression and constipation. The excitatory effects include convulsions, release of antidiuretic hormone and vomiting.

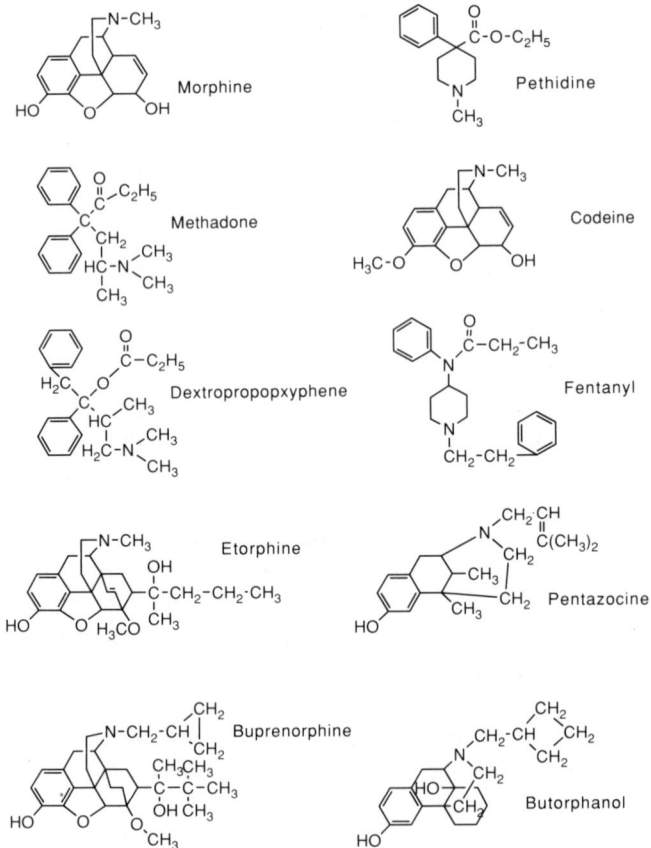

Figure 8.4 Opioid analgesics.

Some of the opioid analgesics are partial agonists; one of the most important of these is pentazocine. If pentazocine is given alone it produces typical agonist effects. If it is given after a pure agonist (e.g. morphine) its antagonistic activity will be apparent. Naloxone, a pure opioid antagonist, competitively antagonizes the actions of a pure agonist such as morphine or the endogenous opioids.

Opioids are drugs of addiction and as such are subject to strict controls according (in the UK) to the Misuse of Drugs Act.

Morphine

Morphine is the principal alkaloid found in opium and is the most powerful naturally occurring analgesic drug. It is an agonist at both μ and κ opioid receptors. Amongst the domestic animals it is used mainly in dogs, where it is said to have the most reliable action. In this species, analgesia is accompanied by sedation. Larger doses may induce sleep or even coma. Considerable debate surrounds its use in the cat. In the past, the recommended dose produced profound excitement, and was probably too large. The use of low doses avoids this problem and effective analgesia is achieved. The action of morphine is considered to be unreliable in horses, cattle and pigs, although there is not a great deal of information available on its effects in these species.

As morphine is rapidly absorbed from the gut it can be given by the oral route, although it is normally administered by injection. The peak analgesic effect is observed about 20 minutes after intravenous injection and at about 90 minutes after intramuscular injection.

The major disadvantage associated with the use of morphine is its respiratory depressant effect. This is the main reason that it is not widely used for anaesthetic premedication in animals. Extreme care should be taken in the administration of morphine to animals showing any degree of respiratory depression. Vomiting, which results from stimulation of the chemoreceptor trigger zone by morphine, is not often a problem in sick animals. Similarly, although the gastrointestinal effects of morphine cause constipation in humans, this is not usually a significant problem in dogs and cats. Tolerance to the action of morphine is quickly acquired.

The main use of morphine is in the treatment of pain, either in the postoperative period or following road traffic accidents. However, it should not be administered in cases of head injury as it has been shown to produce a rise in intracranial pressure.

Pethidine (meperidine)

Pethidine has about one-tenth the potency of morphine and there is little species variation in response to its depressant action. Its spectrum of actions indicates that it may be a relatively good agonist at κ receptors. Vomiting is rarely seen after the administration of pethidine and it does not cause excitement in cats or horses. Pethidine is relatively rapidly metabolized in most species of domestic animal and hence the dose may have to be repeated at intervals of 1–2 hours. In equianalgesic doses, the respiratory depressant effect of pethidine is comparable to that of morphine. It is probably more widely used in veterinary anaesthesia than is morphine, but the indications for its use are similar.

Methadone

Methadone is a synthetic analgesic which provides good analgesia but does tend to cause respiratory depression. Methadone is less sedative than morphine. It is widely used in the mainland of Europe, but is not commonly used in the British Isles.

Codeine

Codeine occurs naturally in the opium poppy. It is similar to morphine in its actions, but has only a quarter the potency. Respiratory depression is also very much less than that with morphine and it does not induce vomiting. It may, however, produce constipation. Codeine is particularly useful in combination with aspirin or paracetamol in the treatment of less severe pain. Although it is an alkaloid of opium, most preparations containing codeine are included in schedule 5 of the Misuse of Drugs Regulations in the UK and are thus largely exempt from restrictions under the Act.

Dextropropoxyphene

This is not a very potent analgesic but is useful in that it does not produce constipation and has only a very slight respiratory depressant effect. It is available in combination with paracetamol and this preparation is probably one of the most suitable oral analgesics for use in small animals.

Fentanyl

Fentanyl is primarily a μ agonist and is one of the most potent synthetic opioid analgesic drugs. It is said to be about 500 times more potent than pethidine and it is normally used in conjunction with a butyrophenone tranquillizer (e.g. droperidol) to produce the state of neuroleptanalgesia in dogs, primates and some laboratory animals (see page 135). Fentanyl reduces sensitivity to pain but causes respiratory depression in some species. This can be reversed with nalorphine, but the analgesic effect will also be reduced. The administration of fentanyl produces defecation in most dogs within a few minutes, but unlike morphine it does not elicit vomiting in this species. It often produces a bradycardia, which can be counteracted by the administration of atropine, without affecting the analgesic response. High doses of fentanyl have a profound and deleterious effect on renal function in dogs. Administration is by intramuscular or intravenous injection.

Etorphine

Etorphine is also a synthetic, potent analgesic agent with about 1000 times the strength of morphine. It is only available commercially in neuroleptanalgesic combinations (see page 134); with acepromazine for large animals and with methotrimeprazine for small animals. It is not suitable for use in cats. The analgesic part of the combination can be reversed by the specific antagonist diprenorphine. In view of its extreme potency, etorphine needs to be handled extremely carefully—a number of human fatalities have occurred following accidental and deliberate administration of the drug combination. Its potency does, however, make it extremely useful for the immobilization and capture of wild animals, using small volumes of drug which can be administered with a blow pipe, dart gun or other device.

Pentazocine

Pentazocine was developed during attempts to produce an opioid antagonist but was found to be a partial agonist at κ receptors. It is classified (in the UK) as a schedule 3 controlled drug by the Misuse of Drugs Regulations. The potency of pentazocine is approximately one-third that of morphine. The side-effects of vomiting, constipation and respiratory depression are also comparatively reduced. Pentazocine does not produce excitement in any species and there is also no evidence that it causes the dysphoric effect in animals that may occur in humans. High doses in horses tend to produce ataxia and muscle tremors. It has mainly been used in dogs and horses.

Buprenorphine

This agent is also a synthetic analgesic with partial agonist activity at μ receptors. Many aspects of its action are similar to those of pentazocine. Although its abuse potential was formerly considered to be low, it was recently classified as a schedule 3 controlled drug, with a special requirement for it to be kept in a locked receptacle. Respiratory depression is reduced and vomiting and gastrointestinal effects do not occur to any significant extent. Unlike pentazocine, it is about 30 times more potent than morphine.

Butorphanol

Butorphanol is a partial agonist at μ receptors as well as being a κ receptor agonist. As the administered dose is increased, the effect of the drug reaches a plateau and it has been suggested the response may be reduced if the dose is increased further. Butorphanol produces marked sedation and is commonly used in combination with detomidine as a sedative/analgesic in the horse. It is also an effective antitussive in dogs, where it has an elimination half-life of 1.5 hours and a duration of action of about 4 hours. Absorption is very rapid after either intramuscular or subcutaneous administration.

Clinical uses of opioid analgesics

Opioid analgesics are used in situations of severe or acute pain. Their major disadvantage is depression of respiration, and they should not be administered to animals with pre-existing respiratory depression. They are the drugs of choice for the management of pain associated with road accidents and other traumatic injuries and also for pre- and postoperative analgesia. The analgesic response to pethidine and methadone is similar to that with morphine but the hypnotic effect of morphine may be a useful side-effect in many of these cases. Pethidine may be more useful in cases of acute abdominal pain, where its spasmolytic action could provide additional relief.

Opioid antagonists

The only pure opioid antagonist available is naloxone (Fig. 8.5). Two other drugs generally referred to as opioid antagonists are nalorphine (Fig. 8.5) and levallorphan; however, both are partial agonists. Thus they are ineffective in reversing moderate respiratory depression and they do not reverse pentazocine-induced respiratory depression.

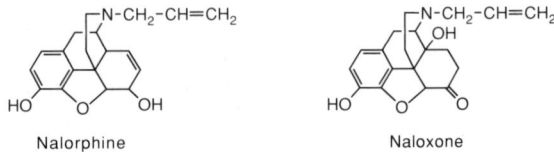

Figure 8.5 Opioid antagonists.

Naloxone

Naloxone is a derivative of oxymorphone and, as a pure opioid antagonist, will reduce or prevent both the analgesic effects of opioids and their side-effects. It is the drug of choice for the reversal of opioid-induced respiratory depression, but has not been widely used in veterinary medicine. A dose of 0.4^{-1} mg/kg is recommended for the reversal of etorphine. The duration of action of a single dose of naloxone is short, both in humans and dogs. Further doses are often required at 15-minute intervals, or an infusion can be used.

Nalorphine

This is an opioid antagonist with marked analgesic activity. It reverses both the analgesic and respiratory depressant effects of opioid analgesics. The degree of antagonism is dose dependent. It does not reverse the respiratory depression produced by the barbiturates or other general anaesthetic agents. It has been specifically recommended for use in dogs for the reversal of morphine and related compounds. A dose of 2.2 mg/kg s.c. is recommended for dogs.

Doses

morphine
cattle and horse	up to 60 mg i.m.
pig	up to 20 mg i.m.
dog	0.2 mg/kg i.m., i.v. or s.c.
cat	0.1 mg/kg s.c. or i.m.

pethidine
cattle and horse	up to 1 g i.m.
pig	up to 0.5 g i.m.
dog	up to 3.5 mg/kg i.m. or s.c.
cat	up to 5 mg/kg i.m. or s.c.

methadone
horse, dog	0.2 mg/kg i.m. or 0.1 mg/kg i.v.

codeine
dog	2 mg/kg p.o.
cat	1–2 mg/kg p.o.

dextropropoxyphene
dog	up to 32.5 mg p.o., t.i.d.
cat	32 mg/day p.o.

fentanyl
    dog   200–500 μg/kg i.v. or i.m.

pentazocine
    horse   0.33 mg/kg i.m. or slow i.v.
    dog   up to 3 mg/kg i.m., i.v. or s.c. every 3 hours
    cat   up to 3 mg/kg i.m., i.v. or s.c. every 3 hours

buprenorphine
    dog   0.01 mg/kg i.m., s.c. or i.v.
    cat   0.01 mg/kg i.m., s.c. or i.v.

butorphanol
    dog   up to 0.05 mg/kg s.c. or i.m. 2–3 hourly; up to 0.5 mg/kg p.o. 2-4 times daily.
    cat   up to 0.75 mg/kg s.c., i.m. or i.v. 4–8 hourly
    horse   0.1 mg/kg i.v. 4-hourly

Non-steroidal anti-inflammatory drugs (NSAIDs)

NSAIDs are used mainly in the treatment of pain and inflammation in muscle or joints in various species of domestic animals. Occasionally they may be used for their antipyretic effects. The group includes aspirin, one of the most widely used drugs in the world, and a number of others, some of which, like aspirin, have analgesic and antipyretic activity. The structures of some of the drugs in this class are shown in Fig. 8.6. The actions of the NSAIDs are due to their ability to inhibit the enzyme cyclooxygenase and thus prevent the biosynthesis of prostaglandins and thromboxanes. Prostaglandins also appear to sensitize pain receptors to other noxious substances such as bradykinin and histamine. In some instances, an inhibition of the production of bradykinin, stabilization of lysosomes and inhibition of the migration of polymorphonuclear leucocytes and macrophages into the site of inflammation may also contribute to the response. Thus the NSAIDs act by interfering with the initiation of pain impulses rather than on the central nervous system. A number of the drugs in this group are known to be nephrotoxic in dogs, in humans and possibly in other species. Most of the drugs are liable to produce ulceration of the gastrointestinal tract.

Acetylsalicylic acid (aspirin)

Salicylate is an ancient remedy for pain, inflammation and fever, originally used in the form of powdered willow bark. Aspirin has been used since the turn of the 20th century and is probably one of the most widely

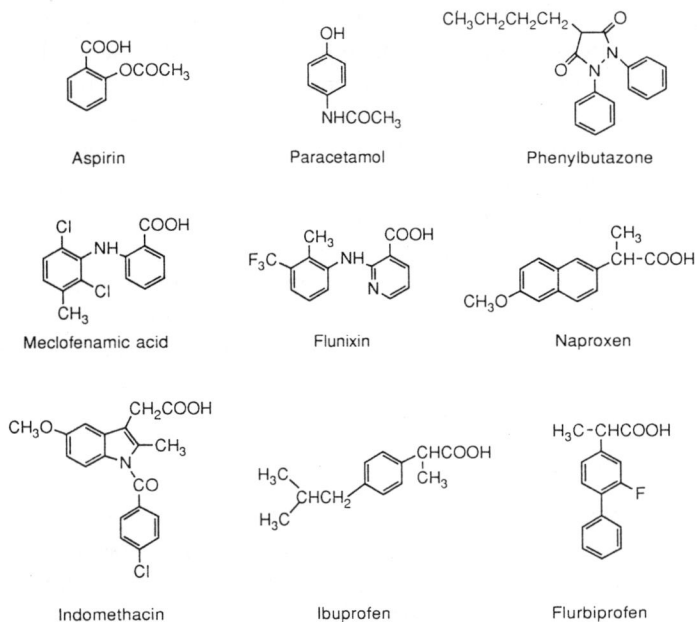

Figure 8.6 Non-steroidal anti-inflammatory analgesics.

employed drugs in human medicine. It has been used in the management of inflammatory and degenerative orthopaedic diseases and postoperative pain in dogs. Although it has no effect on normal body temperature, it has an antipyretic effect in the presence of fever. It has a long-lasting inhibitory effect on platelet aggregation, which is due to the inhibition of thromboxane synthesis. Due to its antiplatelet activity, it has been used to reduce the vascular complications associated with heartworm therapy in dogs. In cats, aspirin is a useful anti-inflammatory, analgesic and antipyretic. It has also been used to treat thrombotic disorders.

Being an organic acid, aspirin is largely un-ionized in the stomach, from which it is rapidly absorbed. Although the upper small intestine is more alkaline, the large surface area for absorption compensates for the greater degree of ionization and the rate of absorption is thus maintained. After absorption, hydrolysis by esterases results in the production of salicylate, also effective as an anti-inflammatory and analgesic. Binding of salicylate to plasma proteins varies between species, but is usually between 50 and 70 per cent. The drug is conjugated and excreted in the urine. Excretion is significantly increased in the presence of an alkaline urine and administration of sodium bicarbonate is of benefit in the management of toxic overdoses.

The enzymes that catalyse the conjugation of salicylate occur at a particularly low level in cats and thus aspirin has a plasma elimination half-life of approximately 40 hours in this species (compared to 1 hour in horses and 8.5 hours in dogs). Thus accumulation of the drug is a significant risk, especially in kittens less than 30 days old (and probably old cats as well), which are even less able to clear aspirin. It follows that the use of aspirin should be avoided in old cats and kittens, or in any animal with impaired hepatic or renal function.

The most common side-effects associated with aspirin use are in the gastrointestinal tract, where irritation of the gastric mucosa by the undissolved drug or inhibition of the protective effect of prostaglandins may both contribute to gastritis.

Paracetamol (acetaminophen)

Paracetamol has been extensively used in humans but its use is somewhat limited in domestic animals. It has negligible effects on peripheral cyclooxygenase, thus it has no anti-inflammatory action. The major advantage of paracetamol is that it causes less gastric irritation than aspirin, although it is considered to be a less effective analgesic than aspirin and is rapidly excreted. When used in high doses, the toxic effects are similar to those of aspirin, with cats being particularly liable to develop haemolytic anaemia and liver necrosis. Paracetamol has been shown to be nephrotoxic.

Ibuprofen

Ibuprofen has been used extensively in humans but in domestic animals its use is limited to dogs. Gastric irritation and nephrotoxicity are the most common side-effects. Although it has been suggested that these are unlikely to occur with therapeutic doses, recent data indicate that dogs may be particularly sensitive to the ulcerogenic and nephrotoxic actions of ibuprofen. Additional care should be exercised in its use due to its long elimination half-life.

Phenylbutazone

Phenylbutazone was withdrawn from human medicine (in the UK) when the development of fatal blood dyscrasias was associated with its use. It is thought to be less toxic in animals and it is still available to the veterinarian for use in horses and dogs. It is more effective as an anti-inflammatory agent than an analgesic and is considered to be most effective in the management of pain associated with the locomotor system. The mechanism of action of phenylbutazone is similar to that of aspirin; it inhibits the action of cyclooxygenase.

Phenylbutazone can be administered either orally or by intravenous or intramuscular injection. Its absorption from the gut is rapid and peak concentration occurs in the plasma within 2 hours of oral administration. Absorption is delayed after intramuscular injection, due to fixation of the drug to muscle protein, and it may take 6–10 hours to reach peak plasma levels. It is highly bound to plasma proteins (99 per cent) and thus is capable of interactions with other drugs which are highly protein bound. In the treatment of navicular disease in horses (see page 205), for example, phenylbutazone is contraindicated when warfarin is being used as an anticoagulant because of the risk of haemorrhage. Metabolism in the liver produces an active metabolite, oxyphenbutazone. In horses, both the parent drug and oxyphenbutazone reach high concentration in inflammatory exudate. The metabolism of therapeutic doses of phenylbutazone is more rapid in horses and dogs than in humans and hence there is less likelihood of cumulative toxicity. When higher doses are administered to horses, the elimination half-life increases and so does the possibility of accumulation. There is a long elimination half-life in cats (approximately 18 hours) and thus the risk of toxicity in this species is increased. Phenylbutazone and its metabolites are excreted via the kidney.

Gastric irritation, similar to that caused by aspirin, is the most likely side-effect. Although less common than in humans, blood dyscrasias have occurred with use of phenylbutazone in animals. Tachyphylaxis is a serious problem with long-term administration.

Meclofenamic acid

Meclofenamic acid is an extremely potent anti-inflammatory analgesic, indicated for the oral treatment of acute or chronic inflammatory conditions involving the musculoskeletal system in horses. In these cases, it is the drug of second choice (after phenylbutazone). After initial dosing for 5–7 days, the animal's condition should be reassessed and dosing adjusted accordingly. The mechanism of action of meclofenamic acid and its adverse effects are similar to the other drugs in this class.

Flunixin

Flunixin is a relatively new anti-inflammatory analgesic which is approximately four times more potent than phenylbutazone. It has primarily been used in horses and cattle and, more recently, in dogs. It is a potent analgesic and is particularly useful in the management of pain associated with equine colic. It is not yet recommended for use in cats. Flunixin is also available in combination with the antibacterial oxytetracycline, for use in the treatment of respiratory disease and acute mastitis in cattle.

Flunixin has side-effects similar to other drugs in this group. Like phenylbutazone, it is concentrated in inflammatory exudate where it has a much longer duration of action. Particular care should be exercised if it is to be used to treat the signs of abdominal pain in the horse; i.e. proper diagnosis should be made before administering the drug as it may mask the signs of a potentially fatal condition.

Naproxen

This is an anti-inflammatory which also has analgesic and antipyretic activity. It is used in horses and dogs. It has a particularly long half-life (74 hours) in dogs (which may be due to extensive enterohepatic circulation) and should be used with extreme caution in this species. It is not recommended for use in cats at any dose. Once-daily administration is adequate in horses. The most likely side-effects are in the gastrointestinal system.

Flurbiprofen

Flurbiprofen has some structural similarities to ibuprofen and may be quite toxic in the dog.

Doses

aspirin
  dog   30–60 mg/kg/day p.o. in 2 or 3 doses; dose at the low end of the range for analgesia and at the higher levels for anti-inflammatory effects.
  3 mg/kg every 6 days to reduce platelet aggregation.
  cat   10–40 mg/kg p.o. in a 48-hour period; at the low level for analgesia and the high level for anti-inflammatory effects.

paracetamol
  dog   25–30 mg/kg 4 times daily
  cat   25 mg/kg, once daily

ibuprofen
  dog   30 mg/kg/day, loading dose 20–30 mg/kg/day in divided doses initially, 10–15 mg/kg/day after a few days.

phenylbutazone
  horse   up to 4 g/day p.o. for 3 or 4 days then 1 g/day on alternate days. 1–2 g/day i.v. not more than 3 successive days.
  (Note: Administration of the drug should cease not less than 8 days before racing.)

dog   2-20 mg/kg/day p.o.; reduce after a few days

cat   10 mg/kg/day p.o. (or up to 20 mg/kg/day for a few days, if necessary).

meclofenamic acid

horse   2.2 mg/kg/day mixed in the food for 5–7 days

(Note: Administration of the drug should cease not less than 8 days before racing.)

flunixin

cattle   2.2 mg/kg i.v. 24-hourly, up to 5 days

horse   1.1 mg/kg i.v. or i.m. 24-hourly, up to 5 days

dog   1.1 mg/kg i.v. or p.o. 24-hourly

flurbiprofen

dog   loading dose 30 mg/kg then 15 mg/kg after 2 days.

(Note: $\geqslant$50 mg/kg may be fatal.)

Corticosteroids

The naturally occurring glucocorticoids, hydrocortisone and corticosterone are secreted by the adrenal cortex under control of the hypothalamic-pituitary-adrenal axis. Release of the hormones is controlled by diurnal rhythms, stress and feedback inhibition by circulating levels of hydrocortisone. The glucocorticoids have important effects on carbohydrate, protein and fat metabolism and are potent anti-inflammatory agents (see page 89). The mineralocorticoid, aldosterone, also secreted from the adrenal cortex, under the influence of the renin angiotensin aldosterone system, plays an important role in the control of sodium, potassium and water excretion (see page 243).

Endogenous and synthetic corticosteroids have varying combinations of glucocorticoid : mineralocorticoid activity (see Table 3.2). Those used as anti-inflammatory agents are relatively selective glucocorticoids. The anti-inflammatory activity of these drugs is due to their effects on leucocytes and to their ability to inhibit the action of phospholipase A_2.

The response to glucocorticoids includes a decreased number of neutrophils at the site of inflammation. Furthermore, movement of lymphocytes, monocytes, eosinophils and basophils from the vascular bed to lymphoid tissue, reduces the number of these cells. The activity of leucocytes and macrophages, especially their ability to phagocytose and kill microorganisms, is reduced. By inducing vasodilation and reducing capillary permeability, corticosteroids reduce plasma extravasation. The suppression of fibroblast activity reduces collagen and mucopolysaccharide formation. The inhibition of phospholipase A_2 activity by corticosteroids is mediated by the action of lipocortin, produced by leucocytes in response to glucocorticoids. Thus the synthesis of prostaglandins and leukotrienes is inhibited. Release of mediators is also reduced by the action of glucocorticoids, and the cell membranes of lysosomes and mast cells are stabilized.

Clinical use of corticosteroids

Corticosteroids inhibit the inflammatory response, regardless of the inflammatory stimulus. It is important to note that they do not influence the cause of inflammation. Thus important signs and symptoms may be masked and the condition of the patient, while appearing to improve, may in fact be deteriorating. By reducing the pain in a damaged organ or limb, the natural instinct to protect the affected part or avoid using the limb no longer functions, and further damage may result. The chance of further degenerative changes is increased because of the suppression of repair processes by the corticosteroids.

Inflammation and immune responses are closely linked and are both non-specifically suppressed by glucocorticoids, but the inflammatory response will recur after ceasing palliative therapy if the cause persists. Inflammation is a defence mechanism against infection and appropriate chemotherapy must be used concurrently if glucocorticoids are used in infective inflammatory episodes.

The continued presence of high levels of corticosteroid in the blood exerts a constant negative feedback effect on the hypothalamus and pituitary. Thus, endogenous production of cortisone is inhibited. Given over periods longer than about 1 week, pituitary and adrenocortical suppression become a potentially serious clinical problem, such that sudden withdrawal of the hormone may be lethal. Alternate-day therapy with drugs that have a short half-life may reduce the severity of pituitary adrenal suppression. In any event, withdrawal of glucocorticoids should be gradual and the use of long-acting depot preparations should be avoided where possible. The hypothalamic pituitary adrenal (HPA) axis may remain depressed for months and, in animals so affected, supplementary therapy with steroids is necessary during times of stress. The inhibition of the ability to counter infection and the retardation of wound healing (both of which are a direct result of the fundamental anti-inflammatory actions of the drugs) are serious problems associated with corticosteroid therapy. The catabolic actions of the glucocorticoids lead to muscle weakness, thinning of the skin and hair loss. Osteoporosis, diabetes mellitus and gastric ulceration may also occur.

A variety of different preparations are available for oral, topical or parenteral administration. Production of esters allows modification of the speed of absorption, particularly from an injection site. Thus formulations which slowly release the active substance can be administered by intra-articular injection and provide long-term therapy. Different esters can be combined to yield drugs with a rapid onset of action and a depot effect.

Musculoskeletal conditions

Musculoskeletal disorders are commonly treated by intra-articular injection or oral dosing with glucocorticoids. They have been used in the treatment of myositis, tendonitis, bursitis and arthritis. Such therapy produces marked remission but there are potential hazards. The relief of pain may allow the patient to resume activity too soon and thereby strain an injured limb. The repair phase of the inflammatory reaction is also suppressed and healing may be prolonged. Long-term use may cause degenerative changes associated with inhibition of articular cartilage synthesis. Calcification of soft tissues around the joint may also occur. Glucocorticoids have been reported to be of little sustained benefit in the treatment of equine joint disease. Although there may be initial dramatic improvement in signs, acceleration of the disease process can occur. Where possible, it is better to use alternative measures to remove the underlying cause of the disease.

Intra-articular injections of preparations that combine rapid onset of action and prolonged duration have been used in horses, dogs and cattle. The technique should only be used to decrease pain and swelling from injury to periarticular soft tissues or synovial membrane where the articular cartilage is not damaged. Contraindications for intra-articular injection include sepsis in or around the joint, intra-articular fracture (where repair will be inhibited) and degenerative bony lesions. A novel formulation of the potent glucocorticoid flumethasone in dimethyl sulphoxide is available. It is sufficiently rapidly and well absorbed through the skin to be used as a topical application in horses for the treatment of acute musculoskeletal conditions.

Inflammatory skin conditions

Such conditions respond well to systemic or topically applied corticosteroids, which are of particular value in the treatment of hypersensitivity reactions such as flea-bite allergy, where they reduce the itch associated with the allergic reaction and thus reduce self-inflicted damage. Topical application is rational for dermatoses, to reduce the possibility of side-effects associated with the metabolic actions of the glucocorticoids and suppression of the HPA axis. However, the drugs are absorbed into the circulation and over-enthusiastic use can measurably suppress the HPA axis. Acetonides are well absorbed into skin, where they are bound, thus reducing the risk of systemic effects. Many of the preparations for topical application include an antibacterial such as neomycin.

Corticosteroids are contraindicated in pyodermas and in demodectic mange, where they enhance the existing immunosuppression, thus favouring multiplication of the pathogens already present.

Eye and ear conditions

Glucocorticoids reduce the inflammatory response and subsequent corneal opacity in allergic blepharitis, conjunctivitis and non-ulcerative keratitis. Their use should be avoided if there is corneal ulceration because re-epithelialization and vascularization may be retarded. Antibiotics should be administered concurrently in cases where local infection is also a problem.

Glucocorticoids are invaluable in the treatment of otitis externa to break the cycle of inflammation, irritation and self-trauma. Drops or ointments usually incorporate antibacterials, which must be used in conjunction with the steroids if infection is present.

Comparison of steroidal anti-inflammatory agents and NSAIDs

NSAIDs, unlike corticosteroids, only inhibit cyclooxygenase and have no effect on the lipoxygenase pathway. Thus, the levels of leukotrienes are not decreased (and may even increase) with NSAIDs and the responses to these mediators are not influenced by NSAIDs. The NSAIDs are potentially able to completely inhibit cyclooxygenase activity. The consequent removal of the protective effect of prostaglandins on the bowel renders them more likely than the steroids to induce gastrointestinal ulceration. Advantages associated with use of NSAIDs are that the healing process is not reduced, nor is resistance to infection compromised.

Gold

Gold-containing compounds for the treatment of rheumatoid arthritis were introduced about 70 years ago. Initially there were fears that accumulation of gold would give rise to toxic reactions but the demonstration that this does not occur and the introduction of an oral formulation have increased the use of gold. In veterinary medicine, gold salts are used in the management of immune-mediated joint diseases in dogs and immune-mediated skin disease in dogs and cats. They may be used where corticosteroid therapy produces intolerable side-effects. The gold-containing compounds differ from the previously described anti-inflammatory agents in that they appear to arrest the progress of rheumatoid arthritis and they have only minimal anti-inflammatory activity in other circumstances. Sodium aurothiomalate (Fig. 8.7) and auro-thioglucose are injectable preparations of gold, widely used in animals. The orally effective formulation of gold, auranofin, is a relative newcomer and its use in veterinary medicine is less well documented.

Aurothiomalate and aurothioglucose are only poorly absorbed after oral administration and are more usually administered by deep intramuscular injection at weekly to monthly intervals. The drugs are concentrated in synovial membranes and also in liver, kidney, spleen, adrenal glands, lymph nodes and bone marrow and are excreted mainly via the kidneys (70 per cent). Elimination of gold is slow and it may take 1 month to eliminate 75–80 per cent of a single intramuscular dose.

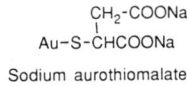

$$\text{Au–S–} \overset{\displaystyle CH_2\text{-COONa}}{\underset{|}{\text{CHCOONa}}}$$

Sodium aurothiomalate

Figure 8.7 Sodium aurothiomalate.

Auranofin has a different pattern of serum protein binding and different tissue distribution from the injectable gold salts. Relatively less auranofin is found in the kidney and this may account for the fact that only a small proportion of the dose (15 per cent) is excreted in the urine. The major portion is excreted in the faeces.

The mechanism of action of the gold compounds is unclear. A variety of actions have been observed but it is not known which, if any, of these is responsible for the therapeutic response to gold. The inhibition of the function of mononuclear phagocytes and consequent suppression of immune responsiveness may be important here.

Side-effects and toxicity

Treatment with gold salts may be lifelong and, because of the potentially serious nature of the side-effects, animals require careful monitoring. Complete blood count (CBC), platelet count, serum biochemistry and urinalysis should be performed before instituting treatment, and then (except for serum biochemistry) every 2 weeks for the first month, monthly for 3 months and every 3–4 months thereafter. Serum biochemistry should be checked every 4–6 months.

The most serious side-effect of the injectable gold compounds is nephrosis. Transient and mild proteinuria is frequent. Adverse effects in the renal system are not a common problem with auranofin. Mucocutaneous lesions, often involving the mouth, are relatively common side-effects. Dermatological side-effects (rash, pruritus) are common in humans, especially with auranofin.

Thrombocytopenia may develop but is usually reversible. It has been suggested that an immune mechanism which results in an accelerated degradation of the platelets, may be responsible for this in dogs. Bone marrow depression (agranulocytosis and aplastic anaemia), pulmonary fibrosis and corneal ulceration have also been observed. In dogs an increased faecal volume and altered faecal electrolytes may occur with auranofin therapy. This results in an increased volume of fluid remaining in the intestine. Diarrhoea often responds to a reduction in dose.

Dose

auranofin
  dog   0.05–0.2 mg/kg p.o., b.i.d. to a maximum of 9 mg/day.

sodium aurothiomalate
  dog   administer a small test dose first, to test for adverse reactions
         then 5–40 mg (depending on size), i.m. weekly (usually
         10–20 mg) for 6 weeks. Can be repeated if necessary.

CHAPTER 9

THE HAEMATOPOIETIC SYSTEM

Drugs used in the treatment of anaemia

Transport of oxygen to the tissues is the most important function of the blood. This is achieved by binding of oxygen to haemoglobin, a protein in red blood cells. Any disease state in which the quantity or function of red blood cells is deficient is classified as an anaemia.

Iron is a vital component of haemoglobin, and as such is necessary for transport of oxygen. The body stores of iron are controlled by absorption from the small intestine, so that in states of iron deficiency the rate of absorption is increased. In healthy animals very little iron is lost from the body and only a small fraction of dietary iron is absorbed. Two-thirds of the total body iron is found in the red blood cells. The rest circulates bound to transferrin, a plasma globulin, or is stored (in combination with a protein) as ferritin in hepatocytes and other cells. Generally iron absorption is inhibited when storage sites are saturated, although the control mechanism may break down when excessive amounts of iron are ingested.

The efficient utilization of iron requires the presence of a number of cofactors (notably copper). In their absence, formation of haemoglobin may be affected, even if iron levels are adequate.

Vitamin B_{12} (cyanocobalamin), a cobalt-containing vitamin, is necessary for DNA synthesis, and is therefore vital for cell formation. Since red cells are constantly being produced, vitamin B_{12} deficiencies result in malformed red cells. This is not normally a problem in ruminants, because ruminal bacteria synthesize vitamin B_{12}. Many non-ruminant species also have enteric bacteria capable of synthesizing vitamin B_{12} and thus dietary deficiency of the vitamin is not a common clinical problem. More commonly (especially in cattle, sheep and goats), a deficiency in the dietary intake of cobalt results in vitamin B_{12} deficiency states.

Types of anaemias

Acute blood loss

In these cases the bone marrow is still capable of red cell production and the real problem is hypovolaemia. The consequences of the anaemia are not immediately apparent. If the blood volume is replaced, even with plasma, the red cells can cope with the load until new ones are synthesized. A healthy animal will usually make up the loss within 1 week to 10 days. If blood loss is extensive, or occurs over a short period of time (e.g. during surgery) it may be necessary to transfuse whole blood or red cells.

Chronic blood loss

It is important to identify the cause of the blood loss and initiate treatment. If blood is being lost chronically, it is quite possible that more iron is lost each day than can be replaced by absorption. Thus an iron-deficient anaemia will eventually occur. Cattle that are heavily infested with sucking lice, or horses carrying heavy burdens of blood-sucking strongylid worms, are liable to become anaemic. After treating the cause, the iron deficiency must also be treated. It may also be necessary to give packed red blood cells by transfusion.

Haemolytic anaemias

Haemolytic anaemias are associated with a number of factors, including infections, poisoning and genetic defects. The cause should be identified and treated. Medications which stimulate haematopoiesis may be of value. Vitamin B_{12}, cobalt and iron supplementation will assist recovery. It may be necessary to give whole blood by transfusion.

Hypoplastic anaemias

Hypoplastic anaemias are also associated with drugs, infections, neoplasms, etc. In these cases the bone marrow production of one or more blood cell type is reduced. Treatment is as for haemolytic anaemias.

Nutritional anaemias

Most animals do not suffer from problems associated with inadequate ingestion or absorption of the essential nutrients for blood cell formation. The addition of iron to veterinary 'tonic' preparations probably does little to improve the state of health of the recipient.

Suckling pigs are most liable to develop iron deficiency anaemia. Occasionally veal calves and rarely young lambs and kids may also be affected. Piglets are born with very low iron reserves and grow rapidly in the early weeks. They need to absorb approximately 300 mg iron in the first 3 weeks of their lives and only about 1 mg per day can be suckled from the sow. Where the animals are raised on soil, iron in the soil provides the extra iron needed. In farms where the piglets are raised in more hygienic conditions, often indoors, this is not possible and supplementation with iron is essential.

Treatment of iron deficiency states

The preparations available are suitable for either oral or parenteral administration. The simple salt, ferrous sulphate, provides an adequate source of iron for oral treatment. The more complex chemical formulations, with elaborate claims for reduced toxicity, offer no real advantage. They should never be mixed in solution with other drugs as there are many chemical incompatibilities.

Iron dextran is the most common preparation for parenteral administration. Deep intramuscular injection is required. After absorption via the lymphatics, the compound is broken down and free iron enters the bloodstream. Absorption of iron is increased in iron deficiency states, but as the deficiency is corrected absorption will return to normal (i.e. <10 per cent). It may take weeks to months of iron therapy to correct a severe iron deficiency, and if the underlying cause has not been treated, relapse is likely. Gastric irritation or vomiting may occur but can be reduced if iron is administered parenterally. Injections may also be required in animals where malabsorption limits the amount that can be absorbed, or where very large amounts are required.

Dose

horse	0.5–1 g iron (as iron dextran) per week as a divided dose at 2 sites
horse and cattle	2–4 g/day p.o. for up to 2 weeks

Treatment of iron-deficiency anaemia in piglets

The injection of iron dextran provides a slow-release source of iron, with most of the iron being absorbed within about 1 week of the injection. The animals are injected at 3–5 days. There is a risk of damage to the sciatic nerve or spinal cord if injections are administered earlier.

Dose

piglet   100–200 mg Fe (as iron dextran) i.m.

Iron toxicity

Iron has a relatively high margin of safety and it requires the ingestion of large amounts before toxic effects occur. With the exception of piglets, which are most frequently treated with iron, toxicity in animals is rare. The signs include lethargy and dyspnoea, which may be followed rapidly by death. This is most likely where the sow has received a diet which is rich in polyunsaturated acids and low in vitamin E, which sensitizes the piglets to iron.

For orally ingested iron, treatment consists of inducing emesis, followed by gastric lavage with sodium bicarbonate solution (1–5 per cent). Desferrioxamine specifically chelates iron and increases its rate of excretion, and can also be used.

Treatment of vitamin and mineral deficiencies

Vitamin deficiencies *per se* are relatively rare in domestic animals (see Chapter 4). The most common of these are due to inadequate intake of either cobalt or copper. Cobalt is an essential requirement for the synthesis of vitamin B_{12}, which in turn is necessary for erythropoiesis. One of the important functions of copper is its role in the absorption of iron from the gastrointestinal tract. In the absence of adequate supplies of copper, reduced iron absorption may lead to an iron-deficient anaemia. Further details of the effects of and treatment of cobalt and copper deficiencies can be found on pages 111–112.

Drugs which affect blood coagulation mechanisms

Haemostasis is the name given to the events whereby blood flow from a damaged vessel is arrested. It is a complex process, which consists of three distinct phases. Immediately the vessel is cut the precapillary sphincters contract to reduce blood flow through the affected vessel. Within seconds, exposure of the platelets to the collagen of the vessel wall activates the second phase, the adhesion of platelets to each other and to the vessel wall. The consequent formation of a platelet plug controls the blood loss for the short term. The final phase consists of a series of reactions which result in the generation of strands of fibrin which strengthen the platelet plug. The coagulation process involves a number of clotting factors, which are referred to either by names or by roman numerals (Table 9.1).

Table 9.1 Nomenclature of clotting factors

Clotting factor	Common name
I	Fibrinogen
II	Prothrombin
III	Tissue thromboplastin
IV	Calcium ion
V	Labile factor
VII	Proconvertin, stable factor
VIII	Antihaemophilic globulin (AHG)
IX	Christmas factor, plasma thromboplastin component (PTC)
X	Stuart-Prower factor
XI	Plasma prothrombin antecedent (PTA)
XII	Hageman factor
XIII	Fibrin-stabilizing factor

Clotting factors are activated and then catalyse the conversion of the next substrate. Thus an amplifying 'cascade' of reactions occurs (Fig. 9.1). There are two pathways which result in the formation of activated Factor X (Factor Xa). The intrinsic system, in which all components are present in circulating blood, is the slower pathway, requiring some minutes for the formation of Factor Xa. The extrinsic system, triggered by factors released from injured tissues or by contact with foreign surfaces, by-passes some of the early reactions and is completed within seconds.

Lysis (Fig. 9.1) of the clot begins to occur within 24–48 hours after its formation. The first step in this process is the conversion of plasminogen, incorporated in the clot, to plasmin. This can be achieved by a variety of activators which are found in blood, vessel walls and many tissues. The clot is broken down by the action of plasmin.

Drugs may be required to stimulate the coagulation process or to inhibit it. Because of the complexity of the reactions involved in the cascade, there are many sites at which drugs may act to interfere with normal coagulation processes.

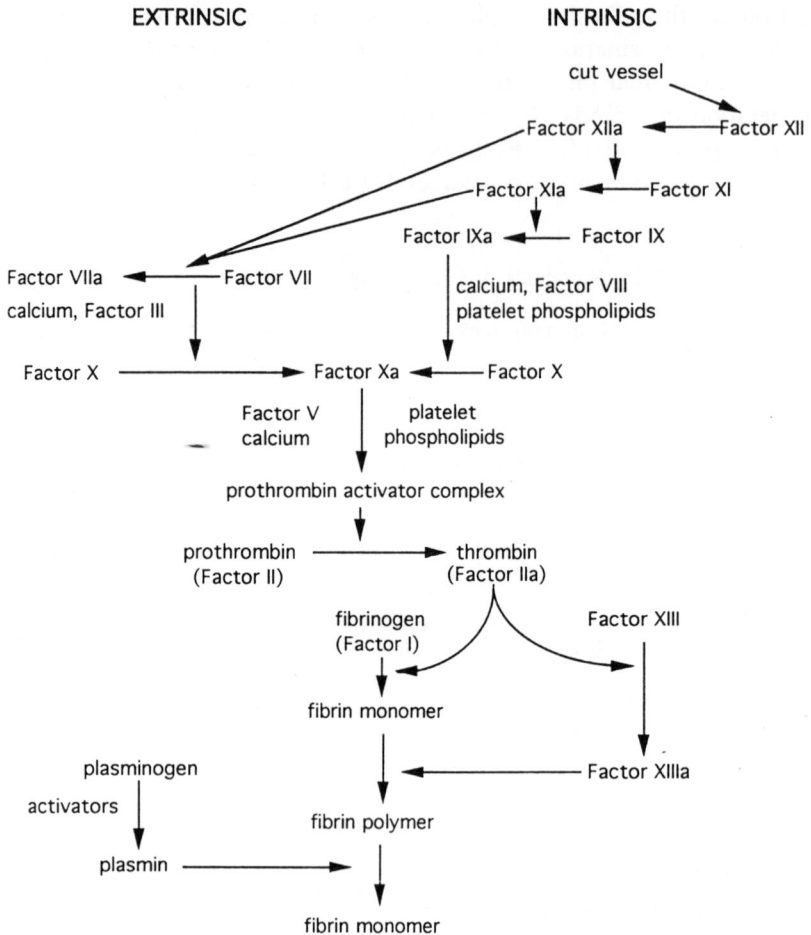

Figure 9.1 Formation and lysis of blood clots. Activated factors are designated 'a'.
Intrinsic system: Factor XII is activated by contact with the cut vessel. Factor XIIa
activates Factor XI, which in the presence of Ca^{2+}, activates Factor IX. Factor IXa,
together with Ca^{2+}, platelet phospholipids and Factor VIII, activate Factor X.
Extrinsic system: Factors XIIa and XIa, formed in the intrinsic system, activate
Factor VII. Factor VIIa, in combination with Ca^{2+} and Factor III (thromboplastin)
released by tissue trauma, activate Factor X.
Common pathway: Factor Xa, Factor V, Ca^{2+} and platelet phospholipids form a
prothrombin activator complex which converts prothrombin (Factor II) to thrombin
(Factor IIa). Thrombin catalyses the conversion of fibrinogen (Factor I) to soluble
fibrin monomers and also activates Factor XIII. Factor XIIIa then crosslinks the
fibrin monomers, producing an insoluble mesh of fibrin in which blood cells, platelets
and plasma are trapped to form the clot.
Lysis: Activators, including thrombin, fibrin and kinases, convert plasminogen to
plasmin. The proteolytic activity of plasmin converts the fibrin chains to soluble
polypeptides.

Anticoagulants

Chelating agents

Since Ca^{2+} is an absolute requirement for coagulation, any substance which removes Ca^{2+} from blood has anticoagulant activity. Chelating agents, particularly sodium edetate (EDTA) and sodium citrate, are used as anticoagulants for blood which is stored for analysis. Sodium citrate can also be used as the anticoagulant in blood collected for later transfusion because the citrate ion is metabolized by the recipient. The addition of sodium fluoride and potassium oxalate to samples of blood for laboratory analysis prevents enzyme activity and coagulation.

Heparin

Heparin is a naturally occurring substance, so named because it is found in quantity in the liver. It consists of a heterogeneous group of straight-chain anionic mucopolysaccharides of variable length. Commercial preparations have alternating sequences of sulphated disaccharide units; the sulphate groups render the molecule strongly acidic. The most common sources of heparin are bovine lung and porcine intestinal mucosa.

The anticoagulant effect of heparin is due to its antithrombin activity. It binds to antithrombin III, a plasma α-globulin which inactivates thrombin, thus inhibiting the conversion of fibrinogen to fibrin. The change in conformation of antithrombin III which results from the binding increases the velocity of the inactivation of thrombin. This effect is reinforced by the binding of heparin to thrombin, bringing it into proximity with heparin-bound, activated antithrombin III. Furthermore, it inhibits activated Factors IX, X, XI and XII in the coagulation cascade. The multiple sites of action of heparin insure prompt and effective anticoagulation of blood both *in vivo* and *in vitro*.

Because heparin is degraded in the gut, it must be administered parenterally. The intravenous route is the one of choice since other routes often lead to the formation of haematomas at the injection site. Heparin is metabolized by liver enzymes and therefore has a relatively short duration of action. Thus, it is administered most commonly by slow intravenous infusion.

Side-effects of heparin are minimal. The greatest problem associated with its use is that of overdose and consequent haemorrhage. Treatment of severe overdose is with protamine sulphate, a low molecular weight protein. The strongly basic protein reacts with heparin to form a stable complex devoid of anticoagulant activity.

Oral anticoagulants

The anticoagulant effect of this group of drugs was first discovered when a haemorrhagic disorder occurred in cattle which had consumed spoiled sweet clover. The active principle was found to be bishydroxycoumarin (dicoumarol) (Fig. 9.2). This substance is still used as an anticoagulant. Many other coumarins have been synthesized in the search for clinically useful compounds which may offer some advantage over dicoumarol. Perhaps the best known of these is warfarin (Fig. 9.2), which is widely used as a rodenticide. Warfarin is of interest to the veterinarian as a potential poison in domestic animals and as an anticoagulant in the treatment of navicular disease.

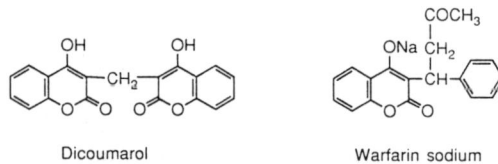

Dicoumarol   Warfarin sodium

Figure 9.2   Oral anticoagulants.

The major difference between the coumarin derivatives and heparin is that the coumarins are ineffective *in vitro*. Their anticoagulant effect is due to the inhibition of the synthesis of a number of clotting factors. Vitamin K is an essential cofactor for the synthesis of prothrombin and Factors VII, IX and X. The coumarins act as anti-vitamin K agents and coagulation is prevented. Their onset of action is slow, since time is required for the breakdown of circulating clotting factors before the effects of inhibition of synthesis are seen. Similarly, their effect may persist for some days after the last dose of drug, while adequate levels of clotting factors are synthesized. The coumarins are very strongly bound to plasma albumin (approx. 99 per cent) and therefore the response may be modified by concurrent administration of other drugs which are protein bound. In particular, non-steroidal anti-inflammatory drugs or corticosteroids should not be used with warfarin because of the serious risk of inducing haemorrhage.

Single doses of warfarin are unlikely to be lethal to domestic animals unless very large amounts are consumed. Toxicity is more likely when intake occurs over a few days or when the concurrent administration of another protein-bound drug, such as phenylbutazone, results in an increase in the plasma level of unbound warfarin. In these cases all efforts to control bleeding must be made. Pharmacological antagonism of the effects of an excessive blood level of a coumarin-based anticoagulant requires the administration of large doses of vitamin K_1. Administration of 1 mg/kg i.v. usually induces an increased plasma prothrombin concentration within 30 minutes. Synthetic analogues of vitamin K are cheaper but are less potent and have a significantly delayed effect. In severe cases, transfusion of whole blood may be necessary.

Therapeutic uses of anticoagulants

Anticoagulants are widely used in human medicine in the prevention and treatment of thromboses and emboli. A similar application in veterinary medicine is the treatment of navicular disease in horses. This condition is thought to cause about 30 per cent of all cases of chronic forelimb lameness in horses, generally in animals 6–12 years old and not regularly worked. One theory of the aetiology is that occlusive vascular changes—arteriosclerosis and thrombosis—occur in the blood supply to the navicular bone and that these lead to ischaemic necrosis and erosion of the flexor cartilage. Nonsteroidal anti-inflammatory drugs relieve the associated pain, but do not treat the condition. Medical treatment in current use includes isoxsuprine to effect vasodilation and anticoagulant therapy to counteract the progressive thrombosis.

Warfarin is the drug of choice but there is a risk of haemorrhage and it should only be used with facilities for monitoring the one-stage prothrombin time (OSPT). This is particularly important since, unlike isoxsuprine, warfarin therapy is continuous. The dose for each patient must be individually determined, with the object to lengthen the OSPT by about 25 per cent of its pretreatment value. Since OSPT values may vary markedly between animals, it is important to obtain consistent data for pre-dosing coagulation status before therapy is commenced. If clinical improvement is unsatisfactory after 6–8 weeks, further prolongation of OSPT to 50 per cent of the pretreatment value may be necessary. Frequent measurement of OSPT must be performed while the dose is being determined and then continued, at increased time intervals, for the duration of the therapy.

Dose

warfarin
horse   Start with 1 mg/50 kg bodyweight p.o. If necessary, after 10 days this may be increased by up to 20 per cent. Final dose may be up to 8.5 mg/50 kg. Careful monitoring of coagulation status needs to be maintained during the period of dosage stabilization and thereafter.

Antiplatelet drugs

The formation of a platelet plug in the early stages of clot formation is associated with the release from the platelet of substances which induce adhesion and aggregation of the platelets. Adenosine diphosphate (ADP) is released initially. Its effects are reinforced when the activity of cyclooxygenase results in the release of thromboxane A_2 (TXA_2), a powerful inducer of platelet aggregation. Aspirin and other non-steroidal anti-inflammatory drugs which inhibit the cyclooxygenase pathway are potent inhibitors of platelet aggregation. These effects are irreversible and persist for the life of the platelet.

Thrombolytic drugs

Streptokinase, a protein obtained from streptococci, activates endogenous plasminogen, stimulates the production of plasmin and so promotes lysis of clots. It is available in combination with streptodornase, which liquefies viscous exudates. The use of this combination in veterinary medicine is limited to local application to wounds where removal of blood clots and exudates is desirable.

Coagulants

Coagulants are agents which stimulate the clotting process and thus assist in the arrest of blood loss.

Thromboplastin (Factor III, thrombokinase), isolated from animal sources, is available for direct application to wounds. It initiates the cascade of reactions involved in clot formation and thus accelerates haemostasis.

Thrombin, the enzyme which converts fibrinogen to fibrin, is also useful for the control of bleeding. It is administered by local application of powder, solution or sponge containing thrombin.

Fibrinogen (Factor I) is isolated from human sources and is available in powder form. The powder is dissolved in normal saline before use. Endogenous thrombin converts the applied fibrinogen to fibrin.

Fibrin foam, in the form of a fine sponge, contains human fibrin. Pieces of sponge, applied directly to wounds, provide a frame for clot formation. Soaking the sponge in thrombin solution before application hastens the rate of clot formation.

Absorbable gelatin sponge, a water-insoluble sponge, can absorb many times its own weight of fluid. It may be soaked in thrombin solution prior to use to accelerate clot formation. If implanted, it is absorbed over approximately 6 weeks.

Oxidized cellulose, in a gauze or sponge, interacts with blood, producing a matrix for clot formation. It is absorbed if left *in situ*.

Therapeutic applications of coagulants

The coagulants are only suitable for local application to the site of bleeding and are effective only for the arrest of capillary oozing. Bleeding from large vessels will not be reduced by these agents. They should never be injected intravenously or allowed to enter large vessels.

Both absorbable gelatin sponge and oxidized cellulose may be allowed to remain at the site of bleeding and will eventually be absorbed. However, oxidized cellulose should not be left *in situ* when fractures are involved since it interferes with bone regeneration.

Topical application of adrenaline or noradrenaline has also been used in the control of capillary bleeding. The effectiveness of these drugs is associated with their vasoconstrictor activity. The presence of volatile hydrocarbon anaesthetics such as halothane and, to a lesser extent isoflurane and enflurane, may sensitize the heart muscle to the arrhythmogenic actions of adrenaline and noradrenaline and extra care must be taken in these circumstances.

CHAPTER 10

THE CARDIOVASCULAR SYSTEM

A number of drugs are used in veterinary medicine for their actions on the cardiovascular system. The most commonly used are those which stimulate the failing heart or relieve its workload and those which correct cardiac arrhythmias.

Cardiac failure

Heart muscle has the capacity to regulate its force of contraction with changes in muscle length. This most important mechanism, known as the Frank–Starling law of the heart, enables the muscle to contract more forcefully when there is an increase in left ventricular muscle fibre length at the end of diastole, i.e. stretching of the muscle immediately prior to contraction. The Frank–Starling law of the heart is illustrated in Fig. 10.1, where the relationship between end-diastolic length and force of contraction in the normal heart is shown. In the presence of positive inotropic drugs or sympathetic stimulation, the relationship moves to a different curve and at any given starting length the force of contraction will be greater than in the untreated heart. Failing heart muscle, on the other hand, functions on a depressed Frank–Starling curve, with reduced contractility at any end-diastolic length, when compared to the normal heart.

In congestive heart failure (CHF), the myocardial contractility is so low that cardiac output fails to meet body requirements. Compensatory mechanisms are invoked and these provide extensive reserves, although as the disease progresses, they exacerbate the failure (Fig. 10.2).

1. Increased activity of the sympathetic nervous system occurs in an effort to increase cardiac output. The enhanced sympathetic activity increases myocardial contractility and heart rate and thereby increases the oxygen demand of the myocardium. Cardiac output may actually fall because

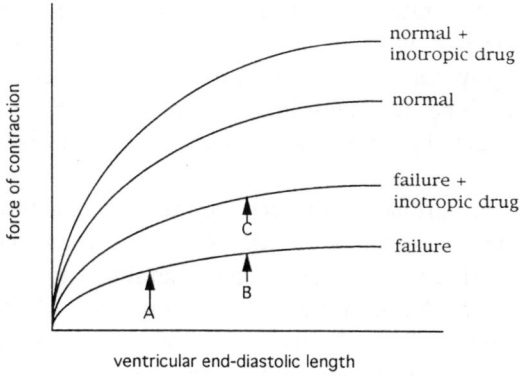

Figure 10.1 Relationship between ventricular end-diastolic length and force of ventricular contraction, also referred to as the 'Frank-Starling curve'. Each curve represents a different 'inotropic state'. Failing heart muscle operates on a depressed Frank-Starling curve, so that at any end-diastolic length, the force of contraction is considerably less than that in healthy heart muscle. One method of compensation in heart failure is movement of the operating point along the curve from A to B, so that the muscle is able, by starting with increased length, to contract more forcefully. The use of inotropic agents shifts the Frank-Starling curve for failing heart muscle towards normal and the operating point moves to C. Note that inotropic agents also affect the curve for healthy heart muscle.

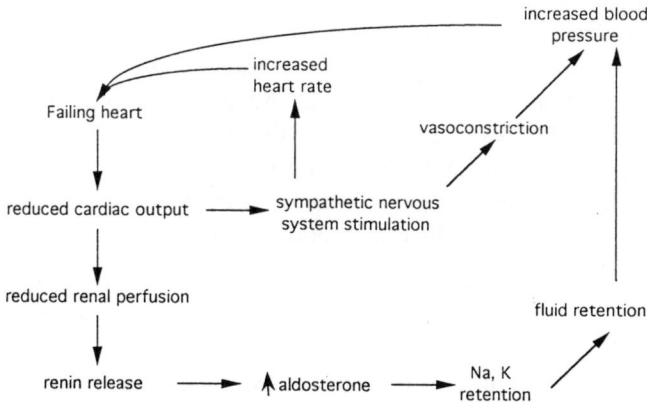

Figure 10.2 Compensatory mechanisms in heart failure (for explanation see text).

at higher heart rates there is reduced time in diastole for ventricular filling. Selective vasoconstriction maintains the blood supply to the brain and myocardium at the expense of the peripheral and visceral circulation. The resultant increase in peripheral resistance impedes ventricular ejection and further increases myocardial work and oxygen demands.

2. The reduced cardiac output reduces renal blood flow and the kidney responds by releasing renin which, by the consequent generation of angiotensin II, further increases peripheral resistance and the workload on the heart. Aldosterone release from the adrenal cortex is also increased by renin and there is a consequent increase in the renal distal tubular reabsorption of Na^+ and water.

3. The increased retention of Na^+ stimulates the release of antidiuretic hormone from the anterior pituitary and there is further retention of water.

4. Venous return increases as a consequence of the fluid retention and the myocardial fibres are stretched. In the initial stages of heart failure, Frank-Starling's Law operates and the force of contraction of the heart is increased. This is shown in Fig. 10.1 as the movement along the heart failure curve, from the point marked A to the point marked B.

With increasing severity of the underlying cardiac abnormality, excessive exercise, increased dietary sodium intake or simply the positive feedback effects of the compensatory mechanisms themselves, compensation fails and treatment is required. There are two different approaches to the treatment of CHF. The contractility of the cardiac muscle can be increased by the use of cardiac stimulants. This will return the Frank–Starling curve for the failing muscle towards normality (Fig. 10.1). This increased contractility is represented by the movement of the operation of the heart from the point marked B to the point marked C. The second approach to therapy is to reduce the workload of the heart. In this case, the compensatory mechanisms that mediate vasoconstriction and fluid retention are inhibited; vasodilators are used to reduce the pressure against which the heart has to work and diuretics (Chapter 12) are used to reduce the volume of fluid.

Cardiac stimulants

The main cardiac stimulant substances in use for the management of chronic heart failure in veterinary medicine are the digitalis glycosides and the xanthine derivatives. The glycosides have been employed in the treatment of heart failure for more than 200 years and, although alternative approaches to the treatment of heart failure are increasing in popularity, glycosides are likely to be commonly prescribed for the foreseeable future.

Digitalis glycosides

These substances are derived from plant sources, the most common being *Digitalis purpurea* (the common foxglove), which contains digitoxin, and *Digitalis lanata* (the woolly foxglove), which contains lanatosides A and C, from which digitoxin and digoxin are extracted. The early use of digitalis was by the administration of relatively crude plant extracts, but pure glycosides are now readily available and their use is preferred. The term 'digitalis' is commonly used to refer to all drugs having actions like the naturally occurring compounds. Ouabain, a glycoside extracted from the seeds of *Strophanthus gratus*, is sometimes used in experimental studies because it is more rapidly acting than either digoxin or digitoxin. In clinical practice, although others are available, the choice of drugs is between digoxin and digitoxin.

Each glycoside molecule consists of an aglycone (or genin), which is responsible for the activity of the drug, linked by an oxygen atom to up to four molecules of sugar, which influence its water and lipid solubility. The chemical structures of the commonly used glycosides are shown in Fig. 10.3.

Mode of action

The action of the cardiac glycosides is shown diagrammatically in Fig. 10.4. The primary receptor for the therapeutic and toxic effects of the cardiac glycosides is believed to be Na^+,K^+-activated adenosine triphosphatase (Na^+,K^+-ATPase) in the cell membrane. It has been shown that the glyco-

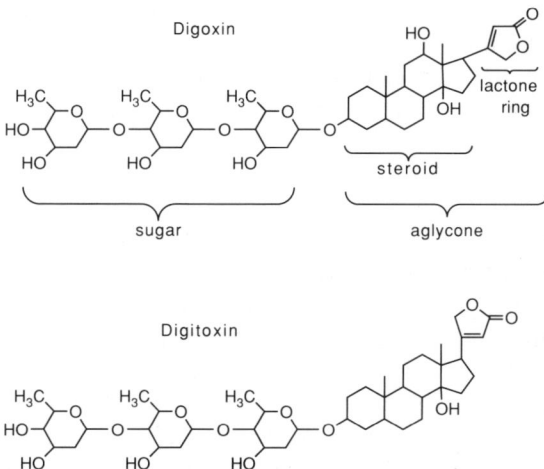

Figure 10.3 Digitalis glycosides.

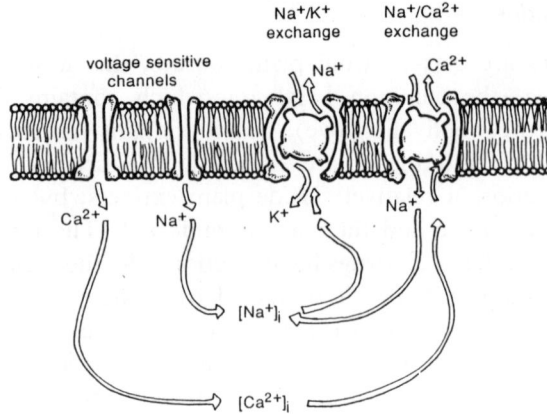

Figure 10.4 Mechanism of action of digitalis glycosides.

sides inhibit this system, which is normally responsible for pumping K^+ into the cells and Na^+ out of them. The inhibition of the pump results in an increase in the intracellular concentration of Na^+ ($[Na^+]_i$) and a decrease in the intracellular concentration of K^+ ($[K^+]_i$). Another transport mechanism in cardiac muscle fibres exchanges intracellular Ca^{2+} for extracellular Na^+. The glycoside-induced increase in $[Na^+]_i$ reduces the concentration gradient of Na^+ across the cell membrane and thereby reduces the extrusion of intracellular Ca^{2+} by this pump. Thus $[Ca^{2+}]_i$ increases and with each action potential there is an increased release of Ca^{2+} from the sarcoplasmic reticulum to activate the contractile apparatus. In addition, an increase in the movement of Ca^{2+} into the cell during the plateau of the action potential, further increases the availability of Ca^{2+} for the contractile process.

Actions
A positive inotropic effect is the most important action of the digitalis glycosides. Thus they enable the heart to contract more forcefully without disproportionately increasing energy requirements or increasing heart rate. Improved emptying and a reduction in the size of the dilated failing heart occur as a result of this main effect. The positive inotropic effect can be demonstrated in both normal and failing heart muscle (but is more obvious in failing muscle). With the increase in the force of contraction of the heart, the requirement for compensation by the sympathetic nervous system is reduced and heart rate falls. This effect on heart rate is enhanced by the actions of the glycosides at various sites within the central nervous system, which result

in an increase in efferent vagal impulses to the SA node. The slower heart rate increases the time in diastole, allowing improved diastolic filling and increased coronary blood flow, which occurs during diastole. In addition to the cardiac slowing, the increased vagal tone reduces the velocity of conduction of impulses through the AV node. Although digoxin and other glycosides are able to directly depress AV conduction, it is not likely that any direct action on the AV node occurs at the plasma levels of drug found in normal clinical practice.

The cardiac glycosides, by their effect on cardiac contractility, correct the basic deficiency in cardiac function which is responsible for the development of the various signs and symptoms of heart failure. As a result, the compensatory mechanisms described above are no longer needed to maintain function, or are needed to a lesser extent. The effect on heart rate has already been mentioned. The bradycardia is accompanied by a diuretic response which is secondary to the improved perfusion of the kidneys and consequent fall in the secretion of renin. The increased Na^+ excretion is associated with loss of fluid and a reduction in the secretion of antidiuretic hormone. Although digoxin has no diuretic effects in a healthy animal, loss of excess fluid in a dog with heart failure may account for the loss of approximately 10 per cent of its bodyweight during the initial 7–10 days of therapy. A further result of the loss of fluid and general improvement in the circulation is a fall in peripheral venous pressure.

Digitalis glycosides have been shown to cause contraction of smooth muscle in arterial resistance vessels and smooth muscle in veins. This vascular activity has little clinical significance because, in a patient with heart failure, the reduction in sympathetic tone which occurs when the cardiac contractility is improved overcomes the vasoconstriction directly induced by the drug.

While it is clear that the positive inotropic effects of the digitalis glycosides are independent of any effect at β-adrenoceptors, there is less consensus about the general interaction of these drugs with the sympathetic nervous system. Some research results suggest that there is increased efferent sympathetic nervous system activity in the presence of therapeutic levels of the cardiac glycosides; others have found the opposite response. It is generally accepted that the cardiac arrhythmias which occur in response to toxic doses of glycosides are partly due to enhanced sympathetic activity. Within the parasympathetic nervous system the picture is clearer and the increased activity of this system in the presence of glycosides is well documented.

Toxicity
Digitalis glycosides have a very low margin of safety and only remain in use because they are effective in the management of a life-threatening disease. Cases of poisoning of livestock after eating foxglove are rare, probably because

of the odour and bitter taste of the plant. The earliest signs of toxicity often involve the gastrointestinal tract and include anorexia, vomiting and diarrhoea. These effects are initiated in the central nervous system rather than directly on the gastrointestinal tract. Vomiting is due to the stimulation of the chemoreceptor trigger zone in the area postrema of the medulla, although local irritation of the gastric mucosa may also contribute to the response.

All types of cardiac arrhythmia have been known to occur in response to toxic doses of digitalis glycosides. Vagal stimulation causes slowing of the SA node and slowing of conduction along AV junctional tissue. This is seen electrocardiographically as prolongation of the P-R interval. Furthermore there is increased sympathetic drive, diminished SA and atrial refractory period, increased AV refractory period and slowed impulse conduction. Thus overdosage commonly causes initial AV lengthening and then AV block or marked sinus bradycardia. Inhibition of cardiac Na^+,K^+-ATPase, by reducing $[K^+]_i$, reduces resting membrane potential to a less negative value, which leads to an increase in excitability. Thus the incidence of cardiac arrhythmias is increased in patients with hypokalaemia. The most frequent ventricular arrhythmias associated with digitalis toxicity involve premature depolarizations, which result in a bigeminal (or trigeminal) rhythm or ventricular tachycardia. Increased automaticity in the ventricular conduction system leads to ectopic ventricular beats. Ventricular fibrillation may follow. Propranolol and lignocaine (see below) are used to treat glycoside-induced arrhythmias.

Kinetics

Absorption of both digoxin and digitoxin from the gastrointestinal tract is quite variable, although digitoxin is generally better absorbed than digoxin. Administration of the drugs in elixir form generally results in more uniform absorption than from tablets. Since the formulation of the drug (either elixir or tablets) is of major importance in achieving a reliable degree of absorption, it is especially important that a particular brand is selected and adhered to. Distribution of the glycosides is complete within about 10 hours. Digitoxin is extensively bound to plasma proteins (about 90 per cent), digoxin much less so (about 25 per cent).

Plasma levels of digoxin in the range of 1.4–3.1 nmol/l (when the sample is taken 8 hours after last dose) have been found to be associated with therapeutic effects, but maintaining plasma levels of 2.1–2.9 nmol/l should give adequate effects without risk of toxicity.

Metabolism of digitoxin and, to a lesser extent, digoxin occurs after uptake into the liver. The metabolites and parent glycosides can then undergo enterohepatic recycling where they are excreted into the bile and subsequently reabsorbed. Biliary excretion appears to be important for the elimination of digitoxin whereas excretion of digoxin is through the kidneys. In the presence of renal disease, excretion is greatly diminished and the dose of drug needs to be adjusted accordingly.

The half-life of digoxin varies considerably but is usually found to be between 24 and 40 hours. This gives rise to serious risks of cumulative toxicity and also means that once toxic blood levels of the drug are reached, it may take some time before they fall significantly. Although some research suggests that the half-life of digitoxin is about 13 hours, results from other studies indicate that it may be as long as 48 hours. This variation may reflect the technical difficulties associated with such experiments, but also emphasizes the need for awareness of significant differences in the responses of different animals to the cardiac glycosides and the need for careful monitoring of each individual patient.

Dose

Digoxin

Digoxin has a narrow therapeutic ratio and furthermore there is considerable biological variation in patient response, thus a precise dose has to be determined for each patient. Doses are usually quoted in mg/kg and, because of the fluid retention associated with heart failure, it is important to use the lean bodyweight of the animal in the calculation of dose.

Paediatric elixir of Lanoxin is most uniformly absorbed and allows more accurate dosing for small animals. Otherwise 62.5 μg tablets allow most accurate dosage.

Rapid oral digitalization

In order to hasten the onset of effect, 'digitalization' or 'loading' can be practised. This involves the administration of large doses of drug, divided into several smaller doses and administered at frequent intervals over 1 or 2 days. The patient should be at cage rest and under close supervision. Except in extremely urgent cases, loading is of doubtful value and the practice of giving the drugs to toxicity and then reducing the dose is unnecessary and dangerous.

dog   0.02 mg/kg every 8 hours until digitalization is achieved, which is usually within 2–3 days. This is indicated by a slowed heart rate, diuresis and amelioration of cough and dyspnoea. Administration should cease for 24 hours and then be resumed on a maintenance level of approximately 0.01 mg/kg twice daily.

horse   Approximate digitalizing doses of digoxin for horses are 0.07 mg/kg p.o. or 0.014 mg/kg i.v.

Maintenance

The glycosides are only slowly excreted and therefore the daily dose required to maintain adequate plasma levels is relatively small. When therapy is initiated with the maintenance dose (0.01 mg/kg every 12 hours), it may take up to 10 days for the blood levels to reach steady state and for the full effect of the drug to be manifest. However, this dosage technique is much safer and is adequate in the majority of cases, since initial therapy with frusemide is usually instituted. Digoxin may then be used concurrently, after assessing the response to frusemide (see 'Therapy of congestive heart failure' below).

dog	0.01 mg/kg p.o. every 12 hours. A lower dose is suggested for giant breeds. It is important to note that in all cases, due to the low margin of safety and the natural variation in response between animals, dosage must be adjusted for each patient and the figures quoted here are a guide only. It may be preferable to calculate dosage according to body surface area, at a rate of 220 μg/m^2 b.i.d.
cat	cats are more sensitive to the toxic effects of digitalis glycosides. They require approximately half the dose rate in dogs (i.e. 2–4 μg/kg/day, or 10 μg/kg every 48 hours) and not more than a total dose of 0.05 mg/day.
horse	0.007 mg/kg/day i.v. 0.035 mg/kg/day p.o.

Digitoxin

The doses quoted in the literature vary considerably, with the lower end of the range at about 0.005 mg/kg/day and the upper end of the range at 0.1 mg/kg/day. A starting dose of 0.05 mg/kg/day should be used in the first instance and the patient observed carefully for about 10 days until the full effect develops. If there has been no improvement, and in the absence of toxicity, the dose can be slowly increased to 0.1 mg/kg/day. Unlike digoxin, digitoxin is distributed in body fat and thus the dose should be calculated on true bodyweight.

Xanthine derivatives

The xanthine alkaloids caffeine, theophylline and theobromine are all capable of producing some degree of cardiac and central nervous system stimulation as well as having bronchodilator and diuretic effects. Theophylline is the most potent cardiac stimulant but, like the other members of the group, it has a low solubility and various derivatives have been developed and are available for veterinary use. Aminophylline is the product of the complex of theophylline and ethylene diamine. Other derivatives of aminophylline include etamiphylline and diprophylline.

Mode of action

The mode of action of the methylxanthines as both cardiac stimulants and bronchodilators is still a matter for debate. There are a number of known actions of these drugs which could account for their observed effects. Theophylline is known to increase cyclic AMP levels, to alter the movements of intracellular Ca^{2+}, to inhibit the cardiac depressant actions of adenosine and to increase the release of catecholamines from the sympathetic nervous system. It may be that one or more of these actions will eventually prove to be responsible for the clinical effects of the drugs.

Actions

Theophylline administration results in an increase in heart rate and force of cardiac contraction which, in animals with heart failure, increases cardiac output. The positive inotropic effect is augmented by a reduction in peripheral resistance, due to the vasodilator action of the drug. Blood flow to most organs is increased while the work of the heart is decreased. Relaxation of smooth muscle at other sites also occurs, notably the bronchioles. The peripheral bronchodilator effect is accompanied by some degree of respiratory stimulation associated with stimulation of medullary respiratory centres. Although there is some doubt about the effect of the methylxanthines on renal perfusion in animals with heart failure, it is quite clear that they exert a clinically significant diuretic effect, with appreciable losses of Na^+ and Cl^-.

Dose

aminophylline
  dog, cat   5–10 mg/kg p.o. or i.v. 2–3 times per day

etamiphylline camsylate
  horse, cattle   900 mg p.o., t.i.d.
                      1.4 g s.c. or i.m.
  calf, sheep   300–600 mg p.o.; repeat 4-hourly if necessary
                      0.7–1 g s.c. or i.m. up to 3 times per day
  dog, cat   100–300 mg p.o.; repeat 8-hourly if necessary
                      140–700 mg s.c. or i.m.; repeat 8-hourly if necessary
                      200–500 mg p.r.

diprophylline
  small animals   125–500 mg i.m. or slow i.v.; repeat 8-hourly
                      200–400 mg p.o.; repeat 4–8 hourly
  large animals   1–2 g i.m. or slow i.v.; repeat 8-hourly

β-*Adrenoceptor agonists*

Although both adrenaline and isoprenaline are potent cardiac stimulants and are useful for resuscitation after cardiac arrest, there are a number of reasons why they are of little use in the management of chronic heart failure. Being catecholamines, they are rapidly metabolized by monoamine oxidase in the gut and hence they need to be parenterally administered. They have a short duration of action, they increase heart rate and oxygen consumption and are likely to cause arrhythmias. In the case of adrenaline there is the added hazard of an increased peripheral resistance adding to the load on the failing heart muscle.

Dobutamine, a synthetic adrenoceptor agonist, stimulates the force of contraction of the heart with less chronotropic effect. Furthermore, it is less arrhythmogenic than adrenaline and isoprenaline. Dobutamine must be administered by intravenous injection so long-term use is impractical. It is useful for emergency treatment of heart failure and particularly in human patients with acute myocardial infarction who also have congestive heart failure. There are numerous reports of the effects of dobutamine in experimental animals (especially dogs) but little information about its use in veterinary clinical situations.

Alternative approaches to the treatment of cardiac failure

Angiotensin-converting enzyme inhibitors

Increased activity of the renin-angiotensin system is a well-recognized factor in the body's response to heart failure. It is clear that elevated plasma renin activity is associated with generation of increased amounts of angiotensin II, which then increases peripheral resistance and, by the release of aldosterone, increases Na^+ and water retention. These changes impose an increased workload on the already compromised heart and hasten the deterioration of cardiac function. In recent years there has been a change in the approach to the treatment of heart failure and it is becoming more common to attempt to reduce the load on the heart, rather than to try to stimulate the failing muscle. An effective way to reduce cardiac work is to reduce the activity of the renin-angiotensin-aldosterone system. Cage rest alone may reduce activation of the system but if this is not sufficient, the production of angiotensin II can be inhibited by compounds known as angiotensin-converting enzyme (ACE) inhibitors. At the time of writing, three compounds with clinically useful actions are available—captopril, enalapril and lisinopril. Although the use of ACE inhibitors is still relatively new to veterinary medicine, because of promising results from human studies, their use in humans is increasing and it is quite likely that a similar trend will occur in veterinary medicine.

Mode of action

The inhibition of ACE reduces levels of angiotensin II, thus peripheral resistance is reduced and cardiac workload decreases. Lower angiotensin levels also reduce the release of aldosterone and thereby reduce renal Na^+ reabsorption. The ACE inhibitors have no effects on any other component of the renin–angiotensin system.

Actions

The drugs have no direct effect on the heart or blood vessels; their beneficial effects are due to the reduced cardiac load and increased Na^+ excretion which result from the inhibition of formation of angiotensin II. Plasma renin activity may rise as the renin–angiotensin system attempts to restore homeostasis. Since ACE is also responsible for the hydrolysis of bradykinin, the actions of this autacoid may be prolonged. It is doubtful whether the enhanced actions of bradykinin are of clinical significance.

Side-effects

The most common problem associated with the administration of ACE inhibitors to patients with heart failure is a marked fall in blood pressure, usually associated with the first dose. This is likely to be worse in patients which have been previously treated with diuretics which can stimulate activity in the renin-angiotensin system. The risks can be reduced by starting treatment with small doses and slowly increasing the dose levels.

Dose

captopril   0.25–2.0 mg/kg p.o., t.i.d.

Vasodilators

Other ways to reduce the workload of the failing heart are reduction of cardiac preload, by use of venodilators, or reduction of afterload, by the use of drugs which dilate arterioles. As in the case of ACE inhibitors, the use of these drugs is becoming more common, both in human and veterinary medicine. The clinician can choose between drugs which have a direct effect on the blood vessels, like hydralazine, or those which exert their effect by inhibiting the vasoconstrictor effects of noradrenaline, like prazosin.

Mode of action

Hydralazine acts as a vasodilator, directly on the smooth muscle of blood vessels, and is more effective on the arteriolar side of the circulation. Prazosin is a selective, competitive antagonist at α_1-adrenoceptors, found in both veins and arteries.

Actions

The arteriolar vasodilation produced by hydralazine causes a reduction of peripheral resistance. Compensatory responses to this action include tachycardia and increased plasma renin activity. Prazosin produces a fall in both arteriolar and venous resistance. This is achieved by inhibiting the vasoconstrictor effects of noradrenaline, released by the sympathetic nervous system in an attempt to compensate for the reduced cardiac output. Although there is some reflexly mediated effort to restore blood pressure, prazosin is less likely to increase heart rate than hydralazine. Vasodilator therapy must be instituted carefully, since it has been observed in dogs, as in humans, that the first dose may cause sudden collapse.

Dose

| hydralazine | 0.5–2 mg/kg b.i.d. |
| prazosin | 0.02–0.1 mg/kg b.i.d. |

Diuretics

The pharmacology of the diuretics is described in Chapter 12. They are used in the management of congestive cardiac failure because the loss of water that they induce reduces the load on the failing heart muscle (see below). Frusemide is the preferred drug.

Dose

frusemide
   dog   initially 2–5 mg/kg daily, in divided doses, for several days, followed by gradual reduction to the minimal dose required to limit signs of congestion.

Therapy of congestive heart failure

The treatment of congestive heart failure is generally restricted to dogs, and occasionally horses and cats, but treatment of food animals is not considered to be economically viable. Restriction of exercise, in some cases with enforced cage rest, is an important aspect of therapy as animals with congestive heart failure may be restless and dyspnoeic with cardiac output requirements beyond the compensatory reserves. Where sedation is indicated, morphine appears to be the narcotic of choice in the dog (0.2–0.5 mg/kg s.c. up to 3 times per day) and it has been suggested that it may increase cardiac output. It will also aid in suppressing a persistent cough if this is not relieved with proper use of cardiac stimulants, diuretics and bronchodilators.

The owner should be educated to feed the appropriate diet to restrict the animal's sodium intake; canned and dried food should be avoided. An appropriate diet would be home-cooked skeletal meat, vegetables and rice or pasta. Salt-free seasonings can be added if unpalatability is a problem.

In addition to dietary management and restriction of exercise, most patients with decompensated congestive heart failure will require treatment with one or more of the drugs described above. It will be appreciated that the pharmacology of some of these drugs is complex and somewhat controversial. Similarly, there are differing views about the therapeutic management of these patients and the following summary is intended to provide guidelines based on a consensus of opinion.

1. In relatively mild cases, one of the xanthine derivatives (etamiphylline or diprophylline) is used by some clinicians. They are less potent inotropic agents than the digitalis glycosides and, indeed, many clinicians consider them to be rather impotent in practice. However, in the emergency treatment of heart failure, slow intravenous injection of a xanthine derivative will produce an immediate, although transient, increase in cardiac output. They are effective bronchodilators and are widely used for this effect in the treatment of more severe cases of congestive heart failure, in conjunction with drugs which have more potent actions on the cardiovascular system.

2. When the patient is more severely decompensated, the use of diuretics is the first line of treatment of many clinicians. Frusemide and the less potent thiazides promote loss of Na^+ and water, which rapidly reduces the circulatory volume overload. Cardiac efficiency is thereby improved and some patients do not require additional therapy. This is particularly useful when digitalis glycosides are poorly tolerated (especially in cats).

   Thiazides cause K^+ loss which reduces $[K^+]_i$ and thereby potentiates the therapeutic effects and the potential arrhythmogenicity of digitalis glycosides used concurrently. The more potent drug, frusemide, is favoured by many clinicians. K^+ loss does not appear to be a problem using the drug at the recommended oral dose of 2–5 mg/kg daily in divided doses and reducing this to the minimum necessary to maintain an improved cardiac performance. However, frusemide may also potentiate the therapeutic and toxic effects of digitalis glycosides by increasing the plasma concentration of the glycosides, apparently by interfering with their excretion.

   Frusemide, administered intravenously, is effective in the emergency treatment of congestive heart failure, as an alternative to an intravenous xanthine derivative. The rapid diuresis reduces the circulatory overload, but the prompt effectiveness is probably also due to venodilation and consequently reduced preload induced by the drug.

3. Although there is still some debate about the value of the digitalis glycosides in the management of animals with heart failure, they are still the most commonly used drugs for this condition in dogs and horses, with digoxin being the drug of choice from this group. Cats are particularly sensitive to the toxic effects of the glycosides and their use is best avoided in this species. Treatment with diuretics is preferred.

The major problem associated with the use of digoxin and like drugs is the very low margin of safety; the veterinarian needs to monitor patients carefully, especially during the initial weeks of therapy while dosage is being adjusted to suit individual animals. Digoxin is often used with frusemide after the effects of the initial therapy with diuretics have been assessed. As explained above, the potency of digoxin is thereby increased and dosage must be carefully adjusted according to the response. With proper monitoring, this combination of drugs is effective and is probably the most common approach to the therapy of congestive heart failure.

Problems of digoxin toxicity can be minimized with careful practice and awareness of factors that predispose to toxic reactions. In addition to the potentiating effect of concurrent diuretic therapy, old age, myocarditis, severe heart disease, renal failure, hypothyroidism, anoxia, hypernatraemia, hypercalcaemia (by increasing Ca^{2+} entry into the cells and so facilitating excitation contraction coupling), hypomagnesaemia, alkalosis and corticosteroids may also exacerbate toxicity.

If toxicity does occur, the drug should be withdrawn and cage rest instituted. These measures are usually effective in controlling cardiac arrhythmias and other signs of intoxication. If these procedures are unsuccessful, specific anti-arrhythmic therapy is indicated.

4. β-Adrenoceptor antagonists have been used together with cardiac glycosides for the control of tachycardia, especially where there is atrial fibrillation or suspected cardiomyopathy. In dogs, propranolol is the drug most commonly used (up to 1 mg/kg t.i.d., p.o.). The reduction in oxygen consumption which results from reduced contractility may also be beneficial. Furthermore, since the sympathetic nervous system plays a permissive role in the arrhythmias which occur with digitalis toxicity, blockade of the β-adrenoceptors may protect the heart from this toxic effect. However, it should be remembered that blockade of cardiac β-adrenoceptors reduces the support from the sympathetic nervous system and there is a risk of exacerbation of congestive heart failure. This problem can be minimized by ensuring that diuretics have been administered to reduce fluid accumulation and that the animals are adequately digitalized.

5. The alternative and relatively new method of management of congestive heart failure does not utilize cardiac stimulants to induce the failing,

overloaded myocardium to work harder. Restriction of exercise and salt intake and the use of diuretics to reduce the circulatory overload are part of the modern therapeutic approach. In addition, further reduction of the workload of the failing heart is achieved by the use of vasodilators or ACE inhibitors as described above.

The results achieved by some veterinary cardiologists using these techniques are extremely encouraging, but more clinical evidence is required before they can be properly assessed against traditional lines of therapy.

Acute cardiac emergencies

Rapid responses are required when cardiac arrest, partial or complete AV block or Stokes–Adams syndrome occur. The potent β-adrenoceptor agonists are generally used in these cases. Because they are rapidly metabolized, administration by slow i.v. drip is necessary. In cases of cardiac arrest, where physical means are unable to start the heart, intracardiac injection may be necessary. Once the heartbeat is restored, adrenaline or isoprenaline infusion can be commenced. When the patient is stable and a satisfactory level of cardiac performance has been achieved, further doses can be given by intramuscular injection.

Dose

Cardiac arrest
  adrenaline
    dog   50–100 μg intracardiac
  isoprenaline
    dog   20–40 μg intracardiac

Acute cardiac failure
  adrenaline
    horse, cattle   4–8 μg/kg s.c. or i.m.
                 2–4 μg/kg slow i.v.
    dog   0.5–15 μg/kg s.c., i.m. or slow i.v.

  dobutamine
    dog   2–7 μg/kg/min

Treatment of cardiac arrhythmias

Cardiac arrhythmias may arise from disturbances in the rate, regularity or site of origin of cardiac impulses or from abnormal conduction which alters the sequence of atrial and ventricular activation. One of the main factors involved in the genesis of arrhythmias is increased activity in pacemaker cells. This is often associated with changes in autonomic activity, electrolyte disturbances, trauma, disturbances of acid–base balance and a number of disease states.

The action potential from spontaneously depolarizing cells exhibits a characteristic slow depolarization which, by convention, is called Phase 4. When the membrane potential reaches threshold, rapid depolarization, Phase 0, occurs. The mechanism by which this depolarization is effected relies on a sudden, brief increase in the permeability of the cell to Na^+, which then enters through the 'fast Na^+ channels'. Repolarization of the cell occurs during Phases 1, 2 and 3 and is associated with movement of K^+ out of the cell. During Phase 2 there is also movement of Ca^{2+} into the cell through the 'slow' channels. During repolarization the cell is refractory until it has repolarized below the threshold potential.

Similar action potentials can be recorded from cells in atrial conduction fibres, the AV node and Purkinje fibres. These automatic cells are normally dominated by the pacemaker cells of the SA node, which reach threshold potential first. Where the rate of firing of the automatic cells at other sites exceeds that of the SA node, an ectopic pacemaker is established and the normal rhythm is disturbed.

Abnormal impulse conduction can also cause arrhythmic contraction. Circus movement may cause re-entry phenomena when the combined circumstances of action potential duration, conduction velocity and refractory period allow the impulse to continuously re-excite an area of heart muscle. These changes result in irregular contractions which, in the case of ventricular function, cause haemodynamic instability. Drugs used in the treatment of cardiac arrhythmias should, ideally, block the abnormal initiation and propagation of impulses without significantly affecting normal cardiac function.

Drugs with anti-arrhythmic activity are divided into four classes. The division is based on their mechanism of action.

Class 1 anti-arrhythmic drugs

The anti-arrhythmic action of the drugs in this group is associated with their ability to reduce the rate of entry of Na^+ into the cell, restricting the sodium-dependent component of the inward current and thus the maximum rate of depolarization (Phase 0). They also slow the rate of diastolic depolarization

(Phase 4), which will reduce the rate of firing of pacemaker cells. The beneficial effects are enhanced by the increase in refractory period that occurs with the administration of these drugs. Some of the drugs in this group are also used as local anaesthetics and it is most likely that similar effects on the Na$^+$ channels in nerves are responsible for this action.

Quinidine

Quinidine (Fig. 10.5) is the dextrorotary isomer of quinine, a naturally occurring alkaloid from the bark of the cinchona tree. Quinidine has anti-malarial activity similar to that of quinine, but its anti-arrhythmic activity is greater.

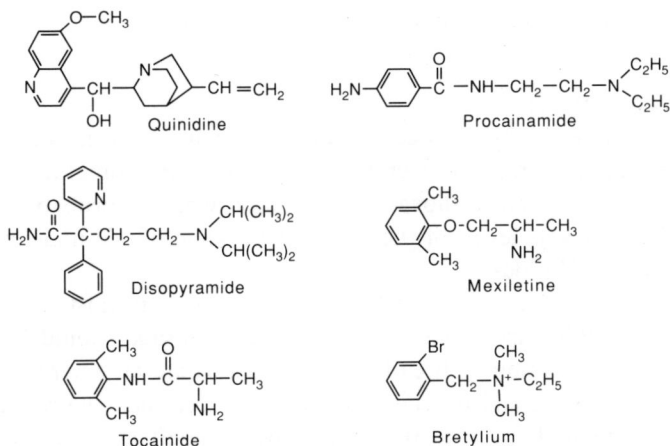

Figure 10.5 Anti-arrhythmic drugs.

Actions

Quinidine is the prototype of Class 1 anti-arrhythmics and as such it slows the rate of diastolic depolarization and the maximum rate of depolarization in the action potential. Membrane responsiveness is reduced, thus the threshold for depolarization is raised. The effect on the spontaneous depolarization of the SA node is less marked than that at other sites and ectopic pacemakers can therefore be controlled with little effect on the normal pacemaker. Conduction through the AV node and the bundle of His is slowed and this is reflected in an increase in P-R interval and wider QRS complexes in the ECG. Quinidine also produces some degree of vagal blockade. It increases the effective refractory period and this direct effect is enhanced by its vagolytic activity.

Heart rate changes induced by quinidine are variable. In the treatment of atrial flutter or fibrillation there may be an increase in ventricular rate as atrial rate is slowed and more effective impulses can enter the ventricles.

Paroxysmal atrial or ventricular tachycardia and multiple ventricular ectopic beats in dogs may be treated with quinidine. The drug converts only occasional cases of atrial flutter and fibrillation (of very recent onset) to normal sinus rhythm. Quinidine appears to be more effective in the therapy of atrial fibrillation in horses.

Kinetics

After oral administration the peak effect is reached after 1–3 hours. Peak effect can be reached at 30–90 minutes after intramuscular injection. The rates of metabolism and excretion vary between species. The duration of action is between 6 and 8 hours.

Side-effects and toxicity

In dogs, gastrointestinal side-effects include anorexia, vomiting and diarrhoea. Because the drug is rapidly excreted large doses are sometimes required. These may cause sudden cardiovascular collapse, which is probably associated with very high plasma levels of the drug. Depression of AV node conduction can progress to AV block.

Erythema and oedema of the nasal mucosa occurs in most horses treated with quinidine. The reaction is dose-related and dosage should be adjusted accordingly or restriction of breathing may necessitate an emergency tracheostomy. Laminitis may also occur and requires treatment with cortisone to prevent permanent damage to the feet. Other side-effects in horses include gastrointestinal disturbances, similar to those seen in the dog, and urticarial wheals.

Quinidine is contraindicated in cases of SA, AV or intraventricular block. The negative inotropic effect of quinidine exacerbates the problems of decompensated congestive heart failure and it should not be used in cases of severely depressed myocardial function. No Class 1 anti-arrhythmic is safe for use in cats.

Plasma concentrations of digoxin have been shown to increase when quinidine is added to the dose regime of animals previously stabilized on digoxin, giving rise to the possibility of the development of toxicity.

Dose

dog	6–10 mg/kg every 4–8 hours p.o.
horse	A test dose of 5 g is administered on day 1. If the drug is tolerated, 10 g, 3 times daily is administered on day 2. The

10 g dose is given 4 times daily on days 3 and 4. This dose should be sufficient in most cases, but can be increased to 10 g, 7 times daily, on days 5 and 6 and, if necessary, to 10 g, 8 times daily, for the next 2 days. Quinidine has an extremely bitter taste and, after suspending the powder in water, needs to be administered by stomach tube.

Procainamide

Procainamide is similar to the local anaesthetic procaine, but it has an amide link (Fig. 10.5) which reduces metabolism in the blood and allows a more prolonged duration of action.

Actions

The electrophysiological effects of procainamide are very similar to those of quinidine, although it may have less myocardial depressant effect at high doses. As with quinidine, a paradoxical increase in left ventricular rate can occur in the treatment of atrial flutter and fibrillation. Procainamide also has a slight parasympatholytic effect and can cause some degree of ganglion blockade in the dog.

Side-effects and toxicity

If the drug is administered intravenously, care should be taken to monitor blood pressure as the vasodilator activity can cause hypotension. Noradrenaline can be used to maintain blood pressure in these cases. Besides hypotension, toxicity may be manifest as gastrointestinal effects (nausea, anorexia and vomiting), central nervous system depression or ventricular tachycardia and asystole. The dosage should be discontinued if gastrointestinal side-effects occur. The use of procainamide is contraindicated in SA, AV or intraventricular block.

Kinetics

After oral administration there is complete absorption of the dose and maximal effects occur within 1 hour. Excretion occurs via the kidneys and dose reduction may be necessary in cases of renal impairment.

Dose

dog   125–500 mg every 4–6 hours p.o.

Lignocaine

Lignocaine is commonly used as a local anaesthetic and many of the commercially available preparations contain adrenaline, which prolongs the duration of action of the local anaesthetic by virtue of its vasoconstrictor activity. It is most important that solutions of lignocaine *without* adrenaline are used in the management of cardiac arrhythmias.

Actions
Lignocaine depresses the excitability and automaticity of ventricular tissue, with much less effect in atrial tissue. There is an increase in the effective refractory period relative to the action potential duration. Cardiac depressant activity has been demonstrated, although this may not be clinically significant at therapeutic blood levels. Its rapid onset of action makes it a most useful drug for dealing with emergency situations.

Side-effects and toxicity
Toxic doses of lignocaine may cause central nervous system stimulation, with convulsions in extreme cases. In the cardiovascular system, bradycardia and hypotension may occur. SA, AV or intraventricular block, or excessive prolongation of P-R interval or QRS complex, represent contraindications for the use of lignocaine.

Kinetics
Although lignocaine is well absorbed after oral administration, the first-pass metabolism by the liver results in low and variable blood levels. Furthermore, gastrointestinal side-effects are more likely after oral dosing and therefore intravenous administration is generally used. The metabolites of lignocaine are excreted by the kidneys.

Dose

Lignocaine is always administered by intravenous injection or infusion. An acute bolus dose of 2–5 mg/kg is administered over 1–2 minutes; it may be repeated at 20-minute intervals. For infusion, the rate is 25-75 μg/kg/min.

Disopyramide

Some of the actions of disopyramide (Fig. 10.5) are similar to those of quinidine; others are like lignocaine. The anti-arrhythmic efficacy of disopyramide is similar to that of quinidine but it is less likely to cause loss of appetite and disturbance of gastrointestinal function. It is more effective in ventricular arrhythmias.

Dose

dog   50–200 mg t.i.d.

Phenytoin

Like lignocaine, phenytoin increases the duration of the effective refractory period relative to that of the action potential. Automaticity of the Purkinje fibres is depressed.

Side-effects and toxicity
Toxic doses may cause hypotension, reduced heart rate or even cardiac arrest. Central nervous system manifestations of toxicity include drowsiness, ataxia and nausea.

Dose

dog   4–8 mg/kg, 3-4 times daily
       up to 5 mg/kg i.v. over several minutes

A number of newer drugs, which by their mode of action are classified as Class 1 anti-arrhythmics, are available for human use. Mexiletine and tocainide (Fig. 10.5) have actions very similar to those of lignocaine. Tocainide has been used in dogs (10-20 mg/kg t.i.d., p.o.) but, as yet, there is insufficient evidence to assess its usefulness. Encainide and flecainide selectively depress the fast Na^+ channel and produce marked depression of Phase 0, more so than any other drugs of this group. It is possible that these new agents may find a place in veterinary medicine.

Class 2 anti-arrhythmic drugs

β-Adrenoceptor antagonists exert anti-arrhythmic activity in situations where the activity of the sympathetic nervous system contributes significantly to the arrhythmia. Although the prototype drug of this class, propranolol, has local anaesthetic activity, this is only significant at very high doses and the clinical usefulness of these drugs as anti-arrhythmics is clearly due to blockade of β-adrenoceptors.

Actions

Blockade of cardiac β-adrenoceptors substantially increases the refractory period of the AV node and reduces automaticity of the Purkinje fibres, particularly when this is increased by catecholamines. The effective refractory period relative to the action potential duration is lengthened. In high doses propranolol has some ability to block Na^+ channels but this, like its local anaesthetic action, is probably not clinically significant.

Side-effects and toxicity

Large doses may cause severe cardiac depression, hypotension or bradycardia. These problems are increased in the presence of heart or lung dysfunction. Where pulmonary disease occurs, even the use of selective β_1-adrenoceptor antagonists should be carefully considered as these agents are selective, rather than specific.

Dose

propranolol   0.1–1 mg/kg p.o., t.i.d.

Class 3 anti-arrhythmic drugs

Drugs which prolong repolarization and thus prolong the action potential are grouped in this class.

Bretylium

The classification of bretylium (Fig. 10.5) as an adrenergic neurone-blocking agent is based on its ability to inhibit the release of noradrenaline from sympathetic nerve terminals. Its anti-arrhythmic activity, however, is thought to depend on the prolongation of the action potential and of the refractory period it induces, rather than its anti-adrenergic effects. The drug is not widely used in veterinary medicine.

Amiodarone

This drug has anti-arrhythmic effects similar to those of bretylium.

Class 4 anti-arrhythmic drugs

This group includes the drugs which are described as 'calcium antagonists'. Their anti-arrhythmic activity depends on the blockade of the entry of Ca^{2+} into cardiac cells through the slow Ca^{2+} channels. Drugs of this type have been used in dogs, but with little obvious success.

Verapamil

Verapamil inhibits the transmembrane flux of Ca^{2+} through the slow Ca^{2+} channels. Because the normal function of the SA and AV nodes depends on this movement of Ca^{2+}, the rate of discharge and conduction velocity in these tissues is depressed. The refractory period on the AV node is increased.

Verapamil is liable to depress force of contraction, thus great care is needed in patients with left ventricular dysfunction. AV nodal effects of verapamil are potent and therefore patients with AV block should not receive it.

Dose

dog   0.05–0.15 mg/kg i.v. over 2 min

           1-5 mg/kg p.o. t.i.d.

Cardiac glycosides

The cardiac glycosides have a variety of actions which contribute to their anti-arrhythmic effects. The most important of these is probably the action of the drugs on conduction through the AV node. By increasing the AV nodal refractory period, fewer atrial action potentials are allowed to reach the ventricles and the ventricular rate is reduced. This effect is of benefit in atrial flutter and fibrillation. The increase in vagal tone and reduced sympathetic activity in animals with heart failure which have received digitalis also reduces the tendency to arrhythmias. Irrespective of the type of arrhythmia, these are the drugs of first choice where congestive heart failure is involved.

Therapeutic applications of anti-arrhythmic drugs

Supraventricular arrhythmias

Sinus bradycardia can be considered to occur when the heart rate is significantly below that which would be expected in an animal of that size and breed. In horses these low heart rates may be accompanied by second degree partial AV block or sinus node exit block, which usually disappear when heart rate increases. Such arrhythmias require no treatment, since there are no other clinical signs. When patients are presented with associated signs of weakness or syncope, atropine or glycopyrronium have been used successfully to antagonize excessive vagal tone. Since atropine and glycopyrronium have other parasympatholytic effects, some clinicians prefer to use a sympathomimetic such as isoprenaline when longer-term treatment is necessary. It should be noted, however, that occasional sudden deaths (possibly due to ventricular fibrillation) have been reported with long-term use of isoprenaline.

Heartblocks (sino-atrial or atrioventricular) may be associated with digitalis intoxication and the first line of treatment is withdrawal and adjustment of the dose. Where specific anti-arrhythmic therapy is necessary, isoprenaline or atropine would again be the drugs of choice, although atropine appears to be less effective than in sinus bradycardia. In patients with congestive heart failure, isoprenaline is the drug of choice.

Severe bradyarrhythmias in dogs have been successfully controlled by the permanent implantation of cardiac pacemakers.

Dose

dog

atropine	0.05–0.1 mg/kg s.c.
glycopyrrolate	0.01 mg/kg i.m.
isoprenaline	5–10 mg up to 3 times daily, p.o.

Supraventricular tachycardias can often be temporarily relieved by applying pressure to the carotid sinus or eyeball, which increases vagal tone. When the tachycardia is due to congestive heart failure, treatment of the underlying condition, as previously described, is likely to restore normal rhythms.

Atrial or sinus tachycardia, in the absence of heart failure, can be effectively treated with propranolol, which will increase the refractory period of the AV node and decrease the automaticity of the SA node.

Atrial fibrillation is not catastrophic *per se*, but it reduces ventricular filling and therefore cardiac output. In dogs it is not readily restored to sinus rhythm and is commonly associated with signs of congestive heart failure. Initial therapy is aimed at relieving the heart failure with digoxin and diuretics. Digoxin, besides increasing the force of contraction, slows the ventricular rate by vagal and extravagal mechanisms, but does not cure atrial fibrillation. Propranolol may be used with digoxin if the latter does not sufficiently reduce the ventricular rate. By itself, propranolol may induce heart failure by preventing sympathetic support to a compromised myocardium. Dogs with atrial fibrillation may survive usefully for several years with this therapy, even though the fibrillation persists.

Quinidine is used, probably more commonly than any other drug, to attempt to restore sinus rhythm. Although the success rate in dogs is low (the arrhythmia must be of very recent origin for the drug to be effective), it is more effective in horses. It is important to note that a paradoxical increase in ventricular rate may occur when the atrial rate is decreased to the point when more of the atrial impulses can be conducted by the AV node to the ventricles. This effect is exacerbated by the vagolytic effect of quinidine, which causes an enhancement of AV conduction. It is usual, therefore, to 'protect' the ventricles by pretreatment with digoxin, which depresses AV conduction.

Electrical defibrillation causes conversion to sinus rhythm in some cases, but atrial fibrillation usually recurs. Some clinicians administer quinidine before electrical defibrillation and maintain therapy for several weeks if conversion is successful.

Ventricular tachyarrhythmias

These require careful assessment (including ECG) to determine the cause and to treat that if possible, before attempting specific anti-arrhythmic therapy. Ventricular tachycardia is a serious arrhythmia because it may be prefibrillatory. The arrhythmia may be associated with congestive heart failure and respond to therapy previously described for that disease. It may be a sign of endocarditis, congenital cardiac defects or cardiomyopathies. Extrinsic systemic conditions such as hyperthyroidism (thyroid tumour or iatrogenic), hypokalaemia (losses from the gut or prolonged therapy with thiazides), hypocalcaemia and hypoxia may all induce ventricular tachycardia. Toxic doses of digitalis glycosides can induce ventricular tachyarrhythmias, in which case the drug should be withdrawn for reassessment of dosage.

Documented clinical evidence on the relative efficacy of drugs in suppressing ventricular tachyarrhythmias in dogs is rather limited, but the following points give some guidelines for drug selection.

Lignocaine (without adrenaline) is the drug of choice for acute arrhythmias. It must be administered i.v. and is only effective for about 20 minutes, so that other drugs must be used where a long-term effect is required. Of these, procainamide and quinidine have been the most widely used, the former apparently being the more common choice. These may be superseded by the newer drugs disopyramide and tocainide if further clinical reports are favourable.

Phenytoin, lignocaine and β-adrenoceptor antagonists are useful in the management of digitalis-induced arrhythmias and it has been suggested that phenytoin does not interfere with the positive inotropic action of the glycosides.

β-Adrenoceptor antagonists can be effective in extrasystoles and tachycardia of ventricular origin. In cases where excessive sympathetic nervous system activity or sensitization of the myocardium to catecholamines is known to contribute to the arrhythmia (e.g. in the presence of halogenated anaesthetics, myocardial infarction, digitalis overdose), these agents are obviously of use. It has been suggested that propranolol is the only anti-arrhythmic agent which is safe for use in cats and is therefore recommended for the treatment of feline idiopathic cardiomyopathy.

CHAPTER 11

FLUID THERAPY

Two-thirds of bodyweight is composed of water, although this varies with the fat content of the body and with age. Of the total body water, two-thirds is intracellular and one-third is extracellular. The extracellular fraction comprises that which is intravascular (plasma), accounting for one-quarter, and the interstitial fluid, which accounts for the other three-quarters. There is a distinct difference between the chemical composition of extracellular and intracellular fluids. In the plasma and interstitial fluids (i.e. extracellular) the main cation is Na^+ and here HCO_3^- and Cl^- are the main anions. In the intracellular fluid K^+ is the main cation and organic PO_4^{3-} is the chief anion (Table 11.1).

Table 11.1 Electrolyte composition of body fluids

	Na^+	K^+	HCO_3^-	Cl^-	PO_4^{3-}
	(mmol/l)				
Plasma	135–145	3.5–5	24–28	98–106	1–2.5
Intracellular fluid (for muscle cell)	10	150	10		75

Water intake is controlled mainly by thirst, which is probably under the control of the hypothalamus. Water output occurs in four ways:

1. A significant amount of water is lost from the respiratory tract in animals which pant, such as the dog. In other species a variable amount of water is lost from the respiratory tract.

2. Water is lost from the skin, both by diffusion from its surface and through sweat. The amount lost from sweat varies from species to species and depends on the number of sweat glands in the skin.
3. Loss from the faeces—again this shows species variation and reflects the type of diet.
4. Loss of water from the kidneys—this is under the control of antidiuretic hormone, which is released from the neurohypophysis. Urinary losses in dogs, cats and most other domestic species amount to 20 ml/kg per day.

The water loss which occurs from the respiratory system, skin and faeces is known as the *inevitable loss* and amounts to about 20 ml/kg per day.

The healthy animal is able to maintain its fluid and electrolyte balance within the narrow limits of normality. Disease processes produce disturbances of both electrolyte and fluid balance, and the aim of therapy is to restore and maintain levels of water and electrolytes within normal limits.

The control of the main electrolytes, Na^+ and K^+, is less critical than that of water. It is mainly carried out by the kidneys, under the control of aldosterone, which regulates reabsorption of Na^+ and the excretion of K^+.

Assessment of fluid and electrolyte disturbance

There are a number of different disturbances of water and electrolyte metabolism which can occur in disease states in animals. In veterinary practice with a scarcity of laboratory facilities, the diagnosis of body fluid deficits is usually made on the case history and physical examination. Laboratory examinations can be carried out to confirm a diagnosis. The history of the food and water intake of any animal which is presented with suspected body fluid abnormality is essential. Urinary output and loss from the gastrointestinal tract should also be ascertained. A careful clinical examination is important in achieving a correct diagnosis.

No clinically detectable signs accompany losses of water of up to 5 per cent of total bodyweight. As the loss increases above about 7 per cent, the eyes sink into their sockets and skin elasticity is reduced. The severity of these signs increases with the degree of water loss. Examination of the state of the mucous membranes and the degree of filling of the peripheral veins and estimation of capillary refill time are also useful in assessing the clinical status of the animal. Circulatory collapse occurs as the loss approaches 15 per cent; a 20 per cent loss results in death.

Laboratory tests involve the examination of blood and urine. Routine haematology should be carried out to estimate the haemoglobin and packed cell volume (PCV). Measurement of blood urea concentration provides valuable information, provided that renal disease can be excluded. The concentrations of plasma electrolytes should be measured, but it should always be remembered that these may not reflect total body content. Acid–base parameters measured in anaerobically collected heparinized arterial blood provide the most reliable information. The laboratory examination of urine should include estimation of its specific gravity and preferably of its rate of production per hour.

Measurement of the central venous pressure is extremely desirable in animals suffering from water and electrolyte disturbances. Normal values vary from species to species but values of 6 cmH$_2$O are considered to be normal for dogs and 15 cmH$_2$O for horses. It should be emphasized that relative changes in these parameters during therapy are of greater significance than absolute values.

Water depletion

This is seen where intake is insufficient to meet the needs of the body. Thirst, which is usually marked, and dryness of the mucous membranes are early signs of water depletion. Death occurs when about 20 per cent of the body water has been lost. Treatment is based on supplying water, e.g. by the administration of an isotonic solution in 5 per cent dextrose. This contains no electrolytes and free water remains after metabolism of the carbohydrate substrate.

Sodium depletion

Sodium depletion arises mainly when Na$^+$-containing body fluids are lost and replaced by water only. Clinical signs develop rapidly and the animal appears very ill, with muscular weakness and excessive fatigue after minimal physical effort. Circulatory collapse occurs relatively early. Treatment is with either isotonic or hypertonic salt solutions.

Potassium depletion

Potassium depletion becomes evident only when losses have occurred for more than 10 days. Clinical signs are related to muscular disturbances and include muscular weakness, particularly of the respiratory muscles, intestinal atony with consequent abdominal distension and cardiac changes. Electrocardiographic examination will indicate bradycardia with prolongation of the QT interval and small biphasic T waves. Treatment of K$^+$ depletion is by oral administration of potassium, if this is possible. Where intravenous administration is necessary, the dose rate should not exceed 0.05 mmol/kg/hour.

Acid–base disturbance

Disturbance to the acid–base balance can be produced by losses of electrolytes; these cause changes in the pH of body fluids. Treatment of either a metabolic acidosis or alkalosis is rare in veterinary practice, as most animals soon correct their own acid–base abnormalities when fluid and electrolyte disturbances are corrected.

Treatment of electrolyte and fluid disorders

There are three main aims in treating electrolyte and fluid disorders: to restore the circulating blood volume; to replace existing deficits and abnormal losses; and to supply normal current requirements. It is usually possible to calculate the deficit; an example of this, in the dog, is shown below.

A dog weighing 30 kg is off food and water for 4 days. It has vomited six times per day for 2 days. Very little urine has been passed for 4 days. The deficit is calculated as follows:

4 days' inevitable water loss at 20 ml/kg/24 hours	= 2400 ml
1 days' urinary production at 20 ml/kg/24 hours	= 600 ml
Loss in vomit at 30 ml/vomit, 12 times	= 360 ml
Total loss of water	= 3360 ml
The total extracellular fluid loss is one-third of the total	= 1120 ml
The deficit of circulating volume is one-quarter of the extracellular fluid (one-twelfth of the total)	= 280 ml

As soon as a diagnosis is made, a crystalloid solution should be administered by the intravenous route. If at all possible a blood sample should be taken for cross-matching and laboratory estimations. If the haemoglobin is low then whole blood should be administered. If the plasma protein values are low then plasma or plasma substitutes (see below) should be administered. They should be administered relatively rapidly at a rate of 5 ml/kg in a 20-minute period. If no satisfactory response is obtained then further assessment of the animal's condition is necessary.

Once an improvement has been observed, the rate of fluid administration should be slowed to 70–80 drops per minute, depending on the size of the animal. If the central venous pressure is not being monitored, observation for signs of pulmonary oedema or venous congestion should be maintained and, if necessary, the rate of administration of fluid slowed or even stopped for a short period of time. The bladder should be catheterized to prevent distension and to enable urinary output to be measured.

Any abnormal losses, such as vomiting and diarrhoea, should be replaced on a volume-for-volume basis until such losses cease. Existing deficits should be repaired within a 48-hour period. In most animals the deficits can be replaced with relatively simple fluids and, if renal function is normal, adjustment will be performed by the kidneys.

During fluid therapy it should always be remembered that the animal still has normal daily requirements of 40 ml/kg/24 hours of water and 1.0 mEq/kg/24 hours of Na^+. This is best supplied by the administration of N/5 saline.

Fluids available for therapy

Blood

Arterial or venous blood can be collected from an animal of the same species. The blood group pattern varies from species to species. In dogs, donors should be A-negative. Ideally, blood should be cross-matched before it is administered but under practical conditions, in most species, it is possible to give a transfusion without producing a reaction. Blood for transfusion should be collected into an anticoagulant; dextrose phosphate is the most suitable. It should not be stored for longer than 1 month at 4°C as red cell viability is seriously affected after this time. Blood unused after this period should have the plasma removed for deep-frozen storage.

Plasma

Whilst blood is used to provide red cells and hence haemoglobin, it also contains plasma proteins which are important in maintaining circulation. Hence, despite the absence of oxygen-carrying capacity, plasma is still an important fluid as it remains in the circulation for a relatively long time. It also poses no cross-matching problems and can be stored in the frozen state for up to 2 years.

Plasma substitutes (plasma expanders)

A number of plasma substitutes, either gelatins or dextrans, are available.

Gelatin products

These are available for both medical and veterinary use. Modern products are purified preparations of large molecules formed by cross-linking of the gelatin peptide chains and are very much less likely to cause the histamine release seen with earlier substances. There are two compounds generally available which are relatively similar. Haemaccel is available for both medical and veterinary use and consists of polygeline (molecular weight 30 000) 35 g/l plus sodium chloride, potassium chloride and calcium chloride as an isotonic solution of pH 7.3. Gelofusine is available for human use but can be used in veterinary practice. It is modified gelatin 4 per cent (molecular weight 30 000) in saline with added calcium.

Glucose polymers

Dextrans are polymers of glucose with oncotic properties similar to plasma. They are available either in normal saline or in 5 per cent dextrose solution. Dextran 70 (molecular weight 70 000) is used mainly for volume expansion of the circulation. Dextran 40 (molecular weight 40 000) is used to improve peripheral blood flow by lowering the blood viscosity. It also has an osmotic effect and draws water into the circulation, hence it should be administered with a crystalloid solution. It should be used with caution in animals with renal disease as it can produce renal failure. Dextran 110 (molecular weight 110 000) and dextran 150 (molecular weight 150 000) increase the viscosity of the blood and are rarely used.

The dextrans are slowly metabolized and the smaller molecules are excreted via the kidney. They therefore remain in the circulation for variable periods of time, depending on their molecular weight. Dextran 70 has a duration of action of 4–5 hours while that of dextran 40 is only 2–3 hours.

Dextrans may interfere with cross-matching and biochemical estimations; hence blood samples for these purposes should be obtained before the administration of dextrans.

Hydroxyethyl starch, Hetastarch, is derived from a waxy starch and consists of polymerized glucose units with introduced hydroxyethyl groups. The average molecular weight of the polymer units is 450 000. As with the dextrans, after metabolism the smaller molecules are excreted via the kidney. The starch is effective for 24–36 hours.

Electrolyte solutions

A large number of electrolyte solutions of varying composition are available for intravenous administration to animals. However, in practice only a few of these are commonly used and they will be discussed here. The electrolyte composition of these solutions is shown in Table 11.2.

Table 11.2 Composition of solutions for intravenous administration

Solution	Composition (mmol/l)						Tonicity
	Na^+	K^+	Ca^{2+}	Cl^-	HCO_3^-	Lactate	
5% dextrose	–	–	–	–	–	–	Isotonic
0.9% sodium chloride (normal saline)	150	–	–	150	–	–	Isotonic
N/5 saline (0.18% saline with 4.3% dextrose)	30	–	–	30	–	–	Isotonic
Hartmann's solution (lactated Ringer's)	131	5	2	111	–	29	Isotonic
Sodium bicarbonate 8.4%	1000	–	–	–	1000	–	Hypotonic
Ammonium chloride (M/6)	–	–	–	168	–	–	

Normal saline

This is used mainly to replace a deficit of Na^+. Whilst it contains an excess of Cl^-, these chloride ions will be excreted by the kidney, provided renal function is normal. Saline is generally used to replace prepyloric losses.

Dextrose 5 per cent

This is used to treat water deficits.

Saline N/5 with dextrose 4.3 per cent

This is used to provide maintenance requirements of both water and Na^+.

Hartmann's solution

Hartmann's solution is relatively similar to extracellular fluid in its composition. Hence it is recommended for treatment of extracellular fluid loss. The lactate is metabolized to bicarbonate.

Acidifying solution (ammonium chloride M/6)

This is used in the treatment of alkalosis. Its action depends on the conversion of NH_4^+ to urea in the liver and the consequent liberation of H^+.

Sodium bicarbonate

Sodium bicarbonate is used in the treatment of metabolic acidosis. This is likely to occur after cardiac arrest and in association with a number of other clinical conditions.

Route of administration

A number of routes have been suggested for the administration of fluids to sick animals. Ideally, fluids should be administered by the oral route because the alimentary tract is able to exercise control over the absorption of electrolytes and water. However, a considerable number of animals which require therapy are suffering from disorders of the alimentary tract (e.g. colic in horses, foreign bodies in dogs). It is often impracticable to administer large volumes of fluid by stomach tube. Under some circumstances a pharyngostomy tube may be inserted surgically. The rectal route has not been found to be very satisfactory. The subcutaneous route may be used, particularly in small and young animals. Absorption is slow and any circulatory abnormalities are definite contraindications for the use of this route. Large volumes of fluid can be given intraperitoneally, particularly in smaller animals, but there is always the danger of producing peritonitis. Despite some of the theoretical disadvantages, the intravenous route is the method of choice in most situations.

Shock

The word 'shock' is probably more abused in veterinary and medical parlance than any other. Although it is difficult to define precisely, it is true to say that it is a state of progressive circulatory failure in which the cardiac output is insufficient to meet the requirements of the tissues for oxygen, nutrition and excretion; hence, cellular damage and death may ensue.

There are a number of different types of shock, classified according to aetiology. These include: hypovolaemia after haemorrhage; sepsis, where the release of an endotoxin results in profound vasodilation and hypotension; and anaphylaxis, where the release of naturally occurring vasodilators dramatically lowers blood pressure. It is often difficult in veterinary practice to establish a proper aetiology. The underlying disease may complicate the clinical picture of shock, which varies from species to species. However, signs generally include pallor of the mucous membranes, tachycardia, cold extremities, impaired consciousness and a low central venous pressure (except in cardiac failure).

Treatment of shock

Treatment is directed at the restoration of tissue perfusion and therefore involves the transfusion of fluid, usually blood plasma or plasma volume expanders. This is best carried out under conditions where the central venous pressure is monitored.

Several other supportive measures should be taken. Oxygen therapy is a valuable adjunct in shock as pulmonary function is often impaired. Broad-spectrum antibiotics should be administered in adequate dosage in cases of shock where sepsis or trauma have occurred (but note that the tetracycline antibiotics are specifically contraindicated in horses).

Since the sympathetic nervous system reaction to shock induces profound vasoconstriction and consequent reduction in tissue perfusion, treatment with α-adrenoceptor antagonists has been advocated. The most useful agent is the α-adrenoceptor antagonist, phenoxybenzamine, which can be administered intravenously at a dose of up to 1 mg/kg. If such an approach is used, adequate fluid replacement is essential. A moderate degree of α-adrenoceptor blockade can also be produced by tranquillizing drugs such as haloperidol and chlorpromazine.

Vasoconstrictive agents such as adrenaline or noradrenaline should not be used in shock since, although they may increase the arterial blood pressure, they reduce tissue perfusion. However, the inotropic agents dopamine, dobutamine or isoprenaline may be used, together with adequate fluid replacement. Dopamine has the advantage of maintaining blood flow to the kidneys. All three substances need to be administered by intravenous infusion, up to 20 μg/kg per minute of dobutamine and dopamine, and up to 0.5 μg/kg per minute of isoprenaline.

Corticosteroids have been used in the therapy of shock, although the exact mode of their action is not known. It is suggested that they stabilize the cell membrane, reduce platelet aggregation, restore normal capillary permeability, stimulate the myocardium and produce vasodilation of arterioles and venules. Endogenous levels of glucocorticoids are raised in shock and large doses, administered intravenously as early as possible, are required. The risk of complications with high doses is negligible with short-term administration. When administered in conjunction with fluids, they increase survival rate in haemorrhagic shock. Hydrocortisone succinate has been recommended in the treatment of Gram-negative septic shock but the effectiveness of corticosteroids in the management of septic shock is a matter for debate.

CHAPTER 12

THE URINARY SYSTEM

A number of different classes of drugs are used in veterinary medicine to treat disorders of kidney and bladder function. Some of these produce their effects by altering the release of renin, an enzyme secreted from the kidney, or by interfering in some way with the function of the renin-angiotensin-aldosterone system. One of the largest groups of drugs that alter kidney function comprises the diuretics; these are used to increase the output of salt and water. Other drugs, less widely used in veterinary medicine, may alter urinary pH and influence the excretion of organic compounds. Bladder function can also be altered by drug action, most commonly by those drugs which act via the autonomic nervous system. Chemotherapeutic agents, used to treat infections of the urinary tract are described in Chapter 18.

The renin-angiotensin-aldosterone system

Experiments conducted around the turn of the 20th century showed that extracts of kidney produced marked elevations in blood pressure when injected into anaesthetized animals. The name 'renin' was given to the active principle, the nature of which was quite unknown. In the years that followed the initial discovery of renin, the system illustrated in Fig. 12.1 was eventually described.

It is now known that renin itself is not the active pressor substance, but that it is a proteolytic enzyme released from the juxtaglomerular apparatus of the kidney in response to a variety of stimuli. Indicators of hypotension or

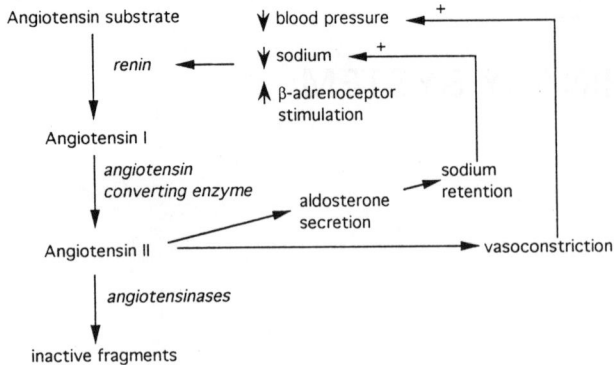

Figure 12.1 Homeostatic role of the renin-angiotensin-aldosterone system. The release of renin is stimulated by a fall in blood pressure, sodium or by adrenoceptor stimulation. The subsequent formation of angiotensin II increases the release of aldosterone which reduces Na^+ excretion. Angiotensin II is also a potent vasoconstrictor and thus increases blood pressure.

hypovolaemia, i.e. a decrease in renal arterial pressure, decrease in the Na^+ load at the level of the macula densa or stimulation of renal β-adrenoceptors all stimulate the release of renin. The enzyme catalyses the formation of angiotensin I, a decapeptide, from the blood-borne substrate, angiotensinogen (or angiotensin substrate).

Another enzyme, angiotensin-converting enzyme (or peptidyl dipeptidase) removes a further two amino acid residues and the remaining octapeptide is called angiotensin II. Large quantities of angiotensin-converting enzyme (ACE) occur in the lungs but its distribution is not limited to the pulmonary bed. (Bradykinin is also a substrate for ACE.) Angiotensin II is an extremely potent vasoconstrictor and is the substance which was ultimately responsible for the marked pressor response observed in the early experiments. The vasoconstrictor action of angiotensin is mediated directly on the (predominantly) arterial smooth muscle. It also facilitates activity in the sympathetic nervous system by peripheral effects and a centrally mediated increase in sympathetic nervous tone.

Angiotensin II has other important actions in the maintenance of circulatory homeostasis, namely the stimulation of the secretion of aldosterone from the adrenal cortex, which increases the reabsorption of Na^+ and water in the distal tubule. Thus the combined effects of angiotensin and aldosterone restore blood pressure and volume. The homeostatic response may be reinforced by an increased intake of water associated with the angiotensin-induced release of antidiuretic hormone.

Angiotensin II has a short half-life in the circulation. It is readily broken down by a variety of enzymes, referred to as angiotensinases.

There are a number of sites where drugs may act to interfere with the normal function of the renin-angiotensin-aldosterone system. Drugs which inhibit the actions of aldosterone are effective diuretics (see below). The efficacy of β-adrenoceptor antagonists in the treatment of hypertension in human medicine is thought to be due, in part, to a reduction in renin output. More recently drugs which are competitive angiotensin antagonists have been developed for similar applications. To date they have been less successful than the β-adrenoceptor antagonists or the newer ACE inhibitors. The latter are becoming increasingly popular in the management of hypertension and congestive cardiac failure in humans. Their use in heart failure in veterinary practice is discussed on page 218.

Diuretics

The vital functions of the kidney include the excretion of waste products and the regulation of salt and electrolyte content and volume of the extracellular fluid. The kidney also exerts some influence in the regulation of acid–base balance. At any time the kidneys receive about a quarter of the cardiac output. The excretory process is achieved by the filtration of the plasma through the renal tubule. By the time the filtrate has passed through the tubule, about 99 per cent of the filtrate has been reabsorbed; the remainder is voided as urine.

Diuretics produce their effects by interfering with the normal transport mechanisms in the kidney. Generally the reabsorption of Na^+ is inhibited and this leads to the excretion of increased volumes of water. A fairly large range of diuretics is available for use in human medicine, but in practice only a few of these are commonly prescribed and the rest are seldom used. In veterinary medicine, there are relatively few applications for diuretics and the choice is made from a limited number of preparations. In this chapter, the drugs which have little clinical veterinary application are only briefly mentioned, with the emphasis being on those which are more likely to be of use to the veterinarian. It is also assumed that the reader has an elementary knowledge of the normal mechanisms involved in renal function.

The use of diuretics dates back to the early 20th century when theophylline and the osmotic diuretics were in common use. (The latter group increased water loss because they were filtered at the glomerulus and were not reabsorbed, thus retaining water in the filtrate by an osmotic effect.) Although the osmotic diuretics are seldom used now, theophylline is still used to treat cardiac failure and respiratory disorders. At least some of its efficacy in these situations is due to its diuretic effect. The next drugs to be employed as diuretics were the organic mercurials, which inhibit the reabsorption of Na^+ from the proximal convoluted tubule and of Na^+ and Cl^- from the loop of Henle. Although the newer mercurial diuretics were less toxic than the original drugs, the use of this group of diuretics has been completely superseded.

The chance discovery that sulphonamides had diuretic activity led to the development of other sulphonamide diuretics which exert their effect by inhibition of the enzyme carbonic anhydrase. The most commonly used of these is acetazolamide (Fig. 12.2).

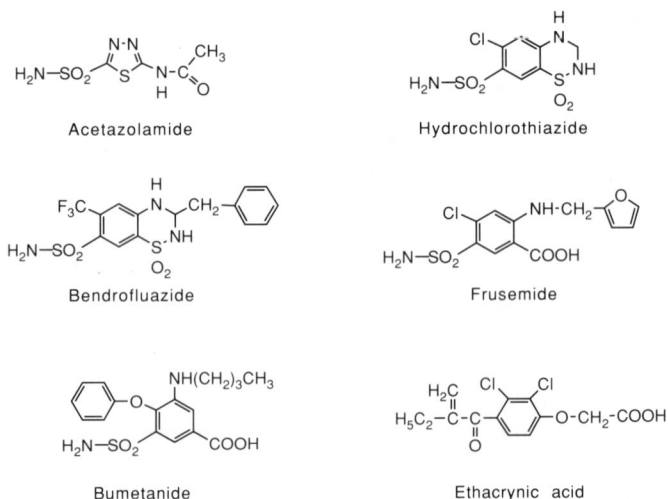

Figure 12.2 The carbonic anhydrase inhibitor, acetazolamide, and structurally related diuretics.

The main action of carbonic anhydrase is catalysis of the reaction

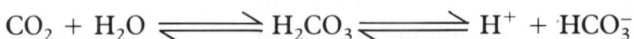

$$CO_2 + H_2O \rightleftharpoons H_2CO_3 \rightleftharpoons H^+ + HCO_3^-$$

The carbonic acid is in equilibrium with HCO_3^- and, in the kidney, the reabsorption of HCO_3^- by the proximal tubule thus depends on the activity of carbonic anhydrase. Inhibition of carbonic anhydrase thus interferes with the movement of HCO_3^- across membranes. Drugs which inhibit enzyme activity cause a relatively mild diuresis, with an increased excretion of Na^+ and HCO_3^-. Elsewhere in the body there is a reduction in the secretion of HCO_3^--containing fluids. In the case of the eye, the reduction in aqueous humour secretion is important in the therapeutic efficacy of the carbonic anhydrase inhibitors in glaucoma (see Chapter 16).

Chemical modification of the acetazolamide molecule resulted in the production of the thiazide diuretics and later those which are known as the 'loop diuretics' (e.g. frusemide) because they exert their effect on the loop of Henle (Fig. 12.2). These two groups of diuretics are the most widely used today. The most recent additions to the available diuretics are those which inhibit the actions of aldosterone and thus have a K^+-sparing action.

Thiazides

The main thiazides used in veterinary practice are hydrochlorothiazide (most common) and bendrofluazide (bendroflumethazide). Although they were originally developed from the carbonic anhydrase inhibitors (Fig. 12.2), the enzyme inhibitory effect is quite weak in the drugs in current use and probably does not contribute significantly to their diuretic effect.

Mode of action

The clinical response is due to the inhibition of the active reabsorption of Na^+, and therefore Cl^-, in the distal tubule, although other effects may occur. The effect of the thiazides on K^+ excretion is a consequence of the primary action on Na^+ reabsorption. Under normal circumstances, K^+ which has been filtered is almost completely reabsorbed in the proximal tubule and the loop of Henle. Secretion of K^+ into the filtrate occurs in the distal nephron by a passive movement, which depends on the electrochemical gradient across the luminal membrane produced by the active reabsorption of Na^+. When, under the influence of the thiazides, Na^+ delivery to the distal nephron is increased, there is a corresponding decrease in luminal membrane potential and an increase in the electrochemical gradient for K^+ from cell to lumen. Thus K^+ excretion is also increased.

Mg^{2+} excretion is increased in the presence of the thiazides, while excretion of both Ca^{2+} and uric acid decreases. The thiazides compete with uric acid for tubular secretion and may thus increase plasma uric acid levels. The response to the thiazide diuretics is independent of acid–base balance.

The thiazides are well absorbed from the gastrointestinal tract. Veterinary preparations of hydrochlorothiazide are available for intravenous or intramuscular administration.

Side-effects

The most common side-effects are those which result from increased K^+ loss or the development of a metabolic alkalosis. The hypokalaemia is not usually of clinical significance with short-term use, unless animals are anorexic and K^+ intake is also reduced. Since hypokalaemia potentiates the toxic effects of digitalis glycosides, special care should also be taken with animals that are receiving one of these drugs concurrently. In general, the thiazides have a high margin of safety.

Uses

Thiazides are used in animals with cardiac failure to prevent fluid retention (see Chapter 10). Fluid accumulation associated with chronic hepatic or renal failure also responds well to thiazides.

Dose

hydrochlorothiazide
horse, cattle	250 mg i.m. or i.v. daily
	500 mg p.o. initial dose,
	250 mg p.o. daily maintenance dose
pig	50–75 mg i.m. daily
dog, cat	12.5–25 mg i.m. daily
	1–2 mg/kg p.o. daily

bendrofluazide
dog	120–250 μg/kg p.o. daily

Loop diuretics

These drugs, which exert their action at the loop of Henle, are also referred to as 'high ceiling' diuretics because they are capable of inducing profound diuresis which follows the excretion of up to 25 per cent of the Na^+ in the filtrate. The group includes frusemide (furosemide), which is the one most widely used in veterinary practice, bumetanide and ethacrynic acid. The chemical structures of these diuretics are shown in Fig. 12.2, where it can be seen that ethacrynic acid is not a derivative of the sulphonamides and is chemically quite different from frusemide and bumetanide. Its mode of action, however, is very similar to that of the sulphonamide derivatives.

Mechanism of action

Active reabsorption of Na^+ and Cl^- takes place in the ascending limb of the loop of Henle, although water is not absorbed. Thus the osmolarity of the tubular fluid is reduced and the interstitial fluid of the medulla becomes hypertonic. This is an important factor in the subsequent reabsorption of water from the collecting tubules. In the presence of the loop diuretics, the transport of Na^+ and Cl^- from the renal tubule to the interstitium is inhibited. This reduces the osmolarity of the interstitium and thus reduces the passive reabsorption of water. Furthermore, the increased osmolarity of the tubular fluid in the distal portions of the nephron results in reduced reabsorption of water. The increased Na^+ load and increased volume of filtrate in the distal tubule also result in increased K^+ excretion. As with the thiazides, changes in acid–base balance do not affect the efficacy of loop diuretics.

It is possible that some of the response to the loop diuretics may be due to the increase in renal blood flow produced by the drugs in this group. This effect is more common after intravenous administration. Because they do not alter glomerular filtration rate, they reduce the filtration fraction, i.e. a smaller proportion of the blood passing through the kidney is filtered. This reduces the concentration of the protein in the peritubular fluid and thereby reduces water reabsorption from the proximal convoluted tubule. Furthermore, the inhibition of the transport of Na^+ and Cl^- is associated with reduced reabsorption of divalent cations. Thus excretion of Mg^{2+} and Ca^{2+} is also increased.

Kinetics

Frusemide is readily absorbed after oral administration. The onset of effect is within 1 hour in single-stomached animals. The duration of action is approximately 3–4 hours. Up to 6 hours may be required for the maximum effect to be obtained after oral administration to cows, and the response may last for up to 24 hours. Frusemide may be administered parenterally. The response begins within minutes of intravenous injection but is much slower if the intramuscular route is used. The drug is strongly bound to plasma protein, therefore it is not filtered at the glomerulus. It reaches the site of action by being secreted into the luminal fluid in the proximal convoluted tubule by an organic acid transport mechanism.

Side-effects

The diuretic response to frusemide is accompanied by an increased excretion of K^+. Hypokalaemia is rarely a clinical problem, but where patients are also receiving digitalis glycosides, the loss of K^+ may precipitate digitalis toxicity during prolonged combined treatment and monitoring of plasma $[K^+]$ is advisable. Furthermore, frusemide potentiates the therapeutic and toxic effects of digitalis glycosides by interfering with their excretion and clearly increasing the plasma glycoside concentration. Marked depletion of Mg^{2+} can occur with prolonged use of loop diuretics. Metabolic alkalosis, due to the increased excretion of H^+ and volume depletion, has also been reported. Ototoxicity is rare and is exaggerated by the concomitant use of an aminoglycoside antibiotic.

Therapeutic uses

Loop diuretics are effective in the management of oedema due to disorders of the pulmonary system, heart failure, liver disease or renal failure. Intravenous frusemide is particularly useful in the treatment of acute cardiac failure (see p. 221). Left-sided failure produces some pulmonary oedema requiring urgent therapy. Benefits after intravenous frusemide may be noticeable within 15 minutes. Loop diuretics are also used to increase excretion of Ca^{2+}, K^+ or halides (which are absorbed in the loop). In these cases, infusion of saline will prevent dehydration. Additional K^+ may also have to be administered.

Dose

frusemide
dog and cat	5 mg/kg p.o. 1–2 times/day
	2.5–5 mg/kg i.m. or i.v. 1–2 times/day
horse	0.5–1.0 mg/kg i.m. or i.v. 1–2 times/day
cattle	0.5–1.0 mg/kg i.m. or i.v.
	2–5 mg/kg p.o.
pig	5 mg/kg i.m. or i.v.

ethacrynic acid
dog and cat	5 mg/kg p.o. 1–2 times/day
	2.5–5 mg/kg i.m. or i.v. 1–2 times/day

Doses for large animals have not been determined.

Potassium-sparing diuretics

These are generally weak diuretics, but have the advantage that they do not induce K^+ loss, as occurs with the more potent drugs.

Spironolactone

Aldosterone regulates the reabsorption of Na^+ and Cl^- in the collecting tubules of the distal nephron. In the presence of high levels of aldosterone, enhanced reabsorption of Na^+ is associated with increased secretion of K^+ and H^+. Spironolactone exerts its action by competitive antagonism of aldosterone. The response includes increased excretion of Na^+ and water, with retention of K^+.

Spironolactone is usually administered in combination with a thiazide or other diuretic to avoid problems of excessive K^+ retention. Thus it is possible to increase the diuretic effect and reduce the side-effects of each of the component substances.

Although it is well absorbed after oral administration, the onset of action of spironolactone is slow and it may take 2–3 days to reach full effect. Administration of high doses of the drug does not hasten the onset of action.

Spironolactone is expensive and prevention of the release of aldosterone, achieved by the administration of angiotensin-converting enzyme inhibitors (see below), may be preferable.

Dose

dog, cat   1–2 mg/kg p.o. daily

Triamterene and amiloride

These agents are also potassium-sparing diuretics, but their diuretic action is not related to aldosterone inhibition. Rather, it depends on the inhibition of Na^+ reabsorption and K^+ excretion in the distal convoluted tubule and the collecting tubules. Triamterene is well absorbed after oral administration; amiloride is only poorly absorbed by this route.

Dose

triamterene   0.5–3 mg/kg p.o. daily
amiloride
   dog and cat   1–2 mg/kg p.o. daily.

Alteration of urinary pH

Regulation of urinary pH may be desirable in some conditions. Alkalinization is commonly used to reduce the signs of inflammation in the urinary tract. The alkaline environment so produced may have some antibacterial effect and enhances the action of sulphonamides and gentamicin used in the treatment of the condition. The solubility of uric acid and cysteine is increased in alkaline urine and the formation of their uroliths is inhibited. Alkalinization can be achieved by the administration of sodium or potassium citrate, acetate or lactate. The cations are excreted with HCO_3^-, thus increasing urinary pH.

Urinary acidification increases the antibacterial activity of tetracyclines, penicillin and nitrofurantoin and is of use in increasing the rate of excretion of basic drugs. The formation of certain types of urinary calculi may also be controlled by the maintenance of an acid urine. Ammonium chloride is the main agent employed for this purpose. Metabolism of ammonium chloride in the liver results in the production of urea, Cl^- and H^+. Acidification of the urine results from the excretion of H^+.

Drugs affecting bladder function

The autonomic nervous system is responsible for the control of normal bladder function. Stimulation of parasympathetic nerves results in the release of acetylcholine, which contracts the detrusor muscle and relaxes the urethral sphincters. Noradrenergic stimulation of the α-adrenoceptors, in contrast, contracts the smooth muscle of the sphincter and prevents urination. Urinary incontinence—the loss of voluntary control of urination—may be due to a variety of factors which may or may not be associated with autonomic dysfunction.

Muscarinic agonists, such as bethanechol, are effective in the management of bladder atony and the avoidance of urinary retention by increasing the strength and completeness of detrusor contraction. Since bethanechol is more effective at the muscarinic receptors in the bladder than at receptors at other sites, cholinergic side-effects can be controlled by the use of low doses. Furtrethonium is another muscarinic agonist with selectivity for bladder smooth muscle and may be of use in alleviating atony.

Some cases of incontinence may be associated with an increased tendency for the detrusor muscle to contract spontaneously. In these animals, anticholinergic drugs (such as propantheline) or mixtures of these may be effective. Propantheline is also used to relax muscular spasm associated with cystitis.

Urinary incontinence occurring in bitches after spaying responds to administration of oestrogens. It is likely that the effect is due to an increased sensitivity of α-adrenoceptors to noradrenaline and a corresponding increase in sphincter tone. Drugs which stimulate α-adrenoceptors (including ephedrine or phenylpropanolamine) can also increase tone, but may have considerable cardiovascular and other side-effects associated with stimulation of adrenoceptors at other sites. Therapy with the α-adrenoceptor antagonist phenoxybenzamine is useful in animals where urinary retention is associated with excessive tone of the urethral sphincter. Although the mechanism is not understood, incontinence due to castration in dogs is effectively managed by administration of testosterone.

CHAPTER 13

THE RESPIRATORY SYSTEM

The majority of respiratory diseases which occur in animals are produced by specific viruses or bacteria. Hence it is possible to prevent most of these conditions by the use of vaccines or to treat them by the use of suitable chemotherapeutic agents (see Chapters 18–22). Other drugs used to treat disorders of the respiratory system include mucokinetic agents, which aid the clearance of airway secretions, antitussives and drugs which interfere with allergic or inflammatory processes. Whilst they may tend to be neglected at the present, the age-old remedies of rest and fresh air are still important in the therapy of respiratory disorders in animals.

Mucokinetic drugs

The drugs in this category are employed to mobilize and evacuate obstructing secretions which otherwise impair ventilation. In veterinary practice, expectorants, mucolytics and bronchodilators are all used to improve the movement of mucus through the airways.

Expectorants

The main effect of expectorants, also referred to as bronchomucolytic drugs, is to increase the volume of secretions produced by the respiratory mucous membranes. In the early stages of inflammation of the lungs and respiratory tract, there is often a decreased volume and increased viscosity of mucus, causing a harsh, dry, non-productive cough. Expectorants are indicated to stimulate mucus secretion. This effect is limited mainly to the trachea, bronchi and bronchioles and may be accompanied by a reduction in the viscosity of mucous secretions. The drugs in this group include potassium iodide, ammonium chloride, ammonium bicarbonate, guaiphenesin, ipecac and squill and they have been grouped below according to their mechanism of action.

Ipecac, squill and ammonium salts

Mucus-secreting cells in the respiratory tract are innervated by parasympathetic nerves and respond to nerve stimulation by increasing the production of mucus. It is believed that expectorants of this type produce their effects by stimulation of afferent vagal sensory receptors in the gastric mucosal membranes. The signals are relayed through a mucokinetic centre in the medulla and this results in the stimulation of efferent vagal pathways leading to the bronchial glands. When administered orally, these drugs are also capable of irritating the stomach and duodenum. The majority of the drugs are also emetics but the bronchomucolytic effect is usually achieved at doses lower than those which are known to induce vomiting.

Volatile oils—menthol, guaiphenesin, etc.

Direct stimulation of bronchial glands increases the volume of mucus secretion. Guaiphenesin may also act as a direct stimulant of the mucokinetic vagal centre.

Iodides

Potassium iodide has been shown to have a number of different actions which could contribute to the increase in the volume of mucus secretion that it induces. It is capable of stimulation of the gastropulmonary vagal reflex as well as direct stimulation of the bronchial glands. Furthermore, it may exert an indirect effect on respiratory function by activating proteolytic enzymes which digest mucoproteins. This action results in a reduction of the viscosity of secretions. Potassium iodide is detectable in bronchial secretions within 30 minutes of oral administration.

Mucolytics

Drugs which alter the viscosity of secretions by altering the organic components are called mucolytics. These include bromhexine, dembrexine, acetylcysteine, carbocysteine and methylcysteine.

Bromhexine

Bromhexine reduces the viscosity of sputum by causing fragmentation of mucopolysaccharide fibres, possibly by the liberation of lysosomal enzymes from the bronchial mucosa.

Dose

dog	1.6–2.5 mg/kg p.o., b.i.d.
cat	1.0 mg/kg p.o. daily
horse	0.1–0.25 mg/kg i.m. or p.o. daily
cattle, pig	0.2–0.5 mg/kg i.m. or p.o. daily

In all species dosage is continued for 5–7 days.

Dembrexine

Although the action of dembrexine on the structure of tracheobronchial mucus has not been reported, experimental data indicate a reduction in the viscosity of secretions, which may be due to an alteration in the sugar side-chains.

Dose

horse	30 mg/100 kg p.o., b.i.d.

Acetylcysteine and methylcysteine

These drugs have free sulphydryl groups which split the disulphide bonds in sputum proteins and thereby reduce the viscosity of the sputum. They are usually administered as aerosols. Since acetylcysteine has a potentially irritant effect on the respiratory tract, bronchospasm and/or severe coughing may follow its administration.

Carbocysteine (S-carboxymethylcysteine)

The action of carbocysteine is probably not the same as that of acetylcysteine and methylcysteine because of the lack of freedom of its thiol group. An effect on the mucoregulatory mechanism in bronchial glands has been suggested. The drug is equally effective when administered by the oral route or as an aerosol in order to facilitate expectoration. It may also have a bronchomucotropic effect after approximately 1 week of therapy. In humans, dosing for some days appears to be necessary before the changes in sputum viscosity are evident.

Therapeutic use of mucokinetic drugs

Whilst the majority of animals resent the application of drugs by inhalation, it is sometimes possible to carry out this type of therapy in cats and more particularly in dogs. This can be done by exposing the animal to the vapour of nearly boiling water. In treating small animals, a steam kettle may be used in a confined space. Alternatively they may be placed in an atmosphere of high humidity such as a shower room.

Since dehydration is known to be associated with difficulty in evacuating airway secretions, in all cases attention should be paid to the state of hydration of the patient. Rehydration with intravenous fluids should be carried out if necessary, in order to discourage the production of sputum of increased viscosity. Aerosols of water may also be produced by either pumps or nebulizers. Other drugs, such as bronchodilators and chemotherapeutic agents, can be added to the nebulizer solution. Volatile substances can also be vaporized in order to give a medicinal smell, although their value is probably limited to just that. Irritant or pungent agents such as menthol are best avoided. The agent of choice is probably still benzoin (Friars' balsam).

A variety of mucokinetic agents are available for veterinary use. Some still include rather outdated mixes of ingredients, including arsenic and strychnine. These are best avoided. It is always necessary, when prescribing drugs which contain a number of components, to be aware of these; e.g. irritant expectorants are not advised for treatment of horses and some of the commercially available preparations contain such ingredients.

Bromhexine has been successfully used in the treatment of acute and chronic bronchitis and chronic cough. When it is administered with oxytetracycline it increases the concentration of the antibiotic in the bronchial mucus by more than 40 per cent. The clinical significance of this action is uncertain. Bromhexine markedly increases the concentration of immunoglobulins A and G in sputum.

Dembrexine is useful in the management of respiratory disease characterized by an abnormal or increased production of mucus in horses. Although improvement is often seen within a few days, treatment should be continued until complete remission occurs, usually in about 2 weeks. One course of treatment should not exceed 4 weeks.

Antitussives

These are drugs which suppress coughing and are only really indicated where coughing is paroxysmal and unproductive, which often causes distress. Although the cough centre is sited in the medulla oblongata in close proximity to the respiratory centre, it is possible to depress the cough centre without depressing the respiratory centre to a great extent. Morphine and other narcotics, including heroin (which are subject to the Misuse of Drugs Act), have been used for cough suppression in the past. At present, codeine phosphate, as a linctus and given orally, is most commonly used for this purpose. Other alternatives, such as dextromethorphan, noscapine and pholcodine, have been developed but have not been shown to be superior to codeine. Butorphanol, an opioid derivative with a spectrum of action similar to that of pentazocine, is an effective antitussive in dogs. Its use is contraindicated in cats.

The locally acting demulcent drugs may also be used in small animals to reduce coughing. These include glycerine, honey and syrup mixtures of these agents which soothe the pain associated with persistent coughing for a short period.

Dose

codeine phosphate
dog   0.5–2 mg/kg p.o. b.i.d.

butorphanol
dog   0.5 mg/kg p.o. 6–12-hourly
          0.05 mg/kg s.c. or i.m. 6–12-hourly

Bronchodilators

Several types of drugs may be used to relieve bronchoconstriction and in the treatment of coughing and dyspnoea.

Muscarinic antagonists

As bronchial muscle contracts in response to stimulation of the parasympathetic nervous system, it is rational to use atropine or other similar drugs to block the muscarinic effects of acetylcholine. However, the reduction of parasympathetic tone to the bronchial glands decreases the volume, and thus increases the viscosity, of bronchial secretions and therefore these drugs are not commonly used as a routine treatment. Other side-effects associated with the administration of antimuscarinics include increased heart rate and decreased activity of the gastrointestinal tract.

Sympathomimetic agents

Bronchodilation results from the stimulation of β_2-adrenoceptors in the smooth muscle of the bronchioles. Increased ciliary beat frequency after the administration of sympathomimetic amines has been observed and it is likely that the enhanced mucociliary transport contributes to the general increase in airway clearance. The ciliary action is also thought to be mediated via stimulation of the β_2-adrenoceptors.

While all β-adrenoceptor agonists with activity at β_2-adrenoceptors are capable of inducing bronchodilation, the side-effects of treatment are, to a great extent, determined by the β_1-adrenoceptor stimulant activity of the drug. Thus, the most common side-effects with non-selective drugs like adrenaline and isoprenaline are tachycardia and increased force of contraction of the heart. Muscle tremor may be associated with the use of large doses of β_2-adrenoceptor stimulants. These drugs also relax uterine smooth muscle.

A number of selective β_2-adrenoceptor agonists are available for respiratory applications. Salbutamol, terbutaline and orciprenaline are most frequently used in human medicine. Clenbuterol is the most commonly used β_2-adrenoceptor agonist in veterinary medicine.

Methylxanthines

In addition to their actions on the central nervous system, heart and kidneys, the methylxanthines are bronchodilators. They include the naturally occurring compounds, caffeine, theobromine and theophylline. All of these substances are active bronchodilators, but theophylline is the most potent. The theophylline derivatives, aminophylline, diprophylline and etamiphylline, are more soluble and can be given by intravenous or intramuscular injection or by the oral route. These are preferred to the older drugs.

The mode of action of the methylxanthines is described on page 217. Recent evidence indicates that adenosine may be one of the mediators of the bronchoconstrictor response. The ability of these drugs to antagonize the effects of adenosine may be of particular importance in their bronchodilator activity.

The methylxanthines stimulate the medullary respiratory centre and may increase the rate and depth of respiration. It has been suggested that if plasma levels are sufficient to inhibit phosphodiesterase, the resultant increase in cyclic 3′,5′-cAMP could inhibit mast cell degranulation and subsequent mediator release. An increase in the beat frequency of the cilia may also enhance mucociliary clearance.

Gastrointestinal problems, including anorexia, abdominal discomfort and vomiting, are the most common side-effects of theophylline and can usually be relieved by reduction in dosage. Toxic effects reflect the activity of the drug on other systems, i.e. tachycardia and arrhythmias, restlessness and anxiety.

Therapeutic uses of bronchodilators

The best response to bronchodilators is achieved after administration by aerosol inhalation. Since the drug is deposited at the site where smooth muscle relaxation is required, an almost immediate response can occur. Furthermore, since the drug is being delivered directly to the site of action, lower doses are required and there is a proportional reduction in the incidence and severity of side-effects. Administration by inhalation can, however, present practical difficulties in veterinary practice. Oral administration is effective (except for adrenaline) and sympathomimetic amines can, in cases of severe anaphylaxis, be given by subcutaneous, intramuscular or even intravenous injection. Side-effects can be reduced by the selection of one of the drugs displaying selectivity for β_2-adrenoceptors.

Clenbuterol is available for the treatment of bronchospasm in horses. It is also recommended for the treatment of chronic obstructive pulmonary disease and acute, subacute and chronic allergies and infections such as equine influenza and bronchopneumonia. Bronchopneumonia in cattle may also be treated with clenbuterol. Muscle tremor and sweating may occur after intravenous injection in horses. These problems are less likely if the drug is injected slowly. Stimulation of β_2-adrenoceptors by clenbuterol causes relaxation of uterine smooth muscle. Furthermore, as the drug antagonizes the actions of both prostaglandin $F_{2\alpha}$ and oxytocin, it should not be administered at the expected time of parturition since uterine contractions may be inhibited. It should not be administered with corticosteroids due to its peripheral vasodilatory effects.

Aminophylline is irritant when given by aerosol or intramuscular injection, hence its use is effectively limited to intravenous infusion or oral administration. Diprophylline is non-irritant and does not give rise to a reaction at the site of injection.

Dose

adrenaline

dog, cat	0.5–15 µg/kg	s.c, i.m. or slow i.v.
horse, cattle	4–8 µg/kg	s.c. or i.m.
	2–4 µ/kg	slow i.v.
sheep, pig	1–3 mg	i.m. or s.c.

clenbuterol

horse	0.8 µg/kg	p.o. or slow i.v., b.i.d.
cattle	0.8 µg/kg	i.m. or slow i.v., b.i.d.

(N.B. Cattle must not be slaughtered for human consumption for 12 days after the last treatment. Three days must elapse after the last treatment before milk, for human consumption, can be taken.)

diprophylline

dog, cat
125–500 mg i.v. or i.m., 8-hourly
200–400 mg p.o., 4–8 hourly

large animals
1–2 g i.v. or i.m., 8-hourly.

etamiphylline

dog, cat
140–700 mg i.m. or s.c., 8-hourly
100–300 mg p.o., 8-hourly

sheep, calf
700–1000 mg i.m. or s.c., 8-hourly
300–600 mg p.o., 8-hourly
(withdraw for 24 hours prior to slaughter for human consumption)

horse, cattle
1.4 g i.m. or s.c., 8-hourly
900 mg p.o., 8-hourly

Corticosteroids

Corticosteroids with glucocorticoid activity may be used to reduce oedema and inflammatory reactions within the respiratory tract. For a description of the mode of action of the corticosteroids see page 191. The anti-inflammatory action of the glucocorticoids is primarily responsible for the effectiveness of these drugs in therapy of respiratory diseases. Oedema is reduced by preventing the usual increase in capillary permeability that occurs with the release of inflammatory mediators. The anti-inflammatory effects are accompanied by an enhanced responsiveness of adenylate cyclase to the actions of β_2-adrenoceptor agonists in respiratory smooth muscle. This has the effect of increasing the response to adrenoceptor agonists administered for therapy as well as the response to sympathetic stimulation.

Therapy with high doses of corticosteroids can lead to the development of Cushing's syndrome or, with suppression of normal glandular activity, a dependence on continued administration of the drugs. These problems are less likely to occur with corticosteroids administered by inhalation, since the dose required is much lower.

Therapeutic uses of corticosteroids

Corticosteroid therapy with dexamethasone or betamethasone may be useful in cases of pneumonia in the horse. Their effect is due to the reduction of the inflammatory response, with consequent reduction of the amount of pulmonary effusion. Concurrent administration of antibiotics is necessary because the immune system will be suppressed by the corticosteroid therapy. Chronic obstructive pulmonary disease also responds to corticosteroid therapy, but long-term treatment is hazardous.

A fulminating, sometimes fatal, pulmonary oedema can result from inhalation of toxic fumes or gastric contents. This can be prevented by prompt intravenous injection of a water-soluble glucocorticoid.

It has been suggested that in bovine respiratory diseases such as shipping fever (*Pasteurella* bronchial pneumonia), animals treated with glucocorticoids and antibiotics recover as well as those which receive antibiotics alone. In calf pneumonia, however, glucocorticoids administered with antibiotics can produce dramatic symptomatic improvement, but the risk of producing chronic disease outweighs any potential benefit.

Dose

betamethasone
  dog, cat   25 μg/kg p.o.
  all species   40–80 μg/kg i.m. or i.v.

dexamethasone
  dog, cat   25–100 μg/kg p.o.
  cattle   20–50 μg/kg i.m. or i.v.

Antihistamines

Although histamine is a powerful bronchoconstrictor, drugs which have the ability to antagonize the effects of histamine in respiratory smooth muscle are of limited value in the treatment of respiratory disorders. The most likely explanation for their lack of efficacy as bronchodilators is that a number of different mediators may be involved in the bronchoconstrictor response and the inhibition of only one of them will do little to relieve the constriction. Some additional benefit may be gained by the antimuscarinic activity that many of these drugs possess, and for this reason they are included in proprietary mixtures.

Trimeprazine tartrate, a phenothiazine derivative with considerable anti-histaminic activity, may be used in dogs and cats to reduce broncho-constriction and coughing.

Dose

trimeprazine tartrate
  dog, cat   500–700μg/kg p.o. daily

Sodium cromoglycate

Sodium cromoglycate (cromolyn sodium, Fig. 13.1) has no bronchodilator activity, nor does it affect the production of respiratory secretions. It does not prevent antigen-antibody reactions, but if it is administered before exposure of an animal to an antigen, it can prevent types I and III allergic reactions. The drug stabilizes mast cells and acts by preventing their degranulation. It has been used mainly to prevent asthma in humans.

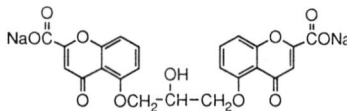

Sodium cromoglycate

Figure 13.1

Therapeutic use of sodium cromoglycate

Sodium cromoglycate is useful in the prevention of allergic respiratory conditions in horses when antigen challenge can be predicted. It appears to be useful in the treatment of chronic obstructive pulmonary disease. The drug is poorly absorbed when administered orally and has to be given as an inhaled powder by means of a nebulizer. Sodium cromoglycate is virtually non-toxic.

Dose

horse   80 mg by inhalation, once daily for 1–4 days.

Acute respiratory failure

Acute respiratory failure, by its very nature, requires rapid and positive treatment. A minimal amount of time should be wasted in assessing the animal's clinical condition. Initially an oxygen-enriched gas mixture, preferably free of carbon dioxide, should be administered. It is usual for this to be administered by mask until an adequate assessment of the animal's condition can be made. If the animal is unconscious or weak it may be possible to pass an endotracheal tube to provide a clear airway and institute positive pressure ventilation. If the upper airway is obstructed then serious consideration should be given to tracheotomy.

Care should be taken in the administration of oxygen over a long period of time and consideration given to adequate humidification of the gas, addition of 4–5 per cent carbon dioxide and the limitation of the oxygen concentration to about 50 per cent. Once an adequate respiratory pattern has been established, consideration should be given to the cardiovascular system. Fluid or drug therapy may be necessary. Drugs used to stimulate respiration, called analeptics, may also reverse circulatory collapse.

Analeptics

Doxapram is the most commonly used analeptic in veterinary practice. Stimulation of respiration is achieved by the stimulation of chemoreceptors in the carotid arteries and aorta and also by stimulation of the medullary respiratory centre. Thus both rate and depth of respiration are increased. Respiratory stimulation is accompanied by an increase in blood pressure, except with high doses of the drug, when blood pressure falls. Doxapram, like other analeptics, is capable of inducing convulsions, but the separation between convulsant and respiratory stimulant doses is considerable.

Prethcamide (Respirot) is a mixture of crotethamide and cropropamide. Respiratory stimulation is probably due to stimulation of chemoreceptors in the carotid and aortic bodies. It is used as a respiratory stimulant in newborn animals and during neuroleptanalgesia or following anaesthesia.

Dose

doxapram

dog, cat	1–10 mg/kg i.v.
dog (neonatal)	1–5 mg i.v., s.c. or sublingual
cat (neonatal)	1–2 mg i.v., s.c. or sublingual
horse	0.5–1.0 mg/kg i.v.
calf (neonatal)	40–100 mg i.v., s.c. or sublingual
lamb (neonatal)	5–10 mg i.v., s.c. or sublingual

prethcamide (Respirot)

calf, foal	up to 5 ml; 1 ml contains 75 mg of each component
lamb, piglet and small animals	up to 2 drops/kg (1 ml=36 drops). This dose is applied to the tongue and repeated (up to 2 times) at 30 sec intervals, until a response is elicited.

Pulmonary oedema

Pulmonary oedema is an abnormal accumulation of fluid within the lungs. It can arise from a number of different circumstances; these can be related to cardiac and non-cardiac causes. Cardiac pulmonary oedema is due mainly to left-sided heart failure associated with such conditions as chronic mitral valve disease or left-to-right shunts. The non-cardiac causes are varied and include such diverse conditions as the inhalation of toxic fumes, systemic toxins, shock (including electrocution) and overtransfusion. Common clinical signs of pulmonary oedema include tachypnoea, dyspnoea and moist rales in the lungs. Coughing may produce a frothy pink mucus, which is also seen in the endotracheal tube when the condition occurs under general anaesthesia. Radiographic diagnosis is helpful, as the condition is typified by the presence of matted and blotchy pulmonary opacities.

The main objective in the treatment of pulmonary oedema is to improve respiratory gas exchange. Therefore animals should be treated as for acute respiratory failure. An attempt should be made to ascertain the aetiology of the condition and at least to differentiate the cardiac and non-cardiac forms. Diuretic therapy with intravenous frusemide (1–2 mg/kg) should be instituted. Oral therapy can be commenced provided a response is obtained. If the animal appears to be restless it should be sedated with a low dose of one of the phenothiazine derivative tranquillizers. If pulmonary oedema is secondary to cardiac failure then the appropriate therapy for the cardiac condition should also be instituted.

CHAPTER 14

THE GASTROINTESTINAL TRACT

Disturbances of normal gastrointestinal function in domestic animals may result in different clinical signs, including vomiting, diarrhoea, dysentery, weight loss, atony, impaction, spasm and manifestations of visceral pain. A variety of drugs which relieve these signs and restore normal function are available. Although gastrointestinal disorders are common, many are self-limiting and manageable with conservative therapy, such as correcting dietary indiscretions. Additional therapy may be used to satisfy 'client demand', but the efficacy of some of the drugs in use is questionable.

In the first instance, an accurate diagnosis is of major importance. For example, vomiting or diarrhoea may be caused by a foreign body, requiring surgical treatment, or an infection, which necessitates specific chemotherapy. On the basis of the diagnosis, with a knowledge of the pathophysiological mechanisms involved and an understanding of the pharmacology of the available drugs, a rational approach to therapy can be achieved.

Drugs which affect appetite

The loss of appetite that is often associated with disease can be treated with a number of 'tonic' preparations. Many of these produce their effects by stimulation of the taste buds, thereby increasing the flow of saliva, and are correctly termed sialogogues (or sialics). Older substances, commonly known as bitters, include gentian, ginger, strychnine and brucine (from nux vomica) and quinine (from cinchona). A number of different commercial preparations are available, all of which contain mixtures of up to five ingredients. Evidence for their therapeutic efficacy is tenuous, except perhaps where they are included in mixtures to stimulate salivary production in ruminants. In this case, the maintenance of a fluid medium in the rumen is important for normal function.

Stimulation of salivary glands can also be achieved by the administration of parasympathomimetic agents or anticholinesterases, but this is of no real therapeutic benefit. Improvement of appetite following the administration of vitamins or steroids to sick animals is unlikely to be due to a gastrointestinal effect, but rather to a general improvement in the feeling of well-being in the animal. It has been claimed that low doses of diazepam or pentobarbitone will induce cats and dogs to eat.

The use of appetite suppressants in the management of overweight animals is not generally necessary. Control of food intake is usually possible and this should correct the problem. Where drug-induced appetite suppression has been tried, particularly in dogs, the response has often been disappointing.

Inhibition of salivary secretion

Inhibition of salivary secretion can be most efficiently achieved by the administration of antimuscarinic drugs. In the ruminant, the secretion of a considerable quantity of saliva is controlled by the sympathetic nervous system and therefore antimuscarinics are less effective in these animals.

Drugs which act on the oesophagus

Surgical removal of oesophageal obstructions in cattle is often hampered by local muscle spasm. Drugs which relax smooth muscle may be useful aids. These include proquamezine (a phenothiazine derivative), hyoscine N-butylbromide (an antimuscarinic) and methindizate (a non-specific smooth muscle relaxant). The commercial formulations of these drugs may also include an analgesic to relieve the pain associated with such obstructions.

Reflux of gastric acid or ingestion of corrosives can cause oesophagitis in dogs. Aluminium hydroxide is useful in the treatment of this condition because of its antacid effects (see below). Metoclopramide (see below), to hasten transit through the stomach, and cimetidine (see page 104), to reduce the acidity of the stomach contents, are also used.

Dose

proquamezine
cattle 240–750 mg slow i.v. total dose

methindizate
cattle (adult)	25–50 mg
calf, pig, sheep	12.5 mg
cat	1.25 mg
dog	2.5–10 mg

hyoscine *N*-butylbromide
cattle 80–100 mg i.m. or i.v.

metoclopramide
dog, cat 0.5–1 mg/kg b.i.d. s.c., i.m. or i.v. daily

cimetidine
dog 5–10 mg/kg p.o. 2–4 times daily

Drugs which affect the stomach

Gastric stimulants

Muscarinic agonists all increase secretions and motility of the stomach but are not generally used for this purpose. Where the activity of the stomach needs to be increased, the dopaminergic agonist metoclopramide is preferable. The response to metoclopramide includes increased gastric contractions and relaxation of the pyloric sphincter, which accelerates gastric emptying. The drug also decreases intestinal transit time. These effects may involve an augmentation of acetylcholine release or an increased sensitivity of muscarinic receptors in the gastrointestinal tract. The antiemetic effect of metoclopramide is due to its dopamine antagonist action in the central nervous system (see below).

Metoclopramide is used to prevent recurrence of gastric dilation and volvulus. It is of benefit as an adjunct to surgery for displaced abomasum and in the management of pylorospasm and associated gastric reflux.

Forestomach stimulation in ruminants is indicated in ruminal impaction, which often follows excessive ingestion of cereals, root crops or autumn grass. It may be achieved by drugs with muscarinic activity (carbachol) or those which inhibit acetylcholinesterase (neostigmine). None of these is ideal, as muscarinic side-effects cannot be avoided. Nicotinic receptors may also be stimulated by large doses (e.g. >4 mg carbachol). In these cases, the consequent stimulation of autonomic ganglia and release of adrenaline from the adrenal medulla inhibits the muscarinic effects on the reticulorumen.

An alternative treatment for ruminal impaction is menbutone, which appears to increase gut motility indirectly by stimulating the flow of bile and pancreatic juices. It is doubtful whether the use of choleretic agents (those which increase the secretion of bile) is of benefit in other situations.

Dose

menbutone   5–10 mg/kg deep i.m. or slow i.v. in all species.

Gastric sedatives

Adrenoceptor agonists and drugs with antimuscarinic effects reduce tone and motility of the stomach. Opium alkaloids also inhibit smooth muscle activity in the stomach and delay gastric emptying. However, their most important gastrointestinal effects are on the intestines (see below).

Agents used to aid expulsion of gas from the stomach (eructation) are called carminatives. Some of these are essential oils (e.g. eucalyptus, peppermint), which are used as flavourings in medicinal products. Their effects include a mild irritant action on mucous membranes and relaxation of the gastric musculature. Release of gas is particularly aided by the relaxation of the cardiac sphincter.

Reduction of flatulence can be achieved by the administration of a defoaming agent such as dimethicone (dimethyl polysiloxane), which disperses mucus-surrounded gas pockets and prevents their further formation.

The use of antacids in veterinary medicine is generally restricted to the treatment of ruminal acidosis. This may occur following grain overload, which results in the production of lactic acid instead of the normal volatile fatty acids. Chemical neutralization of the acid is accompanied by the production of gas which can then be released by eructation. Drugs which are available are systemic antacids, where the compound is soluble and may be absorbed (e.g. sodium bicarbonate), and non-systemic antacids, where insoluble compounds remain within the gastrointestinal tract (e.g. salts of aluminium, calcium or magnesium).

Sodium bicarbonate is useful where systemic acidosis has developed, otherwise it may cause alkalosis. The magnesium salts have a laxative effect (see below), whereas the aluminium salts are constipating. It is common, therefore, to combine these and allow each to counteract the unwanted side-effect of the other. Magnesium and aluminium salts have a longer duration of antacid effect than sodium bicarbonate.

Dose

aluminium hydroxide
| cattle | 30 g |
| dog, cat | 20 mg/kg |

magnesium hydroxide
calf, foal	2.5–5.0 g
pig	1.0–2.5 g
dog	0.3–0.6 g
cat	0.1–0.3 g

calcium carbonate
horse	30–60 g
cattle	60–360 g
sheep, pig	8–15 g
dog	0.5–4 g

Antizymotics

Antizymotics prevent or decrease bacterial fermentation by killing or inhibiting rumen bacteria, so the production of gas ceases. The use of volatile oils, such as cresol, lysol, phenol and chloroform is no longer advised. Oil of turpentine remains as the only volatile oil used as an antizymotic and its use is decreasing in favour of newer preparations. Its actions also include stimulation of salivary secretion and a carminative effect. It has a distinct odour, which may affect flesh and milk, and it should not be administered to animals due for slaughter within 4 days or to those used for milk production.

Silicones consist of alternating silicone and oxygen atoms, with methyl groupings attached to the silicone atoms. They increase the surface tension of liquids and thus reduce foam stability.

Clinical uses of antizymotics

Bloat occurs when the gaseous products of bacterial fermentation cannot be released by the normal process of eructation. In cases of tympany, where the gas is free, it can be removed by stomach tube or trochar and cannula. The use of drugs is necessary when free gas cannot be mechanically removed, such as in frothy bloat. In these cases, often due to a high intake of saponin, the gas is in the form of bubbles, forming a frothy mass. Polymerized methylsilicone, administered by stomach tube or injected directly into the rumen, can be used to treat bloat. Methylsilicone polyrincinate, an organo-polysiloxane, and kaolin (see below), in combination are used for prophylaxis. Low foam detergents of the polyoxyethylene-polyoxypropylene series (e.g. poloxalene) are also effective in prophylaxis and treatment of frothy bloat. Dioctyl sodium sulphosuccinate and nonyl-phenyl-ethoxylate have been of benefit.

Dose

dimethicone
  cattle   100 ml emulsion of dimethicone (25 mg/ml)
  sheep   25 ml emulsion of dimethicone (25 mg/ml)

poloxalene
  cattle   22–44 mg/kg p.o. daily

Treatment of equine colic

Horses with colic should be regarded as potential emergencies where rapid treatment is vital for a good prognosis. A discussion of the differential diagnosis of colic is beyond the scope of this book, but an accurate diagnosis forms the basis of the veterinarian's decision whether to treat the patient medically or surgically.

In the first instance the relief of the acute abdominal pain is of major importance for humanitarian reasons and to aid clinical examination. The ideal analgesic should relieve pain and not depress cardiovascular or gastrointestinal function. To date no such drug is available to the equine practitioner. The drugs commonly used to treat equine colic fall into four categories: non-steroidal anti-inflammatory drugs; narcotic analgesics; α-adrenoceptor antagonists; and spasmolytics. Little is known of the effects of many of these drugs on propulsive motility of the equine gut in health and disease, but as a general rule they tend to depress motility to varying degrees.

Narcotic analgesics are most effective but, because they depress propulsive motility and enhance sphincter tone, they may aggravate the underlying condition. They should be avoided if the colic is due to an intestinal obstruction. In contrast to many other animal species, the use of narcotic analgesics in horses does not appear to cause significant cardiovascular depression.

α-Adrenoceptor agonists or the non-steroidal anti-inflammatory analgesics provide suitable alternatives for use in horses. The use of sedatives may be necessary in distressed animals. Where the α-adrenoceptor agonist, xylazine, is used as an analgesic, additional sedation is not required since it has considerable tranquillizing effects. It reduces intestinal motility and may decrease intestinal blood flow but its short duration of action makes it a useful drug for examination of the patient with severe abdominal pain. It can be combined with butorphanol to prolong the analgesic effect. Detomidine, a new sedative/analgesic for use in horses, has similar actions to those of xylazine but has a longer duration of action. If used in colic cases, it should be administered at the lowest dose rate (see page 127).

Non-steroidal anti-inflammatory drugs (NSAIDs) are peripherally acting analgesics. Flunixin is the most effective NSAID for relief of visceral pain. It does not appear to alter motility or intestinal blood flow. Due to its potent anti-endotoxin effects, it is of particular benefit to the cardiovascular system in the horse with colic. However, it should be noted that, except at very low doses (0.25 mg/kg), flunixin may mask the clinical signs which indicate the need for surgical intervention. Its use, therefore, should be restricted to those patients in which the cause of the colic has been positively identified. Phenylbutazone is not widely used as an analgesic in colic patients because, although it is an effective analgesic for musculoskeletal pain, it has only minor visceral effects.

Acepromazine has no direct analgesic properties. The most dramatic effect in animals with colic is hypotension, which results from α-adrenoceptor blockade and which may lead to complications, particularly if anaesthesia and surgery are subsequently required. Thus, if it is used in these cases, the animal must be well hydrated or the drug may exacerbate hypovolaemic shock.

If the underlying cause of the pain can be determined, it is possible to administer drugs which specifically alleviate the cause. The use of antibiotics to treat colic due to bacterial enteritis is an example of specific drug therapy. More commonly, general symptomatic treatment is instituted.

Liquid paraffin is commonly used as a lubricant and is necessary before the administration of purgatives (see below). Softening of the dry impacted food material requires thorough mixing with the liquid paraffin by intestinal contractions. This should be borne in mind when selecting an analgesic in these cases.

Relaxation of smooth muscle tone with spasmolytics may provide relief, especially in cases where the pain is due to spasm of intestinal smooth muscle. Their use is contraindicated in impactions, where hypomotility may be present. The spasmolytics most commonly used are hyoscine, methindizate and proquamezine. Some of the formulations also incorporate an analgesic.

In cases of flatulent colic a reduction of gas production is indicated. Antizymotics (see above) can be used. Neomycin, an antibiotic, has also been shown to be effective and is regarded by some clinicians as the drug of choice

Some disagreement exists concerning the use of metoclopramide in horses. The drug has been shown, using an experimental ileus model, to be capable of restoring gastro-duodenal co-ordination, thereby virtually restoring transit to normal. Any drug to be used in potential cases of ileus should be administered as a prophylactic measure on completion of surgery, but the possibility that metoclopramide may disrupt intestinal anastomoses has yet to be eliminated. An additional problem which has been encountered during its limited use has been induction of excitement and collapse. Further work is needed to develop a suitable dose regimen that will stimulate and co-ordinate gastrointestinal activity without the risk of these side-effects.

Shock is a serious complication of colic and requires special treatment. The general principles of the treatment of shock can be found on page 242.

Dose

liquid paraffin	up to 15 ml/kg by stomach tube
magnesium sulphate	up to 0.5 g/kg p.o.
dihydroxyanthroquinone	20–50 mg/kg
hyoscine *N*-butylbromide	80–120 mg i.v.
methindizate	25–50 mg i.v. or i.m.
proquamezine fumarate	300–900 mg slow i.v.
neomycin	4–8 g p.o.

Emetics

The ability to vomit is not universal among animals. As far as domestic animals are concerned, ruminants and horses are unable to vomit effectively. Guinea pigs, rabbits and rodents are also limited in this way. In those animals which are able to vomit, this activity is controlled by the emetic centre, located in the medulla (see Fig. 14.1). Input to the emetic centre may be from higher centres (cerebral cortex or limbic system), the semicircular canals and from a variety of sites in the periphery, particularly the gastrointestinal tract and pharynx. The chemoreceptor trigger zone (CTZ) in the area postrema is also connected to the emetic centre and is thought to be involved in the vomiting response to chemicals in the blood. The area is particularly sensitive to drug effects because it is one area of the brain which is not protected by an effective blood–brain barrier. The response of the CTZ appears to involve dopaminergic receptors. Dopamine, applied locally, can induce vomiting and the response can be inhibited by drugs with dopamine receptor antagonist activity. The effects of centrally acting emetics, which act by stimulation of (presumably dopamine) receptors in the CTZ, can be violent.

Serotonin (5-HT) stimulates a subgroup of receptors, 5-HT_3-receptors, in the CTZ and thereby induces vomiting. A peripheral action of 5-HT, which involves stimulation of afferent vagal fibres and consequent CTZ responses, may contribute to vomiting induced by radiation and drugs used in cancer chemotherapy.

Irritation of the gastrointestinal epithelium elicits vomiting. Locally acting emetics capable of producing this effect include warm, strong solutions of

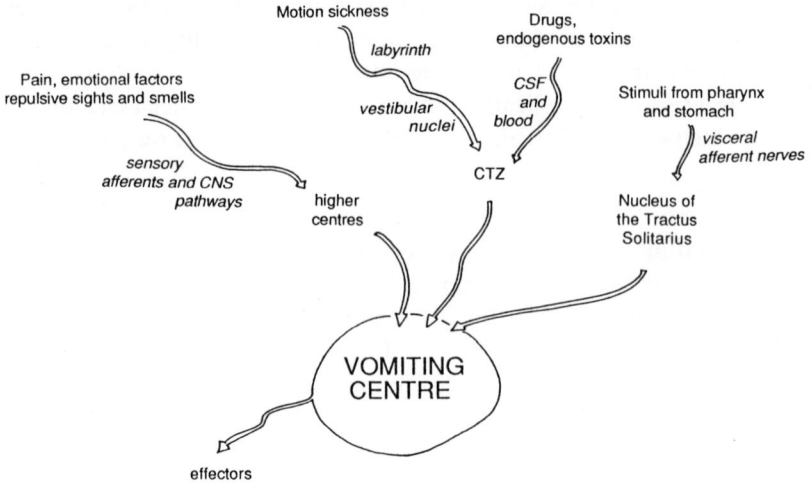

Figure 14.1 Mechanisms in the control of vomiting. For details, see text.

sodium chloride or sodium bicarbonate, 1 per cent copper sulphate or zinc sulphate. The Na^+ salts may also be effective if applied in the crystalline form to the back of the tongue. One crystal of sodium carbonate (washing soda), pushed over the back of the tongue and swallowed, is an effective method of producing emesis. In general, the emetic effect of these agents is less reliable than that of the drugs which have an action in the central nervous system.

Apomorphine is a synthetic morphine derivative which is a potent, rapidly acting emetic. Its action is exerted by stimulation of the dopamine receptors in the CTZ. Since apomorphine is sedative in high doses, it should not be used to induce emesis in cases where there is already some central nervous depression.

Ipecacuanha emetic mixture is prepared from the dried root of *Cephaelis ipecacuanha*. The alkaloid emetine is the active principle. It causes emesis by a combination of a local gastric irritant effect and stimulation of the CTZ. It is a fairly safe and effective emetic, commonly used in the treatment of poisoning in humans and therefore widely available.

Xylazine reliably causes emesis in cats and dogs.

Clinical applications of emetics

The elimination of orally ingested non-corrosive poisons can be aided by the administration of emetics. They should not be used in advanced states of poisoning because it is likely that vomiting would be dangerous for the patient.

Apomorphine can be administered by any route. If it does not elicit a satisfactory response, the dose should not be repeated because profound central nervous system depression may occur. It is also likely that depression of the emetic centre by administration of further doses would reduce the chance of an emetic response. Apomorphine is not recommended for use in cats, since they are relatively resistant to its emetic actions and the high doses required are too depressant.

When locally acting emetics are used, it is preferable to use the sodium salts since, if emesis fails and systemic absorption occurs, these are less toxic.

Dose

apomorphine hydrochloride
    dog   3–6 mg/kg s.c.

xylazine
    dog, cat   0.05–1 mg/kg i.m.

ipecacuanha (as Paediatric Ipecacuanha Mixture B.N.F.)
    dog, cat   1–2 ml/kg p.o. (maximum dose for dogs 15 ml)

Antiemetics

Antiemetics may exert their effects locally, by protection of the gastric epithelium from irritation, or centrally, by depression of the medullary emetic centre or blockade of the dopamine receptors in the CTZ. Centrally acting antiemetics are generally antagonists at muscarinic, histaminic or dopaminergic receptors. New drugs, which are selective antagonists at 5-HT_3-receptors, appear to be effective antiemetic agents, although details of their mechanism of action are yet to be determined.

The antihistamines used as antiemetics include cyclizine hydrochloride, meclozine hydrochloride, buclizine hydrochloride and diphenhydramine hydrochloride. These are most commonly used in the prevention of motion sickness, especially in dogs. The drugs are antagonists at histamine H_1-receptors, but their potency in this regard does not seem to bear a direct relationship to their anti-motion sickness potency. All of these agents are likely to produce sedation, which may be a useful side-effect in the circumstances.

The antimuscarinic antiemetics, hyoscine, dicyclomine hydrochloride and isopropamide iodide, have antiemetic effects which are similar to those of the antihistamines, although of shorter duration. Their action is also centrally mediated. Some drowsiness and antimuscarinic side-effects, such as dry mouth, may occur. Hyoscine is of little use in cats, since it causes central nervous system stimulation.

Dopamine receptor antagonists block the dopamine receptors in the CTZ and, because most of them have some antimuscarinic activity, may also block the emetic centre in higher doses. Drugs in this group include those used as neuroleptics (major tranquillizers) in human medicine, with the phenothiazines and the butyrophenones being the most important groups.

Chlorpromazine, prochlorperazine, triflupromazine and trifluoperazine are some of the drugs which, on the basis of their chemical structure, are classified as phenothiazines. Another member of this group, acepromazine (acetylpromazine), is commonly used in veterinary medicine. The pharmacological profile of members of the group varies. They have dopaminergic antagonist activity, combined with variable antimuscarinic and antihistaminic activity. Many also have adrenoceptor antagonist effects. It is obviously quite difficult to explain the exact mechanism of the antiemetic effect of drugs with such complex actions; no doubt many of them contribute to the overall response. Similar considerations apply to the group of neuroleptics which are butyrophenone derivatives, including haloperidol and droperidol. These may be less useful in veterinary practice since they have been reported to cause 'bizarre behavioural changes' in animals.

Metoclopramide is a more specific dopamine antagonist, with clinically useful antiemetic activity. It is thought to act on both the CTZ and the emetic centre. It is less sedative than other dopamine receptor antagonists. As noted above, metoclopramide also increases the rate of gastric emptying. It is used in small animals as an antiemetic.

Chlorbutol is a central nervous system depressant. It has a local analgesic effect on gastric mucosa which complements its central antiemetic effect.

Clinical application of antiemetics

Vomiting may be exhausting in debilitated patients and can lead to dehydration and profound acid–base disturbance. It is important initially to determine the cause of vomiting and to treat this, wherever possible. This should be done before the administration of antiemetics, which may mask clinical signs and interfere with the diagnosis.

Dose

Prevention of motion sickness — dogs

cyclizine hydrochloride	25–100 mg p.o.
meclozine hydrochloride	2–10 mg/kg up to 10 kg p.o.
	2–6 mg/kg over 10 kg p.o.
diphenhydramine hydrochloride	2–5 mg/kg p.o.
promethazine	2.5–10 mg/kg p.o., b.i.d.

dicyclomine hydrochloride	5–10 m.g. total p.o.
isopropamide iodide	0.2–1.2 mg/kg p.o.
hyoscine	0.03 mg/kg p.o. 4 times daily
acepromazine	0.05–0.25 mg/kg i.m. or slow i.v.
	1–3 mg/kg p.o.
metoclopramide (and cat)	0.5–1.0 mg/kg all routes or p.o.

Drugs which affect the reticular groove

Generally, drugs administered orally to ruminants first enter the forestomach, where dilution and possibly bacterial metabolism take place. However, activation of the reticular (oesophageal) groove reflex allows swallowed material to pass directly into the omasum and abomasum. Some substances, particularly solutions of copper sulphate and sodium bicarbonate, are capable of stimulating the reticular groove closure reflex. Although it is possible that administration of solutions of such salts may increase blood levels of a drug after oral dosing, there is little evidence to suggest that this procedure is of practical benefit.

Laxatives and purgatives

Drugs in this class promote defecation. The response to agents described as 'laxatives' is the passage of soft stools, whereas after purgative (cathartic) administration more watery stools are likely. Some laxatives are capable of causing purgation if the dose is increased.

Emollient laxatives

These agents include lubricant laxatives, mechanical laxatives and faecal softeners. They are long-chain hydrocarbons, resistant to biological or chemical reaction. Since they are not absorbed from the gastrointestinal tract, the effect is exerted locally. As their name implies, drugs in this group soften the faecal mass and lubricate its passage through the intestine. They are eventually excreted unchanged from the gastrointestinal tract.

Liquid paraffin (BP) (mineral oil) is one of the oldest and still one of the most commonly used laxatives. It is a mild lubricant laxative and will not elicit purgation, regardless of increase in dose. There is little likelihood of untoward effects on casual administration. It may interfere with the absorption of fat-soluble vitamins, but this is only liable to be clinically significant if the drug is administered chronically. White and yellow soft paraffin have similar effects.

Dioctyl sodium sulphosuccinate (and the calcium version) is an anionic surfactant which is used as a faecal softener. Increased water retention results in the production of softer faeces. It may be administered by mouth or enema. Poloxalene is a non-ionic surfactant. Accumulated faecal masses in the colon and rectum are broken up, allowing the penetration of water.

Mechanical or bulk laxatives

These laxatives are resistant to digestion in the gastrointestinal tract. They swell on absorption of water and thereby provide increased bulk to stimulate peristaltic activity. The retention of fluid ensures that the faecal mass remains soft. Wheat bran is perhaps the best known member of this group, which also includes agar-agar, sterculia, fruit and a variety of cellulose and hemicellulose preparations.

Osmotic (saline) purgatives

Osmotic purgatives are salts in which the component ions are absorbed only very poorly, if at all, from the gastrointestinal tract. They exert an osmotic effect during their passage through the intestine, drawing water from the tissues into the lumen and resulting in an increase in the faecal mass. The increased mass stimulates peristaltic activity. Since water is vital for their effect, adequate supplies should always be available for animals treated with these purgatives. Furthermore, they should never be administered to dehydrated animals.

Salts of Mg^{2+} are the most common osmotic purgatives. The sulphate (Epsom salts) is the most used; the oxide (hydrated), hydroxide and citrate also have some purgative effect. A small proportion of the Mg^{2+} is absorbed, so repeated administration should be avoided. Sodium salts (phosphate, sulphate) are also effective as osmotic purgatives.

Irritant (contact) purgatives

Irritant purgatives increase intestinal activity by irritation of its mucosal lining. This effect may be augmented by the activation of secretory mechanisms which increase fluid secretion into the lumen. Castor oil, linseed oil and olive oil act as irritant purgatives after they are metabolized by lipases to ricinoleic, linoleic and oleic acids respectively. Of these, the ricinoleic acid is the most irritant and the whole intestinal tract is evacuated. It is then necessary to provide animals with sufficiently bulky feeds to restore normal intestinal function to avoid further constipation. The oleates are the least irritant of the group.

Danthron (dihydroxyanthraquinone) is a synthetic compound related to a group of anthraquinone glycosides which includes senna and cascara sagrada. The naturally occurring substances need to be hydrolysed *in vivo*, with the release of the glycoside sugar, before absorption. The active irritants, emodin alkaloids, are excreted into the large intestine, producing the stimulant effect. This may take some time, which delays the onset of action of the drugs. Danthron does not need to be metabolized before being effective.

Phenolphthalein is chemically similar to the anthraquinones and has a similar mode of action. It provides a good illustration of the increase in duration of action that may occur when a drug undergoes enterohepatic cycling. Some of the phenolphthalein is absorbed, and a proportion of this is excreted in the bile and subsequently reabsorbed. This continues repeatedly, with diminishing quantities excreted in the bile. Because of its unpredictable duration of action it is now rarely used, but may be included in some proprietary mixtures.

Enemas

Enemas exert a local effect after administration *per rectum*. Soapy solutions, sodium chloride solutions and glycerine all cause distension and stimulate defecation when administered this way. They are used to remove impacted material. Dioctyl sodium sulphosuccinate (1 per cent solution) can be used in cases of faecal impaction.

Clinical applications of laxatives and purgatives

In cases of chronic constipation every attempt should be made to determine the cause of the problem and institute appropriate treatment. The most likely cause is dietary mismanagement, and in this case the owner should be advised of corrective measures.

Liquid paraffin is generally free from side-effects but some anal leakage may occur and present problems in pets. It is commonly used in cats, to assist in the passage of hair through the alimentary tract when mild gastritis results from ingestion of hair. Liquid paraffin, administered by stomach tube, is effective in the treatment of impaction colic in horses.

The effect of the bulk laxatives is mild and considered to be the most 'physiological'. Agar-agar and other carbohydrate bulk laxatives are not suitable for herbivores, where fermentation in the gastrointestinal tract would occur. They are most commonly used in small animals and can be combined with liquid paraffin in the treatment of constipation in cats.

The administration of osmotic purgatives results in the passage of more watery stools. They are generally less reliable purgatives in horses; the best response by horses and cattle is to sodium sulphate, usually administered by stomach tube.

Where it is possible that an obstruction may be present, or in cases of enteritis or colitis, irritant purgatives should not be used. Their use should also be avoided in lactating animals because the active laxative principle is excreted into the milk and will affect the young. They are not suitable for adult horses or ruminants but are effective in foals and calves. Linseed oil is used in horses, and castor oil in foals, calves, pigs and dogs. Relatively mild responses occur after the administration of cascara, which is used in dogs and cats.

Danthron is suitable for use in all domestic animals. Although the onset of effects of danthron is relatively prompt in small animals, the agent may take up to 36 hours to be effective in large animals. The onset of action will also vary with fullness of the intestine and is speeded by dilution of the drug. Laxative responses are seen with low doses, purgation with higher doses. Since repeated dosing can lead to drastic catharsis, this should be avoided until it is clear that the effects of the first dose have been seen.

Dose

liquid paraffin (BP)   all species 1–2 ml/kg
　　(Dose in horses may be increased up to 5 ml/kg.)

dioctyl sodium sulphosuccinate
　　cattle, horse　　　5–15 g
　　dog　　　　　　　15–120 mg
　　cat　　　　　　　15–30 mg

methylcellulose
　　dog　　　　　　　0.5–5 g
　　cat　　　　　　　0.5–1 g

magnesium sulphate
　　horse, cattle, pig, sheep　　0.25–1 g/kg

agar
  dog   up to 10 g

sterculia
  dog   200 mg/kg
  cat   120–240 mg

linseed oil
  horse, ruminant   1.5–2 ml/kg

castor oil
  foal, dog, cat   1–2 ml/kg

danthron
  all species   5–15 mg/kg

Other drugs which affect the gastrointestinal tract

Drugs which stimulate muscarinic receptors (e.g. carbachol, bethanechol) increase smooth muscle activity in the gastrointestinal tract. Carbachol is a potent gastrointestinal stimulant and as such may be dangerous in cases of intestinal obstruction, where rupture or intussusception could occur. Bethanechol is preferable. Either bethanechol or pilocarpine are suitable for the management of feline dysautonomia. Anticholinesterases produce similar effects; neostigmine appears to produce fewer side-effects than the other members of the group.

Antimuscarinics have the opposite effect and can be used as antispasmodics. The use of quaternary amines, such as hyoscine N-butylbromide, atropine methylnitrate or the synthetic agent, propantheline, reduces the entry of the drugs into the central nervous system and so reduces the chance of central side-effects. Many commercial antidiarrhoeal preparations contain antimuscarinic agents, e.g. Neutradonna tablets contain sodium aluminium silicate (650 mg) and belladonna alakaloids (calculated as hyoscyamine 48 μg). Pirenzepine, a selective muscarinic M_1-receptor antagonist, reduces the output of acid from the oxyntic cells of the stomach with little other antimuscarinic effect.

Histamine H_2-receptor antagonists selectively inhibit the effects of histamine on H_2-receptors, with little or no effect on H_1-receptors. Thus gastric acid output is reduced. Cimetidine was the first of these to be widely available for clinical use. Others (e.g. ranitidine, nizatidine) are now available. Indications for the use of histamine H_2-receptor antagonists in the dog include chronic gastritis, oesophagitis and peptic ulceration associated with mastocytomas, hepatic disease and uraemias.

Opioids have a constipating effect which may be elicited by different mechanisms in different species. In general, there is a decrease in the propulsive movements of the gut and an increase in the tone of the smooth muscle. These responses are probably exerted on the neurones of the myenteric plexus, although they may be reinforced by some actions in the central nervous system. Morphine and codeine have antidiarrhoeal effects at doses below those needed for analgesia.

Diphenoxylate is a derivative of pethidine, which has potent gastrointestinal effects at doses which do not alter central nervous system activity. Like other opioids, it may be more toxic in the cat. Loperamide, a newer synthetic pethidine derivative, has similar antidiarrhoeal effects and is even less likely than diphenoxylate to elicit central responses. Thus the problems of drowsiness, respiratory depression and the risk of addiction associated with morphine are overcome. Loperamide also has anticholinergic actions and inhibits secretions induced by some bacterial endotoxins. It has a high margin of safety, with large doses being well tolerated, even over long periods of time.

Dose

diphenoxylate
   dog   60 μg/kg p.o. daily

loperamide
   dog   100 μg/kg p.o.

cimetidine
   dog   5–10 mg/kg p.o. 2–4 times daily

Adsorbents and protectants

Solids which bind toxic or otherwise undesirable substances and carry them out of the gastrointestinal tract are called adsorbents. Aluminium hydroxide, silicates (kaolin, magnesium trisilicate), activated charcoal and pectin all act as adsorbents. There is some evidence from *in vitro* studies that they can absorb bacterial endotoxins. Bismuth salts, chalk and activated attapulgite are also commonly incorporated into antidiarrhoeal preparations. The objective is to coat the enteric mucosa and protect it from irritants in the gut contents. Commercial preparations often contain a number of ingredients (e.g. Mucaine is a suspension of aluminium hydroxide gel 4.75 ml, oxethazaine 10 mg and magnesium hydroxide 100 mg in 5 ml).

Kaolin (hydrated aluminium silicate) is the most widely used adsorbent in veterinary medicine. It is a naturally occurring substance which is virtually insoluble and, besides its adsorbent effect, is pharmacologically inert. It is extremely safe and while its effects may not be overwhelming, it is unlikely to cause harm.

Activated charcoal is a most effective adsorbent and is useful in the emergency treatment of poisoning.

Dose

kaolin
    all species   100–500 mg/kg

magnesium trisilicate
    dog, cat   1–5 mg/kg every 4–6 hours

activated charcoal
    20–120 mg/kg mixed in water and given as a drench.

Astringents

Astringents act by causing local precipitation of proteins on skin or mucous membranes, which provide a protective barrier for the tissue beneath. Both Zn^{2+} and Al^{3+} have astringent actions but their use is limited to external surfaces. Intestinal astringent effects can be produced by the vegetable, catechu, which produces its effect by the liberation of tannic acid in its passage through the bowel. Tannic acid has astringent activity which results in a protective coating of precipitated proteins over the bowel mucosa. This may be useful in the treatment of diarrhoea. Catechu is one of the ingredients in antidiarrhoeal drenches.

Treatment of diarrhoea

Diarrhoea results in a net loss of water and electrolytes from the body and, if it persists, the consequent dehydration can be severe. Under normal circumstances there are large fluxes of water from the intestinal lumen to the blood and from the blood to the lumen. In the healthy animal the former is greater, resulting in a net gain (i.e. absorption). The opposite occurs in the animal with diarrhoea, resulting in a net loss (i.e. secretion into the intestinal lumen). The overall therapeutic objective is to restore the fluid balance, either by promoting increased absorption or by reducing secretion, or both.

Ideally, treatment of diarrhoea should be based on an accurate diagnosis of the cause. This is a major topic and only a brief mention of some of the important factors follows; a detailed discussion is beyond the scope of this book. Operative treatment is necessary where the cause is intussusception or a foreign body in the intestine. Anthelmintics are indicated when diarrhoea is due to a heavy worm burden. In small animals, dietary mismanagement is probably the commonest cause of chronic diarrhoea, although the possible presence of specific diseases such as distemper, canine parvovirus disease or feline infectious enteritis (for which vaccines are available) should not be overlooked. Thus the only therapy which may be necessary in small animals is a period of 1–2 days on an appropriate fluids-only intake. Conversely, diarrhoea in young farm animals is commonly associated with a mixture of potential viral, bacterial and protozoal pathogens. Vaccines are available for passive immunization by dam vaccination of calves, lambs and piglets against enterotoxic *E. coli* and more recently against rotavirus in calves. Antibacterials are widely utilized in addition to the non-specific treatments described below.

Fluid replacement

Dehydration and electrolyte loss is the major cause of death in severely affected diarrhoeic young animals. Thus the importance of effective rehydration therapy cannot be over-emphasized. Intravenous rehydration using saline solutions, homologous plasma or plasma substitutes such as degraded gelatin and electrolytes, is only necessary in severely affected, comatosed animals. Suitable solutions are available commercially.

Oral rehydration therapy is simpler and very effective. The technique utilizes the principle that glucose and amino acids continue to be actively absorbed from the gut in the diarrhoeic animal, even in the presence of enteric infection, and the process is accompanied by the absorption of Na^+ and water. Thus there is a net increase in absorption, thereby achieving the therapeutic objective explained above. Commercial formulations (based essentially on Compound Sodium Chloride and Dextrose powder BPC) are available for all species. The manufacturer's directions with respect to withdrawal of solid food should be observed. In scouring calves, temporarily witholding milk is important because lactose digestion is impaired and excessive milk feeding causes undigested milk to reach the large intestine, resulting in fermentive diarrhoea.

Intestinal adsorbents and protectants

These inert substances are commonly incorporated into commercial antidiarrhoeal preparations for oral administration. Despite the evidence from *in vitro* studies, conclusive proof of their clinical efficacy is lacking. However, intestinal adsorbents and protectants have the virtue of being safe and comply with the precept of the Hippocratic school, 'Above all, do not harm'.

Drugs which reduce intestinal motility

Intestinal hypermotility appears to be a common cause of diarrhoea. This may be due to scavenging, leading to irritation of the intestinal mucosa, or to increased secretion stimulated by bacterial enterotoxins, causing dilation and reflex contraction. Less commonly (especially in dogs), the aetiology may be more complicated, because diarrhoea may also be due to intestinal hypomotility. In these cases, hypomotility encourages bacterial overgrowth in the intestine which causes the breakdown of bile salts. The resultant products act on the colon to decrease absorption of water and electrolytes.

In contrast to the non-specific treatments described above, the use of motility-inhibiting drugs is not without risk: reducing peristalsis permits retention of enterotoxin-producing organisms in the gut, thereby increasing the flux of fluid into the lumen. This is particularly relevant in young farm animals and some authorities consider that motility-inhibiting drugs should not be used to treat diarrhoea in these species.

Antimuscarinic drugs such as atropine, hyoscine methylbromide and benzetimide, are constituents of various proprietary formulations, which also commonly incorporate antibacterials. These combinations are thought to be more effective than antibiotic therapy alone. The smooth muscle spasmolytic effect of hyoscine is utilized with the analgesic dipyrone in a parenteral formulation which appears to be useful in the treatment of acute intestinal spasm.

Opioids, which increase smooth muscle tone and decrease peristalsis, have been used for many years in the symptomatic treatment of diarrhoea. Examples of older formulations, still used in species other than cats, include Chloroform and Morphine Tincture BPC (containing chloroform, alcohol and morphine) and Kaolin and Morphine Mixture BPC. Diphenoxylate, a newer drug, is formulated with atropine and is effective in the control of diarrhoea in particular non-responding individuals. Loperamide may be even more effective, especially in the control of secretory diarrhoea.

Specific treatment is indicated for the treatment of diarrhoea associated with idiopathic chronic colitis and exocrine pancreatic deficiency in the dog.

Idiopathic chronic colitis

The drug of choice in this condition is sulphasalazine, normally in conjunction with prednisolone. Corticosteroids are more effective in achieving a remission in mild cases, but sulphasalazine is more effective in preventing relapses. Thus the two drugs are commonly used together.

Following oral administration, sulphasalazine is split by bacteria in the colon to sulphapyridine (an antibacterial) and 5-aminosalicylic acid, which is a non-steroidal anti-inflammatory drug (NSAID). The NSAID is probably the active constituent in treating the disease, but if given independently, both constituents would be absorbed from the small intestine. After sulphasalazine administration, the released salicylate is concentrated in the wall of the colon to produce its anti-inflammatory effect.

Some patients achieve a permanent remission after a few weeks of therapy, but others relapse 4–6 weeks after ceasing treatment and require indefinite, intermittent therapy.

Dose

sulphasalazine	20–25 mg/kg b.i.d., reduced to lowest effective dose after 1 week. Continue for a maximum of 4 weeks.
prednisolone	0.5–1 ml/kg b.i.d. for 5–7 days. Reduce to lowest effective dose administered on alternate days.

Exocrine pancreatic deficiency

This is a common cause of diarrhoea in young dogs (1–2 years old) and therapy is expensive. It is most important to maintain a correct diet. Low-fat and low-fibre diets which incorporate good quality protein and rice should be strictly adhered to, in association with the use of replacement enzymes. Meals should be small and frequent. There is wide variation in the enzyme content of the commercial replacement preparations available, even between different batches of the same brand. Furthermore, a large proportion of the enzyme is inactivated by gastric secretions. In severe cases, it may be advantageous to reduce gastric secretion (which inactivates exogenous enzymes) by the administration of cimetidine (5 mg/kg) about 30 minutes before feeding a meal with added pancreatic extract.

such as changes in vocalization, anabolic and behavioural effects. Effective production of testosterone before and during puberty appears to be important in the subsequent development of normal libido. In sexually mature animals, however, plasma levels of testosterone, above certain threshold values, do not correlate with the degree of libido. Furthermore, there are wide daily variations in plasma levels of the hormone, so that serial sampling is necessary to assess the endocrine status of an animal.

In addition to the virilizing effects described above, androgens have anabolic effects, which stimulate the growth of the musculoskeletal system. These are discussed in Chapter 3.

The oestrous cycle in female animals shows considerable species variation; the bovine cycle is used as an example here (Fig. 15.2). The cow is poly-oestrous, with an average cycle length of 21 days (range 17–24 days).

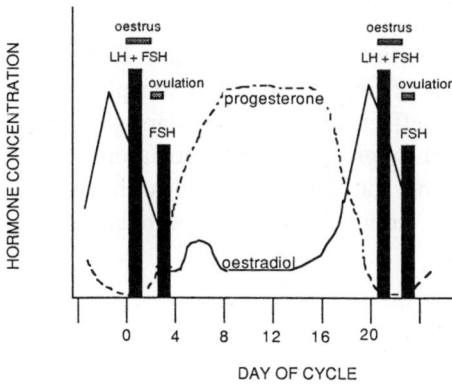

Figure 15.2 Changes in plasma hormone concentrations during the bovine oestrous cycle.

Oestrus, designated day 0, lasts for 6–30 hours and ovulation occurs about 15 hours later (day 1). An increased pulse frequency of release of GnRH a few days before oestrus stimulates the output of gonadotrophins. FSH causes the early growth of the ovarian follicle(s) destined to develop at oestrus. Plasma concentrations of FSH are generally low during the cycle, with a surge at oestrus and a smaller peak concentration about 24 hours later. Similarly, plasma concentrations of LH are low for most of the cycle but begin to rise when stimulated by GnRH. LH causes the final maturation and ovulation of the follicle and secretion of oestradiol (the principal ovarian oestrogen) from the follicle's theca layer. Thus plasma concentrations of oestradiol, which are low for most of the cycle, also begin to increase about 4 days before oestrus, to reach a peak at the onset of heat. The rising concentration of oestradiol in the follicular phase acts on the hypothalamus, causing a positive feedback effect on GnRH release. The resulting pre-ovulatory surge of LH and FSH at the onset of oestrus is believed to cause ovulation and luteinization of the ruptured follicle. After ovulation, plasma concentrations of oestradiol decrease (although there is a second, smaller, unexplained peak on about day 6). During the luteal phase of the cycle, oestradiol is present in low concentrations in the plasma. Progesterone levels, however, are highest between days 8 and 16, when the corpus luteum is mature. These high progesterone levels and low oestrogen levels exert a negative feedback effect on the hypothalamus (at a site distinct from the positive feedback effect seen in the follicular phase). As a result of the inhibited release of GnRH, plasma concentrations of the gonadotrophic hormones, FSH, LH and prolactin, are low during the luteal phase of the cycle. Small fluctuations in these hormones occur during this phase and probably account for the waves of follicular development sometimes observed. Regression of the corpus luteum occurs typically on day 16 of the cycle, due to secretion of prostaglandin $F_{2\alpha}$ from the endometrium. Plasma concentrations of progesterone fall sharply and, with the removal of the negative feedback effect on the hypothalamus, GnRH output increases.

The pineal gland, through its hormone melatonin, plays a role in seasonal breeders by integrating the day length with the breeding season through regulation of GnRH secretion from the hypothalamus.

Hormones and analogues used to control reproductive disorders

Hypothalamic/pituitary hormones

Three synthetic analogues of gonadotrophin-releasing hormone, gonadorelin, buserelin and fertirelin (Table 15.1), are available for veterinary use. Human chorionic gonadotrophin (HCG, chorionic gonadotrophin) is produced by the human placenta and extracted for commercial use from the urine of women in early pregnancy. It is a glycoprotein with molecular weight of 38 000. Although it is structurally different from pituitary LH, it has predominantly LH-like activity.

Pregnant mare's serum gonadotrophin (PMS, PMSG, serum gonadotrophin) is a large glycoprotein molecule (mol. wt. 68 000) produced by the equine chorion and isolated from the serum up to day 80 of pregnancy. It has mainly FSH-like activity, although it has a much greater molecular weight than pituitary FSH. The preparation also has significant LH-like activity.

Table 15.1 Hormones, hormone analogues and antagonists used to control reproductive disorders

Hormone	Non-proprietary name
Gonadotrophin-releasing hormone (GnRH)	Buserelin
	Gonadorelin
	Fertirelin
Gonadotrophins	
Follicle-stimulating hormone (FSH)	Pregnant mare's serum gonadotrophin (PMSG)
Luteinizing hormone (LH)	Human chorionic gonadotrophin (HCG)
Oestrogens	Oestradiol benzoate
	Ethinyloestradiol
	Stilboestrol
Oestrogen antagonists	Clomiphene
	Tamoxifen
Progestogens	Progesterone injection and implants (PRID)
	Fluorogestone acetate
	Medroxyprogesterone acetate
	Altrenogest
	Megestrol acetate
	Proligestone
Prostaglandin $F_{2\alpha}$	Dinoprost
	Cloprostenol
	Luprostiol
	Fenprostalene
	Alfaprostol
Testosterone	Drostanolone propionate
	Methyltestosterone
	Testosterone
	Testosterone phenylpropionate
Testosterone antagonist	Delmadinone acetate

Steroid hormones

The steroid nucleus is common to all naturally occurring androgens, oestrogens and progestogens as well as a variety of other hormones and drugs. Biosynthesis of the steroidal sex hormones depends on enzyme-mediated conversion of cholesterol to progesterone and then to either testosterone or oestradiol (Fig. 15.3).

The mechanism of action of steroid hormones differs from that of most drugs where drug–receptor interactions occur at the cell membrane and responses are often due to changes in membrane permeability. In the case of the steroids, however, the hormone crosses the cell membrane and interaction with its receptor occurs within the cytoplasm of the cell. The hormone-receptor complex then undergoes a conformational change and is transported into the nucleus. Once inside the nucleus, the response to the hormone is mediated by promotion of the synthesis of messenger RNA and the corresponding influence on protein synthesis.

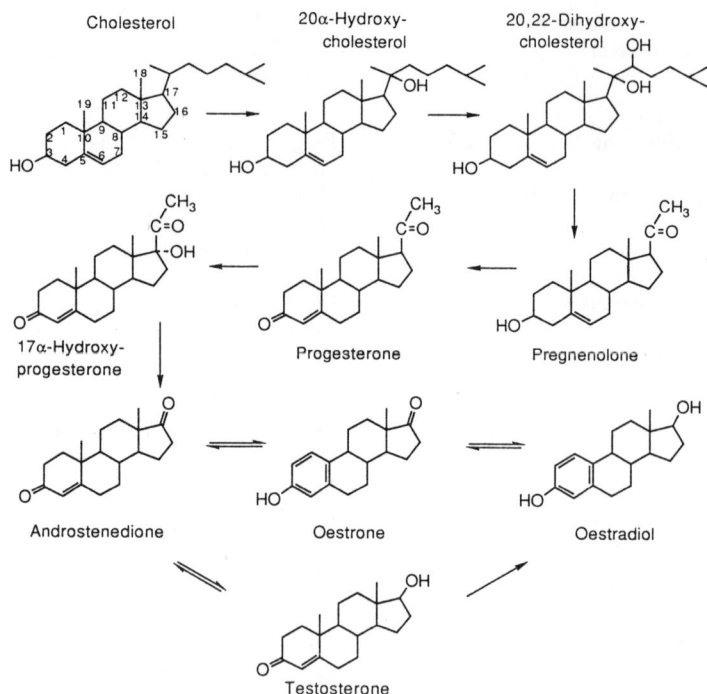

Figure 15.3 Biosynthesis of steroid hormones.

The naturally occurring hormones are all rapidly metabolized in the body and thus have a short duration of action. In many cases, although the hormones may be efficiently absorbed after oral administration, much of the dose is lost on the first pass through the liver. Thus semisynthetic and synthetic compounds have been developed with the aim of producing drugs with selective activity and a variety of pharmacokinetic profiles from which the prescriber may choose the most appropriate.

Addition of an α-alkyl group at C17 reduces the first-pass metabolism of steroidal hormones; most commonly either methyl or ethyl groups are added. Another method of increasing the duration of action of the hormones is esterification of hydroxyl groups on the steroid nucleus. In general, the duration of action of the resulting compound depends on the length and chemical complexity of the attached ester. For example, testosterone propionate needs to be administered three times weekly, while testosterone oenanthate injections are effective for 3 weeks.

The duration of action of the hormones may also be increased by altering the formulation of the preparation. This is usually achieved by reducing the rate of absorption of the active substance. Thus, from an aqueous base, all of the hormone may be absorbed within hours. Increasing the crystal size can extend the period for complete absorption to some days. Suspension of the active ingredient in an oily base can also be used to slow the rate of absorption and thus prolong the duration of action.

The commonly used preparations with veterinary product licences are shown in Table 15.1. In the case of androgens, selection of appropriate preparations gives a choice of initial daily oral dosing, less frequent intramuscular administration or subcutaneous implants, where activity persists for about 60 days. Delmadinone acetate (Fig. 15.4) is a compound with progestogenic activity as well as anti-androgenic activity.

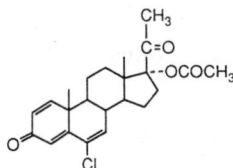

Delmadinone acetate

Figure 15.4   Delmadinone acetate.

Oestradiol benzoate, marketed as such, is the major oestrogen for veterinary use. Some of the synthetic oestrogens do not have a steroid structure but it is not difficult to detect the similarity between their structures and that of oestradiol (Fig. 15.5).

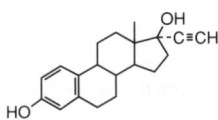

Ethinyloestradiol   Diethylstilboestrol

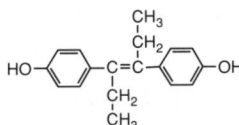

Figure 15.5   Oestrogenic hormones.

The first oestrogen antagonist to be used clinically was clomiphene. It is employed as a fertility drug in women, where it stimulates ovarian activity. Tamoxifen is the other anti-oestrogen used in human medicine, for the treatment of oestrogen-dependent breast tumours. These drugs are not currently used in veterinary practice.

All of the oral contraceptive preparations for women contain a progestogenic component, and a number of different synthetic substances are available. Those used in veterinary practice include fluorogestone acetate, medroxy-progesterone acetate, altrenogest and megestrol acetate (Table 15.1).

Progesterone-releasing intravaginal device (PRID)
Early studies in cows showed that the administration of progesterone for 12 days was effective in some animals in suppressing oestrus and ovulation, but not when begun early in the luteal phase. Later it was found that simultaneous administration of oestrogen shortened the cycle and this led to the development of the PRID. This is a stainless steel spiral covered with an elastomer incorporating progesterone with a gelatine capsule containing oestradiol benzoate attached.

Therapeutic applications of hormones and hormone analogues

Delayed puberty or depressed libido

The manufacturers advocate the use of HCG to stimulate testosterone production in male animals. Even a small dose of HCG can markedly increase plasma testosterone levels for several days and the effect of the drug does not mimic the physiological, pulsatile release of testosterone. The observed response may be due, in part, to a change in testicular capillary permeability (which may cause testicular enlargement due to oedema). Moreover, since libido in mature male animals appears to be unrelated to testosterone levels, some authorities now consider HCG should not be used to treat poor libido. Androgen therapy may be used as an alternative to HCG, but the reservations above also apply to testosterone.

Genital hypoplasia and promotion of the descent of inguinally retained testis

HCG therapy is licensed for use in cryptorchids to simplify subsequent castration, usually advised because of the hereditary nature of the condition and the significant incidence of neoplasia in inguinally retained testes. The success of this treatment is probably due to testicular enlargement associated with oedema rather than the production of a normal testis. Testosterone may be used in cryptorchids as an alternative to HCG.

Since testosterone is essential for the normal development and maintenance of testicular function, it should be rational therapy for hypogonadism after puberty. Although evidence for their efficacy in these cases is equivocal, testosterone and its esters are licensed for this indication.

Impaired spermatogenesis

PMSG is indicated, according to the manufacturers, to treat impaired spermatogenesis. Since the process of spermatogenesis takes nearly 2 months, treatment needs to be carefully monitored. Some consider that the possibility of achieving beneficial results is remote and, since defective sperm output is probably genetic in origin, the use of affected animals for breeding is questionable.

Prostatic hypertrophy and perianal adenomas

These occur quite commonly in older male dogs and appear to be androgen related, although the precise aetiology is unclear. They are usually treated medically, but castration is necessary in some cases to achieve long-term benefit. Prostatic hypertrophy is associated with hyperplasia of the glandular structures. Therapy with oestrogens or progestogens is designed to reduce the output of testosterone by a negative feedback effect on the hypothalamus/pituitary and possibly to counteract the local effects of testosterone on the prostate. Delmadinone acetate, a progestogen with anti-androgen activity, may also be useful. Where there is no response to the initial dose, this should be repeated after 8 days.

Perianal adenomas are not uncommon in old dogs and may recur after excision unless the animal is also castrated. Temporary regression can be achieved with oestradiol or delmadinone.

Dose

oestradiol benzoate	5–10 mg s.c. weekly for 4 weeks, then once per month
delmadinone acetate	1–2 mg/kg s.c. repeated at monthly intervals in animals showing improvement.

Behavioural problems

Behavioural problems, such as certain forms of aggression or vagrancy, may respond to hormone therapy, but behavioural modification training is an important adjunct in treatment. Antisocial behaviour and other behavioural problems are not confined to male dogs and progestogen therapy is used, in addition, in neutered bitches and cats. Delmadinone acetate has proved effective in male dogs and cats in some cases (dose as above).

Megestrol acetate reduces undesirable behaviour in entire and castrated dogs. The initial dose of 2 mg/kg p.o. is administered daily for 1–2 weeks, with subsequent modification of dose according to response. Less frequent drug administration is required if medroxyprogesterone acetate is used. The formulation for depot therapy by subcutaneous injection allows for injection of 10 mg/kg at 3–6-month intervals. Behavioural problems in neutered bitches and female cats and castrated and entire male cats and dogs respond to such therapy.

Anabolic therapy

Methyltestosterone, testosterone or its esters are used in debilitated animals or as supportive anabolic therapy in conditions such as delayed fracture healing. More specific anabolic steroids (hormone growth promoters) are available commercially. Some are testosterone derivatives in which the androgenic potency has been reduced; they are discussed in more detail in Chapter 3. Hormone growth promoters are defined in legislation as substances having oestrogenic, androgenic or progestogenic actions. In the EC there are stringent legal restrictions on the uses of these substances in food animals, including horses, but not in dogs or cats. They may only be administered to food animals to treat infertility, terminate an unwanted gestation, synchronize oestrus or to prepare donors or recipients for embryo implantation. Thus use of these drugs as anabolic agents is legitimate only in cats and dogs.

Hormone alopecia

Since the classical sign of this condition (bilateral symmetry of hair loss) is not always apparent, precise diagnosis may be difficult. In addition to thyroid-, adrenal- and oestrogen-related alopecias, there are ill-defined 'hormone-imbalance alopecias' in dogs and neutered male cats, some of which respond dramatically to androgen therapy. A preparation with the most appropriate formulation can be selected to allow daily oral dosing, less frequent intramuscular injection or subcutaneous implants with activity which persists for about 60 days.

Mammary neoplasia

The growth rate of certain mammary tumours in bitches and cats is oestrogen-dependent and can be reduced with androgen therapy to produce a temporary regression. Megestrol acetate, a progestogen, is also effective in causing regression of oestrogen-dependent mammary tumours in bitches. Subsequent surgery in poor risk surgical patients may be facilitated since progestogen medication often reduces the blood supply to such tumours.

Dose

bitch
testosterone implants   100 mg (duration approx. 60 days)

testosterone esters	40 mg/month
drostanolone propionate	5mg/kg/week, gradually decreasing
megestrol acetate	2 mg/kg/day for 10 days

cat

testosterone esters	12.5–25 mg/month

Treatment of infertility in females

Careful examination and diagnosis is important before using hormones to treat female infertility. For example, acquired lesions in the reproductive tract, for which there is no treatment, may cause fertilization failure. Infections, such as endometritis, need specific antimicrobial treatment. Anoestrus in cows may respond to hormone therapy, but the underlying cause may be an inadequate diet or parasitic infection which requires treatment. The uses of hormones to treat female infertility and to control the oestrous cycle in synchronized breeding are described on a species basis.

Cattle

Treatment of infertility

Infertile cows have calving intervals longer than the normal 12 months and the common presenting signs are either oestrus not apparent or repeated returns to oestrus after insemination.

Oestrus not apparent
A common cause is failure to detect heat (about 20 per cent of dairy cows exhibit oestrus for less than 6 hours) and, when it is a herd problem, commercial heat detectors or milk progesterone assays (which reflect ovarian activity) are useful. In individual animals, to avoid unduly prolonging the calving-to-conception interval, therapy is designed to induce oestrus at a predictable time, as in the first two examples below.

1. There is a palpable corpus luteum or high milk progesterone concentration (it will not be a 'persistent corpus luteum' unless the cow is pregnant—check carefully!—or she has pyometra): the animal is in the luteal phase of the cycle, which is 're-set' by administration of

$PGF_{2\alpha}$, or an analogue, to induce oestrus after 2–5 days. She should be carefully observed and inseminated at induced oestrus. The corpus luteum is not responsive to $PGF_{2\alpha}$ for 5 days post-ovulation, so if no oestrus is observed, the animal should be re-examined and treatment repeated after 11 days.

2. There is no palpable corpus luteum or milk progesterone is low, but the ovaries are round and active: the animal is either approaching oestrus or is in metoestrus. If there has been undue delay since calving, the cycle can be re-set by inserting a PRID for 8 days. $PGF_{2\alpha}$ is administered to lyse any functional corpus luteum 24 hours before removal of the PRID. Oestrus is anticipated within 2–5 days.

3. Anoestrus (true acyclicity) is confirmed by palpably flattened, inactive ovaries on two examinations 10 days apart. This may be treated by insertion of a PRID for 12 days. Six hundred units of PMSG is administered on the day of withdrawal and oestrus should follow in 3 or 4 days. Alternatively, GnRH may induce oestrus within 1–3 weeks.

4. Ovarian cysts, due to anovulation of follicles which do not regress: therapy is indicated if these have not regressed spontaneously by 6 weeks postpartum. The most common are follicular cysts (70 per cent), in which luteinization may be induced with either GnRH or HCG. The cysts should regress after 2–3 weeks but this may be expedited by administration of $PGF_{2\alpha}$ 10 days after the gonadotrophin. An alternative treatment involves the insertion of a PRID for 12 days. When this treatment is successful, oestrus occurs 2–3 days after withdrawal of the PRID. Some claim better results are achieved if the oestradiol capsule is removed from the PRID before insertion. In cases of cysts associated with nymphomania, rather than absence of heat, the signs usually subside about 24 hours after insertion of a PRID.

Results of clinical trials suggest that the efficacy of different types of treatment is about equal; success rates, on the criterion of re-establishment of normal cycles, of approximately 80 per cent have been reported. Conflicting results between some trials may be partly due to the variable extent of fibrosis of follicular cysts. Those with a marked degree of fibrosis are probably unlikely to respond to any treatment.

Luteal cysts (confirmed by milk progesterone levels) are less common (30 per cent). In these animals, cycles are suppressed by the negative feedback effect of progesterone on the hypothalamus. Treatment with $PGF_{2\alpha}$ induces oestrus in 2 or 3 days.

5. Pyometra may be associated with a history of retained placenta or puerperal metritis, and a purulent discharge when presented. A persistent corpus luteum is usually palpable and the enlarged uterus must be distinguished from an early gravid uterus.

If no corpus luteum is present, the condition is probably resolving spontaneously. Prostaglandin administration and the resultant uterine stimulant activity (see below) may expedite recovery. In the presence of a corpus luteum, $PGF_{2\alpha}$ causes regression within 2 or 3 days, with discharge of the uterine contents and return to oestrus. In the small percentage of animals which fail to show clear vaginal mucus after the initial treatment, dosage can be repeated after 7–10 days. Better conception rates are attained following prostaglandin therapy, when breeding is delayed for at least one cycle.

Oestradiol benzoate is an alternative treatment for pyometra, but is considered inferior to prostaglandin therapy. Oestrogens sometimes induce luteolysis with consequent removal of progesterone 'block' and induction of oestrus with uterine evacuation. They also increase uterine tone and contractility (see below) and increase the blood supply to the uterus, thus increasing its resistance to infection.

In addition to either prostaglandins or oestradiol, antibacterial drugs are usually administered to hasten recovery.

Repeat breeders

In contrast to the examples above, in which (apart from some cases of follicular cysts) there is no detectable oestrus, repeat breeders return to oestrus after service or artificial insemination (AI) at normal intervals of 17 to 21 days. The precise cause of this cannot usually be established because of the complex aetiology. Thus empirical treatment is designed to correct those cases which may be due to hormone imbalance.

Either GnRH or HCG (3000 units i.v.) is administered on the day of insemination, with re-insemination after 24 hours using semen from a different animal. This is designed to correct both failure to ovulate (or delayed ovulation) and possible genetic incompatibility. Then 4500 units of HCG is administered i.m. on day 13, to promote a luteotrophic effect, which should prevent potential embryonic loss due to progesterone deficiency.

Controlled breeding

The oestrous cycle may be controlled in suitable sized groups of cows to permit better herd management at service and calving. This facilitates the use of AI and the maintenance of seasonal calving. The cycle is re-set to induce oestrus at a predictable time. Either exogenous progesterone or prostaglandins are used.

Blood levels of oestradiol and progesterone increase within hours after inserting a PRID into the vagina. The PRID is removed after 12 days and the animal inseminated either once, after 56 hours, or twice, at 48 and 72 hours after removal. About 10 per cent of animals may show oestrus

1–4 days after fixed time (56 hours) insemination and failure to re-inseminate reduces fertility because of decreased viability of the spermatozoa. A more recent treatment is to insert the PRID for 8 days and inject $PGF_{2\alpha}$ 24 hours before removal to ensure luteolysis.

The PRID is contraindicated in pregnancy and abortions have been reported following its inadvertent use. Other contraindications are for cows calved less than 20 days, immature heifers and animals with abnormal genital tracts or genital infections.

Luteolysis with prostaglandins

The developing corpus luteum is not lysed by $PGF_{2\alpha}$ or analogues until after day 5 (oestrus = 0) of the cycle and administration of these compounds after normal luteolysis (around day 16) will not affect the timing of the subsequent oestrus. Thus, one commonly used controlled breeding programme is based on the administration of two injections of $PGF_{2\alpha}$, 11 days apart. The first will cause lysis of sensitive corpora lutea and by the time of the second injection, all the group should be in the prostaglandin-sensitive luteal phase. They are then inseminated either on detection of oestrus (within 2–4 days) or once at 72–84 hours or twice at 72 and 96 hours. Double 'fixed-time' insemination appears to give a slight improvement in conception rates compared with single insemination, but this has to be weighed against the increased cost.

Whichever programme is used, animals should be examined to determine that they are not anoestrous or pregnant because $PGF_{2\alpha}$ is ineffective in acyclic animals and induces abortion at certain stages of pregnancy. The drug causes smooth muscle contraction in the myometrium, respiratory tract and gut, which may induce transient abdominal discomfort and increased respiration rate. $PGF_{2\alpha}$ also causes platelet aggregation, thus carrying an increased risk of ischaemia, necrosis and clostridial myositis at the injection site. $PGF_{2\alpha}$ is rapidly inactivated in the body but a semi-synthetic salt is available for therapeutic use. Other synthetic analogues of $PGF_{2\alpha}$, alfaprostol, cloprostenol and luprostiol (Table 15.1), do not induce platelet aggregation and should therefore be less likely to induce reactions at the injection site. The manufacturers' warnings concerning handling all prostaglandins and analogues should be noted. In particular, they should not be handled by pregnant women or asthmatics.

Horses

The mare is seasonally polyoestrous, with a breeding season, in the UK, normally from March to November and anoestrus during the winter months. The ovaries of the anoestrus mare in winter do not respond to endocrine therapy. Oestrous cycles vary in length, with an average duration of 21 days.

The follicles take several days to mature, so that oestrus lasts from 4 to 8 days and ovulation usually occurs 1 to 2 days before the end of oestrus. As in the cow, the corpus luteum develops during the first 5 days or so after ovulation and the total duration of the luteal phase is typically 14 to 16 days. Endocrine therapy in mares is appropriate in a variety of clinical situations.

Induction of ovulation

Because oestrus lasts for 4 to 8 days, several matings may be necessary to ensure that viable spermatozoa are present close to the time of ovulation. When the number of available services is limited, a single i.v. injection of 3000 IU HCG at the time of mating may be administered. If a maturing follicle is present (greater than 4 cm diameter) this will usually induce ovulation within 36 hours. Although administration of HCG is apparently more reliable, GnRH may be administered 6 hours prior to service to stimulate release of endogenous LH.

Irregular oestrous cycles

This condition occurs quite commonly at the start of the breeding season and is believed to be due to insufficient release of pituitary gonadotrophins. The synthetic progestogen, altrenogest, administered in the feed for 10 consecutive days, suppresses cycles by a negative feedback effect on the hypothalamus/pituitary. Most animals return to oestrus and ovulate 7 to 13 days after treatment. This implies that progestogens block the release, rather than the synthesis, of pituitary gonadotrophins. Altrenogest is also used to control the cycles in groups of mares to enable optimal use of the stallion and to suppress oestrus in non-breeders which are difficult to manage when in oestrus.

Induction of oestrus

During the breeding season, administration of a prostaglandin analogue will induce luteolysis of a mature corpus luteum (at least 5 days old); oestrus usually occurs within 2 to 5 days and ovulation 7 to 10 days after injection. Sometimes, at the time of injection, a large follicle is present and this may either ovulate or regress and allow a new follicle to develop. The induction of luteolysis and oestrus in non-pregnant mares during the breeding season is indicated in the following situations:

1. Prolonged dioestrus, due to a persistent corpus luteum, is not uncommon in mares.
2. 'Lactational anoestrus'. Most mares have a corpus luteum by 20 days

postpartum, which may persist ('lactational anoestrus') and good conception rates have been reported following mating at oestrus induced with prostaglandin administration rather than at the natural foal heat.

3. Facilitation of oestrus detection. Induction of luteolysis does not intensify oestrus behaviour. However, when it is difficult to detect, two injections of one of the analogues of PGF$_{2\alpha}$ (Table 15.1) can be given 14 days apart. This is usually followed by the onset of oestrus, 4 to 5 days after the second injection.

Pregnancy failure

Early pregnancy failure, with resorption of the embryo, is associated with a persistent corpus luteum and a similar clinical situation to prolonged dioestrus. Administration of prostaglandin before day 36 of gestation will usually induce luteolysis and an ovulatory oestrus. If pregnancy fails after day 36, the endometrium will be producing PMSG. Although prostaglandin injection usually causes luteolysis, induced oestrus is anovulatory and infertile until the gonadotrophin disappears from the circulation, when it may be too late in the year for another service.

Sheep

The ewe is seasonally polyoestrous and breeding activity is initiated by increasing hours of darkness, which stimulates secretion of melatonin from the pineal gland. This, in turn, stimulates the release of GnRH. Oestrous cycles have an average duration of 16 days and oestrus lasts for 1 to 2 days, with ovulation towards the end of oestrus. The main use of hormones to regulate the oestrous cycle in sheep is for controlled breeding in the normal season and hence synchronized lambing, to advance the breeding season and to improve lambing rates (fecundity). The success of controlled breeding techniques also depends on the quality of animal husbandry and nutrition.

Synchronization of cycles

Daily injections of progesterone are effective, but impractical, to synchronize oestrous cycles. Intravaginal sponges, impregnated with either fluorogestone acetate or medroxyprogesterone acetate, are available for sheep and are analogous to the PRID used in cattle. The sponges are removed 13 days after insertion and most animals exhibit oestrus behaviour 2 or 3 days later. Optimum fertility is achieved with supervised mating with at least one ram per 10 ewes.

Injections of $PGF_{2\alpha}$ analogues have been used, as for cattle, to induce luteolysis and synchronize oestrus. They are not licensed in the UK for use in sheep and results of trials indicate that precision in synchronizing oestrus is poorer than with the use of progestogens.

Out of season breeding

The breeding season can be advanced by about 6 weeks with the use of progesterone-impregnated sponges as described above. In the anoestrous ewe, progestogens alone do not lead to sufficient release of gonadotrophins. Thus an injection of PMSG (300–750 IU) is administered when the sponge is withdrawn.

Other techniques for advancing the breeding season which have been successfully employed experimentally, utilize repeated dosing with GnRH or melatonin. At the time of writing, slow-release melatonin implants are being developed for intravaginal, intraruminal and subcutaneous use in sheep and may soon be available.

Increasing lambing rates

The rate of ovulation can be stimulated by administration of PMSG, but there is an unacceptable variation in the response. An alternative mechanism of action involves the induction of antibodies to the natural ovarian hormone, androstenedione. This hormone is secreted by the ovary with oestrogen and progesterone and, like them, it has a negative feedback effect in the hypothalamus/pituitary to reduce the output of FSH and LH. Ovandotrone albumin (Fecundin) is a steroid protein immunogen, consisting of a combination of ovine androstenedione and human serum albumin. It actively induces the formation of antibodies against androstenedione which, by neutralizing a proportion of the hormone, reduces the negative feedback effect. The consequent increase in the release of gonadotrophins from the pituitary leads to superovulation. The vaccine is administered in two doses, 8 weeks and 4 weeks before tupping (mating). In subsequent breeding seasons, only one injection, 4 weeks before tupping, is necessary. An average increase of about 25 lambs per 100 ewes tupped has been obtained in UK trials. For survival of the extra lambs, treated ewes must be managed as twin-bearing flocks, with provision of adequate nutrition, shelter and supervision.

Pigs

The sow is polyoestrous, with an average cycle length of 21 days. Oestrus lasts for an average of 2 days and ovulation occurs about 36 hours after the onset of oestrus.

Induction of oestrus and ovulation

Anovulation in sows is usually associated with fewer follicles rupturing, which results in smaller litter size. Or, since at least four foetuses are necessary to maintain pregnancy, there may be returns to heat after service. If the underlying cause is not faulty nutrition, rational endocrine therapy is HCG (500–1000 IU i.m. on the day of service).

Postpartum anoestrus is normal during lactation and, provided lactation exceeds 3 weeks, most sows have an ovulatory oestrus about 5 days after weaning. Gonadotrophins are used when it is necessary to induce post-weaning oestrus, particularly when early weaning is practised. The success rate before 40 days postpartum is not marked.

PMSG (1000 IU s.c. or i.m.) at weaning should induce a fertile oestrus within 3 to 7 days. To mimic more closely the physiological endocrine pattern of the oestrous cycle, HCG (500 IU s.c. or i.m.) may be administered after the PMSG. A combination of the two gonadotrophin preparations is available (PG 600) and this single injection may be more convenient.

Oestradiol benzoate (5–10 mg 40 days postpartum) will induce behavioural oestrus, but the possibility of it being ovulatory is less certain. Ovulation is presumably due to the positive feedback effect of oestradiol on the hypothalamus, stimulating a surge of gonadotrophins.

Synchronization of oestrus

The progestogen altrenogest is very effective in synchronizing oestrus in sexually mature gilts. A daily dose of 20 mg (as an oil suspension which is administered as a top dressing to the feed) for 18 consecutive days induces a fertile oestrus 4 to 8 days later in more than 90 per cent of animals. Accurate dosing is important as lower doses may result in the development of cystic ovarian follicles and an unpredictable interval to induced oestrus. There is some evidence, which requires substantiation, that altrenogest slightly increases ovulation rate and promotes embryo survival.

The corpus luteum in the pig is sensitive to luteolysis by prostaglandins during pregnancy, but only between days 12 and 15 of the oestrous cycle. Thus the use of prostaglandins to synchronize oestrus, as described previously for cattle, is not applicable in pigs.

Dogs and cats

The bitch is monoestrous, normally having two oestrous cycles, each divided into four stages, per year. Pro-oestrus lasts, on average, for 9 days (range 2–15 days). A surge of LH initiates the oestrus stage, with ovulation 1–2 days after its onset. Oestrus, when the bitch is sexually receptive, lasts an average of 9 days (range 3–21 days) and is followed by metoestrus. During this period of about 80–90 days, the corpora lutea secrete increasing amounts of progesterone for the first 3 weeks, after which the concentration gradually declines. The fourth stage of the cycle is anoestrus, which lasts 3–4 months before the onset of the next pro-oestrus.

The cat has a very variable pattern of oestrous cycles, which depends to some extent on the breed. The species is unique amongst domesticated animals in that coitus, which stimulates LH release, induces ovulation. Oestrous cycles normally occur from January to September (in the northern hemisphere) with a period of anoestrus in the last three months of the year. Oestrus lasts for 5–10 days and, in the absence of mating, occurs at intervals of about 2 weeks, with waves of follicular development and regression. There are no corpora lutea in the interoestrus periods. Thus, they are not true dioestrus phases, although sometimes they are so called. Following an infertile mating and induced ovulation, the corpora lutea produce an interoestrus period (dioestrus/pseudopregnancy) of about 40 days. By stimulation of the vagina with cotton buds, this can be utilized to keep breeding queens out of call.

Induction of oestrus and ovulation

Induction of oestrus in bitches and cats is more difficult than in other species and the results are variable. Following prolonged anoestrus in the bitch, the most consistent results have been achieved by daily administration of PMSG (50–200 IU s.c.) for up to 3 weeks if necessary. Oestrus usually occurs after 8–10 injections in successful cases and should be followed by the administration of HCG (100–500 IU i.m.) on the day of mating to control the timing of ovulation.

The bitch should not be treated with hormones to induce oestrus within 4 months of the preceding oestrus, since the hyperplastic state of the uterus during this period impairs fertility.

Few published data are available on hormone therapy to induce oestrus in the cat. PMSG (50 IU s.c.) administered daily for 5–6 days, with mating permitted at the onset of oestrus, has been suggested.

Prolonged oestrus (nymphomania) is associated with persistent or slow-growing follicles. A single injection of HCG (100–500 IU i.m.) will usually induce rupture of the follicles in dogs and cats.

Habitual abortion

Habitual abortion, in a minority of cases, is due to deficient secretion of progesterone arising from an inadequate luteal response to gonadotrophins. Progesterone therapy is rational in these cases. The drug may be administered by repeated intramuscular injections or, more conveniently, by subcutaneous implant (up to 100 mg in the bitch). Implants should be removed 2 to 3 days before anticipated whelping to avoid the possibility of delayed parturition.

Other, more common causes of habitual abortion include a variety of maternal diseases, foetal abnormalities and foetal death. Although progesterone, by its stabilizing action on the uterus (see below), may prevent abortion in some of these cases, the end result may not be normal, viable offspring. It can also cause virilizing effects in females and cryptorchidism in males.

False pregnancy

This is such a common condition in adult bitches, occurring 1 to 3 months after oestrus, that it may be considered a normal feature of metoestrus. The animal exhibits behavioural signs characteristic of pregnancy and there is often mammary enlargement and production of milk. Androgens, oestrogens or progestogens may be used to produce a negative feedback effect on the hypothalamus, which inhibits release of GnRH and prolactin. However, it should be appreciated that the response to such therapy is rather erratic and suppression may only be temporary. Affected animals usually recover naturally within a few weeks, so the need for treatment is somewhat questionable. Bromocriptine is a synthetic ergot alkaloid with anti-prolactin activity. It is not licensed for use in bitches, but has been used with equivocal results.

Dose

androgen
    methyltestosterone   5–30 mg daily for 5–7 days

androgen/oestrogen combination
    initially: up to 32 mg methyltestosterone + 0.04 mg ethinyloestradiol
    followed by: 24–32 mg methyltestosterone + 0.03–0.04 mg ethinyloestradiol for 4–9 days

progestogens
    proligestone   33 mg/kg
    megestrol acetate   2 mg/kg for 5–8 days

Pyometra

Pyometra is quite common in bitches over 6 years old (sometimes younger) and occurs during the luteal phase of the cycle. There is an accumulation of breakdown products of uterine secretions under the influence of progesterone (and possibly oestrogens), causing uterine distension. Toxins from the uterine secretions and from secondary bacterial invasion which occurs in some cases, are absorbed into the circulation, causing the characteristic signs of anorexia, depression, vomiting and thirst.

Pyometra may also follow the use of oestrogens after misalliance and after high-dosage or prolonged progestogen therapy. It is recommended that depot formulations of progestogens for postponement of oestrus should only be used during deep anoestrus. The manufacturers' recommendations should be carefully observed whenever progestogens are used in non-spayed bitches since the bitch endometrium is especially sensitive to them.

The treatment of choice is ovariohysterectomy with supportive fluid therapy when required. Medical treatment with antibiotics and prostaglandins is sometimes adopted, but the success rate varies. This has to be balanced against the risk of anaesthesia and surgery on a toxic patient and the potential breeding value of the bitch. There are no prostaglandins or analogues licensed in the UK for use in dogs, but the synthetic $PGF_{2\alpha}$, dinoprost, appears to be used increasingly in the treatment of pyometra and postpartum endometritis. In contrast to most species, the corpora lutea of bitches and cats are not readily lysed by $PGF_{2\alpha}$. The effect is presumably mainly due to the ecbolic action on the myometrium and relaxation of the cervix.

Toxic effects of dinoprost in the bitch may be seen soon after injection and persist for about 3 hours. There is salivation, vomiting, diarrhoea, pyrexia and tachycardia. In cases of closed pyometra, there is risk of uterine rupture or exudate being forced through the oviduct to cause peritonitis.

Dose

dinoprost   0.1–0.25 mg/kg daily for up to five treatments, preferably, only in cases of open pyometra.

Control of the oestrous cycle

The oestrous cycle can be regulated by administration of appropriate hormones. The term 'suppression' refers to therapy during pro-oestrus to abolish the signs of that oestrus. Postponement implies therapy during anoestrus (or interoestrus in cats) to prevent oestrus occurring. Progestogens and, less commonly, androgens are used for these applications. When it is prolonged, oestrus can also be terminated in bitches and cats, for example, by injection of HCG as described above.

Testosterone phenylpropionate is used to suppress oestrus in cats and to suppress or postpone oestrus in bitches. The response is due to a negative feedback effect on the hypothalamus/pituitary which inhibits the release of gonadotrophic hormones. Although the therapy is very effective, the masculinizing side-effects (typically clitoral enlargement and vaginitis) are not acceptable to some owners. However, unlike progestogens, testosterone does not induce endometrial hyperplasia (see below) or impair racing performance and is preferred for use in greyhounds.

A synthetic androgen, mibolerone, is available in some countries for long-term prevention of oestrus.

Dose

testosterone phenylpropionate
    bitch and cat   10 mg s.c. or i.m. every 10–14 days

Progestogens are commonly used to control the oestrous cycle in bitches and, to a lesser extent, in cats, when neutering is not acceptable to the owner. They act by negative feedback on the hypothalamus to inhibit the release of gonadotrophins. They may be administered during anoestrus (or during interoestrus in cats) to postpone oestrus, or during pro-oestrus to suppress the cycle.

Progestogens are contraindicated in bitches less than 1 year old and in animals with uterine disease or mammary tumours. When properly used, progestogens are highly effective, but therapy should never be recommended without cautioning clients about their possible side-effects. They may cause a change in temperament, weight gain and lactation. Subcutaneous injections of progestogens may induce alopecia, so they should be administered at an inconspicuous site. They are diabetogenic, since progesterone is an insulin antagonist.

The most serious potential side-effect is on the endometrium which, in the bitch, is particularly sensitive to the effects of progestogens. High doses or prolonged therapy may cause cystic endometrial hyperplasia followed by pyometra. This effect is claimed to be less common in cats, but it does occur. Therefore it is not considered advisable to extend anoestrus for more than 2 years. The relative potency for the suppression of gonadotrophin release (desired effect) and stimulation of endometrial hyperplasia (unwanted side-effect) differs for different progestogens. Proligestone has comparatively less effect on the endometrium and, despite reports of pyometra associated with its use, it is considered to be the safest progestogen for long-term use. The overall incidence of uterine disorders associated with its use is about 0.3 per cent. Since the duration of therapy is the single most important factor in the development of endometrial hyperplasia, the depot injectable preparations of medroxyprogesterone acetate are recommended for use only during deep anoestrus. The incidence of these side-effects is less when either medroxyprogesterone acetate or megestrol acetate is administered orally and there is the option to cease medication if necessary.

Preparations and dose

progesterone is licensed for temporary postponement of oestrus in
    cats   2.5–5 mg s.c. or i.m., every 3 days.

For prevention of oestrus:

medroxyprogesterone acetate

(not recommended for use in bitches intended for breeding)

bitch	50–75 mg or 3 mg/kg s.c. 6 weeks before oestrus repeated at intervals of 5–6 months.
cat	up to 25 mg s.c. repeated every 6 months.

For interruption of oestrus and subsequent prevention:

bitch	commence therapy when pro-oestral bleeding is evident 10 mg p.o. daily for 4 days, then 5 mg daily for 12 days (Dose should be doubled for animals >25 kg).
cat	2.5 mg p.o. daily, commencing in pro-oestrus.

For postponement of oestrus:

bitch	commence therapy in anoestrus 5 mg daily for duration of postponement (Dose should be doubled for animals >25 kg).
cat	2.5 mg p.o. daily, commence in anoestrus or interoestrus.

proligestone

bitch	up to 33 mg/kg s.c. (consult data sheet for details)
cat	100 mg s.c.

megestrol acetate

Tablets for oral administration are available for suppression or postponement of oestrus in cats and bitches. A number of dosage regimens are recommended by the manufacturers, depending on the species and desired effect. Consult manufacturers' data sheets for details.

Drugs acting on the uterus

The response of uterine smooth muscle to drugs and natural mediators usually depends on the prevailing hormonal status of the animal. High progesterone levels, as found during pregnancy or the luteal phase of the oestrous cycle, inhibit the contractile response of the smooth muscle. In contrast, as progesterone levels decline and oestrogen levels begin to rise at term, the sensitivity of the uterine muscle to stimulants is increased. In general, drugs may be used to either stimulate or relax uterine muscle. Those which induce a contractile response are often referred to as oxytocics, after the naturally occurring uterine stimulant, oxytocin. When they stimulate the uterus at term, they are called ecbolics. Abortifacients are stimulants which are used to induce abortion, i.e. to induce uterine contractions before term.

The uterus has parasympathetic and sympathetic innervation, the responses to which vary, depending on the species and the stage of the oestrous cycle or pregnancy. Both α_1-(excitatory) and β_2-(inhibitory) adrenoceptors are present in the myometrium, but denervation causes little change in uterine motor activity.

The myometrium has a high degree of spontaneous electrical and mechanical activity. As in cardiac and skeletal muscle, the interaction of actin and myosin results in muscle contraction and is instigated by free cytoplasmic Ca^{2+}. This 'activator' Ca^{2+} is in dynamic equilibrium with intracellular, membrane-bound Ca^{2+} stores. Thus, release of stored Ca^{2+} into the cytoplasm, probably triggered by entry of extracellular Ca^{2+} across the plasma membrane during depolarization, causes muscle contraction. When activator Ca^{2+} is bound in intracellular stores, the uterus relaxes.

Female sex hormones

The female sex hormones, oestrogens and progesterone, are small steroid molecules which diffuse freely into most cells, but only affect target tissues such as the myometrium, whose cells have the specific receptor sites in the cytoplasm. The hormone–receptor complex moves from the cytoplasm into the nucleus and promotes the synthesis of messenger ribonucleic acid, which directs the response to the hormone.

Oestrogens promote the synthesis of the contractile proteins and the synthesis and release of prostaglandins. In the presence of oestrogens, Ca^{2+} is less firmly bound in membrane stores than when progesterone is the predominant sex hormone. Under the influence of oestrogens, electrical activity in the myometrium is marked and characterized by regular trains of action potentials. There is also an increase in the number of oxytocin receptors on the cell surface. The oestrogen-dominated uterus thus exhibits a high degree of spontaneous mechanical activity and an enhanced sensitivity to stimulants such as oxytocin.

Progesterone was so named when it was demonstrated, initially in the rabbit, to be the hormone responsible for maintaining gestation. It exerts an overall desensitizing or blocking action on the myometrium. There is an increased degree of Ca^{2+} binding in membrane stores. Electrical activity, recorded as action potentials, is less marked than under the influence of oestrogens and conduction of electrical activity in the myometrium is inhibited. Thus the effect of a stimulus—nervous or hormonal—tends to remain localized rather than inducing an overall contraction.

Cell surface-active agents

There are specific receptors for agents such as acetylcholine, β_2-adrenoceptor agonists, prostaglandins and oxytocin on the surface of myometrial cells.

The effects of these agents culminate in a final common pathway which is either an increase (stimulants) or a decrease (relaxants) in the concentration of cytoplasmic activator Ca^{2+}. However, the intermediary mechanisms for translation of receptor binding into stimulation or relaxation of the uterus are not clearly understood.

Binding of agonists to the β_2-adrenoceptor stimulates a membrane-bound enzyme, adenylate cyclase, which catalyses the conversion of ATP to cyclic AMP. The latter activates specific protein kinases which promote phosphorylation of intracellular proteins and an increased uptake of Ca^{2+} into membrane stores, with a consequent relaxation of the uterus. Although the use of a selective β_2-adrenoceptor agonist reduces the chance of β_1-mediated cardiac side-effects, the vasodilator activity of β_2-adrenoceptor stimulants may be significant.

Oxytocin

This naturally occurring mediator is synthesized in the hypothalamus and then moves along the axons to the posterior pituitary gland where it is stored for release as required. It is a nonapeptide which can be isolated from animal sources. The product of such isolation is usually contaminated to some degree with antidiuretic hormone (vasopressin), so preparation by synthetic chemistry is preferred for therapeutic applications. Oxytocin is involved at different times in normal reproductive processes, including the facilitation of sperm and zygote movement at oestrus and during parturition. The release of oxytocin is under nervous control and is stimulated by teat or genital tract stimulation and by the presence of the foetus in the birth canal.

The uterine smooth muscle stimulant effect of oxytocin is greatest in the presence of oestrogenic tone, so that its actions in oestrus and at parturition are maximal. Under these circumstances it induces frequent, powerful, rhythmic uterine contractions and also causes contraction of the myoepithelium of the mammary gland, causing milk let-down in the lactating animal. The mechanism of action of oxytocin in promoting uterine contraction is not clear. There is some evidence that the pathway may involve release of prostaglandins which then promote release of Ca^{2+} from membrane stores. The duration of action of oxytocin is very short and repeated administration is normally necessary.

Ergot alkaloids

The ergot alkaloids are produced when rye is infected with the fungus *Claviceps purpurea*. A number of alkaloids have been isolated and they produce a range of pharmacological responses including hallucinations, vasoconstriction and stimulation of gastrointestinal and uterine smooth muscle. Ergometrine is one of the most potent uterine stimulants of the naturally occurring alkaloids. The uterine smooth muscle at term is particularly sensitive to ergometrine. It induces powerful, sustained contractions, unlike the rhythmic contractions which occur in response to oxytocin. Ergometrine also has significant vasoconstrictor activity but this is considerably less than some of the other members of the group. Its use is declining in favour of the more potent methylergometrine, which does not have vasoconstrictor activity.

Prostaglandins

Prostaglandins (PGs) are naturally occurring substances, described as local hormones (see Chapter 3). PGs are capable of stimulating a variety of tissues and the nature of the response is often species dependent. PGs appear to be involved in the response to noxious stimuli, allergies, modulation of autonomic nervous activity, blood clotting, renal function and blood pressure control. A role in reproductive function is also most likely.

PGE_2 and $PGF_{2\alpha}$ are potent stimulants of uterine smooth muscle; normally, rhythmic contractions (similar to those with oxytocin) are produced. The sensitivity of the uterus increases as pregnancy progresses. It is possible that $PGF_{2\alpha}$ is partly responsible for the initiation of parturition and that, in combination with oxytocin, it induces cervical dilation and increases uterine motility. It also stimulates the smooth muscle of the gastrointestinal tract, causing nausea, vomiting and diarrhoea and may cause bronchoconstriction by stimulation of bronchial smooth muscle.

$PGF_{2\alpha}$ has luteolytic activity and may be the naturally occurring luteolytic hormone in cows, mares, sows and ewes. PG derivatives have been produced in an attempt to reduce the incidence of side-effects and prolong the duration of action. The enhanced luteolytic activity of these compounds is not accompanied by an increase in uterine stimulant activity.

Therapeutic uses of uterine relaxants and stimulants

Drugs are used either to inhibit or to stimulate uterine contractions in a variety of conditions, but the drug of choice for a particular indication is sometimes dependent on the species. Therapeutic applications are therefore listed under the headings of presenting conditions, rather than according to individual drugs and hormones.

Threatened and habitual abortion

β_2-Adrenoceptor agonists cause relaxation of the myometrium. Clenbuterol is a selective β_2-adrenoceptor agonist and is the most widely used drug of this class. Its use in the treatment of threatened abortion has not been reported, but it is used in cattle at parturition to delay the process for some hours if necessary, to facilitate manipulation of the calf or to relax the uterus prior to Caesarean section.

Dose

clenbuterol
>   cow   0.3 mg i.m. or slow i.v.; repeated if necessary after approximately 4 hours.

Isoxsuprine also induces uterine relaxation. It has been reported to be successful in reducing the incidence of abortion in mares and cows after laparotomy (up to 250 mg every 6 hours for 24 hours after surgery). It is similar chemically to the sympathomimetic amines, but has actions which are not antagonized by β-adrenoceptor antagonists. Furthermore, unlike clenbuterol, it is not selective for β_2-adrenoceptors and is thus more likely to cause tachycardia.

Progesterone therapy is rational when habitual or threatened abortion is due to inadequate secretion of the hormone arising from an inadequate luteal response to gonadotrophins. However, as discussed above, it is questionable whether progesterone therapy is effective in a majority of cases of threatened or habitual abortion.

Dose

mare and cow	up to 800 mg implanted s.c.
bitch	up to 100 mg implanted s.c. (or 2–3 mg/kg s.c. or i.m. daily).

The implants should be removed 2 weeks (in mares and cows) and 2–3 days (in bitches) before the anticipated parturition date.

Misalliance

The treatment of choice in mares and cows is $PGF_{2\alpha}$ or an analogue (see Table 15.1). The drugs induce luteolysis and/or directly stimulate the uterus. In cows, drug administration should be 7–15 days after service; in mares, 10 days after the end of oestrus.

Misalliance in the bitch is effectively treated with oestradiol within 4 days of mating. It appears to act by causing a block at the utero-tubal junction which delays transport of zygotes into the uterus so that the endometrium is not phased for implantation. Treatment is at least 95 per cent effective in preventing pregnancy, but behavioural oestrus may last for several weeks and there is a risk of subsequent cystic endometrial hyperplasia and pyometra.

Dose

bitch   oestradiol benzoate 5–10 mg i.m., s.c.

Induction of abortion and parturition

This is achieved either by luteolysis with $PGF_{2\alpha}$ or an analogue, or by the use of hormones to stimulate one of the succeeding endocrine events of normal parturition.

Some days before parturition (e.g. 10 days in sheep), increased levels of foetal cortisol induce placental enzymes to convert progesterone to oestrogen. Oestrogen reaches the maternal tissues via the placenta, where it promotes secretion of prostaglandins and increases the number of oxytocin receptors in the myometrium. Prostaglandins cause luteolysis, cervical dilation, uterine contraction and the release of oxytocin.

Sheep

The corpus luteum is not essential for the maintenance of pregnancy after 50 days. Prostaglandins are therefore effective for inducing abortion only within this period. They are ineffective for the induction of parturition. Induction of parturition is achieved by the administration of corticosteroids, normally after 140 days of pregnancy. The latency of their effect is 1–4 days.

Oestradiol benzoate has been demonstrated in Australian studies to be effective when used in high doses. Administration between 143 and 148 days of pregnancy induces parturition in virtually all ewes within 24 hours. Oestradiol also prolongs the bonding period, which facilitates fostering.

Dose

dexamethasone phosphate	8–16 mg i.m., i.v., repeat in 3 days if necessary.
flumethasone	2.5–5 mg i.m.
oestradiol benzoate	30 mg i.m.

Dogs and cats

Surgical abortion or elective hysterotomy is the treatment of choice. Prostaglandins are effective but toxic and are not licensed for use in these species in the UK.

Pigs

Induction in pigs is now common practice, to synchronize farrowing at times convenient for supervision. This reduces piglet mortality and enables interfostering within hours of birth to ensure adequate intake of colostrum and optimum matching of litter sizes.

The corpora lutea are essential for the maintenance of pregnancy at all stages in the pig. They are readily lysed by $PGF_{2\alpha}$ or its analogues, which are therefore the drugs of choice. The latency is about 24–30 hours in about 80 per cent of farrowings so the drug is normally administered at 8 a.m. on day 113 in herds with an average duration of pregnancy of 115 days. Parturition should only be induced in herds with good breeding records so that prematurity can be avoided. For example, in herds with an average duration of pregnancy of 115 days, the incidence of stillbirths is about 15 per cent if induced at day 112.

Oxytocin is sometimes administered 24 hours after the $PGF_{2\alpha}$. This ensures that virtually all farrowings occur within 30 hours and it also decreases the duration of the parturition. It is essential to check that injections of oxytocin are preceded by PG administration; otherwise uterine rupture with foetal and maternal deaths can result.

Dose

dinoprost	10 mg i.m.
cloprostenol	175 μg i.m.
oxytocin	up to 5 IU

Goats

The luteolytic effect of $PGF_{2\alpha}$ is utilized because, as in pigs, the corpus luteum is essential at all stages of pregnancy. The duration of pregnancy varies between breeds and reliable records are important. Parturition should be induced as near as possible to the predicted date. If successful, induction of >80 per cent of births will occur within 30–40 hours. Treatment is unsuccessful if not effective within 50 hours.

Dose

cloprostenol	500 μg i.m.

Cattle

Prostaglandins, by causing luteolysis, are effective for induction of abortion in the first half of pregnancy. The latency before delivery is about 3–4 days in early pregnancy but may be about 3 weeks in mid-pregnancy. For the delivery of a mummified fetus, $PGF_{2\alpha}$ is effective at any stage after mating, because a corpus luteum maintains the condition. Corticosteroids are not effective since they require a live fetus to initiate the sequence of hormonal changes summarized above.

Dose

Early abortion
dinoprost	25–35 mg i.m.
cloprostenol	500 μg i.m.

Corticosteroids or prostaglandins are usually used (sometimes in combination) to induce parturition. It should be noted that there is a high incidence of placental retention when parturition is induced by any means. Although the prostaglandins are ineffective in inducing abortion after about day 150 of pregnancy, towards the end of pregnancy (about day 250), sensitivity returns, presumably as placental progesterone production decreases. If given after day 270, about 80 per cent of animals calve within 2 days, but calves born before day 275 may not thrive or even survive. The risk of prematurity is reduced when glucocorticoids are used to induce parturition. Both long- and short-acting formulations are effective, but the latency is different—approximately 2 weeks and 2 days respectively. Use of a long-acting formulation (usually an ester) mimics more closely the physiological time scale of hormonal events and a common technique is to use combined therapy.

Dose

Induction
cloprostenol	500 μg i.m.
dexamethasone trimethylacetate (long-acting)	20–25 mg i.m. 14 days before term, followed 8 days later by either dexamethasone phosphate (short-acting) 20 mg or cloprostenol 500 μg i.m.

Mares
Induction of abortion may be considered necessary in a twin pregnancy. Although one fetus may die spontaneously and the other be carried to term, twin pregnancy in mares is rarely carried to term successfully. $PGF_{2\alpha}$ is effective in causing luteolysis and abortion before day 36 of pregnancy after misalliance or in the case of a twin pregnancy. The response to treatment after that period is less predictable, due to secretion of PMSG from the endometrial cups. The luteotrophic effect renders the corpus luteum refractory to the luteolytic effect of $PGF_{2\alpha}$. Even when luteolysis and abortion are achieved, subsequent heats are unlikely to be fertile until PMSG disappears from the

circulation (when it may be too late in the year for another service), because under its influence maturing follicles luteinize rather than ovulate.

Dose

dinoprost	5 mg i.m.
cloprostenol	125–500 μg i.m.

Induction of parturition in mares can jeopardize the survival of the foal unless the mare is at term. It is generally considered that mares should be induced only in exceptional circumstances. In all cases, the animal must be at least 330 days pregnant with the cervix softened and the udder filling and waxing. A useful index is the concentration of Ca^{2+} in the milk, which rises to exceed 10 mmol/l 12 hours prior to normal parturition. The current technique of choice is oxytocin (5–10 IU) administered by i.v. drip in a dilute solution. Close supervision is essential as the latent period is about 1.5 hours. Signs of colic indicate uterine contractions.

Uterine inertia

Uterine stimulants are indicated to assist delivery in small animals and in pigs where, unlike cattle and horses, extensive manual manipulation is not possible. The drug of choice is oxytocin, administered intramuscularly and repeated, if necessary, at intervals of not less than 30 minutes. Subcutaneous administration may cause skin sloughing or abscessation. Oxytocin is contra-indicated in any form of obstructive dystocia, where it could cause uterine rupture. It may promote placental separation and jeopardize the survival of the unborn foetuses.

Dose

oxytocin
pig	2–10 IU i.m.
bitch	2–10 IU i.m.
cat	2–5 IU i.m.

Oxytocin (10–40 IU) is also used in cows after replacing a prolapsed uterus. Should the prolapse be associated with hypocalcaemia, calcium borogluconate should be administered before manipulation. This procedure will markedly improve smooth muscle tone.

Ergometrine should not be used during second stage labour as it may cause spasmodic contraction of the uterus and delay birth (hour-glass blocking). It is used in bitches during the puerperium to control uterine haemorrhage by inducing involution of the uterus.

Dose

ergometrine maleate
  bitch   0.2–1 mg p.o., s.c. or i.m.

Retained placenta

Cattle

In cattle, retained placenta is a common sequel to premature parturition or uterine inertia caused by hypocalcaemia or dystocia. Manual removal, with consequent risk of damage to the cotyledons, is likely to increase the incidence of metritis and subsequent infertility and should be avoided. There is no agreed treatment and different therapeutic measures are advocated to increase uterine tone and motility.

1. If there is uterine atony due to hypocalcaemia, calcium borogluconate alone may be effective.

   ### Dose

   calcium borogluconate   150–500 ml 40 per cent solution s.c. or slow
   i.v. (warmed to body temperature).

2. Oxytocin is only likely to be effective within about 24 hours of calving, when the myometrium is sensitized by sufficiently high levels of endogenous oestrogens.

   ### Dose

   oxytocin   10–40 IU every 2 hours, up to 4 doses
   Ergometrine (1–5 mg) has been claimed to be more effective than oxytocin but the sustained contractions can cause placental retention if it is administered too early (e.g. when the intention is to prevent or control postpartum haemorrhage).

3. Oestradiol benzoate is sometimes used but, with high doses, there is a risk of inducing anoestrus. In addition to stimulating uterine activity, oestrogens increase the blood supply to the uterus, which enhances resistance to infection.

   ### Dose

   oestradiol benzoate   10–20 mg i.m., repeated after 3 days if necessary.

4. Broad-spectrum antibacterial drugs are usually used in addition to uterine stimulants (see page 415).

Sheep and goats

Treatment is similar to that described for cattle, again avoiding manual removal.

Mares

Foetal membrane retention is much less common in mares than in cattle. In contrast to cattle, because of the different attachment, manual removal of the placenta by gentle traction is normally feasible. The use of oxytocin in this condition in mares is controversial. Intramuscular injection is listed as a contraindication by some manufacturers because of the marked restlessness, straining and profuse sweating which may result. However, it has been used successfully by slow intravenous infusion, but must be administered within 12 hours of foaling.

Dose

oxytocin   50–60 IU in 1 litre of saline by i.v. infusion over 1–2 hours. Intrauterine administration of antibacterials is usual after removal of a retained placenta.

Sows and bitches

Retained placenta in these species is uncommon, but provided that it is recognized and treated within 24 hours of parturition, oxytocin therapy is usually successful. In bitches, gentle massage of the uterus through the abdominal wall 10 minutes after administration of the drug may aid expulsion into the body of the uterus, from which it is easily removed.

Dose

oxytocin   2–10 IU i.m.

CHAPTER 16

DRUGS ACTING LOCALLY ON THE EYE, EAR AND SKIN

Drugs acting on the eye

Although the eye is an extremely complex organ, there is relatively little scope for the therapeutic manipulation of its function. An accurate diagnosis, based on a full history, is essential before instituting treatment. Since ocular signs may reflect systemic disease, a general clinical examination is also essential.

Most drugs used to treat conditions associated with the eye are administered by local application of drops or, less commonly, ointments. In this way, the site of drug action is restricted to the eye and only the small proportion that is absorbed by the conjunctiva enters the systemic circulation. Thus the chances of unwanted side-effects in the rest of the body are reduced. Absorption through the cornea is necessary for the drug to reach its site of action within the eye. The cornea consists of three layers: two have a high lipid content and one is an aqueous structure. For efficient absorption, therefore, drugs must contain both water- and lipid-soluble groupings. The use of concentrated solutions in eye drops aids absorption because the rate of this passive process depends on the concentration gradient.

Drugs for local application to the eye are most commonly formulated either as drops or as an ointment. Although many owners find it easier to administer drops, the constant production of tears limits the contact time of drops with the surface of the eye to some minutes. In many cases, tear production in response to drop instillation may reduce the contact time to less than a minute. Thus, at least in the early stages of therapy, drops need to be applied frequently, up to eight times per day. Ointment formulations are likely to be longer-lasting and could be expected to remain for up to an hour in the conjunctival sac. Their use should be avoided where there are penetrating lesions of the cornea or conjunctiva.

Local injection of drugs, by the episcleral, conjunctival or retrotubular routes, is also theoretically possible. In veterinary practice, however, this method is rarely used.

Drugs administered systemically can enter the uvea, optic nerve and parts of the retina, as these are highly vascular structures. A 'blood–eye barrier', consisting of a blood–aqueous, blood–vitreous and blood–retina barrier, inhibits the penetration of drugs from the systemic circulation to these areas. In the healthy eye, drugs will not enter the anterior chamber unless they are lipid soluble or of small molecular size. However, in the presence of inflammatory conditions, drugs enter both the aqueous and vitreous humour more readily. The conjunctival, corneal and ciliary epithelia are lipid membranes and water-soluble compounds will not pass through these unless they are small enough to pass through the cellular pores.

Muscarinic receptor agonists

Pilocarpine is a naturally occurring alkaloid with potent muscarinic activity. Unlike the natural transmitter, it is not metabolized by acetylcholinesterase and thus has a useful duration of action. When applied to the eye, it produces constriction of the pupil and the lens is focused for near vision. The contraction of the ciliary muscle opens the channels through which the aqueous humour drains and increases its outflow with a consequent reduction in intraocular pressure. Pilocarpine is thus useful in the treatment of glaucoma (see below) and is also sometimes used to reverse the effects of antimuscarinic agents. Increased tear production, due to action of the drug on the lacrimal glands, also occurs and pilocarpine may also be used for this action in keratoconjunctivitis sicca.

A 1 per cent solution of pilocarpine is usually used for eye drops; stronger solutions may cause local irritation. The concurrent use of organophosphates should be avoided, as these may increase sensitivity to the drug. Pilocarpine may be orally administered to dogs that will not tolerate repeated application of eye drops.

Anticholinesterases

By inhibiting the normally rapid breakdown of acetylcholine, drugs in this class have effects similar to those of pilocarpine. Physostigmine and demecarium are reversible inhibitors but their effects in the eye may persist for a number of days. The irreversible anticholinesterase, ecothiopate, has an extremely long duration of action. The intense contraction of the ciliary muscle which follows local application of anticholinesterases (and sometimes the directly acting muscarinic agonists) may produce a painful sensation in the eye.

Muscarinic receptor antagonists

Examination of the retina can be more readily achieved when the pupil is fully dilated, and antimuscarinic drugs are used for this purpose. Dilation of the pupil is accompanied by cycloplegia (paralysis of accommodation), with the lens fixed for distant vision. Atropine, the prototype drug in this class, is rarely used in the eye because, after local administration, its effects are long lasting: in horses the effects of atropine may last for up to 4 weeks. The relatively short-acting antimuscarinics, tropicamide and cyclopentolate (duration of action of about 8–9 hours and 24 hours respectively), are more widely used.

All of the muscarinic receptor antagonists are capable of increasing intraocular pressure. This is due to a reduction in the outflow of aqueous humour associated with the dilation of the pupil and thickening of the iris and is more likely to occur in animals which are predisposed towards narrow angle glaucoma.

Adrenoceptor agonists

Dilation of the pupil can also be achieved by the use of sympathomimetics, which stimulate α-adrenoceptors and thereby cause contraction of the dilatator pupillae. Mydriasis, which follows the administration of sympathomimetic amines, is generally less complete than that following atropine-like drugs because the dilatator pupillae is a less powerful muscle than the sphincter muscle of the iris. The drugs have no effect on the ciliary muscle and so cycloplegia does not accompany the mydriasis. The α-adrenoceptors in the conjunctival blood vessels are very sensitive to sympathomimetics and vasoconstriction and blanching of the conjunctiva occurs at doses lower than those required to produce mydriasis.

α-Adrenoceptor-mediated vasoconstriction of the ciliary body afferent blood vessels decreases aqueous humour formation and thereby reduces intraocular pressure, as long as drainage of the aqueous humour is not hindered by pupillary dilation.

Phenylephrine is used as a mydriatic for routine examination of the fundus and also to break down iris adhesions to the lens which can cause pupil block glaucoma.

Adrenoceptor antagonists

Blockade of the β_2-adrenoceptors in the ciliary body reduces the secretion of aqueous humour and intraocular pressure falls. Blockade of α-adrenoceptors with thymoxamine reduces the effect of the sympathetic innervation to the eye.

Carbonic anhydrase inhibitors

Carbonic anhydrase inhibitors are effective as diuretics (see page 246). Secretion of the aqueous humour, which contains a high concentration of HCO_3^-, depends on the activity of the enzyme carbonic anhydrase. Inhibition of the enzyme reduces aqueous secretion and thereby reduces intraocular pressure.

Treatment of glaucoma

The term glaucoma refers to an abnormal increase in intraocular pressure which, if unchecked, leads to impaired vision or blindness due to retinal damage. Glaucoma occurs occasionally in all species of domesticated animals, but most commonly in dogs. Aqueous fluid secreted by the ciliary body drains into the venous plexus adjacent to the iridocorneal angle and most glaucomas are due to impaired drainage rather than hypersecretion (Fig. 16.1). This may occur with no evidence of intraocular disease (there is a narrow iridocorneal angle drainage defect in certain breeds of dog), but more commonly it is secondary to conditions such as lens luxation or anterior uveitis.

Unlike the situation in humans, with early subjective symptoms of impaired vision, glaucomas in dogs are likely to be relatively advanced and present as an emergency disease problem. In patients with little or no aqueous drainage facility, only surgery is likely to be successful. However, carbonic anhydrase inhibitors are indicated for initial management of acute glaucoma, even when surgical treatment is to be adopted or while the cause is being established.

Carbonic anhydrase inhibitors

Acetazolamide is the carbonic anhydrase inhibitor of choice for the treatment of glaucoma. At the recommended doses, drugs in this category reduce the secretion of aqueous humour by approximately 50 per cent and are often used as adjuncts to therapy with topical miotics. When used for long-term therapy, vomiting and diarrhoea (apparently most common with acetazolamide) are occasional side-effects. Unlike most of the other drugs used for ocular effects, carbonic anhydrase inhibitors are usually administered by mouth, although acetazolamide can be injected intravenously in an emergency.

Dose

acetazolamide	5–10 mg/kg p.o., b.i.d. In an emergency, dilute the preparation in water to 50 mg/ml and administer intravenously.
dichlorphenamide	2–4 mg/kg p.o. 2–3 times/day
ethoxzolamide	4 mg/kg p.o., b.i.d.

(a)

Cornea

Anterior chamber

iris

Ciliary body

Lens

Vitreous body

(b)

Increased intraocular pressure

Impaired drainage

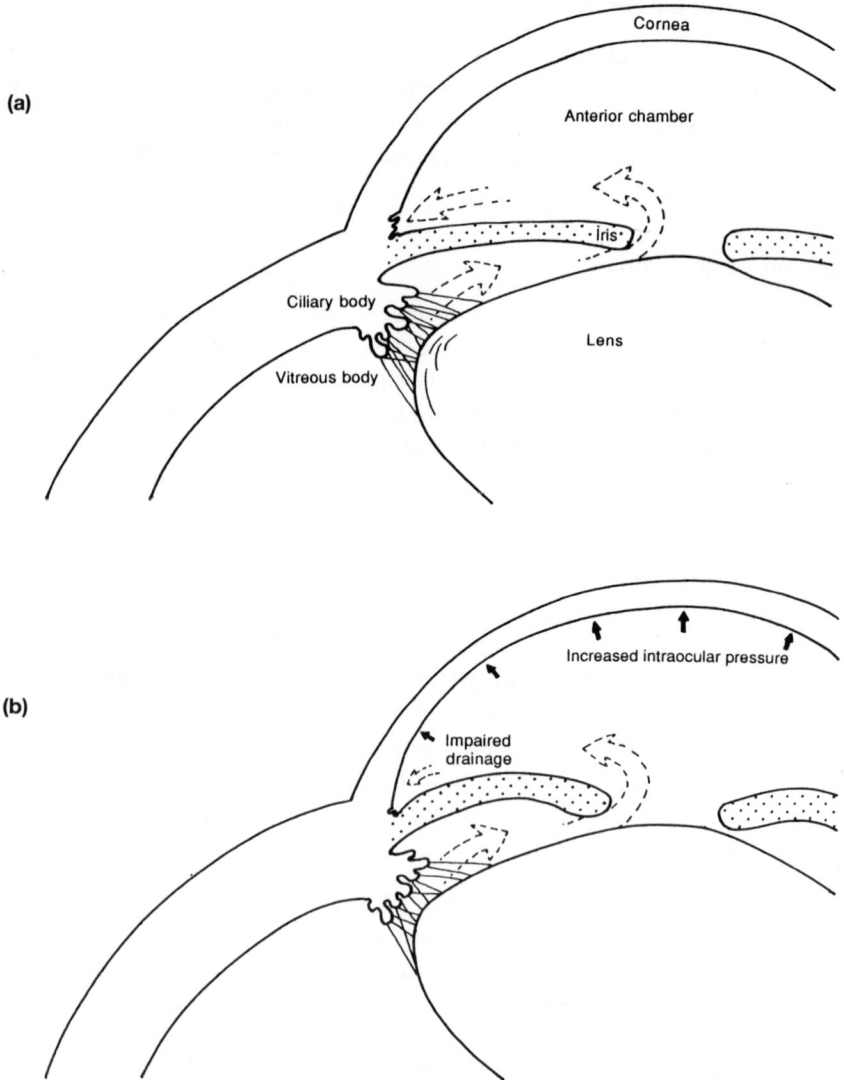

Figure 16.1 Circulation of fluid in the anterior chamber in the normal eye (a) and in the eye with glaucoma (b). Aqueous fluid drains into the venous plexus adjacent to the iridocorneal angle. Impaired drainage, associated with a narrow angle, leads to an increased intraocular pressure and the signs of glaucoma.

Miotics

Agents such as pilocarpine, physostigmine, ecothiopate and demecarium, applied topically, are generally considered to be the most useful miotics for medical control of glaucoma in dogs. They are usually used in conjunction with a carbonic anhydrase inhibitor.

Pilocarpine is commonly used for initial therapy, but only on a short-term basis as it often causes irritation after repeated application. The long-acting anticholinesterases, ecothiopate and demecarium, are generally considered to be the drugs of choice for preventing glaucoma in the fellow eye when there are abnormalities of the iridocorneal angles. They must not be used concurrently with other anticholinesterases, such as organophosphate-impregnated flea collars. Cats are particularly sensitive to these drugs.

Dose

pilocarpine	1 drop of 2 per cent solution every 15 min, 4 times, then 1 drop t.i.d.
ecothiopate, demecarium	1 drop of 0.25 per cent solution once daily, dose adjusted with monitoring of intraocular pressure.

Adrenoceptor agonists and antagonists

Adrenaline or the α-adrenoceptor agonist, phenylephrine, may be used in the treatment of open-angle glaucoma (but not narrow-angle glaucoma). They are generally less effective for treating glaucomas in dogs than miotics and carbonic anhydrase inhibitors. Phenylephrine is contraindicated in patients with narrow-angle glaucoma as the mydriasis may increase intraocular pressure due to obstruction of the iridocorneal angle by the iris root. The α-adrenoceptor antagonist, thymoxamine, is used to treat narrow-angle glaucoma.

Timolol, a β-adrenoceptor antagonist, is widely used in the treatment of open-angle glaucoma. Tear production may be inhibited. It has an additive effect with miotics and carbonic anhydrase inhibitors.

Dose

timolol   0.25 per cent solution 1 drop, b.i.d.

Local anaesthetics

Proxymetacaine, amethocaine and lignocaine are the most widely used of the local anaesthetics for ocular diagnostic and minor surgical procedures or foreign body removal.

Chemotherapy

Antibiotics in ointment or eye drop formulations are administered for local infections in the eye. Further details concerning the pharmacokinetics which apply to such situations, and selection of antibiotics for use in the eye, are on pages 431–432. Idoxuridine, in ointment formulation, is used as an antiviral agent; fungal infections can be treated with pimaricin or miconazole.

Mucolytics

Bromhexine (see page 254), administered parenterally, or acetylcysteine (see page 255) is used to break down the thick mucus over the cornea in cases of keratoconjunctivitis sicca.

Artificial tears

Hypromellose is used to lubricate the cornea in conditions where tear secretion is inadequate, such as keratoconjunctivitis.

Anti-inflammatory drugs

Early and effective treatment of inflammatory conditions in the eye is important to ensure ocular function is not irreparably damaged. Betamethasone and hydrocortisone are the most common corticosteroid components of drops or ointments used as anti-inflammatory agents in the eye. The mode of action of the steroids in inflammation and the indications for their use in the eye are described in Chapter 8.

Local application is effective for superficial lesions. Systemic administration is required for lesions which are posterior to the iris. Subconjunctival injection of repository formulations may provide a depot from which the drug is released for up to 2 weeks. Since the solubility of the drugs determines the degree of corneal penetration, the choice of derivative is important, e.g. acetate derivatives provide higher concentrations of drug in the aqueous and corneal stroma than alcohol derivatives.

Painful conditions of the eye, such as uveitis, can be treated with non-steroidal anti-inflammatory drugs (see Chapter 8). The two drugs in common use are phenylbutazone and flunixin.

Fluorescein

Fluorescein is used as a diagnostic stain to determine the integrity of the cornea and the patency of the nasolacrimal duct.

Drugs acting on the ear

Inflammatory disease of the ear is one of the most common conditions in small animal practice. Despite the variety of therapeutic agents available, effective treatment and cure of these conditions is often difficult. Accurate diagnosis is of major importance. Foreign body involvement is a common cause of inflammation. Neoplastic conditions of the external ear, although rare, should be considered. A number of bacteria, particularly staphylococci and streptococci, may be involved in the early disease process. Secondary contamination with Gram-negative organisms such as *Pseudomonas*, *E. coli* and *Proteus* is common. These organisms are involved in both acute and chronic conditions. Fungal organisms are often present and the yeast *Pityrosporum canis* is the most significant.

Although medical therapy is commonly instituted in aural conditions, its efficacy should not be overestimated. Foreign bodies and excess hair should be removed from the canal. Early surgical intervention may be valuable.

Indiscriminate symptomatic treatment with anti-inflammatory drugs may result in temporary relief but will not influence the underlying pathology and may lead to the development of a chronic, irreversible condition. A similar caveat applies to antibiotic therapy, which if inappropriate may lead to further complications of superimposed fungal infection. Laboratory diagnosis to determine the nature of bacterial and fungal secondary infections should be performed. Appropriate antibiotics should be selected on the basis of the results of these tests. If otocariasis is diagnosed, it should be treated with the appropriate acaricide, such as benzyl benzoate (see Chapter 23).

Corticosteroids are of value in the control of inflammation and oedema (Chapter 8). It is generally recommended that they should be accompanied by appropriate antibiotic therapy and a number of combined preparations are available.

Otitis media occurs as a natural extension of untreated or improperly treated otitis externa. Surgical drainage of the area and irrigation of the tympanic bulla may be sufficient to effect a cure. Cetrimide is the solution of choice.

Drugs acting on the skin

Skin disease is a common presenting problem, especially in small animal veterinary practice, and a full understanding of the therapy of these conditions is important. The skin consists of the hair coat, the stratum corneum and the living epidermis. The hair coat or wool, which has several important functions, including protection from ultraviolet radiation, is made of keratin and presents a barrier to drug absorption. Reactive chemical groups, continuously synthesized, are able to carry drugs away from the surface of the skin.

The stratum corneum or outer layer of the epidermis is covered with dead, keratinized cells which are joined together by an emulsion of sebum and sweat. Alternating layers of lipophilic and hydrophilic substances, punctuated by hair follicles and sebaceous glands, contribute to the multilayered structure of the stratum corneum. The normal skin microflora, which inhibits colonization by pathogenic microorganisms, is located in the outer layers of the stratum corneum and in the entrance to the hair follicles.

Drugs applied to the skin may: (i) be absorbed into the systemic circulation; (ii) penetrate into a particular skin layer; or (iii) remain on the skin surface.

Transport of drugs into and through the skin is a passive process. The stratum corneum or the appendages, such as hair follicles, sweat and sebaceous glands, provide the most significant barriers. Only a few species, including humans and pigs, have a relatively high ratio of stratum corneum : skin appendages. In these cases, the stratum corneum is the rate-determining barrier for systemic drug absorption after topical application. Increased rates of transport may be achieved by a variety of means, including increasing the degree of hydration of the stratum corneum, increasing the area of drug application, increasing the concentration of the drug applied and increasing the local temperature.

In the majority of domestic animals, most of a topically applied drug is absorbed into the circulation relatively rapidly, once the drug reaches the highly vascularized sebaceous and sweat glands, hair follicles and the upper layer of the dermis. Here again, the rate of skin penetration can be increased by increasing the area of drug application, increasing the drug concentration or increasing the local temperature.

There are a number of advantages of topical drug application for systemic delivery. Drugs absorbed this way by-pass the gastrointestinal tract and the liver and thus are not subject to first-pass metabolism. Furthermore, when compared to oral administration as licks or food additives, dosage can be more accurately controlled with topical administration. This route is also less labour intensive than most of the other common routes of administration. Despite these advantages, there are relatively few products which are designed for application to the skin for the purpose of systemic absorption. Most of these are used for the control of internal or external parasites.

A variety of preparations which exert their actions on the skin are available for use in veterinary medicine. Some of these are extremely old and the efficacy of a number of them has been questioned.

Corticosteroids

Corticosteroids are recommended for a number of dermatological conditions, but misuse of these agents can result in serious complications. Preparations for skin application, often in combination with antibiotics and a variety of other compounds, are available.

Emollients

Emollients are usually inert, oily substances which are used to soothe, lubricate and protect the skin or mucous membranes. They may also be used to soften the skin by the formation of an occlusive film over the stratum corneum, thus reducing evaporation of water from the underlying layers of skin. They are generally oils, fats or waxes. Emollients are seldom used on their own and more commonly form the base for administration of, for example, antimicrobial or anti-inflammatory drugs.

Oils which have been used as emollients include olive oil, linseed oil and castor oil. Castor oil has an irritant effect in the gastrointestinal tract, but this depends on its hydrolysis to ricinoleic acid. When applied to the skin, it is bland and soothing.

The animal fat, lanolin, has been used as a base for ointments. The use of synthetic alternatives, including polyethylene glycol and propylene glycol, reduces the incidence of allergic reactions to lanolin. Hydrocarbons, such as White Soft Paraffin B.P. and Liquid Paraffin B.P., are the most common emollient hydrocarbons in regular use in veterinary medicine.

Demulcents

Demulcents are also inert substances, usually water soluble with high molecular weights, such as gums, mucilages or starches. When locally applied, they coat the surface and provide mechanical protection from stimuli associated with the surrounding air or irritants in the environment. Thus they soothe and relieve irritation of skin and mucous membranes.

Glycerol may be used as a vehicle for drugs applied to the skin and as a constituent of teat dips in cattle. It has a disinfectant action and its demulcent effect keeps the surface of the teat supple and reduces the formation of cracks. In high concentration, glycerol will absorb water and it has been used to increase the flow of serum to open wounds. However, it should be remembered that it can be irritant.

Astringents

Astringents are used to precipitate protein on the surface of the skin. Their action is on the surface cells, where they facilitate the formation of a protective layer, under which healing can proceed. They can also reduce surface haemorrhage by precipitation of plasma proteins.

The salts of heavy metals, such as zinc or aluminium, are the most commonly used of a wide variety of available astringent compounds. Solutions of ferric chloride are recommended for control of minor haemorrhage such as that following amputation of tails. Astringents of vegetable origin usually contain tannic acid as the active ingredient.

Protectants and absorbents

Agents used as protectants and absorbents are chemically inert, finely ground, insoluble powders. They cover the skin, preventing contact with irritants, and are usually applied to prevent friction and absorb toxins and exudate. The most commonly used of these compounds are starch and talc. These form the basis of a number of 'wound healing powders', which may also contain antimicrobial, antifungal, anti-inflammatory and/or local anaesthetic agents. Starch is completely absorbed and less likely to cause foreign body reactions. Calamine, a mixture of zinc oxide with ferric oxide impurities, has both protective and astringent properties and is commonly used as a healing powder in humans; it has also been used in animals.

Dextranomer is used to aid debridement of secreting wounds. The cross-linked dextran absorbs water and allows free entry of molecules with molecular weights of less than 1000. Substances with molecular weights greater than 5000 cannot enter and those with intermediate molecular weights enter slowly. Thus the powder efficiently removes exudate and reduces pain, inflammation and oedema. Enhanced formation of granulation tissue is associated with reduced time for wound healing.

Counterirritants

Counterirritants produce local irritation and an acute inflammatory reaction when applied to the skin. This effect increases blood flow to the area and thus increases the supply of endogenous mediators of defence reactions. Removal of waste products by venous and lymphatic drainage is also enhanced. The compounds are said to reduce pain and once the acute inflammation subsides, to promote healing of the underlying tissue.

Counterirritants may cause a mild reaction, which consists of a local reddening of the skin or rubefacient response. (The use of heat may be more effective in increasing blood flow to the skin. Physiotherapeutic techniques have been used in veterinary practice for this purpose, especially in the horse.) More severe counterirritation results in the formation of pustules or vesicles, which are due to exudation following capillary damage. Further irritation has a corrosive effect, with death of skin cells and consequent sloughing.

Counterirritants include volatile oils, cantharides, iodine, mercuric iodide and ammonia. The compounds are applied to the skin where chronic inflammatory conditions exist in tissues just below the surface. The volatile oils, camphor, methyl salicylate and turpentine, have been used as rubefacients. The active principle of cantharides, cantharidin, can cause intense irritation and the therapeutic efficacy of this group of compounds is open to considerable debate. Mercuric chloride has been widely used as a counterirritant, especially in the horse. It is extremely irritant and considerable care must be exercised in its use. Ammonia compounds are most frequently used to elicit a 'rubefacient' action.

Dimethyl sulphoxide (DMSO)

Dimethyl sulphoxide is used as a solvent for a wide variety of compounds. It is remarkable in its ability to penetrate intact skin, so that soon after topical application it can be detected throughout the body. It is also able to carry a number of compounds with it across membrane barriers. Changes in the permeability of the skin, accompanied by reduced electrical potential across the skin, follow topical application of DMSO. It also has antifungal, antimicrobial and anti-inflammatory activity.

DMSO is relatively non-toxic, but toxicity may be increased by general anaesthetics in some species. Only pure compound should be used for topical application, since toxic impurities may be carried through the skin. Use of DMSO must be avoided in animals exposed to anticholinesterase compounds and for some days before and after exposure to these compounds; its use is contraindicated in food-producing or breeding animals. Rubber gloves should be worn by operators applying DMSO. The solvent is hygroscopic and containers of DMSO must be kept tightly sealed.

DMSO has been used to reduce pain, pruritus and inflammation and to aid healing. It is particularly recommended for treatment of racing injuries in greyhounds and horses. The drug is administered 3–4 times per day. The maximum dose should not exceed 20 ml/day for 2 weeks in the dog and 100 ml/day for 1 month in horses.

CHAPTER 17

GENERAL PRINCIPLES OF CHEMOTHERAPY

Most of the disease states which have been discussed so far arise as a result of a malfunction of some body system or the disturbance of a homeostatic control mechanism. Many of these can be treated by drugs. Disease can also be caused by invading organisms or by aberrant tissue growth. There is great variation in the relationship which these establish with the host, ranging from that of neoplastic tissue (which derives from host cells) through viruses (which can only multiply within cells) and bacteria to more complex organisms, which may have more than one host.

Drug treatment of diseases caused by invading organisms is referred to as chemotherapy. There is no difficulty in finding chemical agents which will destroy or prevent the multiplication of invading organisms, but those which are clinically useful exploit differences between the host and the invader, usually at the biochemical level. This concept is known as selective toxicity, and the aim is to eliminate the invader without damaging the host.

The use of benzylpenicillin is a good example of selective toxicity. Benzylpenicillin exerts its antibacterial effect by preventing cross-linkage in the bacterial cell wall; since mammalian cells do not have walls and cannot be acted upon by benzylpenicillin in this way, the selectivity is complete.

It is important to make a clear distinction between the selective toxicity of a chemotherapeutic drug and its therapeutic index (see Chapter 1). With some drugs (e.g. the penicillins), there is close parallelism between these parameters and the drugs are relatively safe. With others, however, (e.g. the aminoglycosides), although selectivity is high, their therapeutic indices are low because they have toxic effects which are completely unrelated to their ability to kill bacteria, hence greater caution is necessary in their use.

Chemotherapy may have biological consequences which extend further than the patient under treatment. For example, bacteria may become resistant to chemotherapeutic agents and this has obvious ecological implications. Therefore the selection of chemotherapeutic agents must be carefully controlled to minimize the spread of resistant organisms among animals and humans.

Chemotherapeutic drugs are usually classified according to the principal purpose for which they are intended, although there may be overlap. Most of the group names are self-explanatory:

1. Antibacterial
2. Antiprotozoal
3. Antifungal
4. Antiviral
5. Anthelmintic (for treatment of infestations by parasitic worms and flukes)
6. Ectoparasiticides
7. Antineoplastic

Antibacterial drugs

Introduction—general principles

The animal body has an extraordinary capacity to deal effectively with bacterial invasion; most infections occur and are eliminated without visible signs or symptoms. It follows, therefore, that most infections do not require chemotherapy. Some do, however, and as discussed previously, the aim of chemotherapy is to employ the selectively toxic effects of a drug to assist the patient to rapidly and efficiently control a bacterial infection without untoward effects on the host.

The principal drugs used in antibacterial chemotherapy are the antibiotics. The concept of antibiosis was first described by Louis Pasteur in 1877 as being diametrically opposed to the more common phenomenon of symbiosis and presumably reflective of competition for survival. At that time, it was known that one microorganism was often capable of inhibiting the growth of another, both *in vitro* and *in vivo,* but the observation that typhoid bacteria failed to grow in filtered media in which other organisms had been grown was critical. *Pseudomonas aeruginosa* (then *pyocyanea*) was particularly effective in this respect and filtered cultures of this organism were the basis of an effective commercial product (pyocyanase) which was assumed to be an enzyme.

Another line of reasoning which led to the development of antibiotics was that since all organic matter is eventually destroyed by soil microorganisms, it was worth examining soil samples for microorganisms which would be likely to contain enzymes capable of attacking pathogens. This approach produced, amongst others, the aminoglycosides, the tetracyclines, erythromycin and chloramphenicol, all of which remain in widespread clinical use.

The first of the true antibiotics, tyrothricin, was obtained from a protein-free isolate from a culture of *Bacillus brevis* in 1939. Tyrothricin consists of two peptides, tyrocidine and gramicidin, and although it protected mice against pneumococcal infection, it proved much too toxic for systemic use and must be used topically. The serendipitous discovery of the antibacterial activity of penicillin by Fleming in 1929 and its introduction into medicine in the early 1940s marked the real beginning of the antibiotic era. A petri dish which contained agar impregnated with staphylococci was left on the bench for 5 weeks and became contaminated by a rare strain of *Penicillium notatum*, which produced relatively large amounts of penicillin. The climatic conditions were such that colonies of staphylococci grew on the culture plate, except in areas where the mould had produced sufficient penicillin to kill the bacteria in its immediate vicinity.

The isolation of 6-aminopenicillanic acid in 1959 was another important step since, although devoid of antibacterial activity, it is the starting point for a whole range of synthetic penicillins which differ significantly from benzylpenicillin. This approach has also been applied to the cephalosporin group to produce a large number of clinically useful derivatives. Thus, in practice, the concept of a necessarily natural origin for antibiotics no longer applies because there are so many synthetic and semi-synthetic antibiotics and the group is often expanded to include drugs such as the sulphonamides. All are better considered as antibacterial drugs.

Antibacterials have no therapeutic uses other than their ability to assist in the destruction of invading microorganisms. Although they are rather inert from a pharmacological point of view, they are not benign and can induce a wide range of toxic effects. It should also be noted at the outset that, although antibacterial drugs often represent the only treatment for a bacterial infection, other measures, such as the administration of antitoxins and other drugs (e.g. fluids and anti-inflammatory agents) to deal with the sequelae of that infection, may also be important.

Chemotherapy is not always successful. The simplest situation is where a powerful drug is given to an animal that is infected by a sensitive organism but is otherwise healthy. Treatment may prove to be more difficult when it is confounded by the debility of the patient and/or the obstinacy of the organism.

Antibacterial drugs are described as being either bactericidal or bacteriostatic. Bactericidal drugs, as their name implies, actively kill bacteria, superimposing their effects on the host defence mechanisms. Bacteriostatic drugs slow the growth of the organisms and prevent the host defence mechanisms from being overwhelmed. The host defence mechanisms play a more important role in the eradication of the infecting organisms when bacteriostatic rather than bactericidal drugs are used. For example, if treatment is discontinued prematurely, the bacterial population may rise again to cause a relapse. In practice, the distinction between bactericidal and bacteriostatic activity may be blurred. For most drugs, the killing rate is proportional to the concentration attained and drugs which are normally considered to be bactericidal may achieve only bacteriostatic activity after inappropriately low doses. Conversely, a bacteriostatic drug may become bactericidal at high concentration (e.g. sulphonamides in urine).

It is possible to classify the antibacterial drugs in a number of ways but the most convenient, from a practical point of view, is according to their mode of action:

1. Inhibition of bacterial cell wall synthesis e.g. penicillins, cephalosporins, vancomycin, bacitracin.
2. Bactericidal inhibition of protein synthesis e.g. streptomycin, kanamycin, neomycin.
3. Bacteriostatic inhibition of protein synthesis e.g. tetracyclines, erythromycin, chloramphenicol.
4. Interference with bacterial metabolism e.g. sulphonamides, trimethoprim.
5. Alteration of bacterial membrane permeability e.g. polymyxins, colistin.
6. Inhibition of DNA synthesis e.g. nalidixic acid.

Requirements for a clinically useful antibacterial drug are as follows:

- Potent and selective.
- Bactericidal rather than bacteriostatic.
- Able to act independently of host defence mechanisms.
- Low incidence of clinically significant bacterial resistance.
- Acceptable therapeutic ratio for both acute and chronic use.
- Minimal side-effects.
- Activity maintained in presence of pus and other tissue exudates.
- Bactericidal concentrations rapidly attained at the infection site and maintained.
- Synergism or additivity (and certainly not antagonism) with other drugs liable to be used concomitantly.
- Activity against a wide range of organisms. (Although it is good practice to use the antibacterial drug with the narrowest spectrum of activity once the nature and sensitivity of the organism has been established, drugs with a wider spectrum of activity are essential when treatment

must be commenced before the organism can be identified, which is the usual state of affairs. Broad-spectrum antibiotics are also used for the management of polymicrobial infections.)

Synergism and antagonism among antibacterial drugs

Much more is written on this subject than applies clinically. A few facts are worth noting. If two bactericidal drugs are used concomitantly at dose levels which would be minimally effective if given alone, the net effect is sometimes dramatically increased—particularly if the drugs have different modes of action and there are effects on two vital processes. A clinical example is the combined use of benzylpenicillin and streptomycin in the prevention or management of infections associated with compound fractures. In most cases, however, it is unnecessary to use more than one drug. There is generally no synergism among the bacteriostatic drugs. In fact, one drug may interfere with the attachment of the other to the bacterial ribosome. If marginal doses are used, additive effects may occur, but usually the weaker drug is redundant. There is a special case, however, for the use of sulphonamides in combination with inhibitors of folic acid synthesis such as trimethoprim. Here, both drugs act at different points in the synthetic pathway to cause a sequential blockade.

The response to a bactericidal drug may be diminished by previous/ concomitant exposure to a bacteriostatic drug. This is because bactericidal drugs are most effective when the organism is actively growing. An exception to this general rule is the interaction between mecillinam and the penicillins (and cephalosporins). Exposure to mecillinam alters the morphology of sensitive bacteria, rendering them exquisitely sensitive to the effects of penicillin.

Causes of failure of antibacterial chemotherapy

Antibacterial chemotherapy is usually, but not always, successful. Causes of failure may relate to the nature of the infecting organism, the diagnosis, the condition of the patient and to the drug which is administered.

Drug resistance

This problem is largely one of bacterial genetics. Antibiotics do not cause bacterial resistance but exert a selection pressure for resistant strains, which may arise by spontaneous mutation, to become dominant. Thus, the ability of an organism to survive in the presence of antibacterial drugs confers an ecological advantage and explains, in part, the prevalence of such organisms in the hospital and agricultural environment.

Intrinsic (natural) resistance

Some bacteria are intrinsically resistant to certain antibacterial drugs. This may be either a species or a strain characteristic and may involve either a single drug or a group of drugs. A good example is the absence of a cell wall in some mycoplasma strains, which renders them completely resistant to the penicillins and cephalosporins. Other organisms achieve intrinsic resistance by not depending on a metabolic process which can be disrupted by the drug, having cell walls or membranes which preclude the entry of the drug, or by elaborating enzymes which degrade the drug.

Acquired resistance

Here, an organism which is initially sensitive to a drug, acquires resistance during the treatment of an individual patient. This has obvious clinical and ecological relevance. A variety of biochemical mechanisms have been shown to operate. There may be decreased uptake of the drug into the bacterial cell (e.g. tetracyclines), or the organism may acquire the ability to destroy the drug (e.g. penicillins) or to produce an increased amount of a metabolite which antagonizes the drug (e.g. sulphonamides). Less commonly, the organism may fail to convert the drug to a growth-inhibiting metabolite, or the affinity of the drug for the receptor in the organism may be altered (e.g. erythromycin).

Drug-resistant strains may not revert to sensitivity although there may be some loss of pathogenicity. Enteric infections in farm animals, however, frequently revert to sensitivity over a period of a few weeks after the antibiotic-induced selection pressure is withdrawn. In practice, this often means that an antibiotic can be changed and then successfully used again in the same situation, provided that a period of a few weeks has elapsed. From a more general clinical viewpoint, it is important to realize that resistance to a drug may be acquired with great rapidity and there is a need for great care in situations where high-risk drugs are used. In some cases, the use of adjunctive therapy may slow or prevent the development of resistance.

Transferred (infectious) resistance

This type of resistance involves the transfer of genetic material which confers drug resistance from one species or strain or organism to another. These may include both pathogenic and non-pathogenic organisms. Resistance to several antibacterial drugs may be transferred at the same time. The mechanism of transfer may involve passage of plasmids down a cytoplasmic bridge (conjugation) or by bacteriophage (transduction). Transferred resistance was first noted among organisms from the human gastrointestinal and upper respiratory tracts but is now known to occur in other species and in the hospital environment.

Bacterial persistence

This term is used to describe a situation where fully-sensitive organisms survive in a concentration of a drug which has killed the great majority of the bacterial population. Bacterial persisters are liable to occur in situations where there are foreign bodies or poor drainage. They are usually regarded as relatively dormant cells which are metabolizing slowly, although sometimes the cell wall may be lost if the environment is hypertonic, such as in the renal medulla of some species. Bacterial persistence should not arise if the infection is treated promptly with adequate doses of an appropriate drug, and if it is suspected, a second drug (acting by some different mechanism) should also be given.

Poor host defences

A variety of circumstances may arise in which the host defence mechanisms become compromised. Most important are the concomitant use of other drugs, such as corticosteroids and immunosuppressants, and disease, particularly of non-infective aetiology, such as diabetes. In these situations it is best to use bactericidal drugs.

Drug factors

The effect of an antibacterial drug depends ultimately on the concentration which can be achieved in the immediate neighbourhood of the bacteria. This depends firstly on the concentration of free drug which can be attained in the blood and thus on the degree of protein-binding, the extent and rate of metabolic inactivation and/or excretion and the extent of inactivation by the host flora. In most cases, biological membranes have then to be crossed. For example, only a few drugs (e.g. chloramphenicol) are able to cross the blood–brain barrier in the absence of inflammation. Even in cases where there is inflammation and penetration occurs (e.g. penicillin), it may be difficult to maintain an adequate concentration of the drug. Although there is little protein in the cerebrospinal fluid and the proportion of unbound drug is commensurately greater, there is an active process in the choroid plexus which returns penicillin to the blood. Cell barriers may also occur. It has been shown by fluorescence microscopy that the transport of tetracyclines across cells occurs with difficulty. Where bacteria are contained in avascular lesions (abscesses), the drug may not be able to penetrate sufficiently to exert a useful effect.

Toxic effects of antibacterial drugs

As will now be apparent to the reader, no drug is free from unwanted effects. These are usually referred to as side-effects—a term which is best restricted to therapeutically undesired, but unavoidable effects. It is an important principle in pharmacology that there is a definite relationship between the severity of a clinical condition and the acceptable incidence and/or severity of side-effects of drugs used to treat that condition. A risk-benefit assessment must be made by the veterinarian before treatment is commenced.

Most of the antibacterial drugs in current use are pharmacologically inert in the classical sense. Nevertheless, they are capable of producing a wide range of toxic effects, some of which can be life-threatening.

Although the acute toxicity of most antibacterial drugs is low and inadvertent overdose is unlikely to have serious consequences in most cases, problems may arise if there is an underlying abnormality in the patient, such as impaired hepatic or renal function. For example, when the renal function is compromised, the antibiotic dosage should be adjusted according to the creatinine clearance or other appropriate index.

The toxic effects encountered with antibacterial drugs are not usually extensions of their therapeutic effects. A notable exception is chloramphenicol, where selective toxicity is incomplete and its effects on mammalian mitochondrial protein synthesis appear to be inseparable from those in sensitive bacteria.

Hypersensitivity to antibacterial drugs, particularly to the penicillins and cephalosporins, may limit their therapeutic efficacy, although this appears to be less of a problem in domesticated animals than in humans. Development of hypersensitivity requires previous exposure to the drug and the formation of antibodies. Tests for hypersensitivity are not very reliable, and it is important that the veterinarian keeps an accurate record of all hypersensitivity reactions which are suspected to have been drug-induced. Subsequent exposure of a hypersensitive patient to the drug may have serious consequences.

Pyrogenic reactions may occur with parenteral preparations of antibacterial drugs if contamination has occurred or bacterial protein has not been eliminated during the preparation of the dose form.

Thus, it is usually recommended that antibacterial drugs should not be employed in the treatment of trivial infections (where a spontaneous cure might be anticipated), undiagnosed febrile conditions or for unnecessary prophylaxis.

Superinfection

Superinfection is said to occur when a patient being treated with an anti-bacterial drug becomes infected by an organism(s) other than those which caused the original infection. The organisms involved are usually residents which, under normal conditions, exist in ecologically balanced communities in the host and are either harmless or perform a useful function. If the ecological balance of the bacterial community is disturbed as the result of drug therapy, overgrowth of certain organisms or invasion by other pathogenic bacteria and fungi can occur. Superinfection is the cause of much of the diarrhoea and external otitis encountered after antibacterial therapy, particularly with broad-spectrum antibiotics.

Controls on the use of antibiotics in animal husbandry

The public must be protected from the potentially harmful effects of the widespread use of antibiotics in animal husbandry. Antibiotics are used for both prophylactic and therapeutic purposes and for so-called 'growth promotion'. In animals raised under intensive conditions (pigs, poultry), disease is a very likely possibility and the prophylactic use of antibiotics may be viewed as being less costly than an attempt to eradicate established disease.

Dangers to humans are considered to lie in the presence of antibiotic residues in milk, eggs and meat, which may lead to the development of antibiotic resistance in human bacterial flora and the possibility of the transfer of resistance to pathogens. The imposition of designated withdrawal periods before the slaughter of animals and birds for human consumption helps to alleviate the problem, but the length of this period must obviously depend on the pharmacokinetics of the drug concerned and familiarity with the regulations for each drug and species is essential. Additional reasons are held to exist for the control of antibiotic residues in milk. These include the possibility of allergic reactions in the consumer and problems in cheese production.

Growth promotion is defined as the stimulation of an animal's growth during early life by the addition of small quantities of substances in the diet which may or may not be antibiotics. Dietary supplementation with growth promoters is considered likely to yield an average 5 per cent increase in daily weight gain and feed conversion efficiency. This is an important economic gain at very low cost to the producer, but the question must be asked whether the totally non-medical use of antibiotics is desirable for the consumer of the product. Some would argue that such use of antibiotics can never be justified.

In the UK it was recommended by the Swann Committee Report (1969) that antibiotics must be clearly designated as either 'feed' (i.e. growth promoters) or 'therapeutic', and that growth-promoting antibiotics should, by definition, have no therapeutic use in humans or animals. This was to preclude the possibility that the administration of sub-therapeutic doses of antibiotics for stimulating growth in animals might confound the treatment of humans or animals by exerting a selection pressure for resistant strains of bacteria. The Swann Committee recommendation has subsequently been incorporated into subsidiary legislation to the Medicines Act, which allows a limited number of antibiotics (e.g. bamberamycin and virginiamycin) to be mixed in animal feeds for growth promotion. Such growth promoters can be incorporated without veterinary direction, but only at specified concentrations and for certain species. Other antibiotics are commonly mixed in feeding stuffs for therapeutic purposes but only under a written veterinary direction to the feed compounder (see Appendix 1).

Current scientific opinion, 25 years after the Swann report, is that sub-therapeutic doses of antibiotics did not exert a selection pressure for bacterial resistance. However, the report usefully focused attention on ensuring that the use of medicated feeds does not result in medication residues appearing in meat, milk and eggs supplied to the public. More recent (1989) United Kingdom legislation was designed to tighten existing controls on medicated animal feeds. Further details of the legal controls of in-feed medication can be found in Appendix 1.

CHAPTER 18

ANTIBACTERIAL DRUGS

Inhibitors of cell wall synthesis

This group of drugs includes the penicillins, the cephalosporins, imipenem, aztreonam, vancomycin and bacitracin.

Penicillins

The penicillins are perhaps the most important group of antibiotics because they combine very high antibacterial activity and very low systemic toxicity and they are relatively cheap to produce. Their use is limited only by the resistance of organisms and hypersensitivity reactions. The latter are much less frequently encountered in animals than in humans. Unlike most groups of drugs, the synthetic possibilities for the penicillins are at an early stage. However, despite the introduction of new synthetic and semi-synthetic derivatives, benzylpenicillin remains the drug of choice for the treatment of infections caused by the organisms sensitive to it.

Penicillins are produced by various *Penicillium* species. Fleming's original strain was *Penicillium notatum*, but modern sophisticated 'brewery' type operations usually employ a mutant of *Penicillium chrysogenum*, which produces a much higher yield.

The penicillin nucleus (Fig. 18.1) is formed by the fusion of a five-membered thiazolidine ring and a four-membered β-lactam ring with a side-chain attached to the peptide linkage of the β-lactam ring. The cephalosporins (see below) also have a β-lactam ring but here it is attached to a six-membered sulphur-containing ring. The intact nucleus is the chief requirement for the biological activity of the penicillins, and the side-chain determines the antibacterial and pharmacological characteristics of individual members.

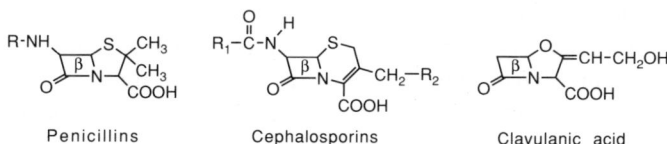

Figure 18.1 Core structures of antibiotics which inhibit cell wall synthesis. The ring marked 'β' is the β-lactam ring.

Three systems of nomenclature are in operation. The oldest assigns an arbitrarily chosen suffix (benzylpenicillin is penicillin G and phenoxymethyl-penicillin is penicillin V). The second uses the chemical name of the side-chain as a prefix (e.g. benzyl- or phenoxymethyl-penicillin). In the third system, penicillins are regarded as 6-substituted derivatives of aminopenicillanic acid, so benzylpenicillin is 6-phenylacetamidopenicillanic acid. This nomenclature lies more in the province of organic chemists.

Penicillin salts are fairly stable in the dry state but are unstable in solution, even when buffered with citrate or phosphate to pH 6.5. Thus, penicillin preparations for parenteral administration usually consist of a dry sterile powder (penicillin plus buffering agents) in a vial plus an ampoule of (sterile) water for injection. The dose form is prepared immediately before administration. A number of penicillin esters have a very low water solubility and can be used to formulate depot preparations.

Three main types of penicillin are available plus some related compounds which are used for adjunctive therapy. These are:

1. Natural: produced by fermentation (e.g. benzylpenicillin).
2. Semi-synthetic: produced by incorporation of precursors into the mould or chemical modification to produce preparations which are clinically useful (e.g. procaine penicillin).
3. Synthetic: synthesized from 6-aminopenicillanic acid (e.g. ampicillin).

The potency of the penicillins is sometimes still expressed in units. This is a relic of a past need for biological assay where each batch was compared with a standard preparation (the international unit is 0.6 μg of the sodium salt of the master standard of benzylpenicillin). This is much too small to be of clinical relevance and the term mega unit ($\times 10^6$) is more common.

Mechanism of action

Most bacteria have a cell wall which reinforces the cell membrane and prevents it from rupturing. Bacterial cell wall synthesis is a three-stage process: (i) formation of precursor units within the cell; (ii) carriage of these units to the exterior, where they are incorporated into the cell wall; and (iii) a transpeptidization reaction which cross-links linear strands to produce a tough, rigid outer coat. The last step is inhibited by the penicillins and cephalosporins, and so fibrous material, unable to cross-link, accumulates on the growing point of the cell. The net result is extrusion of the cell membrane, its eventual rupture due to surface enzyme (autolysin) activity and cell death.

Spectrum of activity

Penicillins are active against certain bacteria but have no effects on protozoa, rickettsiae, fungi or viruses. In considering the spectrum of antibacterial activity of the penicillins, a clear division must be made between drugs like benzylpenicillin, which are very potent but act mainly on Gram-positive organisms, and drugs like ampicillin, which are generally less potent but also act on Gram-negative organisms (these are sometimes referred to as broad-spectrum penicillins). There is little chemical difference between the two types and differences in activity probably represent relative ease of penetration into the bacterial cell and/or differences in the affinity of penicillin binding proteins, which constitute the receptor sites for the drugs.

Resistance

Organisms in which the cell wall impedes entry of the drug are naturally resistant to benzylpenicillin. This occurs mainly with Gram-negative organisms but drugs like ampicillin, which cross the cell wall more readily, may still be effective. More commonly, resistant bacteria have the ability to destroy the drug by producing penicillinase, which is supposed to have evolved from a transpeptidase. Penicillinases are members of the β-lactamase group of enzymes which have different pH optima and immunological profiles. Fourteen groups of β-lactamase, which are divisible into five classes, have been found in Gram-negative bacteria. Class 1 β-lactamases attack cephalosporins; the class 2 enzymes are the penicillinases and classes 3, 4 and 5 are broad-spectrum β-lactamases. They all cause ring-cleavage and thus abolish antibacterial activity. Penicillinases are sometimes released from the organism and these can confound therapy. Occasionally, reduction in bacterial cell permeability, which excludes the drug, has been found to account for penicillin resistance. Reduced activity of autolytic enzymes in the bacteria is also sometimes cited as a cause of resistance.

Under isotonic or hypertonic conditions, cell rupture may not occur and viable organisms without cell walls (protoplasts) are formed. These are resistant to the penicillins and cephalosporins and this is one reason for bacterial persistence. They remain dorhumanst until therapy is stopped, when cell wall synthesis and division begins again. Suspected persisters can be eliminated with other antibiotics such as the aminoglycosides.

Benzylpenicillin

The bactericidal action and low toxicity of benzylpenicillin (Fig. 18.2), and the fact that high concentrations can be obtained in the tissues, make it by far the most reliable and satisfactory of all the antibiotics for the treatment of infections which are sensitive to it. Benzylpenicillin remains the most widely used penicillin in veterinary medicine. It is bactericidal and is most active early in the course of the infection when the organisms are multiplying rapidly. A number of compound preparations are available for specific clinical purposes. These contain benzylpenicillin in combination with other antibiotics which have a completely different mode of action (e.g. dihydrostreptomycin and neomycin) or with another penicillin (e.g. nafcillin).

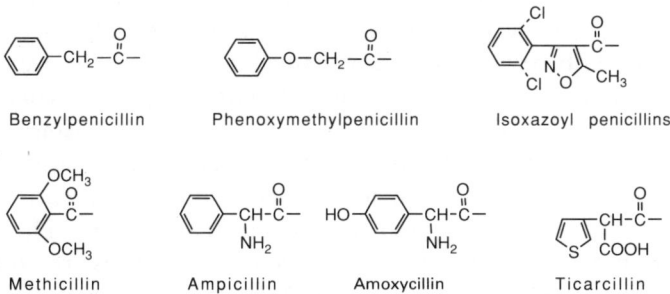

Figure 18.2 Side-chains of penicillins. In the case of the isoxazoyl penicillins, oxacillin has no Cl atoms, cloxacillin has one, dicloxacillin has two and flucloxacillin has one Cl atom and one F atom.

Spectrum of activity
Benzylpenicillin is particularly active against Gram-positive organisms, such as clostridia, streptococci and staphylococci. *Leptospira*, *Erysipelothrix*, *Listeria* and some corynebacteria are moderately susceptible. Although most Gram-negative organisms are resistant, *Neisseria* and *Pasteurella* and some *Haemophilus* species are moderately sensitive. Penicillin-sensitive infections should respond to treatment within 24–48 hours.

Pharmacokinetics
Penicillins are weak acids and are therefore predominantly ionized in plasma (pH 7.4). This hinders their diffusion across membranes. They are also poorly soluble in lipids.

Solutions of the sodium or potassium salts of benzylpenicillin are normally given by injection because gastric acid rapidly destroys the drug. The subcutaneous route is preferable in dogs and cats and the intramuscular route in larger animals. Pharmaceutical variants can be used to control and/or prolong blood levels (e.g. procaine penicillin, crystalline penicillin in oily suspension, benzathine penicillin and mixtures of some or all of these with the soluble salts of benzylpenicillin). Intramammary preparations formulated in various bases are also used to eliminate sensitive infections. Preparations which are introduced into the teat contain a dye which is incorporated as a marker. After giving any antibiotic by any route to lactating cattle, milk must be discarded for the prescribed time. With benzylpenicillin, milk should not be used during dosing and for 24 hours after the last treatment.

Benzylpenicillin is widely distributed in body fluids but there is considerable variation in the concentration attained in various tissues. It becomes 50–65 per cent bound (reversibly) to plasma albumin and the active, unbound, ionized fraction diffuses widely into the extracellular fluid through the fenestrated capillary walls. In the eye and the brain, the capillaries are not fenestrated and penetration of ionized drug is poor. Thus rather low concentrations of benzylpenicillin are attained in brain and the eye and also in nerve, bone marrow, skeletal/cardiac muscle and spleen. Drug concentrations are much higher in blood, liver and kidney. Benzylpenicillin gains rapid access to synovial fluids and there is some transport across the placenta but foetal concentrations are usually much lower than maternal concentrations. The diffusion of benzylpenicillin into abscess cavities is poor. There is little penetration into the cerebrospinal fluid when the meninges are normal, even when the plasma concentration is high. When the meninges are inflamed, although therapeutic concentrations may be attained, this is not reliable. There is less protein in cerebrospinal fluid than in plasma so more benzylpenicillin is unbound, but there is an active transport system in the choroid plexus which returns the drug to the blood.

In horses, benzylpenicillin is more firmly protein-bound than in other species and the plasma concentrations of the free drug are commensurately lower. In practice, this means that the soluble sodium and potassium salts are preferred.

Most of a dose of benzylpenicillin is excreted in a biologically active state in the urine. Some is excreted in the bile and is presumably destroyed by gut microorganisms.

The renal elimination of benzylpenicillin is very rapid and involves both glomerular filtration and active proximal tubular secretion. The presence of benzylpenicillin in the body may be prolonged by administering competitors for the tubular secretion pathway, such as probenecid. The rapid clearance accounts for the short half-life of benzylpenicillin but the high urinary concentrations attained are rarely of clinical significance. This is not the case with the broad-spectrum penicillins, however. The excretion of penicillins is delayed in patients with impaired renal function and they may require a reduction of the dose.

Toxic reactions
Benzylpenicillin is almost non-toxic, in a classical sense, to the larger domesticated animals. Small herbivores, such as rabbits and guinea pigs, however, may exhibit serious reactions to the drug. In these animals, death may occur within a few days of a single dose. This has been attributed to drastic alteration of the normal gut flora and the development, for example, of a pseudomembranous colitis-like condition due to an invasion of *Clostridium difficile*. After large penicillin doses, neurotoxic effects may occur in pigs and horses, which may be humansifested as excitability, incoordination and ataxia. The serious and even fatal hypersensitivity reactions to benzylpenicillin, which are not infrequent in humans, are rare in domesticated animals although both urticaria and anaphylactic shock have been reported in cows which have received intramammary penicillin. Skin sensitization may occur in persons handling any penicillin product and, since this may be of a serious nature, protective measures to avoid contact should always be taken.

Drug interactions
Synergism between the penicillins and the aminoglycosides against Gram-positive organisms normally occurs and this can be utilized in the prophylactic treatment of compound fractures, for example. More recently, mixtures of penicillins with potassium clavulanate, which inactivates β-lactamases, have been shown to interact synergistically.

Dose

Preparations of benzylpenicillin for intramuscular injection.
small animals   100–600 mg daily.
large animals   1.5–6.0 g daily.

Specialized forms of benzylpenicillin
Procaine penicillin   Procaine combines mole for mole with benzylpenicillin to give a product which is poorly soluble and can be formulated into depot preparations. Benzylpenicillin is released slowly from the injection (normally intramuscular) site and peak blood concentrations are reached in about 4 hours and persist for 24 hours. When given to lactating cows, milk should not be used for 48 hours after the last dose. The drug should never be given intravenously as precipitated material can cause the formation

of emboli. Mixtures of soluble and procaine penicillin are also used to achieve a rapid peak and a prolonged effect which can be further extended by inclusion of benzathine or benethamine penicillins. Procaine penicillin-nafcillin preparations are also marketed and there is a plethora of preparations which combine procaine penicillin with other antibiotics (e.g. novobiocin, streptomycin, dihydrostreptomycin, framycetin, chlortetracycline) and other drugs (corticosteroids, histamine H_1-antagonists). The rationale for some of these combinations is difficult to understand.

Occasionally, in pigs, administration of procaine penicillin may cause transient pyrexia and incoordination. A vulval discharge, which has been associated with abortion, may also occur in pregnant sows. Local reactions at the injection site may occur in horses. To avoid the risk of a procaine-positive sample, procaine penicillin should not be given to racehorses for 2 weeks before a race.

Dose

procaine penicillin alone (i.m.)
  all species   10–15 mg/kg s.c. or i.m. 1–2 times daily
  For compound preparations, refer to manufacturers' data

Benzathine penicillin   This is formed by the combination of a N,N'-dibenzyl-ethylenediamine and benzylpenicillin. Again, the solubility is low and the drug remains at the injection site for about 6 days while absorption takes place, and low concentrations of penicillin can be found in the plasma. It may be combined with procaine penicillin and/or benzylpenicillin, but such preparations are often only effective if the infecting organism is highly sensitive to penicillin. Milk from cows which are treated with benzathine penicillin should not be used for 72 hours after the last dose. Benzathine penicillin is also available in combination with nafcillin and dihydrostreptomycin

Dose

Refer to manufacturers' data for dosage of compound preparations.

Penethamate   This is the hydriodide of the 2-diaminoethyl ester of benzyl-penicillin. It enters the cerebrospinal fluid readily and selectively accumulates in pulmonary tissue. Milk from cows which receive penethamate should not be used for 48 hours after the last dose and animals must not be slaughtered for huhumans consumption during treatment and for 6 days afterwards.

Dose

The dose form consists of a vial containing 5 million units of the drug and a 15 ml ampoule of a sterile (0.15 per cent) solution of methylparahydroxybenzoate which are mixed aseptically to give 18–19 ml of suspension. Daily doses are as follows:

horse and cattle   5 million units i.m. daily
sow, sheep   2.5 million units i.m. daily
Repeat for 1–5 days, depending on condition.

Benethamine penicillin   This is the poorly soluble *N*-benzylphenylethylamine salt of benzylpenicillin. It is slowly absorbed from intramuscular injection sites and releases benzylpenicillin into the bloodstream for 4–5 days. It is used in conjunction with procaine penicillin.

Dose

Refer to manufacturers' data for dosage of compound preparations containing benethamine penicillin.

Synthetic penicillins

Acid-resistant penicillins

Phenoxymethylpenicillin (penicillin V) (Fig. 18.2)
This penicillin is produced by a fermentation process and has an antibacterial spectrum which is essentially similar to that of benzylpenicillin. However, it is about four times less active than benzylpenicillin against most bacteria. Its only advantage over benzylpenicillin is that it is acid-stable and hence better absorbed and more systemically available after oral administration.

The absorption of phenoxymethylpenicillin depends on passive migration of the drug across the lipoprotein barrier of the small intestine. Absorption is rapid but incomplete (about 60 per cent passes into the blood) and there may be considerable variation in the extent to which phenoxymethylpenicillin is absorbed. It has been suggested that severely ill patients tend to absorb the drug poorly and, in human medicine, the initial use of phenoxymethyl-penicillin in patients with life-threatening infections is considered to be unwarrantable. In small animals, an initial course of parenteral benzyl-penicillin therapy is sometimes followed by oral phenoxymethylpenicillin.

Peak serum concentrations are attained within about 30 minutes of oral dosing and therapeutic levels are maintained for about 4 hours. The pattern of distribution is similar to that of benzylpenicillin but phenoxymethylpenicillin is more highly protein-bound. Inflammation facilitates distribution. About 50 per cent of a phenoxymethylpenicillin dose is converted to inactive penicilloic acids in the liver and about 30 per cent appears unchanged in the urine. Active secretion in the proximal tubule accounts for most of the clearance and therefore organic acids which compete for the tubular excretion pathway (probenecid and carinamide but also phenylbutazone, indomethacin and aspirin, for example) increase the half-life of the drug.

Dose

cat, dog   8 mg/kg p.o. every 8 hours or 16 mg/kg p.o. every 12 hours will maintain high blood concentrations of the drug.

Penethicillin and propicillin
These are orally active and almost indistinguishable from phenoxymethyl-penicillin in their pharmacokinetic and antibacterial profiles. Claims for their superiority over phenoxymethylpenicillin are often valid only for a particular bacterial strain or species and the data usually derive from *in vitro* observations.

Penicillinase-resistant penicillins

These penicillins have modified side-chains which provide enough steric hindrance to prevent them being used as substrates by penicillinases. They are less active than benzylpenicillin and they have similar narrow antibacterial spectra. They should therefore not be used for infections which can be satisfactorily dealt with by benzylpenicillin. The group includes methicillin, which is not widely used in veterinary medicine, the isoxazoyl penicillins and nafcillin.

Methicillin (Fig. 18.2)
This is destroyed by stomach acid and must always be given parenterally (usually intramuscularly). The incidence of intrinsic resistance to methicillin is increasing steadily. Resistance usually extends to all penicillins with a similar mode of action (i.e. across the group and sometimes to the cephalosporins). The time to peak plasma concentration after intramuscular injection is about 30 minutes and there is then a decline to a low level within 3–4 hours. About 75 per cent of a therapeutic dose is excreted in the urine unchanged and the presence of methicillin in the blood can be prolonged by probenecid. The

drug is about 40 per cent protein-bound and there is little penetration of the blood–brain barrier.

Dose

Usually 25–50 mg/kg i.m. or i.v. every 6 hours.

Isoxazoyl penicillins

These combine resistance to penicillinase with acid stability. They are mainly active against Gram-positive organisms. The group includes oxacillin, cloxacillin, dicloxacillin and flucloxacillin (Fig. 18.2). Of these, cloxacillin is most widely used in veterinary medicine. Resistance, which can occur in stepwise fashion, usually extends to the other isoxazoyl penicillins and it is advisable to establish sensitivity tests before and during therapy. There is at least 50 per cent absorption from the gut within 2 hours, although there is considerable variation among individuals and species. Therapeutic concentrations are maintained for about 4 hours, in spite of heavy protein-binding. These drugs do not cross the blood–brain barrier in the absence of inflammation. Small proportions of the dose are metabolized in the liver to penicilloic acids; the rest is rapidly excreted in the urine as the parent drug.

Apart from occasional hypersensitivity reactions common to all penicillins, flucloxacillin has been shown to be highly irritant to the eye, causing severe inflammation and corneal opacities. Locally applied benzathine cloxacillin has been shown to be effective in bovine conjunctivitis, however. Ideally, these drugs should be reserved for infections due to penicillinase-producing cocci (e.g. 50–70 per cent of those isolated from bovine mastitis) but they are often used less appropriately.

Cloxacillin is used in veterinary medicine mainly as the benzathine salt, both alone and in combination with ampicillin for intramammary infusion. It protects ampicillin against β-lactamases by reversibly inhibiting the enzyme (although less effectively than clavulanic acid). Clinically significant synergism between the isoxazoyl penicillins and ampicillin against Gram-positive and Gram-negative organisms occurs only when the tissue concentrations are high. Such formulations are normally used immediately after the last milking of the lactation to treat existing mastitis and to prevent infection during the dry period. These preparations will maintain effective concentrations in the udder for about 4 weeks. They should not be used in lactating cows and if used, milk must be discarded for 30 days. An intramammary suspension of the sodium salt is used if a persistent effect is not required. Here, dosage is every 12 hours. An eye ointment containing the benzathine salt is also available for treating a variety of infections in domestic animals. The formulation is such that effective concentrations of cloxacillin are maintained for at least 24 hours. Cloxacillin is sometimes given orally to dogs to treat superficial infections.

Nafcillin
This is regarded as the most potent of the penicillinase-resistant penicillins. It is mainly used in combination with dihydrostreptomycin in intramammary suspensions which also contain benzylpenicillin—or procaine penicillin if a longer-acting preparation is required. Milk from treated animals should not be taken for human consumption within 3 days of the last treatment. Large variations can occur in excretion times and when animals calve within 4 weeks of the last infusion, it is recommended that milk be tested for antibiotics at intervals.

Broad-spectrum penicillins

These penicillins, which generally have an amino or carboxyl substituent in the side-chain, have activity against Gram-positive organisms. These organisms are also normally sensitive to benzylpenicillin, which, like the broad-spectrum drugs, can easily reach the target site—the transpeptidase enzyme on the outer surface of the cytoplasmic membrane. The second envelope external to the peptidoglycan wall of many Gram-negative organisms, which excludes benzylpenicillin, is readily permeable to these drugs and thus they also have activity against some Gram-negatives. They have specific clinical indications but are often used inappropriately to gain broader coverage instead of establishing sensitivity before starting treatment. It is appropriate to reiterate that, in most cases, the best chemotherapeutic stratagem is to choose the antibiotic with the narrowest spectrum of activity which is likely to be effective in a given situation. Such treatment reduces the chance of superinfection and decreases selection pressure for the development of resistance. Two families of broad-spectrum penicillins are available—the aminopenicillins (e.g. ampicillin) and the carboxypenicillins (e.g. carbenicillin).

Aminopenicillins

Ampicillin
Ampicillin (Fig. 18.2) was first of the aminopenicillins to be developed. It is derived from 6-aminopenicillanic acid. Although the spectrum of activity of ampicillin is much broader than that of benzylpenicillin, against Gram-positives, ampicillin is only about 25–50 per cent as active as benzylpenicillin.

Despite its wide range of activity, a number of clinically significant organisms are insensitive to the drug. These include *Pseudomonas* spp., *Proteus* spp., penicillinase-producing staphylococci and about 25 per cent of β-lactamase-producing stains of *E. coli*. All strains of *E. coli* produce a β-lactamase which destroys benzylpenicillin but ampicillin resistant strains have an additional enzyme which hydrolyses ampicillin. Ampicillin resistance among Gram-negative organisms is often a component of plasmid-mediated multiple drug resistance.

Ampicillin is acid-stable and is rapidly but incompletely absorbed (30–50 per cent) from the gastrointestinal tract. After oral administration, peak serum levels are attained within 1–2 hours, although there are marked species and individual variations in the rate and extent of absorption. In the dog, bioavailability of ampicillin is about 20–40 per cent. The drug is detectable in plasma for 4–6 hours. A degree of enterohepatic shunting occurs and this makes the rise and fall of the plasma concentration rather slower than with many other penicillins. Plasma protein-binding of ampicillin is about 18 per cent and is mainly to albumin. Ampicillin is widely distributed but concentrations vary among tissues and fluids with kidney and liver having the highest concentrations. Ampicillin penetrates into ocular fluids but passage across the blood–brain barrier is poor in the absence of inflammation. It crosses the placenta and is present in foetal serum and amniotic fluid at delivery. It is also present in milk. Ampicillin is cleared by renal tubular secretion and excreted in the urine in high concentrations. Also, because of incomplete absorption and enterohepatic shunting, considerable amounts are present in the faeces. Ampicillin trihydrate is less soluble than the sodium salt and when given by injection (s.c. or i.m.), low levels of the drug can be detected for 12 hours. Injectable ampicillin stearate formulations can be used to extend activity to at least 48 hours, but they are often painful on (i.m.) injection to dogs and cats and may produce a severe local reaction at the injection site in horses.

Toxicity Apart from the hypersensitivity reactions which are common to all the penicillins, ampicillin and closely related drugs are capable of disturbing the intestinal flora with resultant superinfection. This may cause diarrhoea in calves and horses and a colitis-like state in rodents. Ampicillin should not be given to rabbits, hamsters and guinea pigs. Animals for human consumption must not be slaughtered less than 2 days after completion of treatment; this period must be extended to 14 days if long-acting preparations are used. Milk from ampicillin-treated cows should not be used for human consumption for at least 3 days after treatment is stopped.

Drug interactions The synergistic interaction between ampicillin and cloxacillin has already been discussed. Synergism also occurs between ampicillin and the more specific β-lactamase inhibitors, potassium clavulanate and sulbactam, against β-lactamase-producing organisms, such as *E. coli*.

Dose

Ampicillin

pig, dog, cat	4–20 mg/kg p.o. 1–2 times daily
calf	4–12 mg/kg p.o. 1–2 times daily
all other species	2–10 mg/kg s.c. or i.m. 1–2 times daily

Ampicillin prodrugs   Pivampicillin is an acid-stable pivalloyl ester of ampicillin which is better absorbed after oral administration (in humans) and is then rapidly hydrolysed to ampicillin in the gut wall. Epicillin (the sodium salt of 6[D-α-amino-2-(1,4-cyclohexadien-1-yl)acetamido]penicillanic acid) is claimed to produce high concentrations in blood and urine and can be given orally or parenterally. Hetacillin, talampicillin and bacampicillin are other examples which are claimed to be absorbed almost completely from the intestine, producing higher blood levels than ampicillin, and/or to cause less diarrhoea.

Amoxycillin

Amoxycillin differs from ampicillin in having a hydroxyl substituent in the para-position on the phenyl ring (Fig. 18.2). It has a similar *in vitro* spectrum of activity to ampicillin but is generally more active than ampicillin when given orally. This undoubtedly reflects more complete (70–92 per cent) absorption, which is not influenced by the presence of food. Peak plasma concentrations are attained about 2 hours after oral administration. It is also well absorbed from parenteral sites although parenteral therapy is generally unnecessary. Systemic bioavailability of oral amoxycillin in the dog is 60–70 per cent. Amoxycillin is less ionized than benzylpenicillin and is more lipid-soluble. However, the drug crosses the blood–brain barrier with difficulty. Protein binding is of the order of 17 per cent and about 20–30 per cent of a dose is metabolized into penicilloic acid, which is excreted in the urine. No biotransformation to ampicillin has been reported.

Certain Gram-negative organisms (including *E. coli*) are destroyed more rapidly by amoxycillin than by ampicillin. The effectiveness and spectrum of activity of amoxycillin is enhanced by combination with potassium clavulanate, which inactivates β-lactamases.

Dose

all species	7 mg/kg s.c. or i.m. daily
	10 mg/kg p.o. b.i.d

Carboxypenicillins

Carbenicillin

Carbenicillin is the disodium salt of α-carboxybenzylpenicillin. It is degraded by some but not all β-lactamases. It is active against Gram-negative organisms such as *Pseudomonas, Proteus* and *Salmonella* species but *Klebsiella* species are resistant.

Carbenicillin is not absorbed from the gut and must be given parenterally. High serum concentrations can be maintained with the use of probenecid. It is approximately 50 per cent protein bound and there is 80–100 per cent excretion in the urine in an active form.

Resistance to carbenicillin emerges rapidly, especially with deep-seated *Pseudomonas* infections, and gentamicin or tobramycin is often given concomitantly, both for a synergistic effect and to delay the emergence of resistance. It has been suggested that resistance may not occur so readily when the drug is used to treat urinary tract infections. This may be due, in part, to the very high concentrations which are attained.

Carindacillin

This is the indanyl ester of carbenicillin. It is more lipophilic than carbenicillin and, being acid-stable, it is readily absorbed from the gastrointestinal tract. It is then rapidly hydrolysed to carbenicillin. The antibacterial action of carindacillin is due entirely to its conversion to carbenicillin.

Ticarcillin

Ticarcillin (Fig. 18.2) has a similar chemical structure to carbenicillin, with a thienyl group replacing the phenyl group. The spectrum of activity of ticarcillin is similar to that of carbenicillin but it is more active against certain Gram-negative organisms, including *Pseudomonas aeruginosa, Proteus* spp. and certain strains of *E. coli*. It is not stable in the presence of β-lactamases.

If given by mouth ticarcillin is not absorbed, and the intramuscular or intravenous routes must be used. Ticarcillin is 45 per cent protein-bound and although it becomes distributed into most tissues, it does not penetrate to the CSF in the absence of inflammation. The drug is rapidly excreted in the urine.

Resistance to ticarcillin appears to develop fairly rapidly, especially among Gram-negative organisms. Ticarcillin synergizes with aminoglycosides, such as gentamicin, tobramycin and amikacin, and the β-lactamase inhibitor, potassium clavulanate. The concomitant use of these drugs with ticarcillin reduces the emergence of resistant strains.

Penicillin adjuncts

Mecillinam and pivmecillinam
These are derived from 6-aminopenicillanic acid. Pivmecillinam is the piva-loyloxymethyl ester of mecillinam and is a prodrug which is readily absorbed and then hydrolysed to mecillinam (mecillinam is not absorbed from the gastrointestinal tract). Strictly speaking, these drugs should not be classified with the penicillins because an amidino group is substituted in the β-lactam ring. Moreover, they act in a quite different way to the penicillins, although they synergize with them.

In the presence of mecillinam, morphological changes occur in sensitive organisms (principally Gram-negative) which result in the formation of large osmotically stable cells which are exquisitely sensitive to the penicillins and cephalosporins.

Mecillinam has been used in combination with ampicillin, amoxycillin or co-trimoxazole (trimethoprim/sulphonamide combination) for the treatment of urinary tract and enteric infections.

Potassium clavulanate
Clavulanic acid (Fig. 18.1) is derived from *Streptomyces clavigulerus*. It resembles the penicillins in that it possesses a β-lactam ring, but oxygen replaces sulphur in the thiazolidine ring. Although the antibacterial activity of clavulanic acid is very weak, it irreversibly inhibits most extracellular and intracellular β-lactamases and thus synergizes with the penicillins.

The pharmacokinetic profile of potassium clavulanate is very similar to that of amoxycillin. It is absorbed rapidly from the gastrointestinal tract and the influence of food on absorption is minimal. Clavulanic acid is about 20–25 per cent protein-bound and diffuses readily into most body tissues and fluids but penetrates the CSF poorly. The metabolism of the drug is poorly understood. In humans, about 30 per cent of the drug is excreted as such in the urine but the fate of the remainder is yet to be determined. Unlike the penicillins, it is excreted mainly by glomerular filtration.

The drug is normally used in 1 : 2 or 1 : 4 fixed combinations with amoxycillin. These mixtures have been found to be effective in infections of the human urinary tract, respiratory tract, skin and soft tissues, and have also been used successfully in dogs and calves. Combinations with ticarcillin and gentamicin have also been reported to be effective.

Sulbactam (penicillanic acid sulphone)
Like potassium clavulanate, sulbactam is a β-lactamase inhibitor which has the potential to increase the antibacterial spectra of the amino- and carboxypenicillins.

Newer penicillins

These drugs have different protein-binding sites from the aminopenicillins and penetrate Gram-negative organisms more readily. They include the acylureidopenicillins, azlocillin and mezlocillin, and piperacillin.

Mezlocillin and azlocillin

Mezlocillin is active against both Gram-positive and Gram-negative organisms but remains sensitive to most β-lactamases. It is not absorbed from the gastrointestinal tract and is usually given by the intravenous route. It is 27–40 per cent protein-bound and attains high concentrations in most tissues but there is poor penetration into the CSF unless inflammation is present. About 65 per cent of a dose appears in the urine as the active form and about 25 per cent is excreted into the bile. The drug has a short half-life and has to be given at frequent intervals. It can, however, be given together with other bactericidal drugs such as gentamicin, and synergism has been reported. Mezlocillin has been used to treat lower respiratory tract infections, septicaemia, cellulitis, peritonitis and both bile duct and kidney infections in humans. In particular, infections occurring in patients with reduced defensive capacity (e.g. those on immunosuppressants) have been successfully treated. It is considered that the drug should normally only be used after appropriate culture and sensitivity tests. Despite the potential usefulness of mezlocillin against a wide range of microorganisms, veterinary applications are likely to be limited by cost.

Azlocillin has a close structural similarity and pharmacological profile to mezlocillin. It is especially active against *Pseudomonas* species and also synergizes with the aminoglycosides.

Piperacillin

As its name implies, piperacillin has a piperazine substituent on the nucleus. It has a broad spectrum of activity including both Gram-positive and Gram-negative organisms. It is inactivated by most β-lactamases. It has been combined with a variety of other antibiotics in an attempt to produce a synergistic effect. This has not always occurred and both additivity and (occasionally) antagonism have been reported.

The drug is always given parenterally and becomes widely distributed. There is good penetration to lungs and bronchial secretions of human patients with bronchitis, for example. It has a short half-life and is excreted unchanged (40–70 per cent) in the urine. Piperacillin should be reserved for severe infections where it is the most appropriate drug; again, cost is likely to limit veterinary use.

Cephalosporins

The cephalosporins are a group of antibiotics which are closely related to the penicillins. The original source of cephalosporins was the mould, *Cephalosporium acrimonium*, which was isolated from material collected in a Sardinian sewage outfall and contained several antibacterial substances. These included cephalosporin N or synnematin B and cephalosporin C, which are penicillin-like, and cephalosporin P, which is a steroid related to fusidic acid.

The cephalosporin nucleus is 7-aminocephalosporanic acid (Fig. 18.1), which is analogous to 6-aminopenicillanic acid in that they both have a β-lactam ring joined to an S-containing ring. Two side-chains are also present. As with the penicillins, isolation of the nucleus has allowed for the synthesis of several generations (three at present) of derivatives with different antibacterial spectra and pharmacokinetic profiles.

The cephalosporins have many similarities with the penicillins; they share the same mode of action on the bacterial cell wall and are usually bactericidal. They are active against Gram-positive organisms and also, increasingly, against Gram-negatives as their resistance to β-lactamases is improved through the generations. With few exceptions, the cephalosporins have similar pharmacokinetics to the penicillins. Some are destroyed by gastric acid and must be injected; most are well-distributed but cross the blood–brain barrier with difficulty in the absence of inflammation. Except for cephaloridine, most cephalosporins are eliminated mainly by proximal renal tubular secretion although significant amounts of cefoperazone and moxalactam also appear in the bile.

First-generation cephalosporins

These include: cephacetrile, cephalothin, cephaloridine, cefazolin, cephalonium, cephapirin, cephaloglycin, cephalexin, cefadroxil and cephradine. Although these cephalosporins lack activity against many Gram-negative bacteria, they are the members of the group most active against Gram-positives.

Cephalothin

Cephalothin (Fig. 18.3) is the sodium salt of cephalosporin C. It is not absorbed from the gastrointestinal tract and must be given parenterally (usually i.m.). Peak plasma concentrations are usually attained within 30 minutes and decline rapidly thereafter. The plasma half-life is about 1 hour. Protein binding is about 70 per cent and the drug penetrates well into body fluids but not into the CSF under normal conditions. It is metabolized in the liver to a partially active product, desacetylcephalothin. It is rapidly

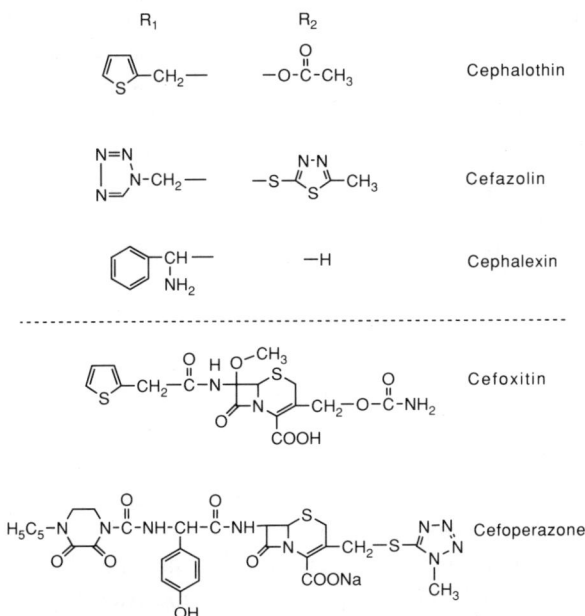

Figure 18.3 Side-chain substituents of the first-generation cephalosporins (cephalothin, cephazolin and cephalexin) and structure of the second-generation cephalosporin, cefoxitin, and the third-generation cephalosporin, cefoperazone.

excreted via the kidneys, by both glomerular filtration and tubular secretion. Probenecid prolongs the presence of the drug in the body. Cephalothin is resistant to destruction by most staphylococcal penicillinases.

Cefazolin
Cefazolin (Fig. 18.3) will almost certainly replace cephalothin for parenteral use. Although the extent of protein binding is rather greater than with cephalothin, the serum half-life is four times that of cephalothin. The renal clearance of cefazolin is slower than that of cephalothin, but adequate concentrations can be achieved in the urine. In severe infections, it is possible to give cefazolin intravenously and then to proceed to oral cephalexin.

Cephalonium
This is a semi-synthetic cephalosporin which must be injected or used as an intramammary preparation. Although it has a broad spectrum and is active against many Gram-positive and Gram-negative organisms, both aerobic and anaerobic, a number of clinically significant infections fail to respond to the drug (e.g. *Pseudomonas aeruginosa*). Cephalonium is resistant to staphylococcal penicillinase.

The intramammary preparation is formulated so that when infused at drying-off, effective levels of the drug will be maintained in the dry udder for up to 10 weeks. It is used to treat existing subclinical infections and to prevent new infections occurring in the dry period or at calving (250 mg/quarter, intramammary infusion). Provided calving occurs more than 4 weeks after the infusion, any cephalonium remaining in the udder is eliminated in the milk within 4 days.

An ointment is also available for the treatment of keratoconjunctivitis caused by *Moraxella bovis* in cattle.

Cephaloridine

Cephaloridine is a derivative of cephalosporin C in which both side-chains are synthetic. It is not absorbed orally and must be injected. After intramuscular injection, peak plasma concentrations are attained within 1 hour and the half-life in the plasma is almost 2 hours. Cephaloridine is only slightly protein-bound (20 per cent) and there is good penetration into body fluids. Cephaloridine readily crosses the placenta, but not the blood–brain barrier.

High levels of cephaloridine appear in the urine after 2–4 hours. Following the observation that probenecid had less effect on cephaloridine excretion than other cephalosporins, it was shown that cephaloridine is cleared largely by glomerular filtration. There is an absolute limit on the amount of cephaloridine which can be cleared and if this limit is exceeded, renal damage may ensue. This has been observed in the rabbit. The dose must be reduced when there is known or suspected impairment of renal function. In humans, the renal toxicities of cephaloridine and some non-narcotic analgesics are at least additive.

Cephaloglycin

Cephaloglycin is a synthetic derivative of cephalosporin C. It is reasonably well absorbed when given by the oral route and peak plasma concentrations are attained within 1 hour and fall to a low level after 6 hours. About 30 per cent of a dose is recoverable from the urine. The modest performance of cephaloglycin has led to its replacement by cephalexin.

Cephalexin

Both side-chains of cephalexin (Fig. 18.3) differ from those in cephalosporin C; the 7-substituent is the same as in cephaloglycin and the 3-methyl substituent is believed to confer stability. Cephalexin and ampicillin have a strong structural resemblance. Although cephalexin is bactericidal, it appears slower to kill than other cephalosporins. It is acid-stable and can be given orally. Therapeutic plasma levels are reached quickly after oral administration and fall to a low level within about 6 hours. Plasma half-life is less than 1 hour. Protein binding is low (15 per cent) and the drug becomes widely distributed. Excretion via the kidneys is rapid; 70–90 per cent of a dose is eliminated, active and unchanged, within 24 hours. Probenecid delays excretion.

Methicillin-resistant staphylococci usually show cross-resistance to cephalexin. Cephalexin is considered to be relatively non-toxic and hypersensitivity is very rare. Renal clearance is reduced in renal failure and the dose should be reduced but cephalexin is not cumulatively toxic like cephaloridine.

Cephalexin is formulated into drops and tablets for oral therapy in cats and dogs and an injection for farm animals.

Dose

cow	7 mg/kg i.m. daily
sheep, pig	10 mg/kg i.m. or s.c. daily
dog, cat	10 mg/kg i.m. or s.c. daily
	10–15 mg/kg p.o. daily

Cephacetrile
The sodium salt of cephacetrile is used to treat both acute and chronic mastitis in lactating cows. Milk must be withheld for 96 hours after the last dose.

Cephradine
Cephradine is a semi-synthetic cephalosporin which is available in both oral and parenteral dose forms. It is used largely for urinary tract infections due to both Gram-positive and Gram-negative organisms.

Second-generation cephalosporins

In second-generation cephalosporins, resistance to β-lactamases from Gram-negative organisms is increased and, in consequence, the antibacterial spectrum is expanded to include organisms such as *Enterobacter* and *Proteus* species. This group includes: cefamandole, cefatrizine, cefoxitin, cefuroxime, cephoxazole and cefaclor.

Cefoxitin
Cefoxitin (Fig. 18.3) is a semi-synthetic derivative of cephalosporin C. It has a methoxy group on the nucleus in the 7-position which confers stability to β-lactamases. The α-methoxy substituent in the 3-position confers resistance to the deacylating enzymes which are responsible for part of the metabolic

inactivation of the cephalosporins. Cefoxitin can be considered to have a broader spectrum of activity against Gram-positive organisms than earlier cephalosporins and to have increased resistance to β-lactamases. It is active against the usual range of staphylococcal and streptococcal species but is inactive against *Streptococcus faecalis* and *Pseudomonas aeruginosa*. Methicillin-resistant bacteria are almost always resistant to cefoxitin.

The absorption of cefoxitin administered by the oral route is negligible and it is given either by intramuscular injection, where absorption is substantially complete, or intravenously. Protein-binding is about 70 per cent but there is good penetration, even into areas of pus and pleural fluid. Cefoxitin penetrates the blood–brain barrier very poorly under normal conditions and it is not recommended for the treatment of meningitis and brain abscess. The half-life in the plasma is just under 1 hour.

Cefoxitin is only metabolized to a very small extent and 80 per cent of a dose is normally recoverable from the urine within 2 hours. Both glomerular filtration and tubular secretion are involved, and renal clearance of the drug is prolonged in renal failure.

Cefuroxime

Cefuroxime is mainly used in an intramammary cerate for treatment of clinical mastitis in milking cows. It is resistant to degradation by β-lactamases from both Gram-positive and Gram-negative bacteria, including all major mastitis pathogens. Milk should be discarded for 60 hours after treatment is stopped. There is a withdrawal period of 1 day before slaughter.

Cephoxazole

This is formulated with procaine penicillin in a quick-release oily base and is used to treat mastitis in milking cows. The base disperses readily in the milk and allows rapid distribution of both antibiotics. Cephoxazole is also believed to protect penicillin against destruction by Gram-negative β-lactamases. The activity of penicillin is thus maintained, even in the presence of Gram-negative commensal organisms. Milk from treated cows must be discarded for 3 days after the last infusion.

Third-generation cephalosporins

These drugs are important in that they have greatly increased activity against *Pseudomonas aeruginosa* and the Enterobacteriaceae. Each member of the group should be considered separately in terms of its specific antibacterial activity and susceptibility to β-lactamases. The rapid development of resistance due to the derepression of inducible chromosomal β-lactamases has been described and indicates a need for restricting the use of these drugs to situations where, on the basis of sensitivity tests, they are the most rational therapy. This group includes: cefoperazone, cefotaxime, cefsulodin, ceftazidime, ceftizoxime, ceftriaxone and moxalactam.

Cefoperazone

Cefoperazone (Fig. 18.3) is normally given parenterally but a formulation is available for the treatment of clinical mastitis in milking cows. Withholding time for milk is 84 hours and for meat 2 days. Unlike other cephalosporins, biliary excretion accounts for 75 per cent of the clearance of the drug.

Carbapenems

Imipenem (N-formimidoyl thienamycin)

Imipenem is a β-lactam antibiotic which was isolated from *Streptomyces cattleya*. It has the widest antibacterial spectrum of any known antibiotic and is highly effective against almost all Gram-positive and Gram-negative organisms and anaerobes, including strains of *Pseudomonas aeruginosa* which are resistant to most other antibiotics. It is also a β-lactamase inhibitor. It is given intravenously to humans in combination with cilastatin, a competitive inhibitor of the renal dihydropeptidase which destroys the drug. It penetrates into most tissues and crosses the blood–brain barrier. It is reserved for the empirical treatment of serious infections in situations where an unpredictable strain of pathogen might be involved. It is particularly useful in immunocompromised patients with multiple infections and in patients with cystic fibrosis. Imipenem is often combined with an aminoglycoside to delay the onset of resistance which can develop rapidly, especially with *Pseudomonas* species. Toxic effects include hypersensitivity reactions and possible neurotoxicity. The efficacy of imipenem in veterinary medicine has not been established.

Monobactams

Aztreonam

Although a β-lactam antibiotic, aztreonam has an antibacterial spectrum which resembles that of the aminoglycosides. It has little activity against Gram-positives or anaerobes but is highly effective against a wide range of Gram-negative bacteria, including *Pseudomonas aeruginosa*. β-Lactamases do not inactivate the drug, which also retains its activity in the presence of pus. The use of aztreonam in veterinary medicine has not been established.

Vancomycin

Vancomycin is a complex tricyclic glycopeptide antibiotic which was isolated from *Streptomyces orientalis* in 1955. It is active against Gram-positive bacteria, including multiply-resistant strains producing β-lactamases, but Gram-negative bacteria are generally resistant. Its use is reserved for the treatment of serious disease caused by these organisms.

It acts to inhibit the second stage of cell wall synthesis, preventing the formation of peptidoglycan from precursors. The function of the cell membrane is also affected and cell lysis occurs. No cross-resistance has been reported to other antibiotics.

Vancomycin is not absorbed from the gastrointestinal tract and must be given by intravenous infusion for the treatment of systemic infections. Oral therapy can be used for serious gastrointestinal infections (e.g. antibiotic-induced). It is about 55 per cent protein-bound and becomes well distributed, crossing to the CSF when the meninges are inflamed. The serum half-life is about 6 hours, with about 80 per cent of a dose being eventually excreted in the urine by glomerular filtration. Cumulation of the drug occurs in renal insufficiency. Vancomycin is often used concomitantly with the aminoglycosides.

The drug is rather toxic and has been found to cause a variety of hypersensitivity reactions, fever, blood dyscrasias, thrombophlebitis, oto-toxicity (often permanent) and nephrotoxicity. Superinfection by Gram-negative bacteria has also been reported. Some of the reactions to vancomycin may be histamine-mediated since they are attenuated by histamine H_1-antagonists in the dog. The toxicity of vancomycin has declined as purer preparations have become available.

Vancomycin is rarely used in veterinary medicine. As in humans, veterinary use should be reserved for serious infections which are unlikely to respond to other drugs. Antibiotic-induced superinfection with *Staphylococcus aureus* or pseudomembranous colitis caused by *Clostridium difficile* could perhaps be treated with vancomycin.

Teicoplanin

This is chemically related to vancomycin. It is considered to be as effective as vancomycin but much simpler to use. It has a long half-life and need only be given once a day in a bolus dose. It is claimed that there is no dose-related toxicity. It is used for the same purposes as vancomycin—serious Gram-positive infections which are resistant to methicillin.

Bacitracin

Bacitracin was first isolated from a strain of *Bacillus subtilis* (Tracy-T strain). The name derives from the fact that it was grown from damaged tissue and street dirt debrided from a compound fracture sustained by a girl called Tracy.

Commercial bacitracin consists of several polypeptides. The structure of bacitracin A, the major component, has been found to consist of ten amino acids in a partially cyclized chain linked to a thiazolidine ring.

Bacitracin is active against Gram-positive organisms, binding to membrane phospholipid and causing a bactericidal inhibition of cell wall synthesis. Most Gram-negative bacteria are intrinsically resistant to bacitracin. Its spectrum of activity is thus similar to that of benzylpenicillin. Bacterial resistance to bacitracin is unimportant clinically. The drug is too nephrotoxic for systemic use but since it is not absorbed from the gastrointestinal tract, it can be used to treat infections by *Clostridium difficile*, for example.

Topical bacitracin is used alone or in combination with a variety of other antibiotics and corticosteroids for infected surgical wounds, eye infections and external ear infections. Hypersensitivity reactions may occur after the superficial use of bacitracin and the rationale for the use of bacitracin-corticosteroid preparations is questionable.

Zinc bacitracin is used as a growth promoter in cattle, pigs and poultry.

Bactericidal inhibitors of protein synthesis

Aminoglycosides

In veterinary medicine, the most widely used aminoglycosides are streptomycin, dihydrostreptomycin, framycetin and neomycin. Newer aminoglycosides, sharing many of the same characteristics, such as kanamycin, amikacin, gentamicin, tobramycin, netilmicin and sissomicin are also available, but cost is the main limitation of their use.

The aminoglycosides are a closely related group with similar chemical structures (Fig. 18.4), antibacterial spectra (mainly against Gram-negatives) and pharmacokinetic profiles. They also share the same toxic effects. The newer aminoglycosides (gentamicin, tobramycin and amikacin) are rather less toxic than the earlier members of the group (streptomycin, dihydro-streptomycin, kanamycin and neomycin) and have tended to replace them

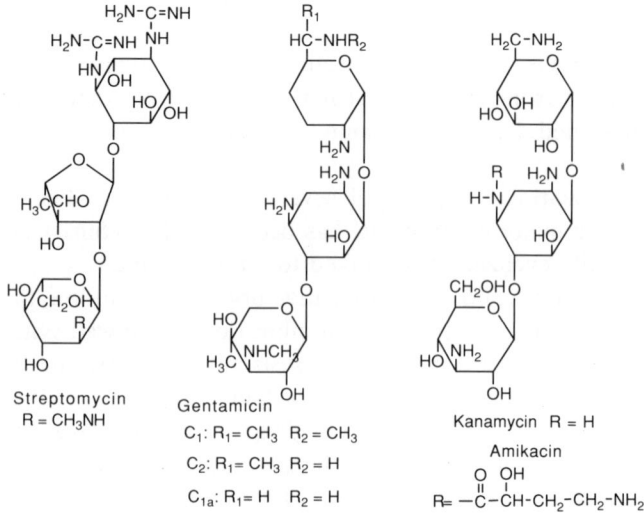

Figure 18.4 Structures of some of the aminoglycosides. Commercial preparations of gentamicin contain a mixture of gentamicin C_1, C_{1a} and C_2.

in human medicine. Streptomycin was isolated from *Streptomyces griseus* in 1944 and the other aminoglycosides have also been obtained from *Streptomyces* species (except for sissomicin, which is obtained from a *Micromonosporum* species, and amikacin, which is synthesized from kanamycin).

Mechanism of action

Aminoglycosides cause a number of changes in susceptible bacteria, including alterations in cell permeability and transport mechanisms. They also inhibit protein synthesis and cause misreading of the genetic code on the mRNA template. This causes incorporation of 'incorrect' amino acids into the peptide. Questions remain about exactly how the aminoglycosides produce their lethal effect and why total inhibition of bacterial protein synthesis kills bacteria whereas the same effect, when induced by other antibiotics (such as erythromycin and the tetracyclines), is only bacteriostatic. It is believed that although all aminoglycosides inhibit bacterial protein synthesis in the same basic manner, there are differences in the way the drugs interact with the ribosomal binding site and cause the conformational changes which disrupt the process. Bactericidal concentrations of aminoglycosides rapidly inhibit protein synthesis in sensitive bacteria which are in the growth phase, the major effect occurring during or shortly after initiation. Aminoglycosides are more active at alkaline than at acid pH.

Antibacterial activity

The aminoglycosides have potent activity against Gram-negative aerobic bacteria but are not generally very active against Gram-positive organisms, except for staphylococci and *Leptospira*, which may respond to gentamicin and tobramycin. Anaerobes are not sensitive to aminoglycosides because they lack the necessary active transport systems for the drug.

Drugs in this group are often used in combination with β-lactam antibiotics (benzylpenicillin, procaine penicillin, benzathine penicillin, nafcillin) and synergism often results. It has been suggested that the inhibition of cell wall synthesis by the β-lactam antibiotic permits greater penetration of the aminoglycoside. Mixtures of aminoglycosides with non-absorbable sulphonamides are used to treat enteritis, and compound preparations of aminoglycosides with chlortetracycline, novobiocin and amphotericin are also available. Aminoglycosides are also available in combination with corticosteroids, histamine H_1-antagonists and anticholinergic drugs.

Resistance to the aminoglycosides

Three mechanisms of resistance may be operative: ribosomal resistance, decreased drug uptake and elaboration of aminoglycoside-modifying enzymes. Ribosomal resistance to streptomycin has been seen clinically and arises as a result of mutations in genes coding for ribosomal proteins which cause an alteration or deletion of the requisite (30S) subunit for aminoglycoside attachment. This type of resistance does not extend to other aminoglycosides. The polycationic nature of the aminoglycosides precludes their passive transport across membranes. Two energy-dependent mechanisms may become modified to restrict the rate of entry of aminoglycosides into bacterial cells. These modifications may be plasmid- or chromosomally-controlled.

The production of drug-modifying enzymes by bacteria is the most common mechanism for resistance to the aminoglycosides. The enzymes are probably associated with the bacterial cell membrane and act to block drug uptake and/or inactivate the drug, thus preventing an effect on ribosomal function. More than 20 aminoglycoside-modifying enzymes have been identified and include those capable of adenylating, acetylating or phosphorylating the drugs. The genes for these enzymes are carried on plasmids and multiple resistance can thus be transmitted by R-factor transfer among Gram-negative bacteria. Apramycin has the important property of resisting most of these enzymes.

Absorption, distribution and excretion

The aminoglycosides have similar pharmacokinetic properties. Their polycationic nature ensures that they are very poorly absorbed, even in the presence of inflammation. Thus oral administration of aminoglycosides is of use in the sterilization of the bowel before surgery and to treat intestinal infections. Often another antibacterial is given together with the aminoglycoside to deal with anaerobes.

Aminoglycosides are usually given intramuscularly. There is good absorption from the injection site and peak plasma concentrations are attained within about 1 hour. Where the infection is severe, they can be given by slow intravenous infusion. Aminoglycosides are often applied topically to treat eye and ear infections. Absorption through the intact skin is minimal but can be increased greatly where open wounds are present.

The volume of distribution of the aminoglycosides is about 25 per cent of lean bodyweight, which is roughly equivalent to the volume of the extracellular fluid. There is little binding to plasma proteins (< 25 per cent). High drug levels are attained in the kidney and, for example, the binding of amikacin in renal tissue probably accounts for the persistence of the drug in the urine. Concentrations of aminoglycosides in the interstitial fluid are generally similar to those in serum. There is good penetration into bronchial secretions, synovial fluid and the pericardium, and bactericidal concentrations are attained after appropriate doses. Penetration into the eye is poor and passage into the CSF is slight, even when inflammation is present. Substantial passage across the placenta occurs and foetal blood concentrations can reach 40 per cent of those in the mother. Aminoglycosides are also excreted in milk and this can be used to clinical advantage in the parenteral treatment of mastitis, usually in combination with penicillins.

Aminoglycosides are not metabolized and are eliminated in the active form by glomerular filtration, with some reabsorption in the proximal tubule. About 80 per cent of a streptomycin dose is eliminated in the urine over 12 hours. The elimination half-lives in normal animals are within the 2–4 h range but they may be greatly extended in patients with compromised renal function. It is possible to adjust the dose in human patients according to the creatinine clearance and thus avoid toxic effects. Aminoglycosides also appear in the bile and are excreted in the faeces.

Toxic reactions

Allergic reactions to systemic aminoglycosides are very uncommon. When applied topically, such reactions occur frequently, especially with neomycin. Contact dermatitis occurs in some persons handling these drugs. Acute toxicity is manifested as an anaphylactoid response, particularly in dogs and cats.

Aminoglycosides can induce neuromuscular blockade, caused by a reduction of acetylcholine output at the motor nerve terminal. There may also be a decrease in the sensitivity of the motor end-plate to acetylcholine. This effect is seen most commonly after intravenous or intraperitoneal administration of aminoglycosides, and it can cause respiratory arrest. General anaesthesia with diethyl ether predisposes patients to neuromuscular blockade after aminoglycosides. Cholinesterase inhibitors or calcium gluconate are effective at reversing the blockade.

All the aminoglycosides are ototoxic and can cause defects in both hearing and balance functions. There are differences among the aminoglycosides as to which function is affected most; streptomycin primarily affects the vestibular system but neomycin, kanamycin and amikacin are primarily toxic to the cochlea. Gentamicin and tobramycin show both vestibular and cochlear toxicity. These toxic effects are exacerbated in patients with renal impairment and those receiving other ototoxic drugs. If the loss of hearing/balance is not extensive, function will usually return to normal when treatment is stopped, but if the loss is more severe, it may be permanent. Aminoglycosides readily penetrate the inner ear fluid, where their half-lives are much longer (10–12 h) than in plasma (2 h). The primary effect is on the peripheral sensory portions of the inner ear and not on the 8th cranial nerve itself. In both animals and humans, it can be shown that the hair cells in the organ of Corti are damaged. With low doses of aminoglycosides, the hair cells in the basal turn of the cochlea are damaged first, with gradual progression to the apex as the dose is increased. The biochemical basis for the damage has not been established. Cats are particularly susceptible to aminoglycoside ototoxicity and these drugs are best avoided in this species.

Acute tubular necrosis, manifested as proteinuria and an inability to concentrate urine, followed by a reduction in glomerular filtration rate and a rise in serum creatinine and blood urea nitrogen, can occur after aminoglycosides. This damage is normally reversible when treatment is stopped. Neomycin is the most nephrotoxic of the group and tobramycin is perhaps the least. It is believed that nephrotoxicity and ototoxicity are related phenomena, involving the binding of the aminoglycoside to membrane constituents. As with ototoxicity, the possibility of aminoglycoside nephrotoxicity is increased by general anaesthesia and other nephrotoxic drugs.

Streptomycin

This was the first of the aminoglycosides. It is available as the sulphate and the hydrochloride and also as a calcium chloride complex. It has widespread use in veterinary medicine and is often combined with the penicillins and other β-lactam antibiotics in the treatment of mixed infections. In humans, streptomycin is still used as a first-line drug in the treatment of tuberculosis, which remains its main indication. Streptomycin is also used for plague and severe cases of brucellosis. In veterinary medicine, streptomycin is frequently combined with procaine penicillin.

Dose

Streptomycin alone
  horse, cow, sheep, goat, dog   10 mg/kg i.m. b.i.d.
Streptomycin is not generally used alone in horses and is toxic to the cat.

Dihydrostreptomycin

This is synthesized by the catalytic reduction of streptomycin. It is no longer used in humans because of its propensity to cause severe ototoxicity, but in veterinary medicine dihydrostreptomycin is often combined with streptomycin because the antibacterial effects appear to be additive and there is reduced toxicity.

Dose

The doses of dihydrostreptomycin are similar to those of streptomycin.

Gentamicin

Gentamicin is the oldest of the 'modern' aminoglycosides. It is used to treat serious infections with Gram-negative bacteria, often in combination with a β-lactam antibiotic. Gentamicin is effective against strains of *Pseudomonas* and *Klebsiella* that may be resistant to other antibiotics. There is also synergism between vancomycin and gentamicin. Dosage is difficult to gauge, however, and after the same dose on a bodyweight basis, gentamicin concentrations in different individuals are liable to vary from subtherapeutic to toxic. Like most aminoglycosides, the effect of gentamicin is greatest at alkaline pH. Gentamicin is incorporated into a number of topical preparations for treatment of superficial infections of the ear and eye.

Dose

dog, cat   5 mg/kg s.c. or i.m. b.i.d. for 1 day, then daily.

Tobramycin

Tobramycin can be considered to be a less-toxic gentamicin. It is often more active than gentamicin against *Pseudomonas aeruginosa* and, sometimes, gentamicin-resistant strains remain sensitive to tobramycin.

Apramycin

This is similar to tobramycin and is principally used for the treatment of enteritis in calves and pigs caused by Gram-negative bacteria. The drug is resistant to most R-plasmid-mediated degradative enzymes so that most pathogenic strains of *E. coli* and *Salmonella* isolated from calves, pigs and poultry are sensitive to apramycin. Apramycin is available as both oral and injectable solutions, a pre-mix formulation and a soluble powder for administration in the drinking water of pigs and poultry.

Dose

calf	20–40 mg/kg daily, by addition to drinking water
piglet	20–40 mg/day p.o.
lamb	10 mg/kg p.o. daily
poultry	25–50 g/100 l drinking water

Long periods must elapse after the cessation of apramycin treatment before animals can be slaughtered for human consumption. These are: calves and lambs (35 days), pigs (14–28 days, according to method of administration), poultry (7 days). In addition, eggs from apramycin-treated poultry should not be used for human consumption.

Kanamycin

Resistance to kanamycin is common and the use of the drug in human medicine has declined. It is more toxic than gentamicin or tobramycin. It can be given orally for the treatment of enteric infections and used topically for ear infections.

Amikacin

Amikacin was produced by the chemical modification of kanamycin and is less active than kanamycin. The isolation of aminoglycoside-modifying enzymes has allowed for the synthesis of new aminoglycosides which are not substrates for these enzymes. There is a low clinical incidence of resistance to amikacin, but resistant organisms are usually also resistant to gentamicin and tobramycin. It has to be given in higher dosage than gentamicin and tobramycin and peak serum concentrations are higher. It is more nephrotoxic and probably more ototoxic than tobramycin. The use of amikacin should be reserved for the treatment of severe infection by *Pseudomonas aeruginosa*, which is resistant to gentamicin and tobramycin. The drug has been used successfully to treat Gram-negative bacterial endometritis in mares.

Neomycin

Neomycin is very toxic and is no longer used systemically in humans because it causes renal damage and is ototoxic. In veterinary medicine, it is used for bowel sterilization, often combined with other antibacterials (e.g. poorly absorbed sulphonamides, such as phthalylsulphathiazole), for the prevention and treatment of intestinal infections, such as scours in piglets, and to treat chronic respiratory disease in poultry. It is also used for topical application, often in combination with bacitracin and other antibacterials and hydrocortisone. Contact irritancy is rare in animals. Neomycin is available in combination with penicillins for intramammary use. Treated animals should not be slaughtered for human consumption for 28 days from the last treatment.

Netilmicin

This is a semi-synthetic aminoglycoside which is also resistant to some of the aminoglycoside-modifying enzymes. It is similar in many respects to gentamicin but is claimed to be less toxic.

Sissomicin

This is also very similar to gentamicin.

Framycetin

Framycetin is similar to neomycin and has almost the same antibacterial spectrum. It is too toxic for systemic use. It is mainly used for the treatment of gastrointestinal infection and for local application, such as external ear infections in the dog.

Clinical uses of the aminoglycosides

Aminoglycosides are used, either alone or in combination, for the treatment of diseases caused by: *Aerobacter* species, *Bacillus anthracis*, *Corynebacterium equi*, *Escherichia coli*, *Klebsiella* spp., *Leptospira* spp., *Mycobacterium* spp., *Pasteurella* spp., *Proteus* spp., *Pseudomonas aeruginosa*, *Shigella equirulis* and *Staphylococcus* spp. They are effective in the treatment of many conditions caused by susceptible bacteria, including respiratory and uterine infections, osteomyelitis, peritonitis, septicaemia, cystitis and mastitis. Dosage is governed by the type and severity of the infection and the species and size of the animal. Since so many compound aminoglycoside preparations are available for specific purposes, the reader is referred to the manufacturers' instructions.

When simple or compound intramammary preparations containing aminoglycosides are used, milk should be discarded for the period of treatment and for 4 days after treatment is stopped. If cerate preparations are used, the discard time is 2 days.

The reader is referred to Chapter 19 for a more detailed rationale of the status of aminoglycosides among the antibiotics.

Bacteriostatic inhibitors of protein synthesis

These antibiotics were originally extracted from soil microorganisms and the group includes chloramphenicol, erythromycin, lincomycin/clindamycin, spectinomycin and the tetracyclines. They have diverse chemical structures (Fig. 18.5) but share the common property of inhibiting protein synthesis in sensitive bacteria. Unlike the aminoglycosides, however, inhibition of bacterial protein synthesis by these antibiotics does not normally result in cell death.

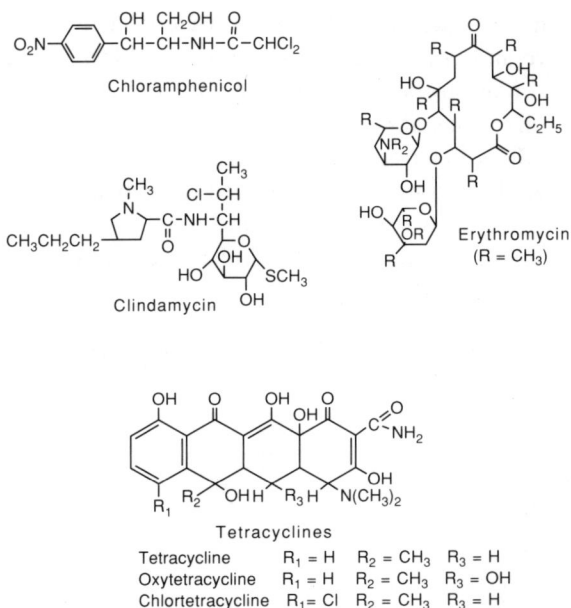

Figure 18.5 Structures of some of the bacteriostatic inhibitors of protein synthesis.

Chloramphenicol

This was first isolated in 1947 from *Streptomyces venezuelae* and was the first of the broad-spectrum antibiotics. It has a relatively simple chemical structure and is now produced by synthetic chemistry. It is chemically stable, neutral and lipid-soluble.

Mechanism of action

Chloramphenicol inhibits protein synthesis in sensitive bacteria. The drug becomes bound to the 50S subunit of the bacterial (70S) ribosome and, by blocking peptidyl transferase, prevents the addition of amino acids to the growing protein chains, which remain attached to the ribosome. The binding of chloramphenicol to the bacterial ribosome is reversible and growth will re-start if a chloramphenicol-treated culture is diluted.

Protein synthesis by mammalian cells occurs mainly on 80S ribosomes, but some protein synthesis also occurs in the mitochondria. Mammalian mitochondrial protein synthesis is inhibited by chloramphenicol and thus the selectivity of the drug is incomplete. It is believed that one of the most serious toxic effects of chloramphenicol in man (bone marrow toxicity, leading to aplastic anaemia) may be explained on this basis.

Antimicrobial activity

Chloramphenicol has a broad spectrum of antibacterial activity, which includes both Gram-positive and Gram-negative organisms. Chloramphenicol is active against all types of anaerobes and also against rickettsial and chlamydial species but not mycoplasmas. Mycobacteria and *Pseudomonas aeruginosa* are also resistant. It is inactive against fungi, yeasts, viruses and protozoa. Chloramphenicol has been traditionally regarded as being a strictly bacteriostatic antibiotic, but more recently it has been found to be bactericidal against some organisms (e.g. meningeal pathogens) in clinically achievable concentrations.

Table 18.1   The *in vitro* sensitivity (MIC*μg/ml) of some bacteria to chloramphenicol

Genus/species	MIC
Bacillus anthracis	2.5–5.0
Streptococcus pneumoniae	1.0–4.0
Staphylococcus aureus	4.0–12.0
Haemophilus influenzae	0.2–0.5
Salmonella spp.	0.5–10.0
Salmonella typhosus	2.0–4.0
Escherichia coli	0.8–8.0
Bacteroides spp.	1.0–8.0
Pasteurella spp.	0.2–10.0
Corynebacterium spp.	0.5–3.0
Proteus spp.	2.5–64
Pseudomonas aeruginosa	50–125

*Minimum Inhibitory Concentration. Adapted from Garrod, Lambert and O'Grady (1981), *Antibiotic and Chemotherapy*, Churchill Livingstone, London.

From Table 18.1 it can be seen that chloramphenicol is particularly active *in vitro* against *Haemophilus influenzae* and salmonellae.

Resistance

Enteric bacteria generally become resistant to chloramphenicol by R-factor transfer which results in the elaboration of chloramphenicol acetyltransferase enzymes. These enzymes facilitate the acetylation of the hydroxyl group which precludes binding to the bacterial ribosome. Although there is no cross-resistance between chloramphenicol and other antibiotics, chloramphenicol resistance is usually acquired as a component of multiple drug resistance.

Absorption

Chloramphenicol, administered in tablets and capsules, is readily absorbed from the gut in cats and dogs, and the plasma concentrations which can be attained are similar to those after injection. Peak plasma concentrations of chloramphenicol are attained in the dog about 30 minutes after an intramuscular injection of chloramphenicol sodium succinate. The hydrolysis of the succinate ester is incomplete, however, and levels of free chloramphenicol are lower than might otherwise be expected. Parenteral administration is necessary for dogs and cats which are fractious or vomiting.

Chloramphenicol palmitate, originally developed for human paediatric use, gives lower plasma concentrations than the free base, particularly in fasted cats. This has been tentatively attributed to a reduced secretion of digestive enzymes and, in consequence, a reduced hydrolysis of the ester. Chloramphenicol palmitate is thus best avoided in cats.

Distribution

Since chloramphenicol is a non-ionized, highly lipid-soluble molecule, it easily crosses membrane barriers to attain effective concentrations in most body tissues and fluids. In domesticated animals, chloramphenicol is 30–46 per cent bound to plasma proteins. A high proportion is therefore in the free state and can readily distribute into extracellular fluids. The apparent volume of distribution is large but there is no evidence for selective tissue binding or sequestration.

Unlike most other antibiotics, chloramphenicol readily crosses the blood–brain barrier, even in the absence of inflammation, with CSF concentrations reaching some 40–65 per cent of the plasma concentration. Concentration in brain tissue also occurs, making this drug particularly useful in the treatment of bacterial meningitis and brain abscess.

The drug also readily crosses into the eye. Therapeutic concentrations are attained in the aqueous humour after local installation of an ophthalmic solution (0.5 per cent) of chloramphenicol. Concentrations can be increased by the use of subconjunctival injections. The placenta is also crossed and toxic effects in the foetus are possible.

Metabolism and excretion

Chloramphenicol is metabolized mainly by glucuronylation in the liver, although some deacetylation and dehalogenation may also occur. These inactive metabolites are excreted in the urine. There is considerable species variation in the half-life of chloramphenicol. Among domesticated animals, it is longest in the cat (6 h) and shortest in the horse (1 h).

Cats are deficient in chloramphenicol-metabolizing enzymes and about 25 per cent of a dose is excreted unchanged in the urine, compared with only about 6 per cent in the dog. Young animals of all species are similarly ill-equipped with metabolizing enzymes and so in these, and in adults with liver disease, there is a danger that repeated dosing may lead to cumulation and toxicity. The extent of glucuronylation increases rapidly during the neonatal period. A small proportion of a chloramphenicol dose is excreted in the bile of cats and dogs.

In ruminants, chloramphenicol is rapidly metabolized by the rumen microflora and little absorption occurs. This is true for calves from about 9 weeks old, and even before that age, the drug is not efficiently absorbed from the forestomach. Chloramphenicol must therefore be administered parenterally to ruminants if a systemic effect is required. In calves, therapeutic plasma concentrations (>5 μg/ml) occur within about 30 minutes of an appropriate intramuscular dosage.

Toxicity

In humans, chloramphenicol can cause two different and potentially lethal toxic effects, but neither of these appears to have been reported in domesticated animals. The first, the so-called 'grey syndrome' in infants is characterized by circulatory collapse with flaccidity, ashen colour and hypothermia. Inefficient metabolizing and excretory mechanisms in the neonate result in abnormally high plasma concentrations of free drug after modest doses of chloramphenicol. The second potentially lethal effect is a non-dose-dependent and irreversible depression of the bone marrow which may be delayed in onset and follow even the smallest dose.

Chloramphenicol also causes a reversible, dose-dependent bone marrow depression in humans and similar effects have been described in the cat. Cats given chloramphenicol (60 mg/kg/day) for 21 days became depressed and dehydrated and there was reversible bone marrow hypoplasia and a decrease in the numbers of circulating neutrophils, lymphocytes, reticulocytes and platelets. Dogs are less likely to develop these effects, which appear to depend on both the dose and the duration of treatment. The drug has caused deaths in young calves from kidney damage.

Drug interactions

The binding of chloramphenicol to its ribosomal binding site *in vitro* may be less efficient in the presence of other antibiotics with a similar mode of action, such as erythromycin. It is believed that the binding sites are not identical but may overlap. The clinical significance of this effect has not been determined.

The undesirability of the concomitant administration of bacteriostatic and bactericidal antibiotics applies to chloramphenicol. Because chloramphenicol inhibits microsomal enzyme activity, other drugs (e.g. pentobarbitone) may be metabolized more slowly and their effects may be potentiated.

Therapeutic uses

Eye
Because of its broad spectrum of activity and its ease of penetration to the inner structures of the eye, chloramphenicol is widely used. It is particularly effective in New Forest disease. Chloramphenicol is often used in combination with hydrocortisone where inflammation is also present.

Central nervous system
Bacterial infections causing meningitis or encephalitis are conditions for which chloramphenicol is often the antibiotic of first choice. This is because such infections are likely to be mixed and selection of a broad-spectrum antibiotic which can easily cross the blood–brain barrier is warrantable even before the pathogen(s) have been identified. Phagocytic activity in the CSF is poor and a drug with bactericidal activity is preferred; chloramphenicol can have bactericidal effects against meningeal pathogens.

Respiratory system
Although the routine use of chloramphenicol in the treatment of respiratory infections was formerly advocated in the data sheets, the drug should only be used in cases where it is clearly indicated. In calves, the use of tetracyclines, the aminopenicillins or tylosin is preferable. If chloramphenicol is used, it should be to treat individual animals rather than on a herd basis, and only sufficient should be left on the farm to treat the animals immediately

concerned. Chloramphenicol is now rarely used in equine medicine in the UK, but is sometimes selected for the treatment of infections of the lower respiratory tract, particularly pneumonia in foals. A notable disadvantage is that the drug has an extremely short half-life in the horse and should be administered every 4–6 hours to maintain therapeutic concentrations. In dogs, cats and pigs, there are alternative broad-spectrum antibacterials (e.g. tetracyclines, amoxycillin, sulphonamide-trimethoprim combinations) which attain therapeutic concentrations in the respiratory tract. Again, infections are likely to be mixed and the use of a broad-spectrum antibiotic is justified, but when the organism(s), particularly mycoplasma, are sensitive to tylosin, this drug should be used because it concentrates in the respiratory tract.

Salmonellosis

Antibiotics are indicated as part of the chemotherapy of suspected systemic salmonellosis. Although the bacteraemia is usually controlled, chronic shedding of pathogens may not be prevented and the carrier state may be encouraged. The injudicious use of antibiotics is therefore to be discouraged except in animals with marked systemic signs, which are usually bacteraemic. Surveys of antibiotic resistance patterns of salmonella serotypes demonstrate that a large percentage are resistant to sulphonamides and streptomycin. Despite the widespread use of antibiotics, most strains remain sensitive to tetracyclines, neomycin, ampicillin, furazolidone, trimethoprim/sulphonamide and chloramphenicol. It is generally accepted that there is no justification in using chloramphenicol as a first choice antibiotic and it should be reserved for cases where there is no equally effective treatment. Dehydration and electrolyte loss are major factors in the pathogenesis of the diarrhoea associated with salmonellosis and fluid replacement is an important component of treatment (see Chapter 14).

Dose

Except in cats, a priming dose of double the values listed below is given initially.

Oral administration
dog	50 mg/kg every 12 hours
cat	25 mg/kg every 12 hours

Parenteral administration (preferably as the sodium succinate)
dog	50 mg/kg s.c., i.m. or slow i.v. every 12 hours
cat	25 mg/kg s.c., i.m. or slow i.v. every 12 hours
horse	30–50 mg/kg every 8–12 hours
ruminant	10–25 mg/kg i.m. every 12 hours
pig	11.25 mg/kg i.m. daily

Status

The Swann Committee (1969) gave special attention to the use of chloramphenicol in veterinary medicine, particularly in food animals. There was concern that the widespread use of the drug might increase the incidence of resistant strains of bacteria (especially *Salmonella typhosus*) in humans. The revocation of the licences for all chloramphenicol preparations intended for oral administration to animals in the UK was considered by the Veterinary Products Committee in 1983. This was based on the possibility that chloramphenicol resistance, acquired by enteric commensals and pathogens in animals, might be passed on to humans and then be transferred to human enteric commensals and pathogens. This proposal has been criticized and was eventually rejected. It is recommended, however, that chloramphenicol should be reserved for ophthalmic and systemic use in situations where clinical and laboratory assessments indicate that no other chemotherapeutic agent would be equally effective.

Lincosamides

Two antibiotics comprise this group: lincomycin, which was isolated from *Streptomyces lincolnensis*, and the semi-synthetic, clindamycin, in which the hydroxyl group in the 7-position is replaced by chlorine. This confers increased activity both *in vitro* and *in vivo*.

Inhibition of protein synthesis by these antibiotics may occur by an effect on chain initiation but it is more likely that peptide bond formation is inhibited. The binding site on the 50S ribosomal subunit is near to, and probably overlaps, those occupied by erythromycin and chloramphenicol. Antagonism between erythromycin and lincomycin has been reported and this may reflect displacement of lincomycin by erythromycin, which binds more avidly to the ribosome.

The antibacterial spectra of lincomycin and clindamycin include Gram-positive cocci, anaerobes (with the exception of some *Clostridium* species) and *Mycoplasma* spp. but not Gram-negative aerobic bacteria.

Resistance to the lincosamides can be induced and resistant bacterial ribosomes fail to bind the drug. There is usually complete cross-resistance between lincomycin and clindamycin and this may extend to the macrolides. The emergence of resistance to the lincosamides is more likely in animals which have received tylosin or virginiamycin as growth promoters. Occasionally, resistance to the lincosamides has been reported during treatment.

Lincomycin and clindamycin, being weak bases with high lipid solubility, are well absorbed after oral (in non-herbivores) or parenteral administration. Lincomycin hydrochloride and clindamycin as the hydrochloride or the palmitate (which is hydrolysed in the gut to the parent compound) are used for oral administration.

Absorption of both drugs is reduced in the presence of food. Lincomycin hydrochloride and phosphate are used parenterally and clindamycin is injected as the phosphate.

These antibiotics are both extensively concentrated in the tissues (e.g. in mammary tissue, where the pH is lower than that of the plasma, and clindamycin in bone). They are extensively protein-bound (60–95 per cent) and there is poor penetration into the CSF. The placenta is crossed readily, however.

About 10 per cent of a dose of either lincomycin or clindamycin can be recovered from the urine of monogastric animals and there is extensive elimination in the bile. Thus, the intestinal microflora is always exposed to high concentrations of lincosamides. Some metabolism to *N*-demethyl and/or sulphoxide derivatives occurs with clindamycin in humans; both of these metabolites have biological activity and have been recovered from urine and bile.

Toxicity

Lincomycin and clindamycin are relatively safe in dogs and cats. Clindamycin may cause local irritation at the injection site and thrombophlebitis has been reported after intravenous injection of the drug. Clindamycin, like the aminoglycosides, can induce neuromuscular blockade, and this is especially likely to occur if other neuromuscular blocking drugs or anaesthetics are used concomitantly.

Serious diarrhoea with haemorrhagic colitis can occur in horses after low doses of lincomycin and clindamycin. Clindamycin is very toxic in guinea pigs, hamsters and rabbits, usually because of the overgrowth of *Clostridium difficile* or *Cl. spiroforme* in the lower bowel. A similar effect occurs in humans and deaths have been reported. Treatment is with metronidazole and vancomycin plus anion exchange resins to bind the bacterial toxins.

Mistaken feeding of lincomycin-containing feeds to cattle has been incriminated in causing milk drop and diarrhoea.

Interactions

Increased activity has been reported for combinations of lincomycin and clindamycin with a variety of other antibiotics including the aminoglycosides, spectinomycin, metronidazole and trimethoprim-sulphonamide combinations. Lincomycin is sometimes given in combination with spectinomycin for the treatment and prevention of mycoplasmal and coliform infections of growing poultry.

Therapeutic uses

In the UK, lincomycin is only licensed for use in dogs, cats, pigs and poultry. Lincosamides are useful in dogs and cats for the treatment of chronic staphylococcal infections and acute anaerobic infections. Because lincomycin and clindamycin accumulate in bone, they have been used in infectious arthritis and osteomyelitis in dogs and cats. Superficial skin infections may also respond to these drugs. Lincosamides should not be used in horses or other herbivores.

In pigs, lincomycin is used (in feed or water) to prevent and treat (whole herd) dysentery and *Mycoplasma* infection. Pigs should not be slaughtered for humans consumption within 24 hours of the last treatment. A water-soluble powder is available for treatment of chronic respiratory disease and coliform infections of growing poultry.

Dose

lincomycin
dog, cat	25 mg/kg every 12 hours or 15 mg/kg every 8 hours orally
	22 mg/kg s.c. or i.m. daily
pig	feed-mix 110–220 g/tonne feed; 4.5–11 mg/kg i.m. daily

clindamycin
dog	5–10 mg/kg, p.o. b.i.d.
	10 mg/kg i.m. b.i.d.

The macrolides

The macrolide group of antibiotics comprises erythromycin, oleandomycin, carbomycin, spiramycin, tylosin and tiamulin, characterized by having macrocyclic lactone ring structures to which sugars are attached. They can be considered as a group because of their similar pharmacokinetic properties and the fact that they inhibit bacterial protein synthesis by binding to the 50S subunit of the bacterial ribosome.

Erythromycin

Erythromycin (Fig. 18.5) is a weak base which binds reversibly to the 50S subunit of the bacterial ribosome at a site which is near to but not identical with the chloramphenicol binding site. In the presence of erythromycin, ribosomal protein synthesis is inhibited, probably at the translocation step. Erythromycin does not bind to mammalian 80S ribosomes but is capable of inhibiting protein synthesis in mammalian mitochondria. In practice, however, the drug probably does not penetrate the mammalian mitochondrial membrane and chloramphenicol-like toxic effects do not occur.

Spectrum of activity

Erythromycin has a spectrum of antimicrobial activity which is similar to that of benzylpenicillin, lincomycin and novobiocin. It is thus more active against Gram-positive organisms (e.g. Staphylococci and Streptococci) and, although humansy Gram-negative bacteria (e.g. Enterobacteriaceae) are intrinsically resistant to erythromycin, others (e.g. *Haemophilus* and *Pasteurella* species) are sensitive. Erythromycin is active against some anaerobic bacteria and some *Chlamydia* and *Mycoplasma* species. It is not actively transported into sensitive bacteria but appears to enter by a passive process and then to be trapped by ribosomal binding. Probably because of greater penetration of un-ionized drug, the sensitivity of Gram-negative bacteria to erythromycin is increased at alkaline pH.

Erythromycin is usually bacteriostatic but can have bactericidal effects in some circumstances.

Resistance

Resistance to erythromycin can develop rapidly as a result of an alteration to the target site and subsequent failure of the bacterial ribosomes to bind the drug. Cross-resistance to other macrolides and lincomycin/clindamycin is common.

Absorption

Erythromycin is formulated for oral administration as the base, the stearate, the ethyl succinate and the lauryl sulphate salt of the propionyl ester (estolate). Parenteral formulations are of the lactobionate and glucoheptate salts. Significant differences exist among the oral formulations as regards absorption and bioavailability. Erythromycin base tends to be inactivated by gastric acid but this can be minimized, either by enteric coating of the tablets or by using erythromycin stearate. Erythromycin stearate escapes destruction in the stomach and is then hydrolysed in the intestine to yield the base. Erythromycin estolate is absorbed from the intestine as the propionyl ester and, although the total erythromycin levels are consistently higher than those attained after the stearate or the free base, there is some doubt as to whether the propionyl ester is biologically active, and thus whether the bioavailability of the active drug is increased. Intravenous administration of erythromycin lactobionate or glucoheptate results in higher blood levels than those attainable after oral dosing. Intramuscular injection of erythromycin is painful and can cause tissue irritation.

Distribution

Erythromycin base is about 65 per cent bound to plasma protein and distributes into most body fluid compartments, but does not cross the blood–brain barrier, even in the presence of inflammation. Low concentrations of erythromycin are attained in the foetus.

Metabolism and excretion
N-demethylation in the liver occurs to some extent, but a large proportion of an erythromycin dose is excreted in the bile and only about 5–10 per cent is excreted in the urine.

Toxic effects
Untoward effects which occur are largely referable to alterations in the intestinal flora following biliary excretion. This effect is particularly serious in horses and the drug may cause fatal diarrhoea; macrolides and lincomycin are not licensed for use in this species in the UK. Erythromycin estolate has been implicated as a cause of cholestatic hepatitis in humans and although the precise pathogenesis of this effect has yet to be established, erythromycin propionate (but not erythromycin base) has been shown to rapidly reduce bile flow in the isolated rat liver.

Therapeutic uses
Penicillin-hypersensitive patients can be treated with erythromycin, although penicillin hypersensitivity is much less common among animals than in humans. It is generally regarded as a drug of second choice in veterinary medicine, but *Campylobacter* infections (e.g. *Campylobacter jejuni* enteritis in dogs and cats) are usually treated with erythromycin.

Erythromycin has been used with success to treat respiratory disease in cattle and sheep caused by *Mycoplasma* and *Pasteurella* species and, often in combination with an aminopenicillin, for *Rhodococcus equi*. The drug is well distributed into the udder and can be used parenterally in staphylococcal mastitis as an adjunct to intramammary therapy. Intramammary use may cause local irritation but the drug is used in both lactating and dry-cow therapy. Milk for humans consumption should not be taken during therapy and three milkings should elapse after the last treatment. Cattle may be slaughtered for humans consumption only after 7 days from the last treatment.

A soluble form of erythromycin (Erythrocin Soluble and Erythrocin Proportioner) is available for water medication of poultry with mycoplasmal infection.

Tylosin

Tylosin (from *Streptomyces fradiae*) is a bacteriostatic antibiotic with a similar structure and spectrum of activity to erythromycin. It is mainly effective against *Mycoplasma*, where it is regarded as being more active than erythromycin. Tylosin is thus often the first choice when *Mycoplasma* species are the major pathogens in respiratory disease. It is used in the treatment of mycoplasmosis in poultry, in particular chronic respiratory disease in chickens and infectious sinusitis in turkeys, respiratory infections in small animals and calves, *Fusiformis necrophorus* infection in cattle and swine dysentery. Tylosin should not be used in horses. Sometimes tylosin is used in combination with sulphonamides (e.g. sulphadiazine, sulphadimidine and sulphathiazole) in the treatment of upper respiratory tract infections in the dog and in various food premix formulations for the control of dysentery in pigs. Tylosin can be given by intramammary injection but is generally not as effective as erythromycin.

Tylosin is a highly lipid-soluble base and is thus well absorbed and distributed, particularly into lung tissue. Local irritation has been reported following parenteral administration of the drug. Bacterial resistance to tylosin has been reported and appears to have about the same incidence as that to erythromycin.

Dose

cattle	4–10 mg/kg i.m. daily
pig	2–10 mg/kg i.m. daily
dog and cat	2–10 mg/kg i.m. daily; 20–45 mg/kg p.o. daily
poultry	50g/100 l drinking water

Chickens must not be slaughtered for human consumption for 24 hours after the last treatment. Eggs should not be used for human consumption. The withdrawal period for turkeys is 5 days.

Tiamulin

Tiamulin is a semi-synthetic antibiotic with a wider spectrum of activity, particularly against Gram-negative organisms and anaerobes, than tylosin. It is used in pigs for treatment of dysentery, enzootic pneumonia and mycoplasmal arthritis. The drug can be given as an oily intramuscular injection or added to the food or water. Accidental injection of oily tiamulin injections can cause serious local reactions and the veterinarian is urged to seek immediate medical treatment.

Dose

pig	10–15 mg tiamulin hydrogen fumarate/kg i.m.

Pigs must not be slaughtered for human consumption within 5 days of the last treatment.

Spiramycin

Spiramycin has a spectrum of antibacterial activity which is similar to that of the other macrolides, but activity is of a lower order. This is more than offset by its ability to concentrate and persist in tissue. In some clinical situations (e.g. chronic respiratory tract infections) this may be an advantage, but when the drug is used to treat bovine mastitis, residues (mostly biologically inactive) are present for prolonged periods after the cessation of treatment. In dry-cow therapy, spiramycin-neomycin combinations have been used effectively. Spiramycin has been added to the drinking water to control *Mycoplasma* infections in poultry.

Dose

calf, pig   20 mg/kg deep i.m. daily for 2–3 days
Withdrawal period for slaughter is 21 days.

Tetracyclines

The tetracyclines are a closely related group of antibiotics (Fig. 18.5). The first to be isolated from a *Streptomyces* species was chlortetracycline, followed by oxytetracycline and tetracycline. The newer members of the group (methacycline, minocycline and doxycycline), are semi-synthetic. These antibiotics have similar spectra of activity, which include both Gram-positive and Gram-negative bacteria and extend to *Mycoplasma, Chlamydia*, rickettsiae and some protozoa (e.g. *Plasmodium* species and some tick-borne species). Minocycline and doxycycline have somewhat broader spectra of activity than the other tetracyclines and are more active against Gram-positive bacteria. This may be associated with their increased lipophilicity.

Mechanism of action

The tetracyclines are bacteriostatic at clinically achievable concentrations. They are actively transported into susceptible bacterial cells and inhibit protein synthesis after becoming strongly bound to both the 30S ribosomal subunit and to mRNA. The net result is an inhibition of peptide chain elongation. Tetracyclines are not actively transported into mammalian cells, apart from those of the gut, liver and kidney, and this appears to be the basis of their selectivity. In mammalian cell-free systems, the tetracyclines are capable of inhibiting protein synthesis.

Most bacteria are slow to acquire resistance to the tetracyclines. Bacterial resistance to the tetracyclines is usually associated with a decreased uptake of the drugs. An increased elimination pathway has also been described in tetracycline-resistant bacteria and the net result is a decreased accumulation of the drug. Bacteria which have become resistant to one tetracycline usually exhibit cross-resistance to the whole group.

Pharmacokinetics

Absorption

In dogs and cats, the tetracyclines are absorbed adequately, but not completely, from the gastrointestinal tract. This is especially true for chlortetracycline, oxytetracycline and tetracycline (about 30 per cent of a dose); minocycline and doxycycline are absorbed more completely (up to 90 per cent). Absorption from the stomach is probably a passive process but an active transport mechanism is believed to be involved in the intestine. Tetracyclines are able to form stable chelates with a number of cations (e.g. magnesium, iron, calcium, aluminium) and this greatly reduces absorption. The presence of food in the stomach delays and reduces the absorption of all tetracyclines, except doxycycline and minocycline. Adult ruminants absorb oral tetracyclines poorly and the drugs should not be given by this route. Moreover, the broad antibacterial spectra of these drugs makes it likely that ruminal fermentation will be disturbed.

Distribution

The tetracyclines are bound to plasma protein to an extent which varies from about 30 per cent (oxytetracycline) to over 90 per cent (doxycycline). They penetrate into most tissues, with the highest concentrations being attained in liver and kidney. The drugs gain access to pleural and synovial fluids but, apart from doxycycline, do not cross the blood–brain barrier, even when the meninges are inflamed. Tetracyclines cross the placenta and are excreted in the milk. Minocycline and doxycycline, being more lipid soluble, penetrate cell barriers more readily and gain better access to abscesses, for example.

The volumes of distribution of the tetracyclines are greater than the total body water, indicating sequestration. They become perhumansently bound to growing bone and teeth but the association of tetracyclines with other tissues (e.g. reticuloendothelial cells) is reversible.

Excretion

It is inferred, indirectly from recovery experiments and from changes in half-life when other drugs are given concomitantly, that some tetracyclines undergo biotransformation, but the mechanism(s) are poorly understood. The drugs in this group, except doxycycline and minocycline, are excreted unchanged in the urine after glomerular filtration. All tetracyclines are actively transported into the bile, however, and are then reabsorbed to a varying extent. Oxytetracycline, methacycline and tetracycline are mainly excreted in the urine; chlortetracycline undergoes both renal and biliary elimination and doxycycline is largely eliminated in the faeces. Doxycycline can thus be used in renal failure.

Toxicity

Although tetracyclines are regarded as being relatively safe drugs, except in horses and young animals, a number of toxic effects have been reported. These are mainly referable to the ability of the drugs to suppress the gut microflora and to chelate metal ions.

The tetracyclines are irritant and small animals frequently appear to experience nausea, and may vomit, after oral tetracycline administration. These effects cannot be ameliorated by calcium- or aluminium-based antacid preparations as chelation renders the antibiotic ineffective. Superinfection with fungi and resistant bacteria (e.g. salmonellae) can then occur. The diarrhoea which sometimes occurs after tetracycline administration can cause malabsorption in calves. Fatal enteritis has been reported in horses, possibly the result of superinfection. There is a definite association between the use of high doses of tetracyclines and serious diarrhoea in horses but this effect has also been reported after therapeutic doses given to animals stressed by anaesthesia (with or without surgery) and travel. Typically, on about the third day of treatment, the horse becomes depressed, with anorexia, diarrhoea, infected conjunctiva, haemoconcentration and jaundice. The syndrome resembles 'colitis X' and appears to be similar to the unusual sensitivity of guinea pigs to antibiotics, where death may result from caecal bloat caused by alterations of the gut microflora.

Parenteral tetracyclines can cause severe irritation at the injection site, which may become necrotic. Pain and irritation can be minimized by appropriate buffering of the preparation and/or the incorporation of a local anaesthetic, an antihistamine or a non-steroidal anti-inflammatory drug.

Tetracyclines are deposited in growing teeth and bones as a bright-yellow fluorescent complex. Administration of tetracyclines to puppies causes discolouration and defective enamel formation of the primary, and sometimes of the permanent, teeth. These effects have also been reported in puppies when tetracyclines were given to the pregnant bitch. The use of tetracyclines during the period of tooth development, including late pregnancy, is discouraged in all species. In newborn puppies, tetracyclines cause a reversible inhibition of the rate of growth of the long bones. Miscellaneous effects attributable to calcium chelation by tetracyclines include prolongation of blood coagulation and acute collapse in cattle after bolus intravenous doses of the drugs.

The tetracyclines should be regarded as being potentially nephrotoxic and hepatotoxic although these effects seldom occur after therapeutic doses. Severe renal damage with proteinuria, glycosuria and occasionally haemoglobinuria has usually been attributed to prolonged storage of tetracyclines under conditions of high temperature and humidity where decomposition to epian-hydro derivatives has occurred. Fatty infiltration of the liver has occurred after the administration of tetracyclines to pregnant humans and has also been described in cattle. Allergic responses to the tetracyclines are occasionally seen in dogs and can be treated with antihistamines.

Clinical uses

Because of their broad spectrum of activity and the difficulties in general practice of accurate bacterial diagnosis, the tetracyclines have been used indiscriminately. They are widely used in the prophylaxis and treatment of bacterial, rickettsial and protozoal diseases in most animals, except horses. The broad-spectrum efficacy of these drugs has been reduced somewhat by the development of resistance, and it is now considered better to treat individual animals than to administer tetracyclines as feed supplements. Some distinction is made among the tetracyclines, usually on the basis of the extent of their absorption and their patterns of distribution and excretion in urine, bile and faeces. For example, oxytetracycline gives higher concentrations in the urine and faeces than chlortetracycline and is preferred for urinary tract infections.

A number of compound preparations containing mixtures of tetracyclines with sulphonamides, penicillins and chloramphenicol are available.

Tetracycline feed supplements are given to ruminating calves for 7–14 days to control pneumonia due to sensitive *Pasteurella haemolytica* strains. They are also given in the food or water of feedlot cattle as a prophylaxis against pneumonias caused by *Pasteurella* and *Mycoplasma* species. Growing pigs are also given tetracycline food supplements to prevent chronic rhinitis caused by *Haemophilus parasuis*.

Intramammary solutions of tetracyclines are used to treat mastitis in lactating cows due to a wide range of organisms, including *E. coli*, streptococci and staphylococci. Milk from treated animals should not be used for 72 hours after the last treatment. The preparations may be irritant, however, and should not be used in the dry cow.

Local application of oxytetracycline pessaries into the uterus has been used successfully in bovine endometriosis. Tetracyclines are used in aerosol form with a dye marker (e.g. gentian violet) specifically for the treatment of foot rot and scald in sheep but also as a topical antibiotic for the prevention and treatment of minor superficial infections. Infectious keratoconjunctivitis (New Forest disease) of cattle and sheep usually responds to a single injection of oxytetracycline beneath the palpebral conjunctiva.

Oxytetracycline is given parenterally to control enzootic abortion in sheep and tick-borne fever in lambs. Parenteral oxytetracycline is used in the treatment of pneumonia caused by *Pasteurella* species in pigs. It is not the first line of treatment for erysipelas.

Urinary tract infections caused by *Pseudomonas aeruginosa* and rickettsial infections in dogs and cats generally respond well to the tetracyclines. Tetracyclines are also used locally in the treatment of otitis externa in the dog and humansy pyogenic skin infections. Prevention of secondary bacterial invasion after viral diseases in small animals can be achieved with tetracyclines.

The tetracyclines are extensively used in the prevention and treatment of a wide range of enteric and respiratory infections of poultry, especially those raised by intensive methods. Dosage is usually in food and water but individual treatment (as a top dressing for immediate consumption by a bird) is sometimes used. The withholding period for poultry is 7 days after the last treatment and eggs from treated birds may not be taken for humans consumption during tetracycline treatment or for one day afterwards.

Dose

oxytetracycline

cattle, sheep	5–10 mg/kg s.c., i.m. or i.v. daily
pig	10–20 mg/kg p.o. b.i.d.
dog and cat	20 mg/kg p.o. b.i.d.; 5–10 mg/kg s.c., i.m. or i.v. daily

chlortetracycline

pig, sheep, cattle	10–20 mg/kg p.o. daily

Animals should not be slaughtered for human consumption until 5–14 days from the last treatment, the period depending on the species and whether a sustained release preparation was used.

dog and cat	20–50 mg/kg p.o. daily

tetracycline

dog and cat	50 mg/kg p.o. daily

Spectinomycin

Spectinomycin is an aminocyclitol antibiotic which was isolated from *Streptomyces spectabilis*. Spectinomycin reversibly inhibits protein synthesis by combining with the 30S ribosomal subunit and interfering with the translocation step of the pathway. It is available as the dihydrochloride. The drug is normally bacteriostatic at clinically achievable concentrations. A bactericidal effect can occur at higher concentrations. Spectinomycin is active against a large number of Gram-negative bacteria but because resistance is so rapidly acquired after exposure to the drug, its use in human medicine is reserved for the treatment of gonorrhoea (a single high dose is used). Resistance is usually acquired by the R-factor transfer of adenylating enzymes. *Mycoplasma* spp. are usually sensitive to the drug but the incidence of resistant *Pasteurella* strains in cattle is increasing.

Pharmacokinetics

Spectinomycin is not absorbed from the gastrointestinal tract and is given by intramuscular injection. Peak plasma concentrations are attained within about 1 hour. There is almost no binding to plasma proteins and the half-life is 2–3 hours. About 80 per cent of a dose is excreted unchanged in the urine. It is often used in combination with lincomycin, where an enhanced effect is claimed.

Toxicity

Few toxic effects have been reported for spectinomycin although, like the aminoglycosides, it is capable of causing neuromuscular blockade. Spectinomycin should be given intravenously, rather than intramuscularly, to the horse because these animals have displayed undue sensitivity to the drug when it is given by the intramuscular route.

Clinical uses

Spectinomycin has been used to treat a variety of bacterial pneumonias and enteric infections, especially those caused by *Salmonella*, coliforms and *Mycoplasma* species in cattle, pigs and sheep. Poultry can be given the drug in the drinking water, intranasally or by subcutaneous injection. Oral spectinomycin is also used for the treatment and control of enteritis in piglets caused by *E. coli*. The drug appears to be particularly effective in the treatment of acute coliform mastitis.

Dose

horse	10–20 mg/kg i.v. daily
calf, lamb	7.5–12.5 mg/kg p.o. b.i.d.
sheep, cattle	10–30 mg/kg i.m. or i.v. daily
pig	10–20 mg/kg i.m. or i.v. daily

piglet	50–100 mg p.o. b.i.d.
dog and cat	100–300 mg i.m. or i.v. daily
poultry	10–20 mg/kg s.c. or i.m. daily

Milk from spectinomycin-treated cows should not be used for human consumption for 48 hours after the last treatment and animals and birds should not be slaughtered for human consumption within 5 days of treatment.

Antimetabolites

The antimetabolite group of antibacterial chemotherapeutic drugs comprises the sulphonamides, the diaminopyrimidines, the sulphones and *p*-aminosalicylic acid. Only the sulphonamides and the diaminopyrimidines are important in veterinary medicine. Before the discovery of the sulphonamides in the 1930s, the management of acute bacterial infections relied on the use of vaccines, antisera and symptomatic treatment and was often ineffective.

Because dyes bind strongly to the protein of wool and silk, it was suggested that they might be able to bind to bacterial protein and so selectively kill the organisms. In 1912, Churchman showed that gentian violet was able to act in this way and acriflavine was used topically to prevent and treat wound sepsis in World War I. In 1927, Domagk commenced a screening programme which involved the administration of dyes to mice which had been inoculated with a highly virulent strain of *Streptococcus pyogenes*. It was already known that sulphonamido substitution in a variety of azo dyes increased the avidity of their binding to wool. A red azo dye of this type, Prontosil (Fig. 18.6), which although inactive *in vitro*, protected mice against an otherwise lethal infection was synthesized in 1932 by Klarer and Meitzsch. The first recorded use of Protosil in man was in 1933, when Foerster successfully treated a 10-month-old boy suffering from staphylococcal septicaemia. The data from animal studies were not published by Domagk until 1935 and, in 1939, he was awarded the Nobel prize for his discovery. In 1936, a clinical trial of Prontosil was carried out in 38 women suffering from puerperal sepsis, which is caused by haemolytic streptococci. Although at that time this condition was invariably fatal, only three of the Prontosil-treated patients died. This was the real beginning of antibacterial chemotherapy.

It was demonstrated in 1935 that the azo bond of Prontosil was hydrolysed *in vivo* to give 4-amino benzene sulphonamide, or sulphanilamide, which was the active part of the molecule. Since that time, over 150 sulphonamides

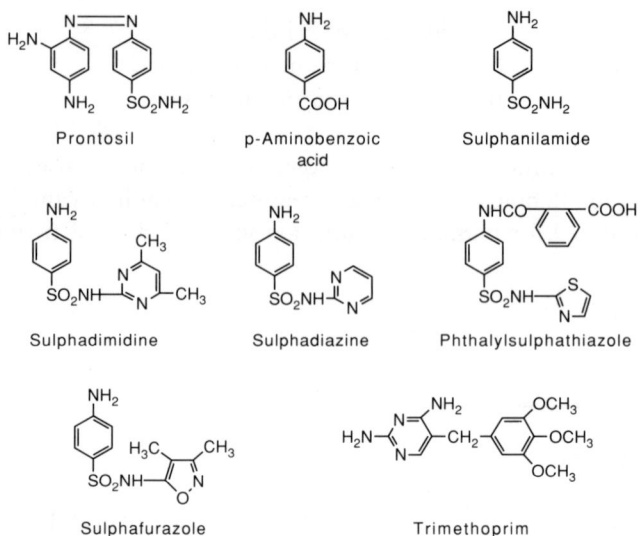

Figure 18.6 Structures of *p*-aminobenzoic acid, some of the sulphonamides and trimethoprim.

have been marketed. Their popularity has declined somewhat over the years, except for certain drugs which are useful in special situations, such as the treatment of urinary tract infections and application to the eye. More recently, it has been found that it is possible to use sulphonamides in combination with other inhibitors of the synthesis of folic acid, the diaminopyrimidines, to produce a sequential blockade of the metabolic pathway. This has greatly extended the usefulness of the sulphonamides.

Mode of action

Sulphanilamide closely resembles *p*-aminobenzoic acid (Fig. 18.6) and has similar bond distances. *p*-Aminobenzoic acid is essential for the synthesis of folic acid by some bacteria. Tetrahydrofolate, formed by the reduction of folic acid, acts as a coenzyme in reactions which result in the synthesis of DNA, RNA, etc. The mechanism of action of sulphonamides, as expressed in the Woods–Fildes hypothesis, envisages competition between sulphonamides and *p*-aminobenzoic acid for the enzyme dihydropteroate synthetase (Fig. 18.7). Blockade of folate synthesis causes profound effects on bacterial metabolism. It should be noted that the only bacteria which are sensitive to sulphonamides are those which must synthesize their own folate. Selective toxicity depends on the fact that mammals obtain *p*-aminobenzoic acid from the diet. Addition of *p*-aminobenzoic acid to a sulphonamide-treated bacterial

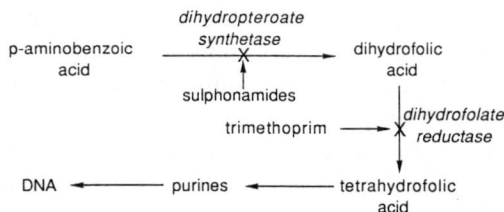

Figure 18.7 Sulphonamides and trimethoprim inhibit the enzymes which catalyse sequential steps in the synthesis of tetrahydrofolic acid.

culture will overcome growth inhibition competitively and addition of folate will act non-competitively to produce the same effect. This is of clinical importance in that pus and necrotic tissue contain p-aminobenzoic acid and amino acids which can antagonize the effects of sulphonamides; therefore wounds must be cleaned before sulphonamides are applied topically. The local anaesthetics, procaine and benzocaine, and procaine penicillin also contain a p-aminobenzoic acid moiety.

Sulphonamides have broad-spectrum activity against both Gram-positive and Gram-negative bacteria and some protozoa and chlamydia. They are regarded as being bacteriostatic under most conditions but they can attain bactericidal concentrations in urine. This usually means that they must be administered for long enough for the body defence mechanisms to be established.

Resistance

Strains of bacteria which are resistant to the sulphonamides are common in animal isolates and usually exhibit cross-resistance to the whole group. Resistance develops gradually and results from an acquired ability to exclude the drug, an altered or additional dihydropteroate synthetase or excessive production of p-aminobenzoic acid. Resistant cells are believed to occur in most susceptible bacterial populations and tend to emerge under suitable selection pressure. It is recommended that a course of sulphonamide therapy should not normally exceed about 7 days and, if there is no clinical improvement after 3 days, a different drug should be selected.

Classification

Figure 18.6 shows some of the sulphonamide family. The members all have the same nucleus and various substituents have been added to the sulphonamido group. The individual drugs differ so markedly in their pharmacokinetics, and thus their clinical uses, that familiarity is essential.

One way of classifying the sulphonamides is into general purpose (systemic) drugs and those which are used for more specific purposes. Examples of general purpose sulphonamides are sulphadimidine and sulphamerazine. Those used for special purposes include sulphacetamide sodium, which is used exclusively for ophthalmic infections; poorly absorbed sulphonamides (e.g. succinylsulphathiazole), which are used to treat intestinal infections; sulphafurazole, which is used to treat urinary tract infections; the long-acting sulphonamides (e.g. sulphamethoxypyridazine); and silver sulphadiazine, which has restricted topical usage.

Absorption

Most sulphonamides are absorbed adequately from the gastrointestinal tract and, except for the long-acting group, reach maximum concentrations in the plasma in 4–6 h. Other exceptions are the gut-active sulphonamides, which are poorly absorbed and exert their effects in the gut.

Solutions of the sodium salts of sulphonamides are highly alkaline and are best given intravenously. Sulphacetamide sodium solutions are an exception in that they have a pH close to neutrality and are essentially non-irritant and can safely be applied to the cornea in concentrations of up to 30 per cent. The topical application of sulphonamides (e.g. sulphanilamide and sulphathiazole) has been considered to cause sensitization and to delay wound healing.

Distribution

Once they are absorbed, the distribution of individual sulphonamides depends primarily on the extent of plasma protein binding, which can vary in a single species from 20 to over 90 per cent. Interspecies variation also occurs. Some sulphonamides (e.g. sulphadiazine) are distributed throughout the body water but others (e.g. sulphafurazole) are restricted to the extracellular water. Most sulphonamides cross readily into the CSF, pass the placental barrier and gain access to ocular, pleural and synovial fluids, inflammatory exudates and milk.

Metabolism and excretion

The metabolism of sulphonamides occurs in the liver and the major products are acetylated derivatives which are excreted mainly by glomerular filtration.

Toxic effects

Although significant toxic reactions are uncommon after normal therapeutic doses of sulphonamides given for less than 2 weeks, these drugs can produce a variety of unwanted effects. Some sulphonamides (e.g. sulphapyridine) are capable of causing methaemoglobinaemia, especially in the cat, and all may alter acid–base balance because of carbonic anhydrase inhibition.

The acetylated derivatives of sulphonamides are inactive and may also be insoluble and tend to crystallize out in the renal tubules causing mechanical damage and even obstruction. This was more of a problem with the earlier sulphonamides but could be minimized by maintaining a high fluid intake and particularly by alkalinizing the urine. Another stratagem was to use sulphonamide mixtures (e.g. sulphadiazine, sulphamerazine and sulphadimidine). Although these drugs behaved in solution as if they were there alone, and were thus less liable to crystallize, their antibacterial effects were additive. Even with the more modern drugs, animals given sulphonamides should always have free access to water and dosing should cease if there are signs of difficulty in urination, cloudiness of the urine or haematuria. Fluids should then be given orally or parenterally. Sulphonamides are contraindicated in dehydrated animals.

Signs of possible hypersensitivity to sulphonamides have been reported in dogs, and adverse effects on the haematopoietic system (thrombocytopenia, leucopenia, aplastic anaemia) and allergic nephritis have also occasionally been noted. Sulphaquinoxaline has caused hypothrombinaemia leading to fatal haemorrhage when given orally to puppies for the control of coccidiosis.

Continuous use of sulphonamides in mammals can cause depression, inappetence and diarrhoea. These effects are probably due to irritation of the gut and, in ruminants, to suppression of the ruminal microflora. Vitamin K production may also be disrupted. Recovery is usually rapid when the drug is discontinued.

In poultry, sulphonamides may cause a decrease in egg production and thinning of shells.

Clinical uses

General-purpose sulphonamides

Sulphanilamide
This is effective against streptococci and *E. coli* but with the availability of better systemic antibacterials, its use is almost entirely confined to local application as a wound dusting powder. It is more soluble than other sulphonamides, dissolving in serum to maintain a steady concentration.

Sulphathiazole
This has the greatest *in vitro* activity of all the sulphonamides, with an antibacterial spectrum similar to that of sulphadiazine. It has a particularly

insoluble acetyl derivative. The main use of sulphathiazole is as the active constituent of some of the 'gut-active' sulphonamides.

Sulphadimidine

Sulphadimidine has a wider spectrum of activity than sulphanilamide, including streptococci, staphylococci, *E. coli*, salmonellae, pasteurellae and some rickettsiae and protozoa. Its pharmacokinetic characteristics, which include virtually complete absorption, low protein binding, good distribution and slow excretion, make sulphadimidine an almost ideal systemic sulphonamide. It is commonly used both orally and parenterally for the treatment of foul-in-the-foot in cattle, enteric, respiratory and septicaemic disease in calves, calf diphtheria and coccidiosis in cattle and sheep. Intestinal and caecal coccidiosis in poultry and atrophic rhinitis in pigs (*Bordetella bronchiseptica* infection) can be controlled by incorporation of the drug into water and food. The withholding period for treated pigs is 7 days.

Parenteral administration of sulphadimidine sodium is by the intravenous or the subcutaneous route. Intravenous injection produces more predictable tissue concentrations in large animals but rapid injection should be avoided as bolus doses have caused ataxia and collapse in cattle. If the drug is injected subcutaneously, then it should be at several sites and each should be massaged to minimize tissue injury.

Dose

It is usual to give an initial loading dose followed by half that dose for daily maintenance. The recommended dose for cattle is 100–200 mg/kg as a loading dose and 50–150 mg/kg for maintenance. The withholding period for sulphadimidine-treated cattle is 8 days.

Sulphadiazine

This has similar effects to its close congener, sulphadimidine, but it is less well absorbed and its elimination half-life is shorter in many species. Sulphadiazine has been used as a growth promoter in pigs and, both alone and in combination with aminopenicillins and tetracyclines, to treat *Nocardia* infections in the dog.

Sulphaquinoxaline

Sulphaquinoxaline has been used for prevention and treatment of intestinal and caecal coccidiosis in poultry. It is given in drinking water, alone or in combination with diaveridine and vitamin K. It is recommended that birds laying eggs for human consumption should not be treated with this drug.

Sulfapyrazole
This is given intravenously for the treatment of sulphonamide-susceptible infections in both small and large animals.

Sulphonamides for ophthalmic use

Sulphacetamide sodium
Solutions of sulphacetamide sodium are instilled into the eye for the treatment of a wide range of ophthalmic infections. It is non-irritant at concentrations of up to 30 per cent and achieves adequate concentrations within the globe. Combination ophthalmic formulations of sulphacetamide with neomycin and/or a corticosteroid are also available.

Sulphonamides for gastrointestinal use

Succinylsulphathiazole, phthalylsulphathiazole and phthalylsulphacetamide
These drugs are completely ionized in the gut and are thus poorly absorbed. They are cleaved in the large intestine to yield the sulphonamide, which is poorly absorbed in this part of the gut. These sulphonamides are incorporated into numerous anti-diarrhoeal formulations (e.g. with kaolin and other anti-bacterials, such as sulphapyridine and neomycin) for oral administration.

Sulphaguanidine
This is often classified as gut-active. It undergoes 50 per cent absorption from the gut and is useful where sensitive pathogens occur in both the gut lumen and the mucosa.

Sulphasalazine
Another special case is sulphasalazine, which is hydrolysed to sulphapyridine and 5-aminosalicylic acid in the large intestine. This 'targeting' of 5-amino-salicylic acid, which has anti-inflammatory activity, is useful in the treatment of idiopathic colitis in the dog. Cats treated with sulphasalazine may develop salicylism.

Sulphonamides for urinary tract infections

Sulphafurazole
Sulphafurazole is rapidly absorbed after oral administration and excreted so rapidly that it is difficult to maintain an adequate plasma concentration. The

very high urine concentrations which are attained make the drug useful in the treatment of urinary tract infections. It is particularly active against coliforms, *Proteus* and *Pseudomonas* species. There is generally no need for a high fluid intake or urinary alkalinization.

Long-acting sulphonamides

The principal factors which determine the chemotherapeutic efficacy of a sulphonamide are: intrinsic activity, concentrations attainable in blood and tissues and elimination half-life. With the long-acting sulphonamides, the tissue concentrations tend to be considerably higher than those of plasma but take up to a week to reach their maximum level. Drugs in this group may not cross the blood–brain barrier. Although acetylation problems do not occur, clearance is slow and these drugs should not normally be used to treat urinary tract infections. If serious toxic effects do occur, elimination of the drug after withdrawal of treatment takes much longer than with conventional sulphonamides. This is reflected in the withholding times.

Sulphamethoxypyridazine
This is well absorbed from intramuscular and subcutaneous injection sites. Peak plasma concentrations are attained within 6–8 hours and since excretion is slow, the drug need only be given once a day. The preparations contain 250 mg/ml and the recommended dose is 200 mg/kg/day.

The drug is unlikely to induce crystalluria but the necessity for an adequate supply of drinking water is stressed by the manufacturer.

Specific indications for sulphamethoxypyridazine include coccidiosis in sheep, metritis and foul-in-the-foot in cattle and diphtheria in calves. Cows and sheep may not be slaughtered for human consumption for up to 21 days from the last dose of sulphamethoxypyridazine. The withholding time for cow's milk is 48 hours and the drug should not be used in sheep producing milk for human consumption.

Sulphadimethoxine
This drug is highly protein-bound and is only slowly eliminated, having an elimination half-life of 11–15 h in large animals. The drug is given parenterally.

Sulphamethoxydiazine
Sulphamethoxydiazine is rapidly and completely absorbed, is only moderately protein-bound and becomes widely distributed. It is slowly eliminated, the withholding time for meat is 15 days, and for milk 7 days. The drug can be given subcutaneously or intramuscularly to most species.

Dose

large animals	initial dose 30 mg/kg (maintenance 20 mg/kg).
calf, lamb, piglet	recommended initial dose 40 mg/kg followed by 20 mg/kg/day.
dog, cat	48 mg/kg followed by 20 mg/kg/day.

Sulphonamides for treatment of burns

Silver sulphadiazine
Silver sulphadiazine was developed for the treatment of severe burns in human patients. It will prevent colonization by *Pseudomonas* spp. of areas intended for skin grafting and will eradicate established infections. The mechanism of action of silver sulphadiazine is not understood. It may be that the principal activity is due to the dissociation of silver ions, which kill the bacteria. In animals, silver sulphadiazine preparations are used to treat otitis externa caused by *Pseudomonas aeruginosa* which does not respond to other treatment.

Diaminopyridines

The Woods–Fildes hypothesis, which explained the antibacterial activity of the sulphonamides in terms of competition with a natural substrate (*p*-aminobenzoic acid) for an essential metabolic pathway, stimulated the synthesis in the early 1940s of a series of potential antimetabolites of purines and pyrimidines. Of these, the 2,4-diaminopyrimidines proved to have antibacterial activity which was later shown to be due to their ability to inhibit dihydrofolate reductase. A series of 5-benzyl derivatives of the 2,4-diaminopyrimidines included the antimalarial, pyrimethamine, and later the more specific antibacterial, trimethoprim (Fig. 18.6).

Trimethoprim has a close structural similarity to the pteridine moiety of dihydrofolic acid and is a very potent competitive inhibitor of dihydrofolate reductase, which prevents the conversion of dihydrofolate to tetrahydrofolate. This, in turn, blocks the synthesis of purines and, ultimately of DNA, RNA and proteins. Thus, a combination of trimethoprim with a sulphonamide is able to cause a sequential blockade of folic acid synthesis (Fig. 18.7), which is an example of true synergism.

Selectivity arises from the fact that bacterial dihydrofolate reductase enzymes are 20 000–60 000 times more sensitive to trimethoprim than the corresponding mammalian enzymes. Other pyrimidines (e.g. pyrimethamine) have similar antimicrobial activity to trimethoprim, but the difference in the sensitivity of bacterial and mammalian dihydrofolate reductases to these drugs is not nearly as great as for trimethoprim. Although a pyrimethamine-sulphadiazine combination has been used successfully to treat toxoplasmosis in humans and a mixture of pyrimethamine and sulphaquinoxaline has been used for coccidiosis in puppies, their use in veterinary medicine is miniscule compared with that of trimethoprim-sulphonamide formulations. It should also be noted that pyrimethamine is teratogenic in the pig.

Spectrum of activity

Trimethoprim has bacteriostatic activity against a wide range of Gram-positive and Gram-negative aerobic bacteria but not usually against anaerobes. It has negligible activity against chlamydiae, mycobacteria, mycoplasmas and *Pseudomonas aeruginosa*.

Resistance

Microorganisms which lack the metabolic step that is inhibited by trimethoprim are intrinsically resistant to its effects. Acquired resistance to trimethoprim usually involves the elaboration by the organism of an altered dihydrofolate reductase enzyme which is not inhibited, possibly because of reduced affinity for the drug. An acquired ability to exclude the drug and increased production of dihydrofolate reductase have also been described in trimethoprim-resistant bacteria. The incidence of trimethoprim resistance is increasing, especially among the Enterobacteriaceae. Often, trimethoprim-resistant organisms are also resistant to the sulphonamides.

Absorption

Trimethoprim is a weak base with low water solubility. It is readily absorbed from the gastrointestinal tract. It should be noted, however, that trimethoprim is degraded in the rumen and is thus not effective if given by mouth to animals with a functional rumen.

Distribution

Therapeutic plasma concentrations are generally attained about 1 hour after oral administration and are maintained for 2–6 hours. Trimethoprim is about 65 per cent protein-bound but, being lipid-soluble, the drug readily penetrates cellular barriers to become widely distributed. There is no evidence of tissue binding. The highest concentrations of trimethoprim occur in the liver, kidneys, lungs and prostate. Trimethoprim readily crosses the blood–brain barrier and antibacterial concentrations are attained in the CSF. High concentrations of trimethoprim also occur in milk.

Metabolism and excretion

Trimethoprim is partly oxidized and conjugated in the liver, and the metabolites, together with unchanged trimethoprim, are excreted in the urine. There is considerable species variability in the extent of metabolism, which ranges from about 50 per cent of the dose in humans to 80 per cent in the dog and almost 100 per cent in the cow. The half-life of trimethoprim is also variable among the species—10 hours in humans, 4 hours in the horse, 2 hours in the pig and 1 hour in the cow.

Toxicity

Trimethoprim is a relatively non-toxic drug but, like pyrimethamine, it can cause folic acid deficiency if high doses are administered for long periods.

Clinical uses

Trimethoprim is seldom used alone in veterinary medicine. Because the drug concentrates in prostatic tissue it has been used alone to treat infection of the prostate, but even here there seems little reason to use trimethoprim rather than a trimethoprim-sulphonamide combination.

Trimethoprim-sulphonamide combinations

The combination of trimethoprim with a sulphonamide inhibits two sequential steps in the synthesis of folic acid and thus of the purines required for DNA and RNA synthesis. This truly synergistic action usually results in a bactericidal effect as opposed to the bacteriostatic effects seen when either trimethoprim or a sulphonamide is used alone. Synergism can be demonstrated *in vitro* and in animals with experimental infections. Synergism generally occurs when the microorganism is sensitive to both drugs and may still occur when the organism is resistant to one of them. A clinical effect is sometimes seen even when the organism is resistant to both drugs.

In humans, trimethoprim is usually given in a fixed (1 : 5) combination (co-trimoxazole) with a single sulphonamide, sulphamethoxazole. This predictably produces a 1 : 20 concentration ratio in plasma (but not necessarily in other tissues or in urine) and the clinical efficacy of co-trimoxazole has been satisfactorily demonstrated. The reason for the use of a single fixed combination is that the two drugs have similar half-lives (10–11 h) and can be given on a twice daily regimen.

Given the wide interspecies variability in the half-lives of both trimethoprim and sulphonamides, such an approach is clearly impossible in veterinary medicine. There is evidence however, that pharmacokinetic matching of the two compounds is not essential and that synergism occurs over a wide range of dose ratios. If a background bacteriostatic concentration of the sulphonamide can be maintained, then this effect will be increased for a variable time after each dose by the presence of trimethoprim.

The principal trimethoprim-sulphonamide formulations in current veterinary use are a 1 : 5 combination of trimethoprim with sulphadiazine (a 'general purpose' systemic sulphonamide), or with sulphadoxine, which has a much longer half-life than sulphadiazine. Combinations of trimethoprim with sulpha-troxazole, sulphadimidine, sulphafurazole and sulphaquinoxaline are also available.

Spectrum of activity

Trimethoprim-sulphonamide combinations have bactericidal activity against a wide range of Gram-positive and Gram-negative aerobic and anaerobic bacteria, including staphylococci and streptococci, *Actinomyces* species, *Bacillus anthracis*, *Bordetella* species, *Corynebacterium* species, *E. coli*, *Haemophilus* species, *Klebsiella* species, *Pasteurella* species, *Proteus* species and *Salmonella* species. Activity is also manifested against some chlamydiae and protozoa, such as *Toxoplasma*, *Pneumocystis carinii* and some malarial parasites. *Mycoplasma* species, *Erysipelothrix*, *Leptospira* and *Pseudomonas aeruginosa* are commonly resistant.

Resistance

The consideration of resistance to trimethoprim-sulphonamide combinations is complicated by the fact that two types of drug are involved. Resistance to sulphonamides was so widespread when trimethoprim was introduced that their clinical efficacy was seriously compromised. The incidence of resistance to trimethoprim-sulphonamide combinations was very low at first but is now increasing rapidly, especially among enteric bacteria which have become resistant to both trimethoprim and the sulphonamides.

Toxicity

Trimethoprim-sulphonamide combinations have a wide safety margin. Apart from the possible induction of folic acid deficiency (which has been reported in humans but not animals) and teratogenesis in the pig, any adverse effects of trimethoprim-sulphonamide combinations are likely to result from the sulphonamide component. However, the fact that thrombocytopenia has occasionally been seen in dogs points to a need for caution.

Transient oedema and pain at the injection site can be reduced in small animal formulations by the inclusion of a local anaesthetic. Intramuscular injection in the horse may cause pain and minor tissue damage.

Hypersalivation and vomiting may occur in cats after oral dosing. Sometimes, the animals also may appear to be depressed and disorientated and may become ataxic or convulse. These effects can be minimized by using coated tablets and advising that the tablets should not be broken or crushed. Vomiting and diarrhoea have also been reported in dogs with jaundice and biochemical evidence of hepatotoxicity. Transient polyarthritis, accompanied by joint pain and pyrexia, has been reported in some large breeds of dogs; it appears to be a hypersensitivity reaction.

Trimethoprim-sulphonamide mixtures should not be used in anaesthetized horses. Fatal cardiac arrhythmias have been reported in horses whose hearts have been sensitized with detomidine or halothane. Deaths, apparently due to respiratory failure, have occasionally been reported in horses after intravenous injection of the combination.

Clinical indications

The clinical advantages of trimethoprim-sulphonamide combinations are referable to broad-spectrum bactericidal activity and good distribution into all body compartments and tissues, including the eye and the CSF, where bactericidal concentrations are attained. The mixture is thus useful for the treatment of meningitis and meningoencephalitis caused by a number of organisms, including *E. coli*. High concentrations of trimethoprim and the sulphonamide (particularly of sulphadiazine) are attained in the urine, which is useful in the treatment of urinary tract infections. The use of trimethoprim-sulphonamide combinations is limited primarily by the resistance of the infecting organisms, particularly to the sulphonamide component. For many infections, the trimethoprim-sulphonamide combination has a similar efficacy to an appropriately selected antibiotic.

Coliform mastitis in cows is treated by high doses of the drug combination, which are administered intravenously rather than locally. Parenteral or intrauterine administration of trimethoprim-sulphonamide combinations can be used to treat postpartum metritis in cattle, sheep and pigs. Abortion in sheep due to *Toxoplasma* and *Chlamydia* infections has been prevented by the timely use of these drugs.

Trimethoprim-sulphonamide combinations have been used to treat acute respiratory infections in horses (including strangles), urinary tract infections and infected wounds. Respiratory infections in cattle and urinary tract infections caused by members of the Enterobacteriaceae and mixed aerobe/ anaerobe infections by sensitive organisms also respond well to these drugs.

In neonatal calves and piglets, undifferentiated diarrhoea usually responds well to oral doses of the drugs. A wide range of superficial and systemic infections in dogs and cats can be treated successfully with potentiated sulphonamides. Coccidiosis in dogs and cats is an indication for the use of these drugs. Trimethoprim and sulphonamides are added to the food or drinking water of piglets to prevent and treat atrophic rhinitis and also to prevent or treat a variety of bacterial infections in chickens and turkeys.

The withholding times for milk and meat in animals which have been treated with trimethoprim-sulphonamide mixtures are complex and depend not only on the nature of the combination but also on the species and the route of administration.

Trimethoprim + sulphadoxine

An injection is available for small animals which contains sulphadoxine (62.5 mg) and trimethoprim (12.5 mg) per ml plus lignocaine (1.0 mg). It is used for the treatment of acute and subacute infections caused by susceptible organisms and for prophylaxis against secondary bacterial infection after viral infections. Doses are expressed as sulphadoxine + trimethoprim.

Dose

dog, cat, piglet   15 mg/kg s.c. or i.m. daily
                     The withholding time for meat is 4 days.

The large animal injection contains sulphadoxine (200 mg) and trimethoprim (40 mg) per ml.

horse   15 mg/kg i.v. (preferred route) or i.m. daily
cattle   15 mg/kg s.c., i.m. or i.v. daily
pig   15 mg/kg s.c. or i.m. daily

The withholding time for meat is up to 8 days. Milk from treated animals must not be used for human consumption

Tablets contain sulphadoxine (250 mg) and trimethoprim (50 mg). In most cases, a single dose is sufficient but it can be repeated, if necessary, after 24–48 h.

Dose

calf and foal   3–10 tablets. For foals, dissolved tablets are administered by a nasopharyngeal tube.

piglet	0.25–1 tablet
lamb	1–3 tablets
dog	0.25–3 tablets

The withholding time for meat is 7 days.

Trimethoprim + sulphadiazine

Bolus formulations containing trimethoprim (200 mg) and sulphadiazine (1.0 g) are available for the treatment of calves. The recommended dose is 1 bolus/ 40 kg/day. The withholding time for meat is 28 days. This formulation should not be used for animals with functionally mature rumens.

The injectable preparations contain trimethoprim (40 mg) and sulpha-diazine (200 mg) per ml.

Dose

expressed as trimethoprim + sulphadiazine

cattle, sheep, pig, horse	15–24 mg/kg/day i.m. or slow i.v.
dog, cat	30 mg/kg day

The withholding time for milk is 60 h, and for meat 18 days.

The drug combination can be given orally to horses as a paste containing trimethoprim (2.6 g) and sulphadiazine (13.0 g) in a graduated syringe. Each syringe provides a daily dose for a 500 kg horse.

The piglet suspensions contain sulphadiazine (50 mg) and trimethoprim (10 mg) in a volume of 1.1 ml. The recommended dose is 1.1 ml/2 kg/day for up to 5 days. The withholding time is 28 days after the last treatment.

Tablets or capsules containing trimethoprim (20 mg or 80 mg) and sulpha-diazine (100 mg or 400 mg) are also available. The recommended doses are: cats 1 small tablet/day; dogs 1 small tablet/4 kg/day or 1 large tablet/16 kg/day.
Dose forms for cats must be given whole.

Suspensions for use in poultry contain trimethoprim (80 mg) and sulpha-diazine (400 mg)/ml and are administered in the drinking water (15 mg/kg/day). The withholding time for meat is 5 days and eggs from treated birds should not be used for human consumption.

Trimethoprim + sulphaquinoxaline
The poultry formula contains trimethoprim (165 g) and sulphaquinoxaline (500 mg). The recommended dose is 30 mg of active ingredients per kg body weight administered in the drinking water. The withdrawal period in meat in broiler chickens is 7 days and in turkeys, 9 days.

Trimethoprim + sulphatroxazole
The injectable formulation contains trimethoprim (40 mg) and sulphatroxazole (200 mg) per ml. The recommended dose is 3 ml/50 kg/day i.v. or i.m. for up to 5 days in cattle, sheep and pigs. The withholding times for meat are: cattle i.v. 10 days after last treatment; cattle i.m. 16 days after last treatment; pigs 9 days; sheep 16 days. The withholding time for milk from cows is 60 hours.

A bolus formulation contains trimethoprim (133 mg) and sulphatroxazole (667 mg). The dose is 1 bolus/40 kg/day to calves for not more than 5 days. The withholding period is 10 days.

Miscellaneous antibacterials

Novobiocin

Novobiocin has been isolated from *Streptomyces niveus* and related organisms. It is a derivative of coumarin. Unlike other antibiotics produced from actinomycetes, novobiocin is a weak dibasic acid which forms salts with bases. The monosodium salt is soluble 1 in 5 in water but the calcium salt is poorly water-soluble. Novobiocin has a rather narrow spectrum of activity which resembles that of benzylpenicillin. It is very active against almost all strains of *Staphylococcus aureus* and less active against streptococci and Gram-negative bacteria. It is thus a candidate for the treatment of infections due to penicillin-resistant staphylococci.

The mechanism of action of novobiocin involves the inactivation of the β subunit of DNA gyrase and it is usually bacteriostatic, but bactericidal effects can occur at high concentrations with sensitive bacteria. Resistance develops fairly readily *in vitro* and has been reported *in vivo*. Cross-resistance to other antibiotics does not appear to be a problem.

Oral doses of novobiocin are readily absorbed in monogastric animals and the drug has a half-life of 2–4 hours. It does not cross cell membranes easily and penetration into tissues is poor. The drug is excreted in the bile and enterohepatic shunting occurs.

Novobiocin may be hepatotoxic and a number of blood dyscrasias have been reported. Skin rashes may occur in cows which are treated locally for mastitis.

Clinical uses

Novobiocin can be used, both systemically and locally, to treat staphylococcal infections which are resistant to other antibiotics. The drug can be used to treat urinary tract infections caused by *Proteus vulgaris* and activity is increased if the urine is alkalinized. Although novobiocin has been used successfully to treat cellulitis and anthrax, it is mainly used for the local treatment of bovine mastitis due to *Staphylococcus aureus*. The withdrawal period for milk is 14 days, and for slaughter it is 10 days. It is often considered prudent to use a mixture of novobiocin and procaine penicillin in an oily suspension for dry-cow therapy (not less than 28 days before calving). The withdrawal period for milk and or slaughter is then increased to 28 days. An intramammary formulation containing prednisolone, neomycin, novobiocin, dihydrostreptomycin and chlorbutol has been claimed to produce an earlier return to normal function in both acute and chronic bovine mastitis. Novobiocin has also been used in combination with tetracyclines to treat non-specific upper respiratory tract infections in dogs. Combinations of novobiocin and quinolones have been claimed to be synergistic.

Dose

cow   400 mg per infected quarter

Polymyxins and colistin

Polymyxin is the generic term for a group of closely related antibiotics (polymyxins A–E) which are produced by various strains of *Bacillus polymyxa*, an aerobic spore-forming soil bacterium. Colistin, which is identical to polymyxin E, was first isolated from a strain of *Bacillus colistinus* found in a Japanese soil sample.

The polymyxins are cyclic polypeptides with molecular weights of about 1000. The molecules have a hydrophobic and a hydrophilic portion and, at normal physiological pH, they behave as cationic surface-active compounds. They are basic and able to form acid salts (e.g. sulphates) which are stable in aqueous solution. Colistin is also available as the methanesulphonate for parenteral use. Polymyxin B and colistin are the least toxic of the group.

The polymyxins and colistin share the same narrow spectrum of bactericidal activity. They are highly active against many Gram-negative organisms including *Brucella* spp., *Escherichia coli*, *Haemophilus* spp., *Klebsiella* spp. and *Salmonella* spp. *Pseudomonas aeruginosa* is inhibited at slightly higher concentrations of the drugs but *Proteus* species are generally resistant. Gram-positive bacteria are intrinsically resistant to the polymyxins, perhaps because the drugs cannot penetrate the cell wall. The polymyxins are able to chemically inactivate the endotoxin of Gram-negative bacteria.

The polymyxins are cationic surface-active agents which bind strongly to the cell membrane phospholipids of susceptible bacteria causing structural disruption which results in cell lysis, even in a hypertonic environment. Membrane transport mechanisms are also disrupted and essential cell constituents (e.g. phosphate and nucleosides) escape. The binding of the polymyxins to bacterial cell membranes is competitively inhibited by a number of metal ions (Ca, Fe, Co, Mg, Mn) and the effects of the drugs are opposed by anionic surface-active agents (e.g. soaps). These agents should not be used concomitantly with the polymyxins. Some cationic detergents (e.g. chlorhexidine) increase the topical activity of the polymyxins.

Perhaps because they disorganize bacterial cell membranes, the polymyxins synergize with a large number of other antibiotics including the cephalosporins, chloramphenicol, clindamycin, erythromycin, fusidic acid, novobiocin, the penicillins and the tetracyclines. Synergism between sulphonamide/trimethoprim combinations and the polymyxins extends activity to resistant strains of enterobacteria, including *Pseudomonas aeruginosa*.

Resistance is rare, but when it occurs it extends to all members of the group but not to other antibiotics. Resistant strains of *Pseudomonas aeruginosa* acquire an ability to exclude the drugs.

Their cationic nature ensures that the polymyxins are not absorbed from the gastrointestinal tract, even after large doses. Colistin methanesulphonate is given intramuscularly when a systemic effect is required. The polymyxins are highly protein- and membrane-bound and diffusion to the tissues is poor. After a delay, the polymyxins are slowly excreted in the urine, mainly by glomerular filtration. Cumulation of these drugs is always liable to occur, especially when there is renal impairment. Colistin is excreted more rapidly than polymyxin B.

The structure and function of some mammalian cell membranes is disrupted by the polymyxins. This is especially true for renal tubular epithelial cells which come into contact with relatively high concentrations of the drugs. Nephrotoxicity is manifested as albuminuria and increased non-protein nitrogen excretion, but sometimes there is haematuria and renal casts occur. These effects have been described in the dog after low doses of polymyxin B. In this respect, colistin appears to be less toxic than polymyxin B, although co-toxicity with other potentially nephrotoxic agents (e.g. aminoglycosides) remains a possibility.

Polymyxin B sulphate causes pain at the injection site and release of histamine which can proceed to tissue necrosis. Colistin methanesulphonate is much less irritant. In humans, peripheral neuropathy and non-competitive neuromuscular blockade have been reported after administration of the polymyxins. Ataxia has been reported in calves after systemic administration of polymyxin B, and deaths from respiratory failure have occurred in sheep.

Clinical uses

Cattle
The polymyxins and colistin are useful in the oral treatment of *E. coli* and *Salmonella* enteritis in calves and the local treatment of *Klebsiella* and *Pseudomonas* mastitis in cows. Polymyxin B and colistin are often given in combination with sulphonamide/trimethoprim for the treatment of enteritis and with tetracyclines for mastitis. The ability of the polymyxins to interact chemically with bacterial endotoxin confers an added benefit. Colistin methanesulphonate and polymyxin B can be given intramuscularly to treat mastitis but transfer of the drugs from blood to udder tissue is poor.

Pigs
Oral polymyxin B has been used to treat *E. coli* enteritis in young animals.

Horses
Polymyxins are used locally for uterine infections by resistant strains of *Klebsiella* and *Pseudomonas*. Polymyxins are also often included in compound preparations for application to the eye. A topical formulation containing polymyxin B sulphate, miconazole, bacitracin and prednisolone is marketed for the treatment of skin infections in horses, dogs and cats.

Dogs and cats
Polymyxins are used in the topical treatment of external ear infections. Many formulations are available which variously contain chlorhexidine or EDTA, insecticides (e.g. pyrethrins), other antibiotics (e.g. neomycin), local anaesthetics (e.g. lignocaine) and corticosteroids (e.g. dexamethasone). Compound eye formulations are also available which contain in addition to polymyxin B sulphate, neomycin sulphate, chloramphenicol, sulphacetamide and prednisolone or hydrocortisone.

For doses, see manufacturers' instructions.

Rifampin

Rifamycin B was originally isolated from *Streptomyces mediterranei* in 1959. There are a large number of semi-synthetic derivatives of rifamycin-B, of which the most important is rifampin. Another is rifamycin SV, which has much lower antibacterial activity and was used in an intramammary formulation to treat bovine mastitis.

Rifampin is a complex macrocyclic antibiotic which is soluble in water at acid pH and in organic solvents. It has broad-spectrum activity against most Gram-positive and many Gram-negative bacteria, including anaerobes. It is particularly active against most strains of *Mycobacterium tuberculosis*, which represents its principal use in humans. It also has antichlamydial, antiviral and antifungal (in combination with amphotericin B) activity. Because resistance develops readily, rifampin is seldom given alone and is usually combined with another antibacterial drug (e.g. trimethoprim, vancomycin, isoxazoyl penicillins, aminoglycosides or erythromycin).

Rifampin is bactericidal and binds tightly to the DNA-dependent RNA polymerases of sensitive bacteria, inhibiting RNA synthesis. This mode of action is unique to rifampin. Selectivity arises from the fact that much higher concentrations of the antibiotic are required to inhibit mammalian mitochondrial enzymes.

Bacteria, including mycobacteria, readily develop resistance to rifampin both *in vitro* and *in vivo*. A one-step chromosomal mutation to an RNA polymerase which no longer binds rifampin produces a high level of bacterial resistance. There is, however, no cross-resistance with other antibiotics.

Rifampin is well absorbed from the gastrointestinal tract of monogastric animals and peak blood concentrations are attained within 2–4 hours. Due, in part, to its high lipid solubility, rifampin diffuses rapidly into most tissues, including the CSF and abscess cavities, often reaching higher concentrations than those in plasma. Importantly, rifampin gains access to cells and can kill phagocytosed bacteria which may be a source of persistent staphylococcal infections. The plasma half-life of rifampin is about 8 hours in the dog and about 6 hours in the horse. Rifampin is metabolized by deacetylation in the liver, a pathway which is subject to enzyme induction, so that there is a progressive decrease in half-life. The drug is excreted in the bile, with enterohepatic shunting, and also in the urine.

Untoward effects are very uncommon in animals. It should not be given to patients with liver dysfunction. Rifampin may have teratogenic potential. Owners should be warned that the animal's urine, faeces, tears and saliva may be an orange-red colour. Rifampin, as an enzyme inducer, may reduce the half-life of drugs which undergo hepatic metabolism (e.g. corticosteroids and digoxin) and this may be a potential source of drug interactions.

Clinical uses

Rifampin has been used in combination with erythromycin to treat pneumonia in foals caused by *Rhodococcus equi*. This is often difficult to eradicate because the organism survives intracellularly. Human brucellosis has been treated with a combination of rifampin and a tetracycline. The ability of rifampin to penetrate cells has been exploited in the treatment of persistent bovine mastitis due to *Staphylococcus aureus* and chronic granulomatous disease complicated by secondary staphylococcal infections. Chronic staphylococcal osteomyelitis, endocarditis, recurrent or deep pyoderma, abscesses and infections resulting from prosthetic implants (e.g. of the hip) have been treated successfully with rifampin. Chlamydial infections also often respond well to rifampin. Disseminated fungal infections are often treated effectively with rifampin and amphotericin B.

Dose

ruminants	0–20 mg/kg/day i.m.
non-ruminants and horses	10–20 mg/kg/day p.o.

Nitrofurans

The nitrofurans are a group of closely related synthetic antibacterial drugs (Fig. 18.8) with activity against some protozoa and fungi. They include nitrofurazone, nitrofurantoin, furaltadone, furazolidone and nifuratel. Nitrofurantoin has the least and furazolidone has the greatest activity.

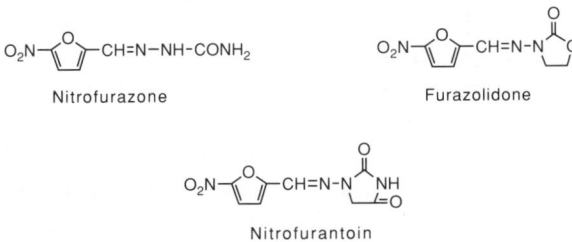

Nitrofurazone   Furazolidone

Nitrofurantoin

Figure 18.8 Structures of nitrofuran antibacterial drugs.

At clinically achievable concentrations, the nitrofurans have bactericidal activity against many Gram-positive and Gram-negative bacteria, but *Pseudomonas* and *Proteus* species are commonly resistant. They are also of value in the control of coccidial and other protozoal (e.g. *Trichomonas* and *Giardia*) infections and were among the first drugs to be used as coccidiostats (Chapter 20).

Mechanism of action

The nitrofurans have a number of adverse effects on bacterial metabolism, but it is their ability to cause DNA damage which leads to cell death. It is believed that reduction of the nitrofurans in bacterial cells gives rise to highly reactive but evanescent intermediates which actually cause the rupture of bacterial DNA strands. Selective toxicity appears to stem from the relative ability of host and bacterial cells to reduce the drugs and the speed with which they are cleared from the host's tissues. Mammalian tissues with high energy requirements (e.g. testicular, nervous, liver and lung tissue) also activate nitrofurans and this may partly explain some of their toxic effects in mammals.

The nitrofurans are all antagonistic to nalidixic acid, which acts at the same site.

Bacterial resistance to the nitrofurans develops in a gradual, step-wise manner. Resistance sometimes involves the acquisition of an ability to exclude the drug, or a loss of appropriate reductase enzymes so that activation of the nitrofurans no longer occurs. Cross-resistance usually occurs among the nitrofurans and can be important clinically.

Although widely used, the nitrofurans have a rather narrow safety margin and they are never administered parenterally. The individual toxic effects of the nitrofurans are discussed separately.

Nitrofurazone

Nitrofurazone (Fig. 18.8) is active against a range of Gram-positive and Gram-negative bacteria. It also has antiprotozoal activity and is used for coccidiosis (see Chapter 20). It is primarily used for the control of enteric infections in farm animals, such as poultry and pigs.

The drug is sometimes used in pigs, usually as in-feed medication, for the control of *Salmonella* infections, but it is poorly absorbed and it is less effective than the more commonly used furazolidone.

A variety of powders, drops, ointments and creams containing nitrofurazone are available. They also contain sulphonamides, corticosteroids, neomycin, phenylmercuric nitrate, retinoin, undecylenic acid, etc. and are claimed to be suitable for specific purposes, usually to aid healing and to prevent colonization by bacteria and fungi.

Preparations are also available which contain nitrofurazone in combination with other antibacterials (e.g. neomycin and polymyxin), lignocaine and an insecticide (e.g. pyrethrins) which are used to control bacterial and parasitic external ear infections and infestations in cats and dogs. A solution of nitrofurazone in water (14 mg/ml) is used for treatment of metritis as a direct application.

Nitrofurazone is normally well-tolerated but there have been reports of toxic CNS effects in calves, consisting of irritability and convulsions, which may have been due to the inhibition of monoamine oxidase.

Furazolidone

Furazolidone (Fig. 18.8) has activity against a wide range of bacteria, including *Clostridium* species, *E. coli*, *Salmonella* species, *Shigella*, staphylococci and streptococci and some protozoa. Thus it is the drug of choice in the treatment of enteric infections in farm animals. It can also be used for the treatment of *Salmonella* infections in small animals, pigs and foals.

The drug is given orally and is poorly absorbed from the gastrointestinal tract. In the UK furazolidone is licensed for use in poultry, rabbits, calves and pigs. Various formulations are available for medication of the drinking water and feed and there are suspensions for administration to individual calves and piglets. The withholding period for meat from treated calves and pigs is 7 days. The drug should not be used in piglets less than 48 hours old. In poultry, furazolidone is incorporated into the feed to prevent hatchery-borne infections. The withholding period for the slaughter of treated birds intended for human consumption depends on the preparation used.

Furazolidone is sometimes used in combination with other antibacterials (e.g. chloramphenicol) for the treatment of enteric infections in calves and foals. Other compound preparations which contain furazolidone in combination with arsanilic acid or morantel citrate are used for piglets raised under intensive conditions. These preparations are claimed to eliminate roundworms and nodular worms (morantel), to control bacterial scours (furazolidone) and *Treponema hyodysenteriae* scours (arsanilic acid).

The drug is also applied locally to the udder, uterus and skin. A preparation containing chlorhexidine and furazolidone in an emollient base is formulated for application to teat skin lacerations, cracks and sores. There appear to be no toxicity problems when the drug is applied locally. A preparation for the treatment of acute (with pyrexia) and chronic (infertility) metritis in cattle contains furazolidone and oxytetracycline as antibacterials, iodohydroxy-quinoline as an antifungal together with α-tocopherol and ethinyloestradiol. A single 20 ml dose introduced by catheter is claimed to be effective.

Toxic reactions, including CNS signs and staggers, have been reported in calves after inadvertent overdosage. Hyperaesthesia and inappetence are common clinical signs; early-weaned animals, those introduced to a high barley diet or debilitated animals seem to be the most susceptible. Treatment should be discontinued if toxic effects are seen; recovery occurs with no apparent long-term effects. Prolonged use of furazolidone is considered likely to encourage the development of resistant *Salmonella* strains. In poultry, inappetence and weight loss can occur.

Nitrofurantoin

Nitrofurantoin (Fig. 18.8) has bactericidal activity against a wide range of microorganisms. Susceptible bacteria generally include many strains of streptococci, staphylococci, *Aerobacter* and *E. coli*. Its pharmacokinetic properties, and hence its clinical uses, are different from those of the other nitrofurans. Nitrofurantoin is readily absorbed after oral administration and is so rapidly excreted that tissue concentrations, except in the lungs, are seldom high enough to exert an antibacterial effect. About 40 per cent of a nitrofurantoin dose escapes metabolism and appears in the urine unchanged over 3–4 hours. Nitrofurantoin is a weak acid and is ionized in acid urine. Thus, renal tubular reabsorption is low and concentrations attained in the urinary tract may be high enough to affect normally resistant *Pseudomonas* and *Proteus* species. It is common practice to co-administer a urinary acidifier to promote drug ionization when using nitrofurantoin to treat urinary tract infections.

The drug is licensed in the UK for use in horses and small animals to treat urinary and upper respiratory tract infections. Its rapid absorption makes it unsuitable for the treatment of enteric infections. Although nitrofurantoin is recommended for the treatment of urinary tract infections in the horse, it should not be used in animals intended for human consumption or those with impaired renal or hepatic function. The efficacy of nitrofurantoin can be improved by making the urine acid.

Higher than recommended doses of nitrofurantoin and/or prolonged treatment with more modest doses can cause toxic effects. These are referable to the CNS and the haematopoietic system (reduced platelet and leucocyte counts). Prolonged bleeding may occur and can be fatal, especially in calves. Inappetence and nausea and vomiting are liable to occur after nitrofurantoin in all species. In the horse, skin reactions are often the first signs of nitrofurantoin toxicity and if these occur, the drug should be stopped.

Dose

dog   4 mg/kg t.i.d.
horse   4.4 mg/kg initially then 2.2 mg/kg every 8 hours for 5 days.

Furaltadone

Furaltadone is usually given in the food or water to chickens, broilers, layers and turkeys to control infections such as septicaemia and infectious bronchitis, caused by susceptible organisms (e.g. *Salmonella* spp., *E. coli*). Caecal coccidiosis and blackhead also respond to furaltadone. It is recommended in ducks only for the treatment of salmonellosis. The clinical uses of furaltadone are limited by its toxicity and it can only be given for relatively short periods (5–7 days). The first sign of furaltadone toxicity is inappetence with consequent weight loss; the drug should then be withdrawn. Tissue residues are not found and there is no withholding period before slaughter for human consumption.

Nitroimidazoles

This group of drugs comprises metronidazole, dimetridazole, ronidazole, tinidazole, niridazole (which has anthelmintic activity) and ipronidazole. They all have similar antimicrobial spectra, which in many ways are similar to those of the nitrofurans, except for niridazole which also has anthelmintic activity. Of the group, metronidazole is the most important.

Metronidazole

Metronidazole (Fig. 18.9) was synthesized in 1967 and was found to have both antibacterial and antiprotozoal activity. It was first used for the treatment of human trichomonal vaginitis. It is also active against a number of other protozoa, including *Giardia lamblia* and *Entamoeba histolytica*. More recently, the use of metronidazole has become popular for the treatment of a wide variety of anaerobic bacterial infections in small animals, birds and horses.

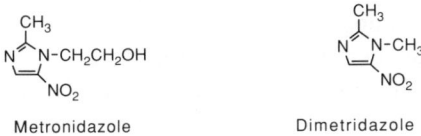

Metronidazole   Dimetridazole

Figure 18.9 Structures of nitroimidazoles.

The bactericidal action of metronidazole is specific for obligate anaerobic and microaerophilic organisms and occurs at clinically attainable concentrations. Like clindamycin, metronidazole can be used for the treatment of a wide range of serious anaerobic infections. For mixed aerobic/anaerobic infections, metronidazole can be combined with other antibiotics, such as the aminoglycosides. Such combinations find clinical application in the management of peritonitis following gut perforation.

To survive and multiply in the absence of oxygen, the mechanisms for energy production and electron transfer in anaerobes must be very different from those of aerobic organisms. Organisms which are sensitive to metronidazole are usually anaerobic (although aerobic bacteria in a hypoxic environment may be sensitive) and have electron transport proteins with a low redox potential. Metronidazole enters these cells with ease and, under anaerobic conditions, the nitro group is then reduced. This is necessary for antimicrobial activity. Several highly, but transiently, active metabolites, which have not yet been identified, are produced and these are believed to become covalently bound to DNA and other macromolecules in the cell. The reactive metabolites of metronidazole inhibit DNA synthesis in both bacteria and protozoa; the helical structure of existing DNA is lost and strand breakage occurs. This usually causes cell death but may also produce cell mutations and the radiosensitization of hypoxic cells. The selective toxicity of metronidazole is largely explicable in terms of the very different redox systems of the cells of the host compared with those of the invading organism.

Metronidazole and the other 5-nitroimidazoles are bactericidal to most Gram-negative and some Gram-positive anaerobic bacteria. The lack of activity against aerobic bacteria can be overcome by combination therapy with a suitable antibiotic. Potent activity is exerted against *Treponema hyodysenteriae*, which is now recognized as a common causal agent of dysentery in swine, and against a wide variety of other protozoa (e.g. *Giardia lamblia, Histomonas meleagridis*).

Acquired bacterial resistance to metronidazole is not encountered frequently but when it does occur it extends to the whole group and sometimes to the nitrofurans. The mechanism appears to involve a reduced capacity of the microorganisms to biotransform the drug to its active metabolites.

Therapeutic drug levels are rapidly attained after oral administration of metronidazole to monogastric species and the half-life is within the range 6–10 hours. The bioavailability of the drug after oral administration approaches 100 per cent. Injections of metronidazole may produce necrosis and abscess formation at the injection site. The drug crosses cell barriers passively and distributes into all body fluids and tissues, including the central nervous system. The liver is the main site of metabolism, where oxidation of side-chains is followed by glucuronylation. About 30 per cent of the drug undergoes metabolism and the remainder is excreted unchanged in the urine.

The most common side-effect of metronidazole in humans is an interaction with alcohol because the drug has disulfiram-like activity. However, apart from local tissue reactions after parenteral administration, side-effects in domestic animals are rare. Nausea and vomiting and signs suggestive of severe central vestibular or cerebellar dysfunction have been reported in dogs after high oral metronidazole doses (>60 mg/kg/day). In laboratory rodents, chronic administration of high doses of metronidazole has produced carcinogenic effects.

Clinical uses

Metronidazole is administered orally or subcutaneously to dogs to treat anaerobic infections such as acute gingivitis and periodontal disease. It is highly effective in *Giardia lamblia* enteritis. Diarrhoea usually stops within 2–3 days but treatment must be continued for 5–7 days. Metronidazole is also used for undiagnosed diarrhoea in dogs. It is the only antibacterial drug with rapid bactericidal activity against *Bacteroides fragilis* infections. Endocarditis and brain abscesses due to *Bacteroides* species have responded to metronidazole where other antibiotics have been ineffective. The drug has been used prophylactically before lower gastrointestinal surgery. Because of possible mutagenic effects, the use of metronidazole is contraindicated in pregnant animals.

Trichomonas infections in bulls have been treated with metronidazole. A solution of metronidazole has also been used topically for this purpose and to irrigate wounds and hoof infections. Intraruminal and genital *Campylobacter* infections have also responded to metronidazole.

Metronidazole has been used in horses to prevent infections after abdominal surgery and to treat pneumonia due to anaerobic bacteria. It should not be used in horses intended for human consumption.

When treating birds and rodents, metronidazole is usually added to the drinking water. Eggs from treated birds should not be used for human consumption.

Dose

dog and cat	20 mg/kg p.o., i.v. or s.c., daily.
horse	20 mg/kg/day slow i.v. infusion daily.
	Oral paste – see manufacturer's instructions.

Dimetridazole

Dimetridazole (Fig. 18.9) is mainly used for the prevention and treatment of swine dysentery and blackhead (*Histomonas meleagridis*) in poultry, turkeys and game birds. Ronidazole and ipronidazole have similar applications. Dimetridazole is usually incorporated in feed (100–200 g/tonne) or water (13.3g/100 l) for prophylaxis. For the treatment of infected birds, a 2–3-fold increase in drug concentration is normally required for 7–14 days. Although tissue residues of dimetridazole cannot normally be found 2 days after treatment stops, withdrawal periods of 6–7 days are specified. If dimetridazole is given to laying birds, their eggs should not be used for human consumption.

For prophylaxis against dysentery in pigs, dimetridazole is given either in the feed (200 g/tonne) or the drinking water (13.3 g/l) and the usual oral dose for treatment is 50–100 mg/kg/day. A withdrawal period of 6 days is specified.

Quinolones

The modern quinolones are derived from their parent compound, nalidixic acid. Nalidixic acid (Fig. 18.10) was developed as the result of the observation that a by-product of a novel synthesis of the antimalarial, chloroquine, had antibacterial activity. Nalidixic acid is an analogue of the original by-product. Oxolinic acid and cinoxacin have similar actions to nalidixic acid, in that they act mainly against Gram-negative organisms and differ only in potency and pharmacokinetic properties. More recently, a number of fluoroquinolones have been developed (e.g. ciprofloxacin and norfloxacin). These have a much broader spectrum of activity, extending to Gram-positive organisms. The fluoroquinolones have a considerable potential for use in veterinary medicine.

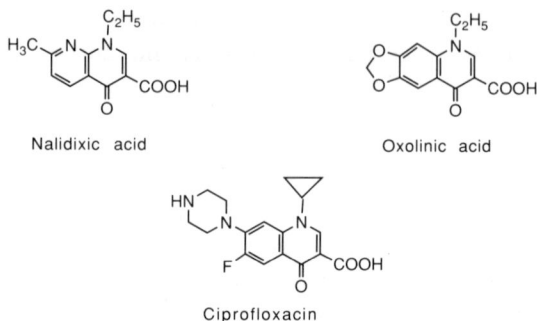

Figure 18.10   Structures of quinolones and the fluoroquinolones.

Nalidixic acid

Nalidixic acid (Fig. 18.10) is a synthetic heterocyclic compound which is stable and almost insoluble in water. It has bactericidal activity against most strains of Gram-negative aerobic bacteria, such as *E. coli*, *Enterobacter*, *Klebsiella pneumoniae* and *Proteus* species at concentrations which can be achieved clinically. *Pseudomonas aeruginosa* strains, aerobic cocci and anaerobic bacteria are usually resistant to nalidixic acid.

The main action of the quinolones is the binding and inhibition of the proper functioning of bacterial DNA gyrase. This enzyme, also known as topoisomerase II, has a number of functions, including supercoiling of DNA which allows it to fit inside the bacterial cell. DNA gyrase is also involved in the interlocking or splitting of duplex DNA rings into daughter rings in the process of DNA replication. Exposure of susceptible bacteria to nalidixic acid results in a rapid inhibition of DNA replication followed by inhibition of RNA and protein synthesis. The bacteria increase in length and the cytoplasm clears from the periphery, followed by lysis.

Resistance to nalidixic acid usually involves a mutation at the gene loci coding for the DNA gyrase subunits. This prevents efficient binding of nalidixic acid to the enzyme. In practice, the emergence of resistant strains can be prevented by combining nalidixic acid with another drug. Cross-resistance with drugs other than the quinolones has not been reported.

Nalidixic acid is well absorbed after oral administration and peak blood concentrations are attained within 2 hours of dosage. It is heavily protein-bound (93–97 per cent). The drug is partially metabolized to an inactive metabolite, 7-hydroxynalidixic acid, and some conjugation also occurs in the liver. The half-life of the drug is 1–2 hours in humans. About 10–15 per cent of an oral dose is excreted unchanged in the urine and about 80 per cent of an oral dose is recoverable from the urine within 8 hours.

Caution should be observed in the use of nalidixic acid as it is capable of causing serious toxic effects on the central nervous system, usually manifested as stimulation and irritability which may progress to convulsions. Fatal seizures have been reported in the dog.

Clinical uses
The clinical use of nalidixic acid is restricted to the treatment of enteric and urinary tract infections caused by Gram-negative bacteria. It is best reserved for infections caused by organisms which are resistant to other antibacterial drugs. Enteritis in calves caused by *E. coli* and *Salmonella* has been successfully treated with nalidixic acid.

Dose

monogastric animals	12 mg/kg p.o., 4 times a day, as an oral suspension and in tablet form.

Other quinolones

Oxolinic acid (Fig. 18.10) has a slightly broader spectrum of activity than nalidixic acid. It is active against *Staphylococcus aureus*. The increased *in vitro* activity of oxolinic acid against Gram-negative bacteria is offset by its more extensive metabolic inactivation and greater toxicity. Cinoxacin is less extensively protein-bound than nalidixic acid and thus smaller doses can be used. This is said to reduce the incidence of adverse effects.

Pipemidic acid and piromidic acid are marketed by Belgian and Japanese manufacturers, respectively. They should both be regarded as having profiles essentially similar to nalidixic acid. Pipemidic acid has been claimed to be effective against some organisms which are resistant to nalidixic acid.

Fluoroquinolones

The major difference between the modern fluoroquinolones and nalidixic acid is the loss of the 8-nitrogen and the substitution of a fluorine at position 6 (see Fig. 18.10). This results in increased activity against DNA gyrase and an extension of the antibacterial spectrum to Gram-positive organisms, including methicillin-resistant strains of *Staphylococcus aureus*. Activity against streptococci, especially enterococci, is more variable. Because the fluoroquinolones have little activity against anaerobes, their impact on the normal gastrointestinal microflora is minimal. Incorporation of a piperazine moiety, as in ciprofloxacin, increases activity against *Pseudomonas aeruginosa*. The older quinolones require dividing cells with intact protein synthesis but this is not necessary for the fluoroquinolones, which also may inhibit transfer RNA synthesis. The toxicity of these drugs is low. A large number of fluoroquinolones are available for human use, including amifloxacin, ciprofloxacin, enrofloxacin, enoxacin, lomefloxacin, norfloxacin and ofloxacin and some of these have begun to be used in veterinary medicine. The synthetic potential of the quinolones is at an early stage, and a new class of antibacterial which combines a cephalosporin and a quinolone has been developed recently (Ro 23-9424). This drug not only destroys the bacterial cell wall but also delivers the quinolone to its DNA target.

Although fluoroquinolones have been used successfully in the treatment of a wide range of conditions in both domestic and farm animals, there is concern that the widespread use of these drugs in food animals might lead to the development of resistance in clinically important human pathogens, particularly those involved in cystic fibrosis.

All of the fluoroquinolones are well absorbed after oral administration to monogastric animals with peak serum concentrations being attained in 1–2 hours. However, the oral bioavailability of these drugs is poor in ruminants. The plasma half-life of enrofloxacin in dogs is 2–3 hours after oral dosage and 3–4 hours in cats after subcutaneous administration. The drugs are minimally protein-bound and become widely distributed in body tissues and fluids (including the CSF), also penetrating macrophages. The drug levels attained in bone, liver, lung and prostate exceed the minimal inhibitory concentration for most staphylococci but not necessarily for streptococci.

The fluoroquinolones are extensively biotransformed to less active metabolites, which undergo renal excretion, and the dose must be reduced if there is renal impairment.

All of the fluoroquinolones exert a significant post-drug inhibition of microbial activity, during which the organisms are unable to divide. This means that the drugs may still be effective if administered less frequently than would be predicted from the half-life.

High doses of fluoroquinolones have been reported to cause the erosion of the cartilage in the weight-bearing joints of immature dogs, resulting in permanent damage. The drugs may also be neurotoxic.

Clinical uses

The fluoroquinolones have proved to be very effective in the treatment of urinary tract infections which are resistant to other antibiotics. They are effective in the treatment of prostatitis, including infections caused by *Pseudomonas* and *Chlamydia* species.

Ciprofloxacin

Ciprofloxacin (Fig. 18.10) has a substituted piperidine ring in the 7-position and a three-carbon ring instead of the methyl group of nalidixic acid. Sensitive organisms include the Enterobacteriaceae, *Haemophilus*, *Pseudomonas aeruginosa* and *Staphylococcus aureus*. Mycobacteria are generally sensitive to ciprofloxacin and there is some activity against rickettsiae.

Ciprofloxacin is absorbed after oral administration and peak concentrations are achieved in monogastric animals within 4 hours. The drug is concentrated in some tissues, including the prostate in man. There is some enterohepatic shunting and the drug has a half-life of about 4 hours in humans. Excretion is mainly by active renal tubular secretion of the unchanged drug (60 per cent) and most of the remainder is passed in the faeces, although a small proportion is broken down to inactive metabolites.

Although there have been reports of antagonism between ciprofloxacin and rifampin, ciprofloxacin has been used in combination with a variety of other antibiotics (e.g. aminoglycosides, penicillins, cephalosporins, imipenem) in the treatment of serious infections in humans. It has been used for the treatment of chronic *Pseudomonas* infections of the urinary tract in dogs. Because high drug concentrations can be maintained in the tissues, oral ciprofloxacin has been effective in the long-term treatment of osteomyelitis.

Dose

7–11 mg/kg p.o.

Norfloxacin

This drug is similar to ciprofloxacin but exerts a greater activity at lower pH than the other quinolones and is concentrated in urine. It is therefore probably best for treatment of urinary tract infections. Norfloxacin also increases the activity of a number of antifungal drugs.

Enrofloxacin

Enrofloxacin is closely related to ciprofloxacin and was specifically developed for use in veterinary medicine. The drug is given orally or by intramuscular injection and has broad-spectrum activity against Gram-positive and Gram-negative bacteria, including clinically important *Mycoplasma* species. When used to treat colibacillosis in calves, 3–5 daily doses (2.5 mg/kg) not only cured the primary infection but prevented the occurrence of bronchopneumonia. *Salmonella* infections in calves have also responded to higher doses (5 mg/kg) of enrofloxacin. Intramuscular injection of enrofloxacin (2.5 mg/kg/day) was effective in the treatment of bronchopneumonia and enzootic pneumonia in pigs. Enrofloxacin-medicated feeds and drinking water have been used to prevent and treat a wide variety of infections in pigs, chickens and turkeys. In dogs and cats, infections of the urinary, digestive and respiratory tracts have responded to enrofloxacin. The drug has also been used both orally and parenterally to treat infections of the skin and external ear.

The only serious toxic effect of enrofloxacin is cartilage and bone toxicity in dogs and horses.

Urinary antiseptics

Hexamine

Hexamine (methenamine) is used to treat recurrent urinary tract infections. It is not active itself but is hydrolysed under acid (pH <5.5) conditions to yield formaldehyde and ammonia. The antibacterial activity of formaldehyde is probably due to bacterial protein denaturation which occurs at concentrations above 2.5 μg/ml. The drug is usually given in enteric-coated tablets or as an elixir. Hexamine is readily absorbed from the gastrointestinal tract but formaldehyde is not released systemically because the pH is too high. Hexamine is usually given with a urinary acidifier such as sodium acid phosphate, ascorbic acid or ammonium chloride. The drug is used for the prophylaxis and treatment of recurrent urinary tract infections in dogs at a dose level of 2.2 mg/kg, three times a day (cats 22mg twice daily). The drug is well tolerated but an adequate urine flow must be maintained to prevent irritation and, possibly, crystalluria.

Mandelic acid

The calcium and ammonium salts of mandelic acid have antibacterial activity in the urine providing that the pH is below 5.5. The drug is given orally to dogs and cats at a dose level of 250 mg/kg/day for not more than 14 days.

CHAPTER 19

SELECTION OF ANTIBACTERIAL DRUGS

Antibiotics are traditionally defined as substances produced by microorganisms which kill bacteria or inhibit their multiplication. They were presumably evolved by lower forms of life to compete with other species. In turn, bacteria evolved defence mechanisms against antibiotics. Collectively, these mechanisms constitute antibiotic resistance, which is of great clinical importance. Because many of the drugs in this group are now produced synthetically, it is simpler to use the term 'antibacterial drugs' which includes the 'traditional antibiotics' together with the sulphonamides, nitrofurans, etc.

The details of the pharmacology of the various antibacterials used in veterinary therapeutics have been dealt with elsewhere in this book. This chapter is concerned with a discussion of the criteria used by the clinician for the selection of an antibacterial drug for a particular patient. In a clinical situation, there is rarely one antibacterial which is clearly superior to all others so that, after narrowing down the field by using the criteria for selection to assess the relative merits of drugs which could possibly be used, an element of personal preference remains.

Before considering the selection of drugs, the first and important question is whether an antibacterial is really indicated. When there is specific or good circumstantial evidence for a non-trivial bacterial infection, antibacterial drugs are valuable, even life-saving, but other infections may effectively be overcome by the body's natural defence mechanisms, with the possible development of immunity. Furthermore, using antibacterials for trivial conditions exposes the patient to possible drug toxicity in addition to exerting a selection pressure for the emergence of resistant bacterial strains. For example, it is not uncommon for *Pseudomonas* to be isolated as the dominant infection in canine otitis externa. The strain is often resistant to the commonly used antibacterials and is probably selected by their injudicious use; thorough cleansing of the ear canal with cetrimide is more effective as a first therapeutic measure, followed by a specific antibacterial drug if it proves necessary.

Prophylaxis is a second major indication for using antibacterials in situations where the development of significant bacterial infection is likely. For example, tissue damage due to contusion of abdominal viscera, wound contamination and impairment of the defence barrier of the respiratory mucosa following virus infections are all rational indications for prophylaxis. However, antibacterials must never be regarded as a substitute for basic surgical principles of cleaning wounds and draining abscesses. Dry-cow therapy and in-feed medication during periods of risk of swine dysentery are other examples of antibacterial prophylaxis.

Criteria for selection

If, on the basis of the considerations outlined above, a decision is made that antibacterial therapy is indicated, the primary objective must be kept clearly in mind—i.e. to attain, at the site of infection, a concentration of drug sufficient to kill the pathogens or to inhibit their further multiplication so that the body defence mechanisms can be effective. Selection is then based on assessing the relative merits of the drugs according to the following criteria:

1. Antibacterial spectrum
2. Pharmacokinetic properties
3. Bactericidal or bacteriostatic action
4. Potential toxicity
5. Relative cost

Antibacterial spectrum

It is not good practice to administer routinely 'good broad-spectrum cover' because this entails a greater risk of upsetting the normal resident bacterial flora and exerting a selection pressure for resistant strains and species to dominate. The problem has been described following oral tetracycline therapy, which may remove normally dominant bacterial flora sufficiently to allow the proliferation of fungi, such as *Candida albicans*. This infection is resistant to most antibacterials and nystatin or amphotericin would then be indicated. Quite distinct from problems associated with selection pressure, a narrow-spectrum drug is the first choice in certain infections. Thus, benzylpenicillin is probably the most effective drug in the treatment of bovine streptococcal mastitis and, furthermore, its activity is less inhibited by milk than that of the other antibacterials. Similarly, although Gram-negative enteric infections are commonly treated with broad-spectrum antibacterials, streptomycin is the drug of choice in *Shigella equiruli* infection in foals.

Selection of an antibacterial on the criterion of spectrum of activity assumes a knowledge of the pathogen(s), but clearly, it is neither practical nor necessary to take samples for laboratory diagnosis in the majority of cases. Diagnosis and drug selection is commonly based on previous experience and logical deduction of the most probable causal pathogen. Thus, where *Mycoplasma* is thought, from experience, to be implicated in calf respiratory disease, tylosin would be a rational choice. *Bordetella bronchiseptica* is commonly isolated from dogs with kennel cough, so a tetracycline might be a first line of treatment for this condition. Urinary tract infections in dogs associated with urine of high pH are usually due to *Proteus mirabilis* infection, and ampicillin or amoxycillin would be rational therapy.

Disc sensitivity tests

Although some organisms, for example streptococci, are quite predictable in their sensitivity to antibacterials, others show a strain variation or may acquire resistance by the transfer of R-plasmids. Hence, appropriate antibacterials should first be determined by sensitivity testing, before considering further criteria for selection. Examples of such organisms are *Staphylococcus aureus*, *E. coli*, *Pseudomonas* spp., *Salmonella* spp. and *Haemophilus influenzae*. Cultures from samples taken during treatment with antibacterials, for example if treatment appears to be ineffective, are confusing and the drug(s) should be withdrawn for 3 or 4 days before sampling.

From the results of a properly conducted sensitivity test, it can usually be concluded that drugs which are ineffective *in vitro* will be no more effective if used clinically. Certain infections of the lower urinary tract may provide an exception to this general rule, for it has been demonstrated in dogs that benzylpenicillin may be sufficiently concentrated in the urine to be clinically effective against *E. coli* which are insensitive *in vitro*.

Conversely, an organism which is sensitive *in vitro* to a particular antibacterial should be susceptible in the clinical situation, provided that the drug reaches the site of infection in adequate concentration and, with certain infections (e.g. *Clostridium perfringens* type D), before the production of lethal amounts of toxin. These factors depend on the pharmacokinetic properties of the drug and will be considered separately below.

Disc sensitivity techniques are not sufficiently precise to relate the degree of sensitivity to the size of the zone of inhibition of bacterial growth.

For example, low molecular weight drugs, such as benzylpenicillin or the tetracyclines, diffuse more rapidly through agar than large molecules, such as erythromycin, which could impose an unwarranted bias in selecting the most suitable drug. Thus the results of disc sensitivity tests should simply be reported as resistant or sensitive for each drug used.

Minimum inhibitory concentration (MIC)

Disc techniques provide a qualitative measure of the sensitivity of an organism to various antibiotics, but a quantitative assessment of sensitivity can be obtained by measuring MIC values. Organisms are grown in a range of dilutions of antibiotics and the lowest concentration preventing visible growth is the MIC value of the drug for that organism. Although the MIC value is quantitative, it is still, like the disc sensitivity technique, an *in vitro* measurement. There is no guarantee that a drug with a low MIC will be clinically effective against the same pathogen, because it may not achieve an effective concentration at the site of infection. Dosage recommendations are commonly based on achieving several times the MIC in plasma, but even then the response will be poor if the drug fails to reach infected tissues in effective concentration. An example can be found in intramammary antibiotic therapy of mastitis. The chosen drug(s) may easily exceed the MIC values in milk for the pathogen(s), yet the clinical response can be disappointing. This is due to failure of the drug to reach the organisms because of associated oedema or inflammatory debris, or because the pathogens are tissue-invasive.

Thus, although the sensitivity of the pathogen(s) to antibacterial drugs is an essential factor in the initial selection of appropriate therapy, it must be considered together with the pharmacokinetic properties and possible toxic effects of the drug before a final selection can be made.

Pharmacokinetic properties

Data on the pharmacokinetic properties of antibacterial drugs are largely derived from studies in normal healthy animals and it should be appreciated that disease processes may alter the situation, sometimes to the patient's benefit. For example, the blood–brain barrier prevents most antibiotics, except when administered intrathecally, from attaining antibacterial concentrations in the cerebrospinal fluid. When the meninges are inflamed, however, permeability is increased and oxytetracycline, for example, may then attain therapeutic concentrations in the cerebrospinal fluid. Similarly, orally administered sulphadimidine is absorbed more rapidly in calves with diarrhoea, thus achieving greater peak concentrations at an earlier time than in healthy animals. Further research is required to provide more pharmacokinetic data in diseased animals, but despite this reservation, a brief description of some pharmacokinetic concepts is appropriate in order to appreciate their importance in selecting appropriate antibacterial therapy.

Pharmacokinetic concepts

When antibiotics are administered for a systemic effect, they are absorbed into the circulation and bound to different extents to plasma proteins. Protein binding is readily reversible and the unbound fraction, which is the active form, diffuses freely into extracellular fluid through the fenestrated capillary walls. In the eye and brain, however, the capillaries are not fenestrated and drugs have to cross intact cell membranes to reach the internal structures of the eye or the cerebrospinal fluid. Similarly, there are intact membrane barriers restricting the passage of drugs across the placenta, the mammary gland and the gut wall. The latter is an important consideration when an antibiotic is administered orally for an intended systemic effect. Thus, in carnivores, chloramphenicol is as well absorbed by oral as by parenteral administration. The situation is quite different in calves where chloramphenicol must be given parenterally for a systemic effect, since after about 1 week of age, there is a rapid decrease in the efficiency of absorption of this drug from the gut.

Membrane barriers consist predominantly of lipoprotein and the ability of an antibiotic to cross an intact (non-fenestrated) biological membrane thus depends largely on its lipid solubility. Most antibacterial drugs are weak organic acids or bases and become ionized in the body to an extent depending on the dissociation constant (pK_a) of the drug and the pH of the surrounding medium. Acidic drugs in an acidic environment are largely non-ionized; the converse is true for bases. Thus, trimethoprim being a weak organic base $(pK_a = 7.6)$, is predominantly non-ionized in the plasma (pH = 7.4) and in this form is more lipid soluble. It therefore passes readily into milk to achieve concentrations several times greater than those in plasma. Judged on the criterion of pharmacokinetic properties, the drug would thus be indicated for the systemic treatment of mastitis.

The details of pharmacokinetics of individual antibacterial drugs can be found with the description of the drugs in question. In this chapter, the pharmacokinetic criteria for antibiotic selection will be discussed, together with that of antibacterial spectrum (see previous section), by considering infections in different body systems, which is how the problem of drug selection is presented clinically.

Bactericidal or bacteriostatic action

The distinction between bactericidal and bacteriostatic antibiotics is not absolute, for some drugs may be bacteriostatic at low concentrations and bactericidal if the concentration is sufficiently increased. In most clinical situations, it probably matters little whether a bacteriostatic or bactericidal drug is selected, for even if the normally effective antibacterial barriers provided by the skin, mucosae and secretions are penetrated, bacteria meet a well-developed system of immune responses. However, when these defence mechanisms are impaired it would be preferable to use a bactericidal antibiotic, provided that it meets the other criteria for selection. Situations where the immune system might be inadequate include those in which the patient is old, debilitated or on concurrent corticosteroid therapy.

Potential toxicity

The basic theme of chemotherapy is selective toxicity, which involves the development of drugs which ideally will kill one type of organism, the parasite, yet produce no toxic effect in the patient. This ideal cannot be achieved absolutely with any drug, but the varying degrees of potential toxicity of antibacterials must be considered when making a selection. For example, the penicillins are remarkably non-toxic, whereas gentamicin should only be administered systemically when the severity of the disease process outweighs the potential toxic effects of the drug. Manufacturers' directions should be observed with reference to dosage, any particular species susceptibility, incompatibility with other drugs and withdrawal periods. Details of the toxicity of individual drugs can be found with the description of the drugs in question.

These criteria for antibacterial selection will now be applied to a discussion of appropriate drugs for use in infections of various body systems.

Skin

Normal skin in the dog is colonized by micrococci as resident organisms, but *Staphylococcus aureus*, *Proteus* spp., *Pseudomonas* spp. and streptococci, which are potential pathogens, are occasionally present in the total population. Pyoderma may occur if predisposing factors such as trauma or ectoparasitism permit the pathogenic bacteria to penetrate subcorneally and to colonize the area in sufficient numbers.

Superficial pyodermas usually respond adequately to topical antiseptics formulated as shampoos, lotions or creams. For example, hexetidine and chlorhexidine have a wide antibacterial spectrum and are much cheaper than antibiotics. Sensitivity tests would be indicated on the relatively small proportion of cases which fail to respond, in order to select an appropriate antibiotic, possibly combined with a corticosteroid, for topical therapy.

Cellulitis and furunculosis are examples of deep pyodermas which require systemic and long-term antibiotic therapy for several weeks to achieve more than a transient remission. The patient should be weighed to make sure that the drug is administered at the recommended dosage. Antibacterial sensitivity tests are necessary, but pending the results, initial therapy may be directed at the most likely pathogens, which are staphylococci and streptococci. If the staphylococci do not produce penicillinase, benzylpenicillin should be effective, but lincomycin and erythromycin penetrate tissues more effectively. If laboratory findings confirm a mixed *Proteus* and staphylococcal infection, broader spectrum therapy is necessary. A trimethoprim-sulphonamide combination has the necessary antibacterial spectrum, including activity against penicillin-resistant staphylococci, and pharmacokinetic data indicate that it should attain antibacterial concentrations in the skin. Amoxycillin has broad-spectrum activity and is superior to benzylpenicillin in penetrating tissues, but it is similarly ineffective against penicillinase-producing strains of staphylococci. This deficiency has now been overcome by potentiating amoxycillin with clavulanate. The drug combination is well absorbed after oral administration and it should be among the first choice of drugs for the long-term treatment of deep pyodermas. More recently, a number of cephalosporins have been successfully used for this purpose.

When *Pseudomonas* is associated with deep pyodermas, it presents a therapeutic challenge, since it is resistant to most antibiotics, including those discussed in the preceding paragraph. Polymyxin B is effective *in vitro* but is too toxic for systemic use and the inadequacy of topical therapy for deep pyodermas was mentioned earlier. Selection of an appropriate drug is effectively limited to gentamicin or carbenicillin. Gentamicin is an aminoglycoside with the usual potential of that group for causing nephrotoxicity. In consequence, gentamicin treatment should be for a maximum of 7 days and it should not be used with other drugs. Carbenicillin is a broad-spectrum penicillin which has yet to be evaluated in veterinary medicine. It is not effective against all strains of penicillinase-producing staphylococci, but most strains of *Pseudomonas* are inhibited. Like gentamicin, carbenicillin is not absorbed from the gut and in human patients large doses of this expensive drug are necessary or resistant strains of bacteria may develop.

Pseudomonas is the organism most commonly isolated from burns, together with staphylococci and *Proteus*. The initial local infection may be followed by septicaemia, which is probably responsible for most of the subsequent deaths in burns patients. Management of burns is a major topic and only the aspect of antibacterial selection will be mentioned here. Silver sulphadiazine has a wide spectrum of activity which includes *Pseudomonas* and yeasts. It has proved effective as a 1 per cent cream in reducing infection in human burns patients and does not appear to interfere with subsequent healing or skin grafts. Mafenide is another sulphonamide of proven effectiveness, but may cause discomfort on application. In treating burns which are already infected, parenteral gentamicin may be necessary to supplement topical therapy.

Eye

Superficial infections of the conjunctiva, cornea or drainage apparatus are commonly due to streptococci or staphylococci and usually respond readily to topical therapy. Infections of the interior of the eye present the usual pharmacokinetic problem of ensuring that the infected site is penetrated by antibacterial drugs. Subconjunctival injection of a concentrated dose of appropriate antibiotic is necessary to achieve this because penetration following topical application is normally minimal unless the cornea has been abraded.

Topical preparations are formulated as drops or ointments. The former allow rapid penetration of the antibacterial drug throughout the conjunctival sac, but it is rapidly removed via the conjunctival vessels and nasolacrimal drainage apparatus, so that drops should be instilled at approximately hourly intervals. Neomycin is suggested as the first line of therapy. Therapy should be re-evaluated after 2 or 3 days so that treatment can be changed if there is no improvement. It is recommended that chloramphenicol should only be used when clinical and laboratory results indicate that there is no equally effective antibiotic. Chloramphenicol is a small, un-ionized molecule which is soluble in both lipids and water; thus it crosses membrane barriers very effectively and is exceptional in that it penetrates the globe following topical application. An ointment vehicle ensures longer retention of antibiotics in the conjunctival sac and ophthalmic formulations of a variety of drugs are available. However, it should be appreciated that in cases with conjunctival abrasions or penetrating corneal wounds, sufficient of the lipid vehicle may penetrate intraocularly to cause a severe inflammatory reaction which predisposes to blindness.

When treating infections of the inner structures of the eye, subconjunctival injection of an aqueous solution of antibiotic is the treatment of choice. A concentrated solution, normally 0.5 ml, is introduced through a fine needle inserted into the anaesthetized bulbar conjunctiva. The drug diffuses from this depot across the sclera into the chambers of the eye where therapeutic concentrations are maintained for up to 48 hours. Doses of some drugs administered in this manner in human ophthalmology are as follows: benzylpenicillin, 0.5 mega units; ampicillin, 100 mg; chloramphenicol, 1 mg; neomycin, 100–500 mg and gentamicin, 20–40 mg.

The pathogens commonly associated with conjunctivitis and keratitis in dogs and cats are *Staphylococcus aureus*, streptococci and, less frequently, *E. coli* and *Proteus* species. Neomycin is a common choice in treatment. Less frequently, *Chlamydia* may cause feline contagious conjunctivitis and a tetracycline or chloramphenicol would be appropriate. Again, chloramphenicol should only be used when clinical and laboratory results indicate that there is no equally effective antibiotic. It is a versatile drug, having a broad antibacterial spectrum and being widely distributed in the tissues. Antibacterial concentrations have been demonstrated in the aqueous humour after local application of ophthalmic solutions, and much higher concentrations are attained following subconjunctival injection.

In horses, bacterial eye infections are usually due to Gram-negative organisms and neomycin is a useful first-line therapy. However, fungal keratitis (*Aspergillus, Penicillium*) is apparently more common than in other species. Treatments used are clotrimazole (1 per cent), miconazole (1 per cent) or natamycin (5 per cent) by local application every 2 or 3 hours.

Keratoconjunctivitis in cattle (New Forest disease) and contagious ophthalmia (pink eye) in sheep can become herd and flock problems, with the infection being spread by flies. Various antibacterials have been used by local application, subconjunctival injection or even parenterally. More recently, cloxacillin and benzylpenicillin/streptomycin (for cattle and sheep), and cephalonium (for cattle) have been formulated as ointments to provide effective and prolonged antibacterial concentrations, sometimes after only one application.

Ear

Most bacterial external ear infections (otitis externa) are mixed; yeasts are not infrequently present with a variety of Gram-positive and Gram-negative organisms, most commonly staphylococci, streptococci and *Pseudomonas*.

Laboratory diagnosis can save time, and ultimately costs, in treating this condition because imprudent use of antibiotics can exert a selection pressure for resistant organisms.

Thorough cleaning of the auditory canal with ceruminolytics and cetrimide is a necessary prerequisite to specific antibacterial therapy. In the absence of laboratory diagnosis, topical neomycin is a logical initial selection, probably in conjunction with a corticosteroid to break the vicious cycle of inflammation and self-trauma. Resistant cases are commonly due to *Pseudomonas* becoming dominant and polymyxin B, although too toxic for systemic use, is very effective topically. Medical therapy of chronic otitis externa can only provide a temporary remission of signs; aural resection is necessary to provide adequate ventilation and drainage of the auditory canal. Following thorough irrigation of the tympanic bulla, the selection and local administration of drugs for the treatment of otitis media is similar to that described for otitis externa.

Urinary tract infections

Bacteria most commonly involved in cystitis are *Proteus mirabilis*, coliforms and *Pseudomonas* spp.; in most cases, one bacterial species predominates. Confirmatory laboratory diagnosis should include bacterial counts (more than 10^5 per ml of urine is considered significant) in addition to cultures. Because urine becomes contaminated on passage through the urethra, it is necessary to ensure that the isolates are from the bladder.

Drug selection is based ideally on the results of sensitivity tests, but pending these, either ampicillin or amoxycillin would be a rational choice for initial therapy. These aminopenicillins have broad-spectrum activity (excluding *Pseudomonas*), and attain a particularly high concentration in urine because they are actively secreted in the proximal nephron. Amoxycillin might be preferred because it attains higher concentrations in the plasma and urine than ampicillin and has a more rapid bactericidal action.

Nitrofurantoin and trimethoprim-sulphonamide combinations are useful alternatives to amoxycillin by virtue of their antibacterial spectrum and their ability to attain effective concentrations in the urinary tract. Trimethoprim has the additional and unusual property of penetrating into the canine prostate, which might make it the preferred drug in cases where the prostate acts as a focus of infection in recurrent episodes of cystitis. Streptomycin attains effective antibacterial concentrations in urine and its antibacterial spectrum would be appropriate for many urinary tract infections (except *Pseudomonas*), but it may well produce toxic effects because of the relatively long-term therapy which is necessary to eliminate infections of the urinary tract.

It is suggested that the selected antibiotic be used for a minimum period of 3 days before considering an alternative if the clinical response is inadequate. Therapy with the most effective drug should then be maintained for a minimum period of 10 days in the first episode of the disease, but chronic or recurrent infections may necessitate at least 4 weeks of treatment. A negative culture from a sample taken 5–7 days after ceasing antibacterial therapy is the only effective test of successful treatment. Clinical evidence in dogs indicates that about 70 per cent of cases should respond to one course of proper antibiotic treatment and about 20 per cent require a further one or two courses. The remainder constitute persistent or recurrent infections and are commonly associated with predisposing factors such as bladder diverticuli, neoplasms or calculi.

When *Pseudomonas* is the cause of cystitis, the previous considerations about duration of therapy require modification, since the range of effective drugs is normally limited to colistin, gentamicin and carbenicillin. Carbenicillin is expensive and has to be administered parenterally; the other drugs are potentially nephrotoxic and therapy should be for a maximum period of 7 consecutive days. Limited clinical evidence indicates that gentamicin is the least toxic. Nitrofurantoin or sulphafurazole may be effective by attaining high urinary concentrations, and recent clinical studies on the fluoroquinolones are encouraging. If gentamicin or nitrofurantoin are finally selected, the pH of the urine should be determined and adjusted if necessary with sodium bicarbonate or ascorbic acid, since gentamicin is most effective at pH 7.5–8.0 and nitrofurantoin at pH 5.5–6.0.

Bacterial infection of the upper urinary tract, leading to pyelonephritis, is normally due to reflux of infected urine from the bladder to the renal pelvis and medulla. Consequently, the principles of selection and use of antibacterials are the same as those outlined for the treatment of cystitis.

Acute interstitial nephritis due to *Leptospira* infection appears to respond most rapidly, and with least risk of carriers developing, to a mixture of benzylpenicillin and streptomycin. A commercially prepared fixed-ratio product is unsuitable; procaine penicillin should be administered once daily and streptomycin at 12-hourly intervals, each at its recommended dosage.

The respiratory tract

The complex aetiology of infectious respiratory diseases, divergent views on the relative importance of viruses and bacteria, the importance of an adequate intake of colostrum and the provision of good ventilation are well documented.

Significant advances have been made in the development of vaccines against certain respiratory viral and bacterial pathogens, but chemotherapy still has an important role. There is no specific treatment against viruses but the clinician has to make a rational selection of antibiotics since the control of secondary bacterial infection has proven benefits when viruses are the primary pathogens. Additional therapeutic measures such as cough suppressants, bronchodilators, expectorants and mucolytics are discussed in Chapter 13. Attention is drawn to the possible value of bromhexine as an adjunct to antibiotic therapy, where it appears to enhance the penetration of antibiotics into bronchial mucus. It is necessary to consider groups of species separately.

Dogs and cats

In dogs and cats, respiratory infections with one bacterial species are rare. Organisms which have been isolated can often be recovered from the naso-pharynx of normal animals: *Bordetella*, staphylococci, streptococci, myco-plasmas, coliforms and *Klebsiella* spp. The use of a broad-spectrum antibiotic as first-line therapy is therefore indicated and there are various alternatives based on the criteria of antibacterial spectrum and pharmacokinetic properties. There is relatively little well-documented clinical evidence on the relative efficacy of the drugs, which is the most important criterion for selection.

Tetracyclines attain effective concentrations in the respiratory tract. The antibacterial spectrum includes *Bordetella bronchiseptica* (which many path-ologists believe to be the most significant bacterial pathogen of the bronchial tree of dogs and cats) and mycoplasmas, but streptococcal resistance is not infrequent. Doxycycline is a relatively new tetracycline which has certain pharmacokinetic advantages over established drugs of that group. It has a higher degree of lipid solubility, penetrates more effectively into inflamed respiratory tissue and absorption by the oral route is not inhibited by food.

Tylosin has a narrower antibacterial spectrum, being mainly active against Gram-positive organisms and mycoplasmas. However, it is highly lipid soluble and concentrates very effectively in lung tissue, so that if the pathogens are sensitive, it is a drug of choice.

Alternative broad-spectrum antibacterials to tetracyclines which concentrate sufficiently in the respiratory tract are trimethoprim-sulphonamide com-binations and broad-spectrum penicillins. Amoxycillin attains higher concen-trations in bronchial tissue than ampicillin.

Whichever drug is used, therapy should be maintained for several weeks when treating pneumonia or pleurisy. In the latter case, thoracotomy and chest drainage may be necessary.

Pigs

In this species, viral infections of the respiratory tract are considered to be less important than bacterial and mycoplasmal infections. The common pathogens are mycoplasmas (causing enzootic pneumonia), *Bordetella* (causing pneumonia and bronchitis in piglets and possibly involved in the aetiology of atrophic rhinitis), *Haemophilus* (causing pleuropneumonia in piglets, sometimes leading to bacteraemia with meningitis and arthritis) and *Pasteurella multocida*, which appears to be secondary to a mycoplasmal or *Bordetella* infection.

Tylosin and the broad-spectrum antibacterials discussed for use in small animals would also be suitable for pigs on the criteria of bacterial sensitivity and current knowledge of pharmacokinetics. There is some clinical evidence to indicate that the administration of tiamulin in drinking water is superior to either tylosin or tetracyclines for the treatment of enzootic pneumonia. When treating large numbers of animals, selection will be influenced by cost and availability of suitable premixes or formulations for medicating drinking water.

Cattle

As in other species, a variety of viruses, mycoplasmas and bacteria are commonly involved in the aetiology of infectious respiratory disease, so again it is logical to select a broad-spectrum antibiotic. Oxytetracycline is probably the commonest first-line therapy on the criteria of bacterial sensitivity, effective tissue distribution, cost-effectiveness and clinical results. When calves are presented in the pre-pneumonic stage, the drug is usually administered in the drinking water for 5–10 days. It should be appreciated that calcium significantly impairs the absorption of tetracyclines, which should not be given with milk. Pneumonic animals are likely to be inappetent and the intravenous administration of oxytetracycline is usually effective, supplemented with a long-acting intramuscular formulation to maintain tissue concentrations.

Alternatives to tetracyclines which have proven efficacy are trimethoprim-sulphonamide combinations or amoxycillin. None of these antibiotics is particularly effective against mycoplasmas. If there is no satisfactory clinical response within about 3 days, or if *Mycoplasma* species are known to be major pathogens, tylosin would be the drug of choice, although recent *in vitro* studies indicate that, as in pigs, tiamulin might be more effective.

If laboratory and clinical data suggest that chloramphenicol is the antibiotic of choice, effective use in calves depends on an appreciation of the pharmacokinetics of the drug. Although it is a small, non-ionized molecule which usually crosses biological membranes easily, after the first few days of life it is not absorbed from the gut in calves and must be administered parenterally. A daily intramuscular dose of 50 mg/kg chloramphenicol succinate is necessary to achieve effective antibacterial plasma concentrations. From the age of 3 months this dose should be administered twice daily because the drug is more rapidly metabolized by older animals.

The use of corticosteroids as adjuncts to antibacterials in the treatment of respiratory infections is controversial. They can produce marked symptomatic improvement in the early stages by suppressing the acute stage of inflammation. However, they also suppress the repair process in the later stages and may thus impair resolution of the parenchymatous tissue. These considerations apply to all species, but there is most clinical evidence from studies in cattle. Corticosteroids as adjuncts to antibiotic therapy are contraindicated in infectious bovine rhinotracheitis and in *Pasteurella* bronchial pneumonia (shipping fever). In the treatment of calf pneumonia, it is generally considered that the risk of producing chronic disease outweighs any benefit which corticosteroids may produce.

Unlike the corticosteroids, non-steroidal anti-inflammatory drugs (see Chapter 8) neither reduce resistance to infection nor impair the healing process. Experimental and clinical evidence has shown that in cases of calf pneumonia, flunixin gives rapid symptomatic relief with a marked reduction in the extent of pulmonary consolidation. It is now used in conjunction with antibiotics for the treatment of this condition.

Horses

The common bacterial pathogens associated with respiratory disease in horses are streptococci, staphylococci, pasteurellae and, in foals, *Corynebacterium equi* as a cause of pneumonia. It is likely that the organisms will be sensitive *in vitro* to benzylpenicillin and this will therefore be the first choice in most instances. When dealing with *Streptococcus equi* (strangles) infections, however, infected lymph nodes should be drained surgically because antibacterials may promote the development of encapsulated abscesses; antibiotics are indicated when there is pulmonary or joint involvement.

Plasma concentrations of benzylpenicillin tend to be lower in horses than in other species, therefore maximum recommended doses of soluble penicillin (sodium or potassium salt) should be administered twice daily and procaine penicillin used only as an adjunct. Long-acting preparations, such as benzathine penicillin, are too slowly absorbed to attain effective tissue concentrations except in the most sensitive infections. Penicillin is water-soluble and distributes freely throughout the body fluids following its absorption.

If subsequent laboratory diagnosis indicates resistance to benzylpenicillin, either amoxycillin or trimethoprim-sulphonamide (assuming that the bacterial sensitivity is appropriate) attain effective concentrations in respiratory tissues and amoxycillin appears to be retained in bronchial mucus. Tetracyclines should not be used in horses because of possible toxic effects.

Clinical evidence indicates that, to avoid relapses when treating severe bacterial infections of the respiratory tract in horses, antibacterial therapy should be maintained for about 10 days after cessation of clinical signs. Some practical problems may be associated with the need for repeated injections.

Central nervous system

Bacterial infections causing meningitis or encephalitis are likely to be mixed; furthermore, treatment should be instituted without delay, which is probably before the pathogen(s) can be identified. For example, in the dog meningitis may be due to the spread of infection from the inner ear or sinuses, or from compound skull fractures. In young calves, it may follow navel infections, coliform septicaemias or pneumonia. In older animals meningitis may occur secondarily to septicaemic salmonellosis, pneumonia or coliform mastitis. Meningitis in foals and piglets is usually due to beta-haemolytic streptococci.

Selection of a broad-spectrum antibiotic is therefore usually appropriate and the field of choice is narrowed on the criterion of pharmacokinetic properties. Apart from the aminoglycosides, most antibacterials will penetrate to some degree into the cerebrospinal fluid (CSF) from the circulation when the meninges are inflamed. Penicillins attain therapeutic concentrations in the CSF in meningitis following parenteral administration of high doses of soluble preparations. Amoxycillin would therefore be a useful choice as it has a rapid bactericidal action and large doses can be administered without danger of toxicity. Chloramphenicol has recently been found to be bactericidal against some organisms (e.g. meningeal pathogens) at clinically achievable concentrations.

However, only a few of the commonly used antibacterials attain therapeutic concentrations in the CSF by standard doses and routes of administration when the meninges are not inflamed. These are chloramphenicol, doxycycline (after repeated doses), trimethoprim and the sulphonamides (especially sulphadiazine, which is commonly combined with trimethoprim). It might be desirable to select from this group, assuming the antibacterial spectrum is suitable, so as to maintain effective concentrations in the CSF and eliminate any residual pathogens after the acute inflammatory phase has subsided. If chloramphenicol is used, the importance of proper dosage and route of administration is emphasized, as explained in the previous section on respiratory infections.

In view of the above factors, a rational selection of first-choice drugs to be given at maximum non-toxic doses should be made. For streptococcal or *Haemophilus* infections, sodium benzylpenicillin given intravenously every 6 hours should be appropriate. An alternative is ampicillin sodium (i.v.) every 6 hours; this would also be a rational choice for treating mixed infections in dogs and cats. For treating Gram-negative meningitis in calves, trimethoprim-sulphonamide could be the drug of choice, given intravenously at 8-hourly intervals. The above dosage intervals and intravenous routes of administration are intended to provide intermittent peak bactericidal concentrations in the CSF, which current evidence suggests is the critical factor in therapy because phagocytic activity in the CSF is poor. However, there is clinical evidence that phenoxymethylpenicillin as in-feed medication is highly successful in the control of streptococcal meningitis in pigs. In human patients, new cephalosporins such as cefotaxime are increasingly used. These have broad-spectrum activity, penetrate into the CSF and are bactericidal at relatively lower concentrations; they are also very expensive.

If two antibiotics are used concurrently in the treatment of meningitis, a combination of bactericidal drugs (e.g. penicillins) and bacteriostatic drugs (e.g. tetracyclines, chloramphenicol) should be avoided. There is both clinical and experimental evidence to show that drug antagonism may result; bactericidal drugs are effective against multiplying organisms but bacteriostatic drugs inhibit multiplication. Theoretically, antagonism could arise when using such combinations to treat bacterial infections other than meningitis, but there appears to be no evidence to suggest that it is of clinical significance.

Bovine mastitis

The principles of the selection of antibiotics for the treatment of mastitis are the same as those discussed in relation to other conditions, but the pathological features of mastitis require that particular consideration be given to the pharmacokinetic properties of the drugs.

Most cases of economic importance are due to staphylococci, streptococci and coliforms, with signs varying from a mild local reaction to severe systemic involvement. Antibiotic sensitivity tests are useful in preliminary selection of drugs but some cases are resistant to treatment even though the pathogens show *in vitro* sensitivity to the drugs used. This is not normally due to selection for drug-resistant strains but to failure of sufficient antibiotic to reach the pathogens. Inflammatory debris and oedema cause compression or blocking of the milk duct system which impedes diffusion of the drug through the milk. Further, staphylococci are tissue-invasive and become walled off by fibrous tissue which the antibiotics may not be able to penetrate.

Intramammary therapy

Following infusion, the antibiotic is released from the formulation and becomes partially bound to proteins in the milk and udder tissue. The unbound fraction is partially ionized, to an extent depending on the pH of the milk and the dissociation constant of the drug. It is the unbound, non-ionized, lipid-soluble fraction which crosses tissue barriers to reach the pathogens.

The ideal properties of a drug selected for the treatment of mastitis include a low MIC value, good tissue penetration, a low degree of protein-binding, low irritancy and a short milk withholding time. Some of these properties, particularly distribution through the udder, can be assessed by measuring the rate of absorption of the antibiotic into the circulation following intramammary infusion. The extent of distribution of some of the available antibacterials is shown below:

Good distribution	Moderate distribution	Poor distribution
ampicillin	benzylpenicillin	bacitracin
amoxycillin	cloxacillin	aminoglycosides
penethamate	cephoxazole	polymyxins
novobiocin	cephalonium	
erythromycin	tetracyclines	
nitrofurans		

Selection of an appropriate drug should be based on the optimum combination of antibiotic sensitivity and ability to distribute throughout the udder.

Systemic therapy

Systemic antibiotic administration is not normally used as the only route, but rather as an adjunct to intramammary infusion to provide better drug penetration of the udder tissue. Bovine plasma has a pH of 7.4 whilst the pH of normal milk is 6.5–6.8. Thus, a basic drug will be largely non-ionized in plasma and, provided that it is not extensively protein-bound, should diffuse through membrane barriers to concentrate in milk. At this acidic pH, a basic drug will be more extensively ionized and therefore 'trapped'. Theoretically, the extent of ion trapping is reduced in mastitic milk because the pH is nearer to that of plasma. However, analogous to the situation in meningitis, the integrity of the blood–milk barrier appears to be reduced by mastitis and antibiotics penetrate more readily.

The extent to which antibiotics penetrate udder tissue following parenteral administration is determined by measuring milk : serum concentrations and the data below should be useful in selecting drugs for systemic therapy.

Good distribution	Moderate distribution	Poor distribution
tylosin	sulphonamides	aminoglycosides
lincomycin	penicillins	
penethamate	tetracyclines	
trimethoprim		

When selection for systemic therapy is based on these pharmacokinetic principles, together with sensitivity of the pathogens, appropriate antibiotics in staphylococcal mastitis would be tylosin, trimethoprim-sulphonamide or oxytetracycline. For systemic treatment of Gram-negative infections, trimethoprim-sulphonamide or oxytetracycline would be the drugs of choice. There is clinical evidence that spectinomycin is effective in treating acute coliform mastitis.

Tylosin is lipid-soluble and, following systemic administration, attains a concentration in milk of about twice that in plasma. A dose of 12 mg/kg maintains milk concentrations greater than 1 µg/ml (the average MIC for streptococci and staphylococci) for 24 hours.

Trimethoprim, like tylosin, is a weak base and distributes readily from plasma to milk, but in solution it is rapidly cleared from the body and a suspension (e.g. Tribrissen 48 per cent), which is more slowly absorbed, must be used to maintain blood levels. A high dose, of the order of 45 mg/kg, which is three times the normal recommended dose, is required to maintain therapeutic concentrations in the milk for 12 hours.

An intravenous dose of oxytetracycline (10 mg/kg) will maintain therapeutic concentrations in milk for 24 hours. This route is recommended as there is evidence to suggest that absorption from intramuscular sites is too slow to achieve adequate concentrations in milk. However, the newer long-acting formulation of oxytetracycline apparently attains peak plasma concentrations within a few hours of intramuscular injection and therefore should be a useful alternative.

The selection of antibiotics for therapy of clinical mastitis has been discussed on the basis of the important criteria of sensitivity of the pathogens and the pharmacokinetic properties of the drugs, but other therapeutic measures are equally important. Fluid therapy is essential in the treatment of acute mastitis where hypotension and metabolic acidosis are associated with absorption of bacterial endotoxins. Secondly, it is generally recognized that bovine mastitis can realistically only be controlled rather than eliminated. In this context, in addition to proper milking machine maintenance and milking parlour hygiene, dry-cow therapy plays an important role. The objectives of dry-cow therapy are to eliminate existing subclinical infection of the udder and to provide prophylaxis during the dry period. Formulations of broad-spectrum antibacterials are available to provide therapeutic concentrations in the udder after a single infusion for the whole of the average dry period.

The use of non-steroidal anti-inflammatory drugs, such as flunixin, as adjuncts to antibiotic therapy was discussed under the heading of respiratory diseases in cattle. More recently, they have been used similarly in the treatment of acute mastitis and early clinical reports are encouraging.

Gastrointestinal tract

The criteria for selecting an antibiotic for treating an enteric bacterial infection are the same as discussed for treating bacterial infections in other sites of the body. However, when treating intensively reared calves or pigs, the decision is complicated by the distinct possibility that the gut microflora will have transmissible resistance to a variety of antimicrobial drugs. In addition, even if rectal swabs are examined for identification of bacteria and antibiotic sensitivity, there may be a poor correlation between the results of the isolates and the true pathogens in the ileum. Consequently, selection is commonly based on previous experience of the most effective treatment on a particular farm.

Farm livestock species

The use of antibiotics is only one aspect of the treatment of infectious diarrhoea in any species. Vaccines are available for passive immunization by dam vaccination of calves, lambs and piglets against enterotoxic *E. coli* and, more recently, against rotavirus in calves. Drugs for symptomatic treatment of diarrhoea are discussed in Chapter 14. In virus-induced diarrhoea, the net loss of water and electrolytes from the body is due to damage of the intestinal villi with consequent malabsorption and net secretion of fluid into the lumen. Enteropathogenic *E. coli*, which are the commonest causes of diarrhoea in neonatal calves and pigs, possess specific cell-surface antigens (adhesion factors) which enable them to adhere to the intestinal mucosa, where the organisms multiply and produce enterotoxins. The enterotoxins stimulate secretion into the intestinal lumen by activation of intracellular enzymes rather than damage to the villi. Salmonellae apparently cause diarrhoea either by enterotoxin production or by damaging the intestinal villi.

It will be apparent from this brief outline of the aetiology of infectious diarrhoea that an adequate intake of colostrum by newborn animals is important. Newborn animals can absorb colostral immunoglobulins through the epithelial cells for approximately one day after birth to provide a massive transfusion of the maternal immunoglobulins. After that time, the epithelial cells lose the ability to absorb protein. In addition to the systemic effects, immunoglobulins can act locally against the *E. coli* adhesion factors and thus prevent colonization.

Although antibiotics are probably the most common treatment when infectious diarrhoea is established, the importance of proper rehydration therapy cannot be over-emphasized, since dehydration is the main cause of death. For example, it has been demonstrated that an oral glucose–glycine–electrolyte formulation was as effective as amoxycillin in reducing the duration of scouring and mortality rate in calves experimentally infected with enteropathogenic *E. coli*, *Salmonella* and rotavirus. However, the best results were obtained by combining both treatments. Thus the rational treatment of bacteria-induced diarrhoea in young farm animals is a combined strategy of ensuring adequate intake of colostrum plus oral rehydration therapy and selective use of antibiotics.

Surveys of antibiotic resistance patterns of *E. coli* isolates from calves and pigs show a high percentage of resistance to tetracyclines, sulphonamides and streptomycin but a lower incidence of resistance to ampicillin and furazolidone. This accords with controlled studies in experimental colibacillosis infections. In both calves and pigs, the following antibacterials were superior to placebos: ampicillin, amoxycillin, apramycin, furazolidone and trimethoprim-sulphadiazine.

The resistance pattern in *Salmonella* serotypes is slightly different from that for *E. coli*. A large percentage of all serotypes are resistant to sulphonamides and streptomycin, but despite the widespread use of antibiotics, most strains are sensitive to apramycin, the tetracyclines, neomycin, ampicillin, amoxycillin, furazolidone, trimethoprim-sulphonamide and chloramphenicol. In mixed infections with salmonellae and coliforms, it should be possible to select an antibiotic which is effective against both.

The systemic use of chloramphenicol should be restricted to situations where clinical and laboratory assessments indicate that no other antibiotic would be equally effective. Caution in using the drug is justified because it is said to be valuable in the treatment of *Salmonella typhi* (typhoid) infections in humans and its indiscriminate use in veterinary medicine might increase the possibility of the development of resistance, which could be transmitted to the human pathogen.

If chloramphenicol is selected to treat systemic salmonellosis in cattle, it should be administered parenterally. The drug is degraded by the rumen microflora and this occurs in calves from about 9 weeks of age. Even before this age, the drug is not effectively absorbed from the gut (in calves) and parenteral administration is essential for generalized systemic infections. Recent studies on the pharmacokinetics of chloramphenicol in calves have shown that in the past there has been a tendency to underdose. To attain effective antibacterial concentrations in plasma (at least 5 μg/ml), a daily intramuscular dose of 30 μg/kg (base) is necessary; in animals over 3 months old this dose should be administered twice daily because the drug is more rapidly metabolized in the liver.

In view of the public health implications of resistance to chloramphenicol, it is recommended that only sufficient be left on the farm to continue treatment of animals immediately concerned.

It has been explained that most *Salmonella* serotypes are sensitive to a range of antibiotics, but a few phage types of *Salmonella typhimurium* have demonstrated multi-resistance to up to eight antibacterials. In calves, these have caused outbreaks of serious disease which are virtually untreatable with antibiotics, but the significant epidemiological factor in the spread of the disease was the movement of infected calves across the country rather than antibiotic selection pressure. Perhaps the well-tried and tested methods of statutory notification, isolation and movement control would be more effective in limiting any future disease outbreaks, rather than proposing limitations on the veterinary use of antibiotics.

Swine dysentery

The anaerobic spirochaete *Treponema hyodysenteriae* is considered to be the primary pathogen in swine dysentery, but it requires the presence of other organisms, commonly *Bacteroides* and *Fusobacterium* to produce the typical signs. The development of effective antimicrobial drugs has reduced mortality and a bacteriological cure can be achieved in animals which might otherwise harbour the organisms in the colon without them being demonstrated by culture from rectal swabs.

Selection can be made from a variety of drugs for treatment or prophylaxis, and formulations are available for in-feed or water medication: dimetridazole, lincomycin, ronidazole, tiamulin, tylosin. Basic hygienic measures must be used in addition to therapy in prevention and control programmes because there is no reliable test to detect clinically normal carrier animals.

Small animals

Antibiotics are not indicated for the majority of cases of diarrhoea in small animals because improper diet is the commonest cause of chronic or recurrent episodes and most acute diarrhoeas are self-limiting. The owner should be instructed to withhold solid food for 24 hours and to encourage the animal to take fluids. Proprietary electrolyte preparations are available, but one teaspoonful of salt per 500 ml of water is often adequate.

The symptomatic treatment of diarrhoea is discussed in Chapter 14, and this conservative therapy may suffice even in cases associated with bacterial infection; antibiotics are indicated in cases which fail to respond or where there is evidence of systemic infection. When there is no evidence of systemic infection, it is rational to select from the drugs which may be administered orally and which are poorly absorbed from the gut, thus attaining a high concentration at the site of infection. The gut-active sulphonamides (phthalylsulphathiazole, succinylsulphathiazole) and neomycin are commonly used antibacterials of this type, and commercial preparations are available which incorporate adsorbents and/or antispasmodics.

When infection is not confined to the gut, there is a choice of various broad-spectrum antibiotics for oral administration which are formulated to produce an effect in the gut but which are sufficiently well absorbed to combat systemic infections. For example, oxytetracycline, trimethoprim-sulphonamide, ampicillin and amoxycillin fulfil this criterion. The broad-spectrum penicillins are particularly useful when the patient is vomiting, since they can be administered parenterally to attain antibacterial concentrations in the small intestine because they are concentrated in the bile and thus secreted into the gut. Erythromycin is the drug of choice for treating *Campylobacter jejuni* enteritis in cats and dogs.

In cases of protracted infective diarrhoea, fresh yoghurt is a useful therapeutic adjunct which provides a source of lactobacilli to aid recolonization of the gut and to discourage colonization by pathogens. When diarrhoea persists after appropriate antibiotic therapy, laboratory diagnosis is advisable as there may be a proliferation of yeasts following suppression of the normal flora. Nystatin (100 000 units every 6 hours) is indicated in this situation, but it is not suggested that it is necessary to use it routinely as a prophylactic whenever tetracyclines, for example, are administered orally.

When either 'gut-active' or 'systemic' antibacterials are used against enteric pathogens, the normal gut flora will also be suppressed and this deprives the patient of B vitamins. If treatment has to be continued for more than 3 or 4 days, a vitamin B supplement would be indicated.

Bacterial endometritis

For the treatment of bacterial endometritis, specific antibacterial drugs may be selected based on the results of sensitivity tests, but in all species infections tend to be mixed, so that broad-spectrum therapy is usually used as first-line treatment.

In the mare, mixed infections of aerobic and sometimes anaerobic organisms are usually present and current clinical evidence suggests that systemic antibacterial therapy alone is rarely effective. For local intrauterine therapy in mares, formulations which are irritant or which contain insoluble constituents (e.g. pessaries) should be avoided and a water-soluble preparation selected. Good results are reported with a water-soluble mixture of neomycin (1 g), polymyxin B (40 000 units), furaltadone (600 mg) and crystalline benzyl-penicillin (5 megaunits) infused daily into the uterus for 3–5 days via a sterile catheter. Successful treatment of endometritis in mares requires that any predisposing factors such as cervical or rectovaginal damage, or pneumovagina are also corrected. Gentamicin is a drug of choice for metritis in mares caused by *Klebsiella* or *Pseudomonas*. It is infused into the uterus at oestrus for 3–5 days (250 ml saline, 10 mg/ml).

Puerperal metritis may occur in cows a few days after parturition and is often associated with difficult calving, uterine inertia or retained placenta. Pathogens commonly isolated are streptococci, staphylococci, *Corynebacterium pyogenes*, clostridia and *E. coli*. Pharmacokinetic studies show that penicillins and tetracyclines reach antibacterial concentrations in the uterus following systemic dosing, which is useful since infection may not be confined to the endometrium. Treatment is usually a combination of broad-spectrum antibacterials, administered both systemically and by infusion (or pessaries) into the uterus. Pessaries may be used prophylactically after difficult calvings. Oxytocin is indicated as an adjunct to antibacterials in cases seen within one or two days of calving when the myometrium is sensitive to its ecbolic action.

Metritis in recently farrowed sows may be associated with retained foetuses or deaths *in utero* arising from systemic bacteraemia or infection via the vagina. The foetuses should be removed if possible. Successful results have been reported with trimethoprim-sulphonamide administered systemically, together with intrauterine infusion of metronidazole for anaerobic infection. At least 7 to 10 days of treatment is usually necessary.

In small animals, metritis is also usually due to mixed infections—streptococci, *E. coli*, *Proteus* and *Haemophilus*—so that broad-spectrum antibacterial therapy is indicated. A trimethoprim-sulphonamide, broad-spectrum penicillin or tetracycline would be a rational choice. Although there are reports of using prostaglandins in the treatment of closed pyometra (see Chapter 15), the drugs are toxic in bitches and surgery is preferred.

Orthopaedic infections

Asepsis is mandatory during orthopaedic surgery because the intervention potentiates colonization by bacteria. There is some degree of ischaemia, and following fracture repair a haematoma forms; both factors contribute to provide a good environment for bacterial growth. Thus antibiotics, commonly benzylpenicillin plus streptomycin, may be used prophylactically, i.e. pre-operatively, and for 3 or 4 days post-operatively to produce inhibitory concentrations in the clot. When infection does occur, surgical drainage and irrigation are necessary, together with sensitivity tests to determine the appropriate drug(s) for local and systemic administration.

Infectious arthritis

The main concern in cases of infectious arthritis is the potential destruction of articular cartilage by the adherence of fibrin clots and the ideal therapeutic goal is sterilization of the joint and removal of debris and fibrin. In septic arthritis (joint-ill) in foals, this usually necessitates drainage of synovial fluid, sampling for sensitivity testing, irrigation with saline and administration of antibiotics locally and systemically. Pending the results of sensitivity tests, a combination of 5 per cent neomycin sulphate locally with benzylpenicillin and streptomycin systemically has proved successful. Treatment for at least 10 days is usually necessary.

Septic arthritis in other species (e.g. joint-ill in young farm animals) is usually treated with systemic antibiotics and, as in foals, requires prolonged therapy. There is often a mixture of Gram-positive and Gram-negative pathogens and in the absence of sensitivity tests results, initial drug selection is usually from benzylpenicillin and streptomycin, amoxycillin or cephalexin. Lincomycin or tylosin are indicated for the treatment of mycoplasmal arthritis in pigs.

Foot infections

The common foot-rot infections of ruminants, caused by *Fusobacterium necrophorum* in cattle and a mixture of *Fusobacterium necrophorum*, *Bacteroides nodosus* and *Corynebacterium pyogenes* in sheep, are sensitive to a range of antibiotics. Selection for systemic administration is usually made from benzylpenicillin or tylosin for cattle, and erythromycin or benzylpenicillin plus streptomycin for sheep. Local aerosol applications of cetrimide in cattle and dichlorophen in sheep are often used in addition, together with footbaths of zinc sulphate in sheep. It is essential, particularly in sheep, that attention is given to basic husbandry such as foot paring and pasture management.

A particular problem in pigs is the condition known as bush-foot. It is associated with tissue necrosis (debridement is necessary) and infection with a variety of anaerobes. Lincomycin and oxytetracycline have been used with moderate success, but metronidazole might prove more effective.

CHAPTER 20

ANTIPROTOZOAL DRUGS

Introduction

Most protozoa are non-parasitic. For example, there are many protozoan species which inhabit the rumen as commensals. These organisms may even have symbiotic effects by facilitating the digestion of cellulose. Nevertheless, infections by pathogenic protozoa are the cause of many diseases in animals, especially in those which are raised under intensive conditions.

Protozoa are unicellular organisms which, unlike most bacteria, do not have a rigid cell wall and have their genetic material located in chromosomes within the nucleus. They also possess an endoplasmic reticulum, mitochondria and a Golgi body and lysosomes. They are generally larger than bacteria and lead an independent existence, feeding on organic material, usually by pinocytosis or phagocytosis. Many protozoa are motile and use a single flagellum (e.g. trypanosomes), cilia (e.g. *Balantidium*) or amoeboid activity (e.g. *Entamoeba*) to effect locomotion. Other protozoa (e.g. some stages of *Eimeria*) have no obvious means of locomotion.

Protozoa often have complex life cycles, which may vary greatly, even in closely related species, and may involve more than one host (e.g. an arthropod vector). Both asexual and sexual reproduction may occur.

The classification of the protozoa is extremely complex. The four main subphyla are grouped according to mode of locomotion. The most important groups are Sarcodina (e.g. *Entamoeba*), Mastigophora (e.g. *Trypanosoma, Leishmania, Trichomonas, Histomonas, Giardia*), Coccidia (e.g. *Eimeria, Isospora, Cryptosporidium, Toxoplasma, Sarcocystis*), Piroplasma (e.g. *Babesia, Theileria*) and Haemosporidium (e.g. *Plasmodium, Haemoproteus*).

Sarcodinal infections

Amoebiasis

The causative organism is *Entamoeba histolytica*, which is primarily a human pathogen. The veterinary significance of human amoebiasis is that infections, without clinical signs, occasionally occur in dogs. Dogs, however, are not believed to constitute a reservoir for human infection.

Infection is by ingestion of viable quadrinucleate cysts, which appear in formed stools. The cyst releases amoeba-like trophozoites which migrate to the large intestine and secrete proteolytic enzymes, which produce ulcers in the intestinal wall and allow the parasites to enter the bloodstream. This often results in the formation of amoebic abscesses in the liver and elsewhere.

Prophylaxis depends largely on adequate human sanitation. Diagnosis depends on identification of motile organisms and cysts in faecal smears.

All forms of the disease can be treated with metronidazole, which enters and is retained in the protozoal cells at concentrations where no uptake into mammalian cells occurs. The drug acts to disrupt energy production mechanisms in the protozoa by preventing the generation of reducing equivalents. It is sometimes used in combination with di-iodohydroxy-quinoline.

Mastigophoral infections

Trypanosomiasis

Trypanosomes are flagellates which live in the blood and tissues of vertebrates. Parasitic trypanosomes infect a wide variety of vertebrate species (cattle, horses, sheep, dogs and pigs), which are the definitive hosts. A few species are of great importance in that they cause widespread sickness and death in both animals and humans in tropical regions. Typically, they have complex life cycles, often involving an arthropod vector (e.g. tsetse flies). In cyclical transmission, the vector becomes infected when it ingests mammalian blood containing infective forms of the parasite. The parasite then multiplies and undergoes changes within the vector before being inoculatively introduced into new hosts (e.g. *Trypanosoma congolense*, *T. vivax*, *T. simiae* and *T. brucei*). Trypanosomes in this group are termed the Salivaria.

Cattle infected by the Salivaria exhibit a disease known as nagana, which is characterized by anaemia, lymphoid enlargement and splenomegaly. The animals lose condition and become progressively lethargic and the condition is usually fatal after some months although some strains of *T. vivax* can cause death within weeks. In horses, *T. brucei* infections are often accompanied by oedema. *T. congolense* infections in pigs are usually mild but infections by *T. simiae* can cause severe pyrexia and are often rapidly fatal. Dogs and cats which are infected by *T. congolense* and *T. brucei* often exhibit fever, anaemia, and corneal opacity and there may also be cardiovascular and neurological signs.

In other trypanosomal species (e.g. *T. melophagium* and *T. theileri*) multiplication and transformation occur in the gut of the host and infective forms of the parasite are voided in the faeces. These parasites (Stercoraria) are transferred from one host to another by flies. Stercorarial infections of cattle and sheep are usually asymptomatic but a related trypanosome (*T. cruzi*), transmitted among humans in a similar way by a bug, causes Chagas' disease, a serious endemic disease found in Central and South America.

In non-cyclical (mechanical) transmission (e.g. *T. evansi*), parasites are transferred from one definitive host to another by biting insects and (in South America) by vampire bats. Carnivores may become infected by eating trypanosome-infected prey. An example of a trypanosomal (*T. evansi*) disease which is transmitted mechanically is surra, which primarily affects horses and may cause anaemia, emaciation and oedema. In the chronic form of the disease there is progressive paralysis of the hindquarters. A related South American organism (*T. equinum*) causes mal de Caderas, which affects the hip.

One exception is *T. equiperdum*, which causes a venereal disease (dourine) in horses and donkeys. The signs generally consist only of abdominal oedema and urticarial swelling but CNS involvement, resulting in ascending motor paralysis, may also occur.

Drugs used in the treatment of trypanosome infections

Arsenicals

Arsenic was used to treat malaria in the 18th and 19th centuries (Fowler's solution—potassium arsenite) and in 1894 it was shown that Fowler's solution would temporarily eliminate trypanosomes from the blood of cattle with nagana and mice with experimental infections. In 1905 it was found that the organic pentavalent arsenical compound, Atoxyl, was trypanocidal, and this stimulated the search for less toxic compounds (e.g. arsphenamine, tryparsamide, melarsen and melarsoprol). They appear to owe their activity to their relative ease of uptake into the parasite and an ability to disrupt glucose metabolism by inhibiting pyruvate kinase. Mammalian tissues rapidly oxidize melarsoprol to pentavalent compounds, which are rapidly eliminated.

Melarsoprol is usually given by intravenous injection. Although organic arsenicals are rather toxic, they penetrate the CNS readily and are thus usually reserved for advanced trypanosomal infections.

Antimonials

In the period from 1906 to 1908, injections of antimony potassium tartrate (tartar emetic) were successfully used to treat human trypanosomiasis (and other protozoal diseases) and experimental trypanosomal infections in cattle. Antimony potassium tartrate is irritant and very toxic, however, and attempts were made to synthesize less toxic organic antimonials. The most important of these is stibophen, a trivalent antimonial compound which is as effective and much less toxic than antimony potassium tartrate. Larger doses can thus be given for longer periods. Sodium stibogluconate is a pentavalent antimonial compound which remains in wide use in human medicine, largely for the treatment of leishmaniasis. The precise mechanism of action of these drugs has not been determined. Sodium stibogluconate is given intramuscularly. Antimony potassium tartrate is still occasionally used in veterinary medicine:

Dose

horses and cattle	3–5 mg/kg i.v.
dog and cat	1–3 mg/kg i.v.

Dyes

Trypan Red and Trypan Blue

In 1904, Ehrlich examined the effects of a series of dyes against experimental trypanosomiasis in mice. The most active member of the initial series was a benzopurin derivative, named Nagana Red, which caused a rapid disappearance of the organisms from the blood and an increased survival time. Further structure-activity studies led to the synthesis of Trypan Red, Afridol Violet and Trypan Blue (Fig. 20.1), which rapidly eliminated trypanosomes from the mice and had a mild action against several trypanosomal species that cause disease in cattle. In 1909, when it was shown that Trypan Blue could also cure piroplasmosis, the drug was introduced into veterinary medicine. Further development eventually resulted in the synthesis of suramin, which remains an effective drug for the prevention and treatment of trypanosomiasis.

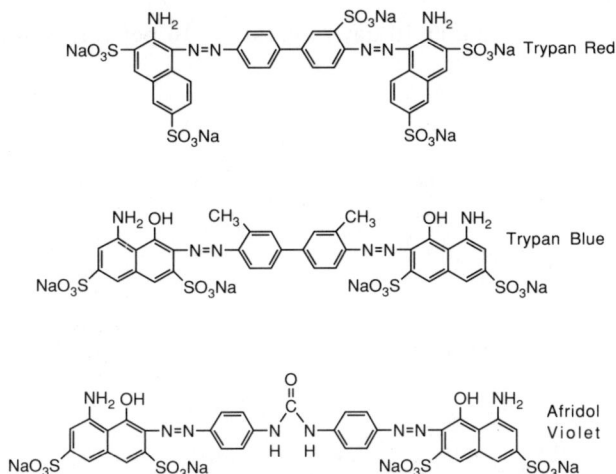

Figure 20.1 Dyes effective against experimental trypanosomiasis.

Suramin

Suramin (Fig. 20.2) is a complex water-soluble derivative of urea. The drug binds avidly to proteins and inhibits so many trypanosomal enzymes that it has proved impossible to establish the locus of the drug's effect, although inhibition of glycerol phosphate oxidase in the parasite has been proposed as a possible mechanism of action. Suramin is slow to act and has a prolonged effect which confers a prophylactic potential. It is extensively tissue-bound and does not cross the blood–brain barrier. Low levels of the drug can be detected in plasma for months after administration.

Suramin can be used to eradicate *T. evansi* infections in horses, cattle and dogs but is less effective as a prophylactic. The drug is rather less active against *T. brucei* and *T. equiperdum*, and is ineffective against *T. vivax* and *T. congolense*. For prophylaxis, suramin has been given at 10-day intervals. *T. brucei* infections in dogs and cats can be treated effectively with suramin. It is usually given by the slow intravenous injection of a 10 per cent solution. The drug has a narrow therapeutic index but cattle tolerate the drug better than horses.

Dose

Treatment
    horse   7–10 mg/kg
    cattle   12 mg/kg

Prophylaxis   1–2 g at 10-day intervals as 10 per cent solution.

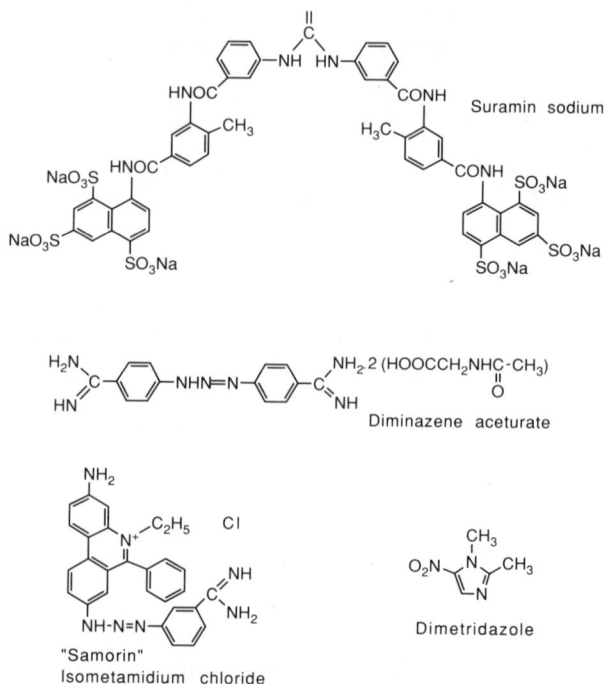

Figure 20.2 Drugs used in the treatment of infections with Mastigophoran species.

Diamidines

The diamidines were developed shortly after suramin. It was noted that trypanosomes required large amounts of glucose to reproduce and that the survival of trypanosome-infected animals could be extended by lowering their blood glucose concentration with insulin. The hypoglycaemic diamidine, Synthalin, was then found to have activity against trypanosomes and other protozoa (e.g. *Babesia*) but since this effect occurred at concentrations which did not lower the blood sugar of mice, the action was presumed to be direct, possibly by binding to DNA. This observation led to the synthesis of a large number of analogues, some of which had potent trypanocidal activity. The most important members of the group are diminazene, pentamidine, phenamidine, propamidine and stilbamidine. They are variously available either as the free bases or as salts.

Diminazene aceturate

In addition to its trypanocidal activity, diminazene (Fig. 20.2) has direct activity against *Babesia* and some bacteria. This drug has been used to treat early human trypanosomiasis with some success and without undue toxicity. In veterinary medicine, diminazene has proved to be effective against *T. vivax* and *T. congolense* infection but in *T. brucei* infections the dose must be doubled. A single injection in cattle will usually produce a complete remission of signs within 24 hours by which time almost complete elimination has occurred, although the effect of the drug on trypanosomes appears to persist for much longer. Diminazene is poorly absorbed from the gastrointestinal tract and it must be given by subcutaneous or intramuscular injection. Diminazene aceturate (7 per cent) is usually formulated with phenazone (8.75 per cent). Local reactions, which may be severe in horses, are liable to occur at the injection site. Central nervous system toxic effects, which include ataxia and convulsions, have also been reported.

Dose

horse, cattle, sheep, dog   3.5 mg/kg i.m. or s.c.

Pentamidine isethionate

This agent has been used in the treatment of early human trypanosomiasis and also at 3–6-month intervals for prophylaxis. In veterinary medicine pentamidine is still occasionally used for the treatment of *T. evansi* and *T. brucei* infections. Other protozoal infections in cattle may also respond to pentamidine. Pentamidine (and the other diamidines) are actively taken up by the parasites, where they become concentrated, but the precise mechanism of action of the drug remains to be determined.

Like diminazene and the other diamidines, pentamidine is ineffective after oral administration but is readily absorbed from intramuscular sites. The drug is heavily tissue-bound, particularly in the liver and kidney, and only a small fraction of the dose appears in the blood. The toxic effects of pentamidine include local reactions at the injection site, and hypotension.

Stilbamidine isethionate

This drug has antiprotozoal and antifungal activity. It has been used in the treatment of early human trypanosomiasis and other protozoal diseases. It appears to be more neurotoxic than pentamidine.

Phenamidine isethionate

Phenamidine isethionate has potent activity against *T. brucei* and *T. evansi* and has also been used to treat *Babesia* infections in dogs, horses and cattle. It also has bactericidal activity. Phenamidine isethionate is readily soluble in water and is usually given by subcutaneous injection.

Dose

horse, cattle	12 mg/kg s.c.
dog	15 mg/kg s.c.

Phenanthridinium derivatives

The first active member of this series, dimidium bromide, was in 1938 found to have trypanocidal activity, but the drug exhibited delayed toxicity and has been replaced by the less toxic homidium and isometamidium chloride (Samorin). The mode of action of the phenanthridinium compounds is not understood. It has been suggested that the drugs are fixed in the parasites and that this inhibits cell division, possibly by an effect on DNA.

Homidium (ethidium)

Homidium is available as the bromide and the more water-soluble chloride salts. Homidium has trypanocidal activity against *T. congolense* and *T. vivax*, some activity against *T. brucei* but it is inactive against *T. evansi*.

Homidium is eliminated fairly rapidly from the body but gives prophylactic cover for about a month. The drug causes severe local reactions at subcutaneous injection sites and since the intravenous route cannot be used, the drug must be given by deep intramuscular injection, where local reactions (e.g. lameness) may still occur. Homidium has toxic effects on the liver but these are generally only transient.

Dose

1 mg/kg i.m.

Isometamidium (Samorin)

Isometamidium (Fig. 20.2) remains in the body for a much longer period than homidium and hence has value as a prophylactic, giving effective protection for up to 6 months. It is currently the drug of choice for the prophylactic treatment of cattle, sheep and goats. The persistence of isometamidium in the mammalian body appears to be mainly due to very slow absorption of the drug from the injection site.

Isometamidium has clinically useful trypanocidal activity against *T. congolense* in cattle and horses, and is of some value in treating *T. evansi* infections. It is usually given by deep intramuscular injection and, like homidium, can cause severe local necrosis at the injection site. Pharmaceutical modification of the formulation has been claimed to reduce local irritancy.

Dose

Treatment   up to 2 mg/kg i.m.

Quinapyramine (Antrycide)

Quinapyramine has moderate trypanocidal activity but also appears to reduce the infectivity of the parasites. A lag period occurs after dosage during which multiplication continues but the parasites are no longer infective. Quinapyramine is thus used for the prevention and treatment of trypanosomiasis. The essentially insoluble chloride salt and the much more soluble methylsulphate salt are often used in combination. This is claimed to produce synergism against the parasites in that the methylsulphate has a short but rapidly acting effect and the chloride salt is absorbed much more slowly from the injection site and exerts a prophylactic effect which may extend for at least 2 months, even in high-risk areas. Quinapyramine is sometimes used concomitantly with suramin or homidium to give greater protection.

Quinapyramine is active against *T. congolense*, *T. evansi*, *T. equiperdum* and *T. equinum*. *T. brucei* is less affected by the drug. Protection against the transmission of *T. equiperdum* during service can be obtained either by maintaining prophylactic treatment of the stallion or by giving a single dose to the mare some 2–3 weeks before service. Trypanosomal resistance to quinapyramine has been reported, which may extend to homidium but not usually to suramin or the diamidines. The drug is given by subcutaneous or intramuscular injection of a 5 per cent or a 10 per cent solution. Local tissue reactions may occur, particularly in the horse, and may result in tissue necrosis and sloughing. Persistent swellings have also been noted at the injection site in the horse. Other toxic effects include salivation, sweating, tremors and gastroenteritis (where fatalities have been reported). In severe cases, there may also be an increase in heart and respiratory rates and collapse.

Dose

A mixture of quinapyramine chloride and methylsulphate is usually used to deliver a total dose of 4–5 mg/kg.

Other Mastigophoral infections

Leishmaniasis

The human leishmaniases are a group of diseases (cutaneous, mucocutaneous and visceral) which affect very large numbers of people in Southern Europe, the Middle East, Asia, Africa and South America. The parasites multiply within macrophages which then rupture and allow for the infection of other macrophages. The diseases are spread from host to host by phlebotomine sandfly vectors; these consume infected macrophages in a blood meal and the parasites undergo multiplication and morphological transformation in the vector before being passed on to other mammalian hosts. Most of these infections are zoonoses involving both domestic and wild animals, especially rodents and dogs, which serve as reservoirs for human infection.

Six main species are recognized and three of these (*Leishmania tropica*, *L. donovani* and *L. braziliensis*) occur in dogs. *L. tropica* causes cutaneous leishmaniasis (oriental sore) at the site of the sandfly bite, and *L. braziliensis* produces lesions which are rather like those caused by *L. tropica*. *L. donovani* invades systemically and causes a visceral form of the disease (kala azar). Dogs which are infected by *L. donovani* typically first lose the hair around the eyes and this is followed by generalized hair loss and eczema. The animals often exhibit intermittent fever, anaemia and adenopathy.

In humans, leishmaniasis was first treated in 1912 with antimony potassium tartrate. Since that time, organic antimonials, the diamidines and, more recently, polyene antibiotics (e.g. amphotericin B), cycloguanil and chloroquine have been used with some success. The canine diseases have not responded well to therapy and the elimination of the sandfly vectors and the euthanasia of infected animals has been considered a more reasonable approach.

Trichomoniasis

Trichomonas infections are common in both animals and humans. In cattle, *T. foetus*, which causes death of the foetus before the fourth month, is of economic importance. The organism is venereally transmitted and causes no signs in the bull which, however, remains permanently infected. Cows appear to recover spontaneously between infective episodes. Pigeons, and occasionally turkeys and chickens, can become infected by *T. gallinae*. The main locus of infection is the crop and the disease can be fatal in young birds. *Hexamita meleagridis* is a biflagellate protozoan which resembles *T. foetus* and can cause enteritis in young turkeys and game birds.

Therapeutic and prophylactic agents

Dimetridazole (Fig. 20.2) has been given orally and intravenously to treat *T. foetus* infections in bulls and also for treatment and prophylaxis of *T. gallinae* infections in pigeons (25–50 g/100 l, for 7 days in the drinking water). Dimetridazole is also used for prophylaxis against and treatment of *Hexamita meleagridis* infections. The related drug, carnidazole (5–10 mg), has also been used for the prophylaxis and treatment of trichomoniasis in pigeons.

Histomoniasis

This is a disease in young turkeys (and occasionally chickens and game birds) which is variously known as blackhead (because of the cyanosis of the head and wattles which may, but does not necessarily, develop) or infectious enterohepatitis. The infecting organism is *Histomonas meleagridis*, which is transmitted among birds in the eggs of the caecal ascarid, *Heterakis gallinarum*. The disease is more likely to occur when the birds are raised intensively. Young turkeys (up to 14 weeks old) develop small ulcers in the caecum which eventually coalesce to involve the whole organ. The liver is also invaded. Young birds invariably die within 1–2 weeks, but in older turkeys a chronic wasting disease may occur, followed by the development of immunity. Chickens may carry the parasite without developing signs and serve as a reservoir for infection. Thus control measures include not allowing turkeys access for at least 2 years to ground on which chickens have been kept.

Therapeutic and prophylactic agents

Dimetridazole
This is a nitroimidazole drug (Fig. 20.2) which can be used for both prophylaxis and treatment of histomoniasis. The drug is mixed with the food or the drinking water. Tissue residues are not detectable after 48 hours but withholding times for slaughter vary from 6 to 28 days according to the preparation; the manufacturer's specifications should be consulted. Dimetridazole should not be given to laying birds or administered concurrently with other histomonicidal drugs. It is also used to treat swine dysentery caused by a variety of bacteria and protozoa.

Dose

poultry
Prophylaxis   13.3 g/100 l drinking water; 100–200 g/tonne feed.
Treatment   26.7 g/100 l drinking water; 500 g/tonne feed.

Furaltadone and furazolidone

Furaltadone can be used to treat histomoniasis in chickens and turkeys. The drug is dissolved in the drinking water (10–40 g/100 l). There is no specified withdrawal period before slaughter. Furazolidone has similar effects and is also administered in the drinking water (15–25 g/100 l).

Nitrothiazoles

Aminothiazole and, more recently, nithiazide and acinitrazole have been used in the prevention and treatment of histomoniasis in turkeys and trichomoniasis in pigeons.

Giardiasis

The causative organism of giardiasis is *Giardia lamblia*, which attaches to epithelial cells in the intestine and can cause both acute and chronic diarrhoea although most infections are asymptomatic. The disease is cosmopolitan and although it primarily occurs in humans, it may also affect domestic animals. Transmission is direct and involves the ingestion of mature cysts from contaminated food or water. Drugs which have been successfully used to treat giardiasis in humans include metronidazole, mepacrine (an antimalarial drug), furazolidone and erythromycin.

Coccidial infections

The causative organisms are a large number of species of organisms which fall into two main groups: the first includes *Eimeria*, *Isospora* and *Cryptosporidium* species, while the second group includes *Toxoplasma gondii* and a number of *Sarcocystis* species.

Coccidiosis caused by *Eimeria* and *Isospora* species

A large number of *Eimeria* and *Isospora* species can infect chickens, turkeys, geese, cattle, sheep, goats, pigs, horses, dogs, cats and rabbits. The organisms mostly infect the epithelial cells of the gastrointestinal tract but the liver (rabbits) and kidneys (geese) may also be invaded. Infections by these parasites are overwhelmingly the most important from an economic point of view but there have been a number of reports of cryptosporidial infections of the upper respiratory tract of a variety of avian species. Immunosuppressed humans can become infected with cryptosporidia. Rodents may serve as a reservoir for coccidiosis in dogs and cats.

The details of the life cycles of the parasites differ among the species but, in general, infection occurs after the ingestion of sporulated oocysts. Unsporulated oocysts are passed in the faeces of infected vertebrates and sporulation, which confers infectivity, occurs under favourable conditions. The sporozoites are liberated from the sporocysts and invade the intestinal epithelial cells of the host where they undergo morphological changes to become trophozoites. The trophozoite divides many times to form a schizont which contains a large number of merozoites. Both the schizont and the host cell then rupture, releasing the merozoites, which are capable of invading other host cells. This process of schizogony may be repeated a number of times (generations) but, eventually, male and female gametocytes are formed. These fuse to form a zygote from which the unsporulated oocyst develops.

The inter-species variations which occur relate largely to the existence of extra-intestinal stages (spleen, liver, lymph nodes) in the life cycles of the parasites. Coccidial infections may cause massive destruction of intestinal epithelial cells and haemorrhage. Infected animals rapidly become anorexic, listless and emaciated. Apart from the use of anticoccidial drugs, treatment of acute coccidiosis may involve rehydration and restoration of the electrolyte balance. Immunity may develop following an infection.

Coccidiosis is particularly important, from an economic point of view, where animals and birds are raised under intensive conditions. The severity of the disease which occurs depends both on the infecting species and the parasite burden. Control measures include good husbandry, as a prime requirement, and the use of anticoccidial drugs for both prophylaxis and treatment. Considerations which apply to the optimal use of anticoccidial drugs are associated with the prevention of the development of resistance by the organisms and the likely effects of the drugs on egg production and food utilization. Potential problems are associated with drug residues in eggs and milk and the need for specified withdrawal periods before slaughter. Resistance has developed to many anticoccidial drugs to the extent that they are now useless in practical terms. Resistance is much more likely to develop in birds reared under intensive conditions than in farm animals. Many therapeutic regimens are employed to maximize the efficiency of treatment and to minimize the possibility of resistance. For example, anticoccidial drugs may be given in sub-therapeutic doses to encourage the development of immunity, drugs may be changed during the growth cycle of a single crop of broilers or between crops, and the use of compound anticoccidial preparations is common. It is likely that effective vaccines will be developed for the control of coccidiosis in the foreseeable future.

Drugs for the prevention and treatment of coccidiosis

Anticoccidial drugs are usually given in the food and water and inhibit the asexual and/or the sexual forms of the parasites.

Sulphonamides

The sulphonamides were among the first anticoccidials and are still used for both prevention and treatment of coccidiosis in poultry, rabbits, cattle and sheep. Considerable variation exists in the activity of the sulphonamides against individual *Eimeria* species and thus they cannot be said to have a broad spectrum of activity. Sulphanilamide was the first sulphonamide to be used for coccidiosis but it has been replaced by other, more active and less toxic sulphonamides.

Sulphaquinoxaline sodium

Sulphaquinoxaline (Fig. 20.3) is a constituent of a compound preparation which also contains the antimalarial, pyrimethamine. The preparation is administered to chickens in the drinking water for prophylaxis against coccidiosis. The withdrawal period for slaughter is 6 days and eggs from treated birds should not be used for human consumption.

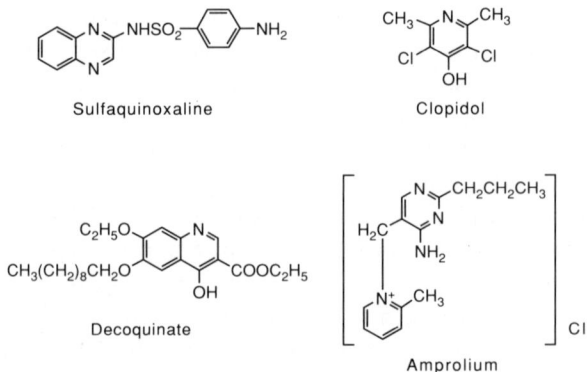

Figure 20.3 Anticoccidial drugs.

Sulphadimidine

This drug is also used for the prophylaxis and treatment of coccidiosis in poultry and for the treatment of coccidiosis in sheep, cattle and rabbits.

Dose

lamb and calf	100–200 mg/kg p.o. or i.v., then 50–100 mg daily
rabbit and poultry	100–233 g/100 l in the drinking water.

The withdrawal period for slaughter varies with species and preparation.

Long-acting sulphonamides

Sulphadimethoxine, sulphamethoxypyridazine, sulphamethoxydiazine and sulfapyrazole have been claimed to be more active against coccidia than sulphaquinoxaline, especially in the treatment of young animals, such as calves. The withholding periods for slaughter following the use of these drugs are generally longer than for the short-acting sulphonamides (e.g. up to 21 days for slaughter and 7 days for milk after sulphamethoxypyridazine.

Dose

sulphamethoxypyridazine
all animals	1 g/50 kg s.c., i.p., i.m. or i.v.

sulphamethoxydiazine
calf, foal, piglet	40 mg/kg initially then 20 mg/kg s.c. or i.m.
horse, cow, sheep	30 mg/kg initially then 20 mg/kg s.c. or i.m.
dog, cat	50 mg/kg initially then 20 mg/kg s.c. or i.m.

Ionophore antibiotics

These complex antibiotics with very low therapeutic indices, are elaborated by various actinomycete species and are widely used in poultry, cattle and sheep but are extremely toxic to horses (a dose of 2–3 mg/kg can be fatal). They are extensively used in the broiler industry and although resistance has been reported, it is not considered to be of importance as yet. These antibiotics are believed to act osmotically by impeding ion transport through the coccidial cell membrane. Activity is mainly against the sporozoite and merozoite forms of the parasites and the drugs must be given continuously in the feed.

The ionophore antibiotics are used mainly for prophylaxis of coccidiosis in chickens and turkeys, but not for treatment, and some are also used to increase food conversion efficiency in cattle and pigs. They should never be given concomitantly with other anticoccidials and can be fatal if given within 7 days before or after a dose of tiamulin.

Monensin

Monensin (*Streptomyces cinnamonensis*) is highly effective in the prophylaxis of coccidiosis in chickens and turkeys and to improve feed conversion efficiency in cattle. It has a broad spectrum of activity but resistance (and cross-resistance to salinomycin) has been reported. Eggs from monensin-treated birds should not be used for human consumption and there is a 3-day withholding period for slaughter.

Dose

chicken	100–200 g/tonne in the feed
turkey	90–100 g/tonne in the feed

Narasin

Narasin (*Streptomyces aurofaciens*) is used for both the prophylaxis and treatment of coccidial infections in broiler chickens. It is not used for egg-laying birds and the withdrawal period for slaughter is 5 days.

Dose

broiler chicken	70 g/tonne in the feed

Salinomycin sodium

Salinomycin (*Streptomyces albus*) is used in the prophylaxis of coccidiosis in chickens, but not turkeys. It is claimed not to cause growth depression or poor feathering of the birds. Salinomycin is also used to improve feed conversion efficiency in pigs, where it has the advantage of not affecting the flavour of the meat. The withholding period for slaughter is 5 days.

Dose

poultry	60 g/tonne in feed

Lasalocid sodium

Lasalocid (*Streptomyces lasaliensis*), like monensin, is used for the prophylaxis of coccidiosis in chickens, turkeys and game birds, being effective against most common avian *Eimeria* species. Lasalocid has also been used to reduce the ruminal Gram-positive population in cows, including those responsible for excessive gas production. This is claimed to improve feed efficiency. The withholding period for the slaughter of turkeys and chickens is 7 days.

Dose

| chicken | 75–125 g/tonne in the feed |
| turkey | 90–125 g/tonne in the feed |

Maduramicin ammonium

Maduramicin (*Actinomadura yumaense*) is much more potent than the other ionophores and is used for the prophylaxis of coccidiosis in broiler chickens. The withholding period for slaughter is 7 days.

Dose

| poultry | 5 g/tonne in the feed |

Quinolones

A number of broad-spectrum quinolone coccidiostatic drugs have been developed but protozoal resistance (and cross-resistance within the group) has limited their usefulness. They act to disrupt electron transport, mainly in the sporozoites.

Clopidol

Clopidol (Fig. 20.3) is used in the prevention of coccidiosis in poultry, game birds and rabbits. It is a broad-spectrum coccidiostatic and acts against the intracellular sporozoites in the host, interfering with the development of the first-generation schizonts. Resistance has steadily increased since the introduction of clopidol. The drug appears to prevent the development of post-infection immunity. It should not be used in laying birds. Overdosage may cause anorexia and it is recommended that the drug should not be given concomitantly with other anticoccidials, although a combination product with decoquinate is available for the prophylaxis of young chickens (to 16 weeks) and turkeys (to 12 weeks), and of rabbits. The withholding period for slaughter is 5 days (game birds, 7 days).

Dose

| game birds, poultry | 125 g/tonne continuously in the feed |
| rabbit | 200 g/tonne continuously in the feed |

Decoquinate

Decoquinate (Fig. 20.3) is given in the food for the prophylaxis and treatment of coccidiosis in chickens, sheep and cattle. There is a 3-day withholding period for slaughter of sheep, and milk from treated animals must not be used for human consumption.

Dose

sheep	50 g/tonne feed
lamb	1.0 g/kg/day; 100 g/tonne feed

Methylbenzoquate

Methylbenzoquate (1.67 per cent) is combined with clopidol (20 per cent) in a pre-mix for prophylaxis of coccidiosis in young turkeys, chickens and rabbits. The withdrawal period for slaughter is 5 days.

Dose

poultry	50 g/tonne in the feed
rabbit	1 kg/tonne in the feed

Dinitolmide

Dinitolmide (3,5-dinitro-*o*-toluamide) is used in the feed for the prophylaxis of coccidiosis in chickens and other poultry. It should not be given concomitantly with other coccidiostatic drugs. The withdrawal period for slaughter is 3 days.

Dose

65–125 g/tonne continuously in feed

Nicarbazin

This drug is an equimolecular complex of *p,p'*-dinitrocarbanilide and 2-hydroxy-4,6-dimethylpyrimidine. It has coccidiocidal activity, mainly against the schizonts which appear after the first generation. It is used mainly for prophylaxis of caecal and intestinal coccidiosis in poultry. Some strains of coccidia which have become resistant to other drugs remain sensitive to nicarbazin. The withdrawal period for slaughter is 9 days. Nicarbazin may reduce both egg production and the proportion of fertile eggs that hatch and should therefore not be used for laying hens.

Dose

poultry   125 g/tonne continuously in the feed.
Nicarbazin is used together with narasin, in a compound coccidiostatic preparation.

Robenidine

This is a broad-spectrum coccidiostatic and coccidiocidal drug which inhibits oxidative phosphorylation in late first-generation and second-stage schizonts. There may also be an effect on the gametocytes. It is used for the prophylaxis of coccidiosis in chickens, turkeys and rabbits. Some resistance has been reported but is not viewed as being serious. The drug has been stated to taint the flesh of birds and strict adherence to the 5-day withdrawal period for the slaughter of poultry (and rabbits) is of obvious importance. It is not used in egg-laying birds.

Dose

turkey and chicken   33 g/tonne continuously in the feed
rabbit   50–66 g/tonne continuously in the feed

Furaltadone

Furaltadone is used to prevent histomoniasis in chickens and can also be used to prevent coccidiosis.

Halofuginone hydrobromide

This agent is used for the prevention of coccidiosis in chickens and turkeys. It has potent broad-spectrum coccidiocidal and coccidiostatic activity against first- and second-generation schizonts. It should only be given to young birds (up to 12 weeks of age for poultry). The withdrawal periods for slaughter are 5 days for chickens and 7 days for turkeys. The drug is not given to egg-laying birds.

Dose

poultry   3 g/tonne in the feed

Amprolium hydrochloride

Amprolium (Fig. 20.3) is used to treat and prevent coccidiosis in pigeons. The drug is thought to act by interfering with thiamin utilization in the parasites. It is dissolved in the drinking water (38.4 mg/l).

Amprolium (25 per cent) is a constituent of a compound preparation with ethopabate (1.6 per cent), a *p*-aminobenzoic acid antagonist, which is claimed to produce synergism and an increase in the spectrum of activity. The drug combination is used to treat outbreaks of coccidiosis in poultry, calves and lambs. The withdrawal period for the slaughter of poultry is 3 days. Amprolium (20 per cent) is also included in a compound preparation with ethopabate (1 per cent) and sulphaquinoxaline (12 per cent), and in another where pyrimethamine (1 per cent) has also been added.

Toxoplasmosis

The causative organism of toxoplasmosis is *Toxoplasma gondii*, which is an intestinal parasite of cats and has a worldwide distribution. The parasite has a complex life cycle with a facultative cystic tissue phase in intermediate hosts, which can include mammals (including cats), birds and man.

Cats generally become infected by eating *Toxoplasma*-infected rodents but infection can also occur from the ingestion of oocysts from the faeces of other cats. Other carnivores (and humans) can become infected by eating raw or inadequately cooked meat. The pathological effects of *Toxoplasma* infections are almost exclusively due to the extra-intestinal phase of the parasite. The parasites travel from the intestine via the lymphatics and the portal system and can invade other tissues. The parasites can also cross the placenta, and in pregnant animals congenital lesions of the central nervous system and the retina may develop. Infections during early pregnancy can cause abortion in ewes, and infections in mid-pregnancy can cause stillbirth. If the lamb is born alive, it tends to be weak.

Toxoplasmosis is not uncommon in humans; serological tests have indicated that about 30 per cent of individuals have been infected at some time. Infection can arise either from the ingestion of oocysts from cat faeces, which can be spread by flies, or by eating inadequately cooked meat containing cysts. Infections in adult humans are usually asymptomatic but where symptoms occur, the condition usually presents as an ill-defined chronic malaise, sometimes with a low-grade fever and swelling of the lymph nodes. Infections during pregnancy are potentially very serious and can result in abortion, stillbirth or congenital damage to the central nervous system (visual impairment, mental retardation, and epileptiform seizures).

Prevention and treatment of toxoplasmosis

General hygienic measures are the first line of defence. Direct or indirect contact with cat faeces appears to be the most common source of infection. Cats should not be given raw meat and pregnant women should limit their exposure to cats and should not assist at lambing time.

Most *Toxoplasma* infections in animals and humans appear to be self-limiting and are often not treated. Ewes which abort as a result of a *Toxoplasma* infection appear to develop a degree of immunity and to produce normal offspring in subsequent seasons.

In humans, a combination of pyrimethamine and sulphadiazine has been used successfully to treat toxoplasmosis but there is dispute over the efficacy of the tetracyclines, except for minocycline which is as effective as the sulphonamide-pyrimethamine combinations. Spiramycin has been found to reduce the ability of the parasite to cross the placenta; clindamycin, since it readily gains access to the eye, can be used to treat experimental retino-choroiditis in rabbits and (with corticosteroids) clinical cases in humans. Clindamycin has also been found to reduce the number of oocysts in the faeces of *Toxoplasma*-infected cats. Monensin-treated (15 mg/head/day) ewes which were exposed to experimental *Toxoplasma* challenge produced more live lambs than a control group.

Sarcocystosis

A number of *Sarcocystis* species employ the dog and the cat as the final host, while two species, *S. bovihominis* and *S. porcihominis*, use man as the final host. The clinical effects of infections in the final hosts are usually limited to mild gastrointestinal symptoms. Infection of the final host occurs after the ingestion of parasites (bradyzoites) which are encysted in meat. These differentiate into gametocytes which conjugate to form oocysts and then sporocysts, which are voided in the faeces. Infection of the intermediate host (cattle, sheep, pigs and horses) is by the ingestion of the sporocysts; these then release sporozoites which are able to penetrate the intestinal wall and, after several asexual cycles in capillary endothelial cells and lymphocytes, finally locate in muscle as mature sarcocysts. This is the infective form for the final host.

The main pathological effects of *Sarcocystis* infection in the intermediate hosts are referable to vascular damage and haemorrhage. The presence of disease may not be apparent, however, until the animals are slaughtered and cysts are identified in the meat. Where the parasite burden is great, the animals may become anorexic, oedematous, listless and emaciated. Pregnant animals may abort. A chronic form of the disease has been described in cattle.

Prevention and control of sarcocystosis

Measures to control sarcocystosis include the separation of dogs and cats from food animals to avoid ingestion of oocysts by food animals; the avoidance of raw meat in the diets of dogs and cats; and the maintenance of general hygiene. There is no really satisfactory drug treatment but in humans the best treatment appears to be sulphonamides together with trimethoprim or pyrimethamine, but the drugs have to be given for long periods.

Piroplasmal infections

Babesiosis

Babesia species are parasites of the erythrocytes of dogs, cats, horses, cattle, sheep, goats and wild animals. They generally cause fever, acute anaemia and severe haemoglobinuria, which is often the first clinical sign. The parasites can be readily identified in blood smears. The condition can be fatal within a few days. Fatal babesiosis can also occur in humans, usually in individuals whose immunity is compromised. The parasites are transmitted from host to host by female ticks (*Ixodidae*) which ingest the infective forms of the parasite in the blood of the host. It is believed that gametocytes are formed in the gut of the tick; these conjugate and undergo schizogony, resulting in the liberation of motile forms of the parasite which then invade the ovaries and eggs of the tick, and hence the salivary glands of the larva. Spread of the infection to the next host is by inoculation. The various species of *Babesia* differ in the severity of the disease which they produce. The effects on the mammalian host also depend on the prevalence of ticks (and thus the parasite burden) and factors associated with the host such as stress and the level of immunity which may have been acquired.

Treatment and control of babesiosis

Reduction of the numbers of vectors by ectoparasite control measures, such as dipping the animals and spraying the pastures, are widely practised but problems with resistance of ticks to insecticides have been encountered. Selective breeding of tick-resistant animals and immunization programmes have also been successful as control measures. One technique is to inject virulent strains of *Babesia* and to control the clinical signs with drugs while immunity develops. In severe cases, blood transfusion may be necessary to restore the haemoglobin level and a number of drugs can also be used. Older drugs include organic arsenicals and antimonials and dyes, such as Trypan Blue.

Pentamidine and diminazene (discussed earlier in this chapter) have also been used in the treatment of babesiosis. In humans, quinine given concomitantly with clindamycin has been reported as effective. The use of amicarbalide and quinuronium has given way to imidocarb, which is currently the most important drug for the prophylaxis and treatment of babesiosis and anaplasmosis in cattle; it can also be used to 'sterilize' cattle before movement to new areas.

Imidocarb dipropionate

Imidocarb is chemically related to amicarbalide and appears to act directly on the parasite and to cause morphological changes. The drug is well absorbed and distributed throughout the body after subcutaneous injection and is detectable for up to 4 weeks after administration, which is the period of effective prophylaxis. Imidocarb is mostly eliminated in the faeces but some is excreted in the urine. It has cholinergic activity which may cause cardiovascular, gastrointestinal and neuromuscular effects. Anaphylactic reactions have been recorded and the therapeutic index of the drug is regarded as being low. There may also be local reactions at the injection site, especially in horses.

Dose

Prophylaxis
   3 mg/kg s.c. as a single dose
Treatment
   1.2 mg/kg s.c.

In the UK the District Veterinary Officer must be informed if imidocarb-treated animals are to be slaughtered or their milk is to be used for human consumption. In Australia, there is a 28-day withholding period for meat, and milk from imidocarb-treated animals is not used for human consumption.

Infections by other protozoa and drugs used in their treatment are shown in Table 20.1.

Table 20.1 Drugs used in the treatment of protozoal infections

Organism	Animal species infected	Drug treatment
Balantidium coli	Pigs	Tetracyclines
Besnoitia besnoiti	Cat (final host)	None effective
	Cattle (intermediate host)	
Hepatozoon canis	Dog, cat	Non-steroidal anti-inflammatory drugs
Haemoproteus spp.		
Plasmodium spp.	Birds	Human antimalarial drugs
Leucocytozoon spp.		
Theileria parva	Cattle	Tetracyclines
Theileria annulata	Cattle	Halofuginone
Theileria hirci	Sheep, goats	

CHAPTER 21

ANTIFUNGAL AND ANTIVIRAL DRUGS

Antifungal chemotherapy

Fungal infections (mycoses) can be divided into two distinct groups—superficial and systemic. The most common superficial mycotic diseases are the dermatomycoses (ringworm). These are caused by various species of *Trichophyton* and *Microsporum*, which affect all domesticated animal species and are often transmissible to humans. Superficial mycotic infections are also associated with otitis externa (*Pityrosporon*) and ulcerative keratitis (e.g. *Aspergillus, Penicillium*), especially in horses. Systemic mycoses can cause brooder pneumonia in chickens (*Aspergillus*), abortion in cattle and sheep (*Aspergillus*) and mastitis in cattle (*Candida*). *Candida* species can also infect mucous membranes (e.g. tongue, pharynx, gastrointestinal tract, genito-urinary tract). Prolonged antibacterial therapy, which eliminates competing bacteria in the gut microflora, can lead to superinfection of the gut with *Candida* species and consequent diarrhoea. Sometimes fungal species, which normally infect superficial sites, can disseminate systemically (e.g. *Candida* species can cause serious disease by invading the bladder, eye, peritoneum and pleura). Fungal infections can often be considered as opportunistic since they can occur in debilitated or immunosuppressed animals and in patients with leukaemia and other cancers.

Antimycotic drugs

The antimycotic drugs are often divided, somewhat arbitrarily, into drugs which are applied topically and those which are used systemically. Such a

Table 21.1   Summary of antimycotic drug indications

Condition	Route of administration	
	Local	Systemic
Systemic mycoses		Ketoconazole Amphotericin B Flucytosine
Dermatomycoses	Natamycin Miconazole	Griseofulvin Ketoconazole
Mycotic keratitis	Clotrimazole Natamycin Miconazole	
Mastitis	Nystatin Clotrimazole Natamycin	
Otitis externa	Miconazole Nystatin Natamycin Thiabendazole	

classification is not mutually exclusive and, in some cases, systemic therapy is used for both systemic and superficial infections (see Table 21.1).

Topical antimycotic drugs

Most antifungal chemotherapy is topical and often involves the use of specific vehicles and keratolytics (e.g. resorcinol, salicylic acid, benzoic acid) to improve the access of other active ingredients to the infection site. This may be of critical importance to the outcome of treatment. A large number of chemical substances have been incorporated into topical formulations for the treatment of dermatomycoses. They are probably best considered as antiseptics and include iodine compounds, dyes (e.g. crystal violet), mercurial preparations, sulphur compounds, chlorbutol, phenol and potassium permanganate. These older topical remedies had only modest efficacy and they have now been largely superseded by more potent broad-spectrum drugs. Thiabendazole, an anthelmintic, and monosulfiram, an acaricide, are also antimycotic and are included in some proprietary broad-spectrum mixed formulations for treating otitis externa.

Nystatin

Nystatin is a polyene antimycotic consisting of a large molecule with a hydrophilic hydroxylated moiety and a hydrophobic moiety containing 4–7 conjugated double bonds. Like the other polyenes it is poorly soluble in aqueous media and undergoes photo-oxidation in solution.

The mechanism of action of the polyenes is discussed in more detail in relation to amphotericin B but, briefly, they occupy ergosterol binding sites in the fungal cell membrane, leading to altered membrane permeability and leakage of intracellular ions. Most bacteria are resistant to nystatin because they lack the necessary cell membrane binding sites. Nystatin has a broad-spectrum antifungal action but is too toxic for parenteral use. However, since it is poorly absorbed from the gut it can be used in dogs to treat *Candida* superinfection of the gut which may occur after prolonged antibacterial therapy. Nystatin has been used in bovine mastitis caused by *Candida* species (300 000 units per quarter, daily for 3 days) but resistant strains occur and clotrimazole or natamycin are preferred.

Dose

dog, cat   100 000 units/kg

Since the drug is effective against *Pityrosporon*, it is incorporated into several proprietary formulations for treating otitis externa, usually with antibacterial, miticidal and anti-inflammatory drugs.

Natamycin

This agent is also a polyene antimycotic with broad-spectrum fungicidal activity. The site of action is on the fungal cell membrane. It has activity against *Candida*, *Cryptococcus* and *Pityrosporon* and some dermatophytes. Ringworm is a common infection of horses and cattle, and rigorous treatment is necessary because the disease is zoonotic and may preclude horses from racing and sale. Natamycin is effective by topical application for treating dermatomycosis (ringworm) in horses and cattle, often in conjunction with griseofulvin, which is administered orally. A suspension of natamycin (0.01 per cent) is sponged onto the affected areas of individually treated animals. For mass treatment, the entire body surface of infected and in-contact animals should be sprayed with the suspension. Patient response must be closely monitored to preclude premature termination of treatment. Furthermore, the spores are viable, mainly within the animals' coats, for several months. Natamycin suspension spray is recommended for disinfection of tack and the immediate environment after clearing gross contamination.

Natamycin (10 ml of a 5 per cent solution in each infected quarter) has been used, as an alternative to clotrimazole, to treat *Candida* mastitis in cows. For keratitis, a 2.5–5 per cent solution is instilled every 2 or 3 hours.

Imidazole derivatives

Clotrimazole

Clotrimazole (Fig. 21.1) was developed from the series of anthelmintics which includes thiabendazole. The drug has activity against a wide range of fungal species including *Aspergillus, Candida, Cryptococcus* and *Microsporum,* and some bacteria. It binds to phospholipids in susceptible fungal cell membranes which causes changes in membrane function, including interference with purine uptake and leakage of essential cell constituents. It is considered to be fungicidal at high concentrations and fungistatic at lower concentrations.

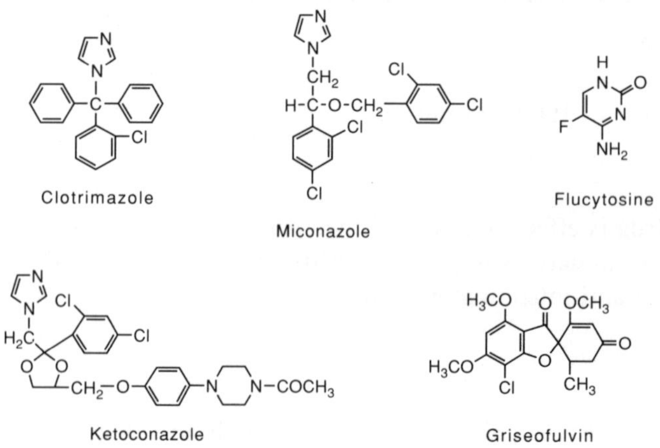

Clotrimazole

Miconazole

Flucytosine

Ketoconazole

Griseofulvin

Figure 21.1 Structures of antifungal drugs.

The use of clotrimazole in veterinary medicine is restricted to local application and intramammary infusion. It is a drug of choice for mycotic (especially *Aspergillus*) keratitis in horses; a 1 per cent cream or solution is instilled every 2 or 3 hours. Good results have been reported in the treatment of bovine mycotic mastitis using 100–200 mg per quarter of 1 per cent solution or cream daily for up to 4 days.

Miconazole

Miconazole (Fig. 21.1) is a fungistatic imidazole, with a similar antimycotic spectrum and mechanism of action to those of ketoconazole (see below). Unlike ketoconazole, it is not absorbed from the gut and intravenous administration is necessary for a systemic effect. It is therefore usually applied topically. Some penetration of the skin occurs after topical application.

Miconazole (as a 1 per cent solution applied every 2 or 3 hours) is used for treating mycotic keratitis (but in *Aspergillus* or *Candida* infections clotrimazole is normally preferred). It is formulated as a 2 per cent cream for treating ringworm in dogs and cats, where treatment is recommended for up to 6 weeks. A 1 per cent lotion is also available. Miconazole is incorporated, together with antibiotics and corticosteroids, into various proprietary preparations for treating otitis externa or dermatophytes, but (since topical dressings may be eaten!) systemic therapy with griseofulvin is generally preferred for treating dermatomycoses in cats and dogs.

Enilconazole
This agent has potent activity against dermatophytes. It is used in a concentration of 0.2 per cent as a fungicidal wash for the treatment of ringworm in horses, dogs and cattle. Spraying the entire animal every 3 days for 4 applications is recommended.

Itraconazole
Itraconazole has recently been introduced into human medicine. It is more lipophilic than miconazole and is heavily tissue-bound. It can be used to treat superficial *Candida* infections since it remains 'locked' in the epidermal cells until they are shed.

Systemic antimycotic drugs

Polyene antibiotics

Amphotericin B
Amphotericin B was isolated from an Orinoco river soil actinomycete, *Streptomyces nodosus*, in 1953. Although very similar to nystatin, actinomycin B can be used systemically but its therapeutic index is low. It is available as a sodium deoxycholate complex which is reconstituted into a colloidal suspension immediately before use with Injection of Dextrose B.P. (5%). The suspension is liable to precipitate and must be protected from light.

Amphotericin B is generally fungicidal with a broad-spectrum activity against systemic mycoses—blastomycosis, histoplasmosis, coccidiomycosis, candidiasis and cryptococcal infections. It is not effective against dermatophytes. Fungal resistance to amphotericin B is rare but has been reported.

Like nystatin and natamycin, amphotericin B binds with high affinity to sterols in the cell membranes of a large number of microorganisms, including fungi, protozoa, algae and yeasts but not bacteria. This alters the permeability of the cell membrane, by producing non-aqueous channels, and a number of its biochemical functions are inhibited. First, potassium ions are lost from the cell and this is followed by the loss of other cell components. The size of the molecules which escape appears to depend on the concentration of polyene. The cell-killing effect of the polyenes does not depend on the active growth of the fungus. Amphotericin B can be either fungistatic or fungicidal, depending on the concentration.

Mammalian cell membranes also contain sterols and after the systemic administration of amphotericin B, erythrocytes lose potassium ions and haemolysis may occur.

Amphotericin B is not absorbed from the gastrointestinal tract and must be given intravenously. The drug is effective in intestinal candidiasis but is seldom used for this purpose. It binds extensively to cholesterol-containing membranes and is heavily protein-bound. Penetration across the blood–brain barrier is poor but may be better if inflammation is present. Amphotericin B has a very long terminal half-life (15 days in humans). Only a small proportion of the dose is excreted in the urine.

Suspensions of amphotericin B are highly irritant to the vein wall and may cause inflammation with the resultant risk of embolism. Amphotericin B is predictably nephrotoxic in dogs and cats. Renal damage is first expressed as low blood potassium and magnesium concentrations and progresses to raised blood levels of urea and creatinine. Later, proteins, blood cells and casts may appear in the urine. These effects are initially reversible, but irreversible damage may occur if treatment is continued. There is recent evidence to suggest that sodium loading may reduce the uptake of amphotericin into renal proximal tubular cells in humans. It is considered prudent to monitor blood urea nitrogen levels at regular intervals during treatment. If values increase to 1.5 times the pre-treatment levels, therapy is discontinued until they return to normal. Fatal cardiac arrhythmias have been reported after amphotericin B in dogs.

Clinical uses Systemic fungal infections are often serious and although amphotericin B remains the drug of first choice, there are many problems associated with its use. The severity of the toxic effects of amphotericin B appears to depend on the total dose; combination therapy with flucytosine (see below) usually results in addition or synergism, enabling the dose of amphotericin to be reduced. There is recent clinical evidence that treatment of dimorphic fungal infections, such as blastomycosis, coccidiomycosis and histoplasmosis, may be more effective when the drugs are used together.

Ketoconazole (see below) was introduced more recently and may largely supersede amphotericin B in veterinary therapeutics by virtue of its broad-spectrum activity, relative lack of toxicity and easier (oral rather than intravenous) administration.

Dose

dog and cat	0.15–1.0 mg/kg as a solution containing amphotericin B (200 μg/ml) slow i.v. infusion, 3 times weekly.
horse	0.5 mg/kg by slow i.v. infusion, every 48 hours.

Flucytosine

Flucytosine (Fig. 21.1) is the 5-fluoro substituted analogue of cytosine and was one of a series of fluoropyrimidines synthesized in the late 1950s and originally intended as anti-tumour drug candidates. It was found to have activity against a number of systemic yeast infections, such as candidiasis and cryptococcosis, which commonly occur in human cancer patients whose immune system has been compromised by chemotherapy.

Flucytosine has a narrow spectrum of activity, mainly against *Candida* and *Cryptococcus* species, and a lower order of activity against some strains of *Aspergillus fumigatus*. Dermatophytes are resistant to flucytosine.

Flucytosine is actively transported into fungal cells and then metabolized by cytosine deaminase to 5-fluorouracil, which is the active compound. Fluorouracil is then converted to an aberrant mRNA but it is not clear exactly how this kills the fungal cell. Selectivity lies in the very small amount of deamination which occurs in the mammalian body. Mammalian cells do not contain cytosine deaminase and it was thought that the very small amounts of 5-fluorouracil detected in the blood of human patients who had received flucytosine arose from the metabolic activity of the gut flora.

Many fungi are intrinsically resistant to clinically attainable concentrations of the drug and some fungi become resistant during treatment. Resistance can arise from a reduction of the active transport mechanism whereby flucytosine is taken up in the fungal cell and/or a decrease in cytosine deaminase activity. To prevent the emergence of resistance, flucytosine is usually given together with another antifungal drug, such as amphotericin B.

Flucytosine can be administered orally or parenterally but the oral route is more commonly used. It is only slightly protein-bound ($\sim$ 10 per cent) and gains access to most body compartments, including the cerebrospinal fluid. The drug is excreted in the urine, largely unchanged.

Flucytosine has been reported to have caused a reversible elevation of liver enzymes in humans and, more seriously, blood dyscrasias which have been fatal.

Clinical uses The main veterinary use of flucytosine is for the treatment of cryptococcal infections in dogs and cats, where it is usually combined with amphotericin B or ketoconazole. It is also used in combination with amphotericin B for systemic *Candida* infections.

Dose

dog and cat   100–200 mg/kg/day p.o., in 3–4 divided doses.

The drug is not generally available in the UK and a written order to the manufacturer is required.

Ketoconazole

Ketoconazole is a fungistatic imidazole derivative and like clotrimazole it acts by disrupting the synthesis of ergosterol and binding to phospholipids in the fungal cell membrane, causing loss of essential cell constituents. It has a broad-spectrum activity, comparable with that of amphotericin B, against the systemic mycoses (blastomycosis, histoplasmosis, coccidiomycosis, candidiasis and cryptococcal infections). Unlike amphotericin B, ketoconazole is also active against dermatophytes and some Gram-positive bacteria and protozoa.

Following oral administration, ketoconazole is well-absorbed, attaining peak plasma concentrations within 2 hours (in dogs) and is widely distributed in the tissues. It is metabolized in the liver and the inactive metabolites are excreted in the bile.

Significant toxicity does not appear to be a problem with ketoconazole, in contrast to amphotericin B, although clinical experience is as yet insufficient to assess any long-term effects. Ketoconazole should be used with caution in animals with hepatic impairment and should not be given during pregnancy because of possible teratogenicity. Otherwise, side-effects reported in dogs and cats are inappetence, diarrhoea and pruritus.

Clinical uses   Ketoconazole has proved successful for treating dermatomycosis in dogs and cats (10 mg/kg daily for about 4 weeks) but griseofulvin is cheaper and its efficacy well proven.

Ketoconazole appears to be effective in treating various systemic mycoses: blastomycosis, histoplasmosis, cryptococcosis, coccidiomycosis and systemic candidiasis. It is much less toxic than amphotericin B, but unfortunately relatively slow acting. Limited clinical evidence suggests that when treating rapidly developing conditions such as blastomycosis, optimum therapy is amphotericin B initially (for its rapid fungicidal action), followed by ketoconazole to avoid prolonged treatment with the more toxic drug.

Ketoconazole has been used in dogs to treat pituitary-dependent hyperadrenocorticism and, before surgery, in adrenal-dependent hyperadrenocorticism.

Dose

For systemic mycoses, the following have been reported:

dog   up to 20 mg/kg p.o. daily
cat   up to 15 mg/kg p.o. daily

Treatment should be maintained for 4 weeks after disappearance of clinical signs.

For canine blastomycosis:

amphotericin B   0.4 mg/kg in 20 ml injection of Dextrose B.P. dextrose, i.v. every 48 hours for 10 doses followed by ketoconazole (10 mg/kg/day) for 2 months.

Griseofulvin

Griseofulvin (Fig. 21.1) was originally isolated from *Penicillium griseofulvum* in 1939 but it was not screened for antibiotic activity at that time. As a result of an investigation into the reason (suspected to be the lack of an appropriate symbiotic fungus) for the failure of conifers to grow in an area in Dorset, UK, a strain of *Penicillium janczewskii*, which produced peculiar distortions in fungal cells and was named the 'curling factor', was found in the soil. The active substance was isolated in 1952 and identified as griseofulvin. It was used originally as a fungicide in plants, then in animals, and has been used in humans since 1958. It is an unusual drug in that it is given systemically to treat superficial mycoses.

Griseofulvin is almost insoluble in water and its bioavailability depends to a large extent on the particle size of the drug in the dose form. Microfining greatly increases bioavailability.

Almost all dermatophytes, such as *Trichophyton* and *Microsporum* species, are inhibited by griseofulvin. Other fungi and bacteria are not affected and the drug has no antibacterial activity. Griseofulvin is taken up into susceptible fungal cells by an energy-dependent process and is concentrated in the cells. Fungal cells must be actively growing to be affected by griseofulvin and some cells become bi- or multinucleate and the hyphae become grossly distorted or 'curled', as originally described. It is suggested that the main effect of griseofulvin is to inhibit fungal mitosis and fungal microtubule assembly. The drug is considered to be fungistatic under most circumstances but fungicidal activity has been demonstrated *in vitro*.

Griseofulvin is given orally. Total absorption is increased by oil and it is suggested that the drug crosses the intestinal wall in the mixed micelles. Corn oil (2–5 ml) is effective as a vehicle and is well accepted by dogs and cats. Although the drug is absorbed through the skin of many species, it only has antifungal activity when given orally.

Griseofulvin binds to keratin and is selectively incorporated into newly formed keratin in the basal epidermal cells (hence systemic administration) and reaches the superficial infected epithelium with progressive maturation of basal cells. Binding to skin keratin is usually reversible but in hair and nails it appears to be non-reversible. It is suggested that keratin with incorporated griseofulvin is no longer a substrate for fungal keratinases.

The drug is demethylated and glucuronylated in the liver and careful dosing is necessary in patients with impaired liver function. It can itself induce liver enzymes and there is a potential for drug interaction if animals are being treated concurrently with hepatic enzyme-inducing drugs such as the barbiturates. It is excreted in the urine.

Griseofulvin is teratogenic in cats and horses and should not be given to pregnant animals of any species.

Clinical uses The mode of action of griseofulvin requires treatment to be maintained until the infected layers are shed; this is cost-effective in cattle and horses if a (less purified) griseofulvin feed additive is used. Tablets are available for small animals.

Diffuse infection is common in cats. In this species and in severely affected dogs, a total body clip (with the clippings burned) is recommended prior to therapy and one month later to reduce the duration of the treatment. Thorough cleaning and disinfection of the environment when treating ringworm was mentioned earlier (see natamycin).

Dose

cattle	7.5 mg/kg daily (normally for 7 consecutive days). Withholding periods for meat and milk vary; consult manufacturer's instructions.
horse	10 mg/kg daily (for infected and in-contact animals). Should not be used in animals intended for human consumption.
dog and cat	15–20 mg/kg daily for at least 3 or 4 weeks (until the lesions are cleared and cultures are negative).

Antiviral drugs

The concept of selective toxicity, exploiting differences in structure and metabolic pathways between host and pathogens, has proved successful in developing anthelmintics, pesticides, antifungal and antibacterial drugs.

Developing antiviral drugs has posed a much more difficult problem. It was believed that viral replication was so closely linked to normal host cell metabolism that antiviral therapy would inevitably be toxic to the host. Viruses are very small obligate intracellular parasites. They penetrate the host's cells, where viral RNA or DNA programmes the host cell ribosomes to replicate viruses, which are then released to invade other cells. Thus, they are completely dependent on the host cell metabolism.

Disinfection and vaccination remain the most important means of controlling viral diseases and very few specific drugs are available for treating infected animals (or humans). The available antiviral drugs are expensive and have a very narrow spectrum of activity. This account is therefore intentionally brief. Selected representative drugs are described according to their site of action on the stages of viral replication.

Drugs which inhibit the entry of viruses into host cells

This approach to the control of viral diseases is normally used for prophylaxis rather than treatment, because clinical signs and symptoms are not usually evident until intracellular viral replication is extensive.

Immunoglobulins

These are protein molecules (IgM, IgG, IgA and IgE) which possess antibody activity and can prevent the entry of viruses into cells. This is achieved by their coating the virus cell-surface receptors which are needed for attachment to and penetration of host cells. The immunoglobulin-coated viruses are also rendered more susceptible to phagocytosis.

Passive immunization is provided by injections of crude or purified preparations of antisera containing immunoglobulins. The antisera are obtained from the blood of healthy animals which have been actively immunized by administration of appropriate antigens, such as attenuated viruses. Passive immunization is effective immediately, but protection lasts for only 2 or 3 weeks. The serum proteins in homologous antisera (donor and recipient of the same species) are destroyed by normal catabolism. The proteins from heterologous antisera (from a different species) are similarly short-lived because the immunized animal is stimulated to make antibodies against them.

There is a danger of hypersensitivity reactions (serum sickness) when using heterologous antisera, which is associated with large quantities of antigen (heterologous protein) in the circulation. This stimulates the formation of antigen-antibody complexes which trigger histamine release from leucocytes, platelets and mast cells. If a hypersensitivity reaction occurs, adrenaline

(4–8 μg/kg s.c.) or a histamine H_1-antagonist should be administered; adrenaline works more promptly and more effectively.

Commercially prepared antisera are more commonly available for control of bacterial rather than viral diseases. A preparation derived from canine serum (Maxagloban P) is available for passive immunization of dogs and other susceptible species against the viruses of canine distemper, canine viral hepatitis and parvovirus; it also contains antibodies against *Leptospira*. The data sheet should be consulted for current recommendations on dosage for prophylaxis and therapy and details of subsequent vaccination programmes.

Antibodies are produced by dams exposed to antigens, either naturally or by vaccination. A natural passive immunization occurs when these maternal antibodies are transferred to the foetus via the placenta (in dogs, cats and pigs) and, to a much greater extent, in the colostrum. Newborn animals can absorb colostral immunoglobulins (IgG, IgM and IgA) through the intestinal epithelium for up to 36 hours after birth to provide a massive transfusion of maternal antibodies. The principle is utilized in the prophylaxis of enteric infections, where vaccines are available for passive immunization (by dam vaccination) of calves, lambs and piglets against *Escherichia coli* and rotavirus in calves (Rotavec K99).

Amantadine

Amantadine (Fig. 21.2) is a water-soluble tricyclic amine which is chemically unrelated to any other antimicrobial drug. This drug inhibits the penetration of sensitive strains of influenza virus into cells of humans and animals. In humans, it is approximately 70 per cent effective by systemic administration in the prophylaxis and treatment of influenza A infection.

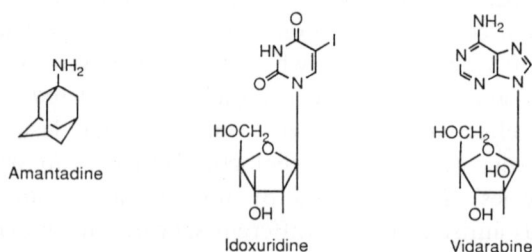

Figure 21.2 Structures of antiviral drugs.

Experimental studies in animals have shown that amantadine, administered via the drinking water to chickens infected with a respiratory virus, reduced the mortality by 50 per cent. Short-term (11-day) prophylactic administration to horses (20 mg/kg) reduced the duration of the virus shedding after experimental challenge with influenza virus. No drug toxicity was observed and it has been suggested that amantadine may be clinically useful for equine influenza prophylaxis.

Drugs which inhibit the replication of viruses

Drugs in this category act after viral penetration of host cells by inhibiting nucleic acid synthesis or subsequent virus assembly and release from cells.

Idoxuridine
Idoxuridine is an iodinated thymidine analogue. This drug is administered only by topical application because of its toxicity. Idoxuridine is metabolized in infected cells and incorporated into viral DNA, giving rise to defective viral proteins. It has been used effectively in ophthalmic drops (0.1 per cent) and ointments (0.5 per cent) to treat herpetic keratitis in cats. Resistance can develop with repeated use.

Vidarabine
Vidarabine (adenine arabinoside) is less toxic than idoxuridine and is used in humans both systemically and locally. Vidarabine binds to DNA polymerase, thus competitively inhibiting the synthesis of viral DNA.

It is reported to be reasonably effective in the treatment of herpes encephalitis in humans, but its main use in human medicine is by topical application for treating herpes simplex keratoconjunctivitis. There are reports of its successful topical use in bovine herpes and vaccinia teat lesions.

Acyclovir
Acyclovir is a newer antiviral drug which is very effective in inhibiting replication of herpes viruses, to which its activity is essentially confined. It acts by inhibiting viral DNA polymerase. The affinity of viral DNA encoded cellular enzymes for acyclovir is much greater than the affinity of normal cellular enzymes, resulting in a several hundred-fold difference in toxicity of the drug to herpes viruses compared to that for mammalian cells.

Acyclovir has not been evaluated in veterinary medicine, but it has been suggested that it may prove useful by topical administration in conditions such as viral keratoconjunctivitis, feline rhinotracheitis and herpes mammillitis in cows. The extent of its use in these conditions may be influenced by the high cost of the drug.

Interferons

The interferons are a group of glycoproteins which are produced in mammalian cells in response to viral infection and are then released to stimulate non-infected cells to resist infection. They are therefore an important part of the body's natural defence mechanism. The mode of action of interferons is complex and involves the stimulation of non-infected cells to produce polypeptides which inhibit the translocation of viral messenger RNA and so block the formation of structural proteins and enzymes.

Interferons antagonize topical or systemic viral infections only in the same or related species, but when they are effective, they apparently protect against a variety of viruses. They have been produced for experimental studies and human clinical trials by tissue culture (which is expensive) and more recently by recombinant DNA cloning techniques.

It has been concluded from preliminary results of human clinical trials that interferon may not be as useful in the therapy of viral infections as was initially suspected. The few published studies of the efficacy of interferons in the treatment of animal diseases indicate favourable resolution of feline leukaemia, feline rhinotracheitis and bovine herpes virus infections.

Immunoenhancers

Levamisole
Shortly after the introduction of this now widely-used anthelmintic, it was observed that the anthelmintic effect was sometimes accompanied by an enhancement of the immune response. Subsequent studies showed that while the immune system is depressed, for example in old or chronically ill animals (or humans), levamisole stimulates cell-mediated immunity and may enhance secondary antibody responses. It enhances the rate of T-lymphocyte differentiation and the activity of phagocytes. It has little effect on animals with a normally active immune system.

In human medicine, there are reports of beneficial effects of levamisole in some patients with chronic bacterial and viral infections, immunodeficiencies, inflammatory diseases and malignant tumours. Administration of levamisole to cows during the dry period has been reported to reduce significantly the incidence of post-calving mastitis. Calves with viral diarrhoea or infectious bovine rhinotracheitis apparently recover more rapidly with levamisole therapy than with symptomatic treatment.

Further clinical studies are necessary to assess the efficacy and optimum dosage of levamisole (and other drugs such as inosiplex) as an immunoenhancer. Overdosing may suppress the immune system. Intermittent dosing appears to be the most effective, and the current tentative recommendation is one-third of the anthelmintic dose daily for 3 days followed by 3 days without treatment. This regimen is continued as necessary to induce remission.

CHAPTER 22

ANTHELMINTICS

Introduction

Worms (helminths) which are parasitic to mammals and birds belong to widely differing taxonomic groups and invade most broadly structures of most species; it should not be assumed that they necessarily remain in the gastrointestinal tract. They are broadly classified into nematodes (round-worms), cestodes (tapeworms) and trematodes (flukes). The complexity of the life cycle of helminths varies greatly; some (e.g. nematodes) generally have only one host (direct cycle) while others (e.g. trematodes) may have two or more hosts and may include an insect vector (e.g. heartworms). Apart from diverting food from the host, which may lead to wasting, helminths have a number of adverse effects which include mechanical injury to organs (e.g. liver flukes), physical obstruction of the gut (e.g. ascarids) and the blockage of ducts, major blood vessels (e.g. heartworms) and lymphatic drainage. Toxic substances may be produced by the parasite and absorbed by the host. The traumas caused by the helminths may be subject to secondary invasion by microorganisms and may predispose to carcinoma.

Anthelmintics are drugs which are used to remove parasitic worms from animals and the term should not be restricted to drugs which merely drive the worms from the gastrointestinal tract. Some drugs, for example certain benzimidazoles, have a very broad spectrum of action, and, although used mainly in roundworm infections, also have some action against tapeworms and flukes. However, anthelmintics are normally selected on the basis of their effectiveness against a particular group of worms (cestodes, nematodes or trematodes) and will be considered in that way for ease of presentation.

Several formulations of an anti-nematode drug combined with a fasciolide are available to treat concurrent fluke infection. The use of such mixtures is not generally considered to be the best therapeutic approach, since control programmes for roundworm and fluke infections may involve using different drugs at different seasons for optimum effect.

Selective toxicity, especially when dealing with systemic infestations, remains a problem, although there has been considerable improvement in recent years. Chemotherapy aims either at the exploitation of biochemical differences between parasite and host or of situational concentration differences, such as the exposure of the worm to a high concentration of the drug for a period which is not long enough for significant absorption by the host.

The clinician must be aware of the different modes of action of anthelmintics, because benzimidazole resistance in nematode species which infect sheep and cattle has been reported and there have also been instances of resistance to levamisole and morantel. When resistance has been confirmed by laboratory diagnosis, it is necessary to use a drug with a different mode of action. However, when drug resistance is suspected only on clinical evidence of unthriftiness of the animal after treatment, other possible causes must be considered. Apparent failure of anthelmintic therapy is most commonly caused by the return of treated stock to a heavily infected pasture, where re-infection can occur within a few days. Except for sustained-release formulations, anthelmintics are normally effective only for the day or two after their administration. Other causes are the emergence of hypobiotic (inhibited) larvae after treatment, resulting in rapid re-infection, and the presence of concomitant disease or nutritional deficiencies. Mass medication in the feed or drinking water, although labour saving, is no guarantee that each animal receives a therapeutic dose, particularly since depressed appetite is a common feature of parasitism. The proper use of anthelmintics is only part of the treatment of parasitism. Attention must also be paid to factors such as adequate diet, hygiene and pasture management, which are outside the scope of this book.

Trematode infections

Liver flukes

Fasciola hepatica is a leaf-like trematode, about 5 cm in length, which is capable of infecting the liver of almost any mammal but is most prevalent in sheep and cattle. It is endemic in many wet regions and causes widespread morbidity and mortality in sheep and cattle. A related species, *Fasciola gigantica*, is found in tropical and subtropical areas but does not occur in western Europe. The eggs of *F. hepatica* are passed in the faeces of infected animals and hatch in about a week to release motile miracidia which penetrate the intermediate hosts, which are snails of the genus *Lymnaea*. The parasite undergoes a three-stage development in the snail and motile cercariae are eventually shed from the snail. These attach to vegetation and encyst. The encysted metacercarial form of the parasite is infective and the metacercariae are released in the mammalian intestine and penetrate the gut wall and liver capsule. They cause considerable damage to the liver parenchyma before migration to the bile ducts. The complete life cycle of *F. hepatica* takes about 18 weeks.

Clinically, fascioliasis in sheep may be acute, subacute or chronic. Acute fascioliasis is due to liver damage caused by the migration of young *F. hepatica* through the liver parenchyma within 6 weeks of infection. The subacute disease occurs 6–12 weeks after infection and is due partly to the same pathological changes of the acute form and also to anaemia resulting from the activity of the adult flukes in the bile ducts. Chronic fascioliasis, produced by liver flukes in the bile ducts, occurs from 12 weeks post-infection. There is a range of flukicidal drugs available to treat chronic fascioliasis, but not all are effective against the acute form of the disease.

The eggs of *F. hepatica* are often present in horse faecal samples, but treatment is rarely necessary. The parasite has occasionally been reported in pigs, but is not normally pathogenic, and fascioliasis is of no significance in dogs, cats or poultry in the UK. In contrast, liver fluke disease in ruminants, mainly due to *Fasciola* spp., causes severe economic loss, particularly following heavy summer rainfall, which enhances the development of infection in the intermediate host.

Cattle apparently have a greater inherent resistance to *F. hepatica* and fascioliasis is seen mainly in the chronic form. Acute fascioliasis is rare and then only affects young calves. Clinical fascioliasis in goats is less common than in sheep and, as in cattle, is usually seen as the chronic syndrome.

Flukicidal drugs

Oxyclozanide

Oxyclozanide (Fig. 22.1) is a chloro-substituted salicylanilide which acts by uncoupling oxidative phosphorylation, thereby decreasing the availability of high-energy phosphates, such as ATP, to the parasites. It has an efficiency exceeding 90 per cent in clearing adult flukes from cattle, sheep and goats, but only of the order of 50 per cent against immature forms. The efficiency of the drug in acute fascioliasis, caused by immature flukes, is improved by a three-fold increase in the dose, but apart from the risk of toxicity, more efficient drugs are available for this purpose. Oxyclozanide has a good safety margin and can be used in young, pregnant and lactating animals; transient scouring and reduced milk yield are the only side-effects which have been reported. It is rare among flukicidal drugs in having a zero milk withdrawal period but treated animals must not be slaughtered for human consumption for at least 14 days. At the time of writing, it is the only flukicide which is licensed in the UK for use in goats. Oxyclozanide is also marketed in various formulations with levamisole for the combined treatment of fascioliasis and nematode infections, although doubts remain about the economic and therapeutic benefits of such formulations.

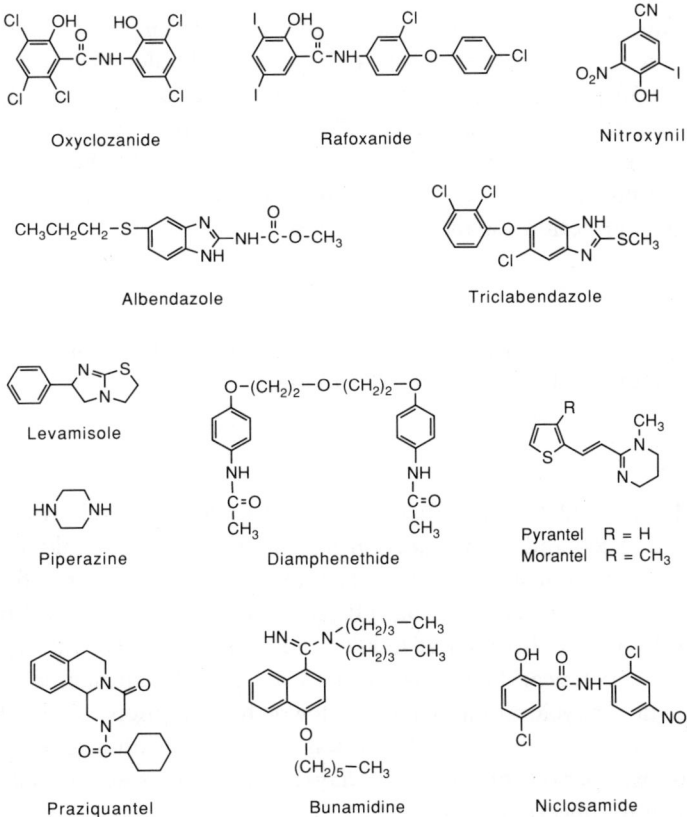

Figure 22.1 Structures of some of the anthelmintic drugs used in veterinary medicine.

Oxyclozanide is well absorbed following oral administration as a drench or in-feed granules and reaches high concentrations in the liver before its excretion in the bile as a glucuronide. It is strongly bound to plasma proteins and adult flukes are affected when they feed on blood and also by the drug or its metabolite in bile.

Dose

cattle	10 mg/kg
sheep and goat	15 mg/kg; acute fascioliasis 45 mg/kg

Brotianide

Brotianide is only available in combination with thiophanate (a benzimidazole for treatment of nematode infections) and is used in sheep. It is structurally related to rafoxanide (see below) and acts in a similar manner to it and to oxyclozanide, by uncoupling oxidative phosphorylation in the parasite and interfering with the production of ATP. Brotianide alone has an efficiency of less than 50 per cent against the young parasite in acute fascioliasis, but in the subacute disease efficiency is 75–90 per cent and increases to over 90 per cent against the adult flukes in chronic disease. At the recommended dose rate, it has a good safety margin and can be used in pregnant animals. The withdrawal period for meat is 21 days.

Dose

sheep   0.25 ml/kg of an oral suspension containing brotianide (22.5 mg/ml) and thiophanate (200 mg/ml).

Rafoxanide

Rafoxanide (Fig. 22.1) is formulated as a suspension for oral administration to cattle and sheep and as an injection for cattle. Like most flukicidal drugs, rafoxanide acts by uncoupling oxidative phosphorylation and interfering with ATP production. It has a good efficacy, similar to that of brotianide, against adult and 6–12-week-old flukes, and toxic effects are rare apart from occasional inappetence. The drug can be used in pregnant animals but, like most flukicides (oxyclozanide being a noteworthy exception), it should not be used in lactating animals where the milk is intended for human consumption. The withdrawal period for meat is 28 days, if the drug is given orally, and 21 days if given by injection.

It is strongly bound to plasma proteins which accounts, to some extent, for its efficacy against haemophagic parasites. The activity of rafoxanide against young flukes in the liver parenchyma is believed to be due to their presence in tracks surrounded by blood containing a sufficient concentration of the drug to destroy them.

Dose

cattle and sheep	7.5 mg/kg p.o.
cattle	3 mg/kg s.c.

Nitroxynil

For use in cattle and sheep, nitroxynil (Fig. 22.1) is marketed only as an injection because orally administered nitroxynil is partly converted to inactive metabolites in the rumen. Nitroxynil uncouples oxidative phosphorylation in the parasite but its activity may also be due to its ability to cause paralysis.

The efficacy of nitroxynil is comparable with that of rafoxanide, being more than 90 per cent efficient in the chronic disease, about 75 per cent in subacute disease and less than 50 per cent efficient against flukes less than 6 weeks old (unless the dose is increased). Nitroxynil can be used in pregnant animals and toxicity is rare at recommended doses. The drug is chemically related to dinitrophenol and has a similar stimulant effect on metabolism, which means that toxic effects are manifested as an increased respiratory rate and a rise in body temperature. The drug is a yellow dye and is not favoured by some sheep owners because it can cause wool staining at the site of injection. The withdrawal period for meat is 30 days and nitroxynil must not be used when milk from treated animals is intended for human consumption.

Dose

cattle and sheep	10 mg/kg s.c.

Albendazole and triclabendazole

The benzimidazoles (see p. 497) are a group of drugs which are highly effective and widely used in the treatment of nematode infections. One of the group, albendazole (Fig. 22.1), also has activity against adult flukes in cattle and sheep at increased dose levels (cattle 10 mg/kg; sheep 7.5 mg/kg) and has activity against tapeworms. It is rapidly and almost completely biotransformed to sulphoxide and sulphone metabolites, which are probably the active forms of the drug.

Triclabendazole (Fig. 22.1) is a remarkable new addition to the benzimidazole group of drugs and although it has little activity against nematodes, it is highly effective in cattle and sheep against all stages of fluke infections, from adult parasite to 2-day-old fluke. Triclabendazole is converted to sulphoxide and sulphone metabolites and the major route of excretion is via the bile. The drug is formulated as a drench and has a good safety margin, being suitable for use in young, pregnant or stressed animals. It must not be used in animals producing milk for human consumption, or in cows within 7 days of calving, and the withdrawal period for meat is 28 days. The drug is toxic to fish; care should be taken to avoid contaminating waterways or dams.

The mode of action and selective toxicity of the benzimidazoles as flukicides is believed to be due to their inhibitory action on the fumarate reductase enzyme of the parasite. The enzyme is necessary for metabolic processes and energy production in the parasite, but not in the host.

Dose

cattle	12 mg/kg p.o.
sheep	10 mg/kg p.o.

Diamphenethide

Diamphenethide (Fig. 22.1) is a substituted phenolic drug which is formulated as a suspension for oral administration to sheep and, in contrast to other flukicidal drugs, it is more potent against immature than against mature flukes. It has an efficiency exceeding 90 per cent against very young parasites in the liver parenchyma and the clinical response in acute fascioliasis is outstanding. Dosage has to be increased to obtain comparable efficacy against adult flukes and the cost of the drug could preclude its routine use in the treatment of chronic fascioliasis. Diamphenethide is safe at the recommended dose rate, but loss of wool and temporary impairment of vision have been reported in overdosed animals. The withdrawal period for meat is 7 days.

The drug is well absorbed from the gut and distributed through the body, reaching high concentrations in the liver and gall-bladder. It is de-acetylated in the liver and the amine metabolite is lethal to immature flukes, which accounts for the particular effectiveness of the drug in the treatment of acute and subacute fascioliasis. The activity of diamphenethide against mature flukes is less clinically useful at normal dose levels because only a small proportion of the active metabolite reaches the bile duct.

Dose

sheep	105 mg/kg

Selection of the most appropriate treatment for fascioliasis

Selection of drugs for the treatment of fascioliasis, or prophylactic control, should be based on a knowledge of their relative efficiency at different stages of the disease. However, particularly for the treatment of chronic fascioliasis, many safe and effective drugs are available and selection will inevitably be based, in part, on personal preference and relative costs. The following summary is intended as a guide in selection.

Goats
Oxyclozanide is the only flukicide licensed for use in goats in the UK and there is no statutory withholding period for milk.

Cattle
Acute and subacute fascioliasis is uncommon in cattle. The drug of choice is triclabendazole, which is also effective in the chronic syndrome. For treating chronic fascioliasis (the most common form in cattle) in late winter and spring, a selection can be made from oxyclozanide, rafoxanide, nitroxynil, triclabendazole or albendazole at an increased dose rate of 10 mg/kg. Oxyclozanide is the only flukicide which can be used in cattle producing milk intended for human consumption.

Prophylactic treatment of unhoused stock is normally carried out in December (in the northern hemisphere) to remove adult and immature parasites arising from pastures affected in the autumn. A second dose in April reduces pasture contamination and consequent snail infection. A single dosing of housed stock with triclabendazole when they are brought in should effectively remove both immature and mature parasites.

Sheep
The two outstanding effective drugs for treating acute fascioliasis, which has a peak incidence from October to January (in the northern hemisphere), are diamphenethide and triclabendazole. For subacute infections, again during the autumn and winter months, selection should be made from diamphenethide, triclabendazole, nitroxynil, rafoxanide or brotianide (marketed as a mixture with thiophanate).

Chronic fascioliasis (which has a peak incidence from January to April in Europe), can be treated with a larger variety of drugs which are effective against mature flukes. Selection for this purpose can be made from oxyclozanide, rafoxanide, nitroxynil, brotianide, triclabendazole or albendazole at an increased dose rate of 7.5 mg/kg. The choice is narrowed if the selection is made from drugs which are also effective against immature flukes.

To reduce pasture contamination with fluke eggs followed by snail infestation, it is recommended that animals should be dosed in March and May (in the northern hemisphere). Diamphenethide and triclabendazole are suggested as the drugs of choice for this purpose.

Other measures
These include a reduction in the populations of the intermediate hosts by the use of molluscicides (e.g. copper sulphate) and/or the removal of snail habitats.

Roundworm infections

Nematodes are cylindrical unsegmented worms, covered with a tough cuticle and possessing a complete gut. The sexes are usually separate. Many nematode species inhabit the stomach and intestines of animals, which may not show clinical signs if relatively few worms are present. It is good practice nevertheless to administer anthelmintics even in these cases, especially when flocks or herds are involved, to reduce pasture infection and to eliminate subclinical infection, which can cause economic losses.

Gastrointestinal nematodes, depending on the prevalent species and degree of infection, can cause enteritis, anaemia, severe unthriftiness and even death in horses, ruminants and small animal species. In the latter, there is an additional problem. If embryonated eggs of *Toxocara canis* from infected dogs are ingested by humans, visceral larva migrans can occur if massive numbers of larvae invade the body; this is called ocular larva migrans if the eye is affected. Although the incidence of such human disease is low, effective worm control in dogs is essential to minimize this zoonotic risk.

A smaller group of nematodes, the lungworms, inhabit the respiratory tract. Such infections have been demonstrated in all domestic species but most research on the pathogenesis and therapy of this condition has concentrated on the disease ('husk') in cattle. This has resulted in the production of the first commercial vaccine against a parasitic worm. Prophylactic use of anthelmintics against lungworms has proved unreliable. It is recommended, therefore, that lungworm vaccine should be used where the disease is endemic and that appropriate anthelmintics be used for treating sporadic disease outbreaks.

When a vaccination programme is adopted, calves must be protected from challenge by the parasite for 2 weeks after the second dose of vaccine. Vaccination does not completely protect against infection and this may result in a low level of pasture contamination. While this enhances the immunity of vaccinated calves, unvaccinated animals are at risk, so that vaccination of each new batch of calves is essential.

In disease outbreaks, the newer benzimidazoles, ivermectin or levamisole are rapidly effective if used before the parasites cause excessive tissue damage.

Treated animals should be returned to a clean pasture because they may not have developed a good immunity. Therapy is less effective in severely affected dyspnoeic animals where the disease is well established and some may remain in poor condition. In a few cases, anthelmintic therapy aggravates the clinical signs, sometimes fatally, but the precise reasons for this await elucidation.

Anti-nematodal drugs

There is a large selection of effective modern anthelmintics which are available for treating nematode infections and many have a wide spectrum of activity which may extend to tapeworms or flukes. The choice of a particular drug is based on relative efficiency, safety, cost and personal preference. Nematodes can develop resistance to anthelmintics and it is generally sound practice to continue to use one drug on a property whilst it remains effective. In horses, resistance to benzimidazoles in small strongyles has been reported. To minimize the problem, the anthelmintic should be routinely changed every 6 months.

Because of the rather daunting list of drugs on the market, the main features of those commonly used are described initially. Tables 22.1–22.6 summarize the relative efficiencies of anthelmintics against nematodes in different domestic animal species and are intended as a guide to drug selection.

Benzimidazoles

This remarkable group of anthelmintics has a very wide spectrum of activity and, in most cases, toxicity to the mammalian host is very low. Nematodes can damage the host in both their larval and adult stages and benzimidazoles are effective against both forms of the parasites.

An exception to the generally low degree of mammalian toxicity is the teratogenicity which can be caused by parbendazole, cambendazole, albendazole and oxfendazole. In sheep treated at about the third week of gestation, the incidence of rib and limb abnormalities in the lambs may be as high as 50 per cent. At the time of writing, the other benzimidazoles are considered safe to use in pregnant animals.

It has been shown that the benzimidazoles inhibit the fumarate reductase enzyme in susceptible parasites, thereby blocking an essential anaerobic pathway (fumarate acts as the terminal electron acceptor) and effecting selective toxicity because this pathway is not used in mammals. Benzimidazoles also bind to tubulin, a protein present in nematodes which is necessary for the formation of microtubules in intestinal cells. The parasites are thus effectively starved. Thiabendazole is also fungicidal *in vivo*.

Table 22.1 Anthelmintics used against gut nematodes in cattle

Drug (formation)	Efficiency			Withdrawal period (days)		Ovicidal	Comments and other activity
	Adults	Larvae	Arrested larvae	Meat	Milk		
Thiabendazole (drench, paste, in-feed)	A	B	Nil	Nil	Nil	Yes	Use at >100 mg/kg
Fenbendazole (drench, in-feed)	A	A	A/B	14	3	Yes	Lungworms and cestodes
Albendazole (drench)	A	A	A/B	14	Not used	Yes	Lungworms, cestodes and flukes (1.3 × normal dose)
Oxfendazole (drench)	A	A	A/B	14	Not used	Yes	Lungworms and cestodes
Febantel (drench)	A	A	A/B	14	Not used	Yes	For arrested larvae use at >10 mg/kg
Thiophanate (drench, in-feed)	A	A	B	7	3	Yes	Double dose in severe infections
Levamisole (s.c., drench, in food or drink, dermal)	A	A	D	3	1	No	Lungworms. Toxic signs may appear
Morantel tartrate (sustained release bolus)	A	B	D	14	0	No	Bolus releases drug over 90 days and prevents larval intake over this time
Ivermectin (s.c.)	A	A	A	21	Not used	No	Lungworms and several ectoparasites

Note: Parbendazole, oxibendazole and cambendazole are also available in some countries and are active against adults and developing larvae of gastrointestinal nematodes. Cambendazole also has activity against lungworms and cestodes.

Key to efficiency A >90%; B 75–90%; C 50–75%; D <50%.

Adapted from Bogan *et al*. *The Pharmacological Basis of Large Animal Medicine* (Blackwell Scientific Publications, 1983) with permission.

Table 22.2 Anthelmintics used against gut nematodes in sheep and goats

Drug (formation)	Efficiency			Withdrawal period (days)		Ovicidal	Comments and other activity
	Adults	Larvae	Arrested larvae	Meat	Milk		
Thiabendazole (drench, in-feed)	A	A/C	A/C	Nil	0*	Yes	Increase dose × 2 for *Nematodirus* and arrested larvae
Fenbendazole (drench, in-feed)	A	A	A	14	3	Yes	Lungworms and tapeworms
Albendazole (drench)	A	A	A	14	Not used	Yes	Lungworms, cestodes and flukes (1.3 × normal dose)
Oxfendazole (drench, in-feed)	A	A	A	10	Not used	Yes	Lungworms, tapeworms, adult flukes (increased dose rate)
Febantel	A	A/B	A/B	7	0	Yes	
Thiophanate (drench, in-feed, feed blocks)	A	A/B	A/B	7	3	Yes	Available in feed blocks
Levamisole (s.c., in feed)	A	A/B	A/B	3	1	No	Lungworms
Ivermectin (oral)	A	A	A	21	Not known	No	Lungworms

*Not used in lactating animals when milk is used for cheese production.

Key to efficiency A 90%; B 75–90%; C 50–75%; D insufficient evidence.

Adapted from Bogan *et al.* *The Pharmacological Basis of Large Animal Medicine* (Blackwell Scientific Publications, 1983) with permission.

Table 22.3 Anthelmintics used against lungworms in ruminants

A. Cattle lungworm *Dictyocaulus viviparus*

Drug	Formulation	Efficiency		Comments
		Adults	Larvae	
Levamisole	s.c. injection, oral	A	A	
Cambendazole	Oral	B	B	In severe infestation repeat treatment in 2 weeks
Fenbendazole	Oral	A	A	
Albendazole	Oral	A	A	
Invermectin	s.c. injection	A	A	

Note: Only fenbendazole and levamisole have been shown to be effective against arrested *D. viviparus*.

B. Lungworms of sheep and goats

Drug (formulation)	Dictyocaulus filaria		Muelleriys capillarus	Protostrongylus rufescens	Cystocaulus ocreatus
	Adults	Larvae			
Levamisole (s.c. injection)	A	A			
Fenbendazole, oxfendazole cambendazole, albendazole (drench, paste, in-feed)	A	A	Few significant results available as yet except that fenbendazole is very effective against *P. rufescens* and *C. ocreatus*		
Thiophanate (drench, in-feed)	A/B	A/B			
Ivermectin (drench)	A	A	★	★	★
Febantel (drench)	A	A	A	A	

Key to efficiency: A 90%; B 75–90%; ★Not yet known.
Adapted from Bogan *et al. The Pharmacological Basis of Large Animal Medicine* (Blackwell Scientific Publications, 1983) with permission.

Fenbendazole, oxfendazole and albendazole are effective at lower dose levels than thiabendazole because they are less soluble and are therefore in contact with the parasites for a longer period. This factor is important when selecting a drug to eliminate hypobiotic (arrested or inhibited) nematode larvae.

The apparently similar mode of action of many of the benzimidazoles means that if nematode resistance develops to one drug, there is usually

Table 22.4 Anthelmintics for nematodes in pigs

Drug	*Ascaris suum* (adults/larvae)	*Hyostrongylus rubidus* (adults/larvae)	*Oesophagostomum* spp. (adults/larvae)	*Trichuris suis* (adults/larvae)	Comments
Thiabendazone	D/D	A/C	A/C	D/D	No withdrawal; ovicidal
Parbendazole	A/D	A/D	A/D	B/U	16 days withdrawal; ovicidal
Cambendazole	A/B	A/C	A/C	D/D	14 days withdrawal, not sows for 5 weeks after service
Fenbendazole	A/B	A/A	A/B	A/D	14 days withdrawal; ovicidal, also active vs. *Metastrongylus*
Tetramisole	A/B	A/C	A/C	B/B	87 days withdrawal, ovicidal also active vs. *Metastrongylus*
Dichlorvos	A/D	A/D	A/D	A/A	No withdrawal
Morantel	A/B	A/C	A/C	D/D	14 days withdrawal
Febantel	A/C	A/C	A/C	A/D	Increased dose rate vs. *Trichuris*. 7 days withdrawal
Thiophanate	A/C	A/B	A/B	A/B	7 days withdrawal, ovicidal

Note: All administered in-feed. Several drugs combined with piperazine to remove *Ascaris*, e.g. thiabendazole. For treatment of clinical parasitism injectable levamisole or ivermectin are used.

Key to efficiency: A 90%; B 75–90%; C 50–75%; D <50%; U insufficient evidence.
Adapted from Bogan *et al. The Pharmacological Basis of Large Animal Medicine* (Blackwell Scientific Publications, 1983) with permission.

Table 22.5 Efficiency of anthelmintics against common internal equine parasites

Drug	Parascaris equorum	Strongy-loides	Large strongyles	Small strongyles	Oesopha-gostomum equi	'Bots'
Piperazine	+	−	−	+	+	−
Thiabendazole	±	+	+	+	+	−
Mebendazole	+	−	+	+	+	−
Fenbendazole	+	+	+	+	+	−
Oxfendazole	+	+	+	+	+	−
Febantel	+	ND	+	+	+	−
Oxibendazole	+	+	+	+	+	−
Pyrantel embonate	+	−	+	+	+	−
Dichlorvos	+	ND	+	+	+	+
Metriphonate	+	ND	−	−	+	+
Ivermectin	+	+	+	+	+	+

Key: + highly effective; ± poorly effective; − not effective; ND no data available.
Adapted from Bogan et al. The Pharmacological Basis of Large Animal Medicine (Blackwell Scientific Publications, 1983) with permission.

cross-resistance within the group. An alternative drug with a different mode of action should then be used.

Thiabendazole
Thiabendazole was the first of the benzimidazoles and because of its very broad spectrum of activity and virtual freedom from toxicity to mammals, its introduction was a tremendous advance in helminth therapy in farm animals. Various formulations are available (see Tables 22.1, 22.2, 22.4 and 22.5) for oral administration to ruminants, pigs and horses for treating gastrointestinal

Table 22.6 Anthelmintics used in dogs and cats: activity claimed by manufacturer

Product	Echinococcus	Taenia	Dipylidium	Toxocara/ Toxascaris	Uncinaria	Trichuris
Nitroscanate*	+	++	++	++	++	0
Fenbendazole	0	++	0	++	++	++
Mebendazole	+	++	0	++	++	++
Bunamidine	+	++	++	0	0	0
Praziquantel	++	++	++	0	0	0
Niclosamide	0	++	++	0	0	0
Piperazine	0	0	0	+	1.5 × normal dose	0

*Not licensed for use in cats.
Activity rating: ++ excellent, + very good; 0 erratic, poor or ineffective.
Adapted from D. Jacobs, In Practice, **6** (1984).

nematode infections. The drug has no activity against arrested larvae and more effective benzimidazoles and other drugs are used for eliminating lungworms.

Thiabendazole differs from other benzimidazoles in being rapidly absorbed from the gut. It is widely distributed in the body and quickly metabolized by hydroxylation followed by clearance in the urine and faeces as conjugation products. Most of a dose is cleared from the body within 2 days. It has proved virtually impossible to determine a median lethal dose for thiabendazole and doses of 20 times the recommended therapeutic dose have not caused significant toxic effects in farm animals. Because of its rapid clearance from the body, thiabendazole, unlike other benzimidazoles, can be used in lactating cows without withdrawing the milk.

Dose

sheep, horse	44–88 mg/kg (depending on parasite).
pig	50 mg/kg
cattle	66–110 mg/kg (depending on severity).

The structure of thiabendazole has been modified to produce a series of benzimidazoles (e.g. fenbendazole, albendazole, oxfendazole, mebendazole, parbendazole and oxibendazole) which, in general, are more slowly metabolized and cleared from the body. Consequently, they are effective in lower doses than thiabendazole and their spectrum of activity is even broader. For example (see Tables 22.3, 22.4 and 22.6), in addition to activity against gastrointestinal nematodes, some are effective against lungworms, tapeworms, flukes and various other parasites in dogs.

Until the introduction of the newer benzimidazoles, hypobiotic nematode larvae could not be eliminated by anthelmintics. This was believed to be due to their low metabolic rate preventing uptake of the drug. It is now known that the most important factor which determines efficacy against arrested (inhibited) larvae is the duration of their exposure to effective concentrations of anthelmintic. Thus at normal dose rates, the less soluble benzimidazoles, fenbendazole, oxfendazole and albendazole, have proved to be the most effective.

Fenbendazole

Fenbendazole is a versatile and commonly used anthelmintic. Like thiabendazole, it is an extremely safe drug and doses of several hundred times the normal therapeutic dosage have been given to sheep without side-effects; furthermore, it appears to be virtually impossible to overdose horses with the drug. Fenbendazole is not teratogenic, unlike some members of the group.

The drug has a wide spectrum of activity against immature and mature nematodes of the gut and respiratory tract of ruminants, pigs, horses, dogs and cats. Fenbendazole is used in pregnant bitches at a daily dose of 50 mg/kg, from day 40 of pregnancy to 14 days post-whelping. This substantially reduces the worm burden in the pups by killing somatic larvae in the bitch (the most important source of infection for puppies).

Dose

Depends on both species and helminth. Refer to manufacturer's instructions.

Fenbendazole has been described to illustrate how altering the structure of thiabendazole produces a drug with useful additional therapeutic applications. Other benzimidazoles will not be so described—albendazole (Fig. 22.1), oxfendazole, cambendazole, mebendazole, parbendazole, oxibendazole—and reference should be made to the tabulated summaries of their clinical applications.

Oxfendazole
Oxfendazole is marketed as a pulse-release bolus formulation. The bolus remains in the reticulo-rumen and delivers five or six doses of oxfendazole at approximately 21-day intervals. Since the first dose is released about 21 days after administration, the bolus provides programmed therapeutic dosing for a period of about 4 months. The oxfendazole bolus is designed for use in cattle when they are turned out to pasture to provide long-term control of parasitic gastroenteritis and lungworm infection.

Pro-benzimidazoles
Febantel and thiophanate (see Tables 22.1–22.5) are not benzimidazoles *per se*. However, febantel is metabolized to fenbendazole and oxfendazole; thiophanate is metabolized to benzimidazole carbamates.

Levamisole

This is one of a group of anthelmintics, also including pyrantel and morantel, which are cholinergic agonists and act at acetylcholine receptors on the surface of the nematode muscle cells and at the neuromuscular junction (see Fig. 22.1). Selective toxicity is not a problem with levamisole at recommended dosage, but it does not have the extraordinarily wide safety margin of the benzimidazoles.

Levamisole is formulated for oral administration and subcutaneous injection in ruminants and pigs. It has a broad spectrum of activity against larval and adult forms of gut nematodes and lungworms.

Levamisole has a depolarizing action on the nematodes which causes a spastic paralysis and expulsion of most of the worms within 24 hours. At higher doses it produces cholinergic effects in mammals, manifested by salivation, defecation, bradycardia and muscle tremors; these toxic effects are rarely seen at normal dosage. Early studies showed that the horse is particularly sensitive to levamisole and the drug is contraindicated in this species.

The rate of T-lymphocyte differentiation and activity of phagocytes is potentiated by levamisole. Beneficial effects of this immunostimulant action have been observed in calves, dogs, cats and human patients with immuno-deficiencies, chronic infection, inflammatory disease and some malignancies. Intermittent treatment with one-third of the normal therapeutic dose for 3-day periods separated by 3 days without dosing seems to provide the optimum response.

Dose

ruminants and pigs   7.5 mg/kg p.o. or s.c.

Morantel and pyrantel

Morantel, which is the methyl analogue of pyrantel (Fig. 22.1) has a broad spectrum of activity against adult gut nematodes in cattle but activity is less effective against immature forms and it is not effective for treating hypobiotic larvae or lungworms. The mechanism of action of both morantel and pyrantel is to produce depolarization blockade of neuromuscular function in the parasite. This is first manifested as a nicotine-like activation followed by paralysis. These drugs thus act in a similar way to levamisole on the parasite, but toxic effects are rarely seen in animals at the recommended dosage, probably because of poor absorption from the gut.

A particular attribute of morantel is its formulation. It is marketed as a sustained-release bolus which provides a continuous release of the drug in the reticulo-rumen for at least 90 days after administration. Administered to ruminating grazing cattle when turned out to pasture, it controls parasitic gastroenteritis for the whole grazing season by reducing the build-up of infective larvae on the pasture. Pyrantel has similar properties to morantel. It is formulated as a paste, suspension and granules for broad-spectrum control of adult gut nematodes in horses and dogs. The drug is effective and has a good safety margin, being suitable for use in young puppies and pregnant and lactating bitches.

Dose

(as pyrantel embonate)

horse 19–38 mg/kg p.o.
dog 14.4 mg/kg p.o.

Organophosphates

Organophosphorus compounds have been used for many years as systemic ectoparasiticides and, subsequently, some were developed as anthelmintics. With the introduction of the broad-spectrum and much safer anthelmintics described above, only two organophosphates, dichlorvos and metriphonate, are currently available as anthelmintics in the UK.

The drugs are anticholinesterases and thus potentiate the effects of endogenous acetylcholine in the parasite. Higher doses induce signs of excessive parasympathetic stimulation in the host and their margin of safety is low. The muscle relaxant suxamethonium should not be used within 10 days of their administration because it is metabolized by cholinesterase and if the enzyme has been inhibited, paralysis will be prolonged. Dichlorvos is available as an in-feed formulation for nematode control in pigs and horses. Metriphonate is formulated as a paste for use in horses. Its spectrum of activity, like that of dichlorvos, includes 'bots' (*Gasterophilus* spp.) which is a useful attribute (see Table 22.5).

Nitroscanate

This anthelmintic is used only in dogs, where it has a remarkably broad spectrum of activity against nematodes (except *Trichuris*) and tapeworms. At the recommended dosage it gives limited control of *Echinococcus granulosus*. Nitroscanate has a wide safety margin and can be used in all dogs, including puppies and lactating animals.

Dose

50 mg/kg

Piperazine

Piperazine (Fig. 22.1) is an old drug used originally in the treatment of gout and later in the treatment of *Ascaris lumbricoides* infection in humans. It has been widely used in veterinary medicine for many years and is still indicated as an inexpensive and efficient treatment for ascarid and other infections (Tables 22.5 and 22.6). Ascarids are not a problem in ruminants in the UK, where the drug is used for the treatment of horses, pigs, dogs, cats and poultry.

Piperazine probably acts by mimicking the inhibitory neurotransmitter action of γ-aminobutyric acid in the worms. Thus, the motility of the parasites is depressed and they are expelled from the gut by normal peristaltic movements (there is no effect on immature stages in other tissues). This is not a simple effect, however; the response of the worm to electrical stimulation is not blocked and the effects of piperazine are antagonized by acetylcholine. It is a pharmacological antagonist of pyrantel and morantel.

The drug is safe at recommended dosage and has a wide safety margin of approximately 1 : 8. There are reports of neurotoxicity in kittens following dosing at several times the recommended level (the drug is widely available in the UK as a General Sales List product); small animals should be weighed to ensure accurate dosing.

Dose

(as piperazine hydrate)
dog and cat	80–240 mg/kg p.o. (according to helminth)
horse and pig	up to 160 mg/kg p.o.
poultry	up to 160 mg/kg p.o.

Ivermectin

This is a relatively recent addition to the range of anthelmintics and, at the time of writing, is licensed in the UK for use in horses, cattle, sheep, goats and pigs. Ivermectin is the most widely used of a group of naturally occurring macrolides, the avermectins, although ivermectin itself is semi-synthetic. The drug has a high degree of efficiency (see Tables 22.1–22.3) against nematode infections in the gut and lungs and canine heartworm. It is also effective against warbles in cattle, and against lice and mange mites in cattle and pigs. Ivermectin has a selective toxic effect on the parasite's nervous system, probably similar to the action of piperazine.

Dose

cattle	200 μg/kg s.c.
pig	300 μg/kg s.c.
dog (heartworm/prophylaxis)	6 μg/kg p.o. monthly
sheep, goat, horse	200 μg/kg p.o.

Nematode control programmes

Cattle

The strategic use of anthelmintics is combined with pasture management in controlling parasitic gastroenteritis. It is mainly young animals in their first grazing season which are affected and anthelmintic treatment should be applied to coincide with peak fluctuations of infective nematode larvae.

Infective larvae overwinter on pasture and infect animals turned out to grass in early spring. It is recommended that animals are dosed at 3 weeks and 6 weeks after they are turned out or at intervals of 5 weeks if ivermectin is used.

A second peak of infective larvae occurs on pastures from about mid-July in the northern hemisphere, arising from animals infected from spring grazing. Anthelmintic dosing should be repeated at this time and continued at monthly intervals if animals are allowed to graze in the same pasture. Alternatively, they should be moved to 'clean' grazing which has not been used by cattle in that year. Any overwintered larvae should have died by mid-summer.

When cattle are housed for the winter, they should be treated with a drug which is effective against hypobiotic larvae which develop in autumn; either ivermectin or one of the long-acting benzimidazoles (see p. 503) would be suitable.

It is more difficult to predict periods of pasture infestation with lungworm larvae and prophylactic use of anthelmintics as outlined for gut nematodes is not considered reliable by some authorities. A rational approach to control is the use of lungworm vaccine where the disease is endemic, and anthelmintics to treat sporadic disease outbreaks. However, since several anthelmintics are effective against gut nematodes and lungworms (see Tables 22.1 and 22.3), strategic use of appropriate drugs to control parasitic gastroenteritis may concurrently control lungworm problems. A recent programme is injections of ivermectin at 3, 8 and 13 weeks after turning out to pasture.

Other species

Programmes for the control of parasitic gastroenteritis in sheep are similar to the strategy outlined for cattle.

In horses, pasture rotation and mixed species grazing combined with routine dosing with a broad-spectrum anthelmintic at 6-week intervals is a rational approach to control worm burdens. The anthelmintic should be routinely changed every 6 months.

Pigs are rarely dosed individually with anthelmintics, but rather are treated by mass-medication with in-feed products (Table 22.4) to alleviate poor productivity. A rational control programme is to dose sows before farrowing and dose the litter at weaning, then at intervals of about 2 months. The nematode burden is controlled in boars by medication twice yearly.

The prophylactic use of anthelmintics in dogs, which is also important for public health reasons, is discussed in the following section.

Tapeworm infections

In most countries, tapeworm (cestode) infection in farm animals is regarded as a minor problem, not requiring treatment with a specific drug. Some of the benzimidazoles (e.g. oxfendazole, fenbendazole and albendazole) which are used to treat nematode infections are also effective against tapeworms. Specific treatment for tapeworms was rarely used in horses, until the evidence of recent reports that *Anoplocephala perfoliata* infection is associated with erosions around the ileo-caecal valve and intussusception. Either niclosamide (200–300 mg/kg) or pyrantel embonate (38 mg/kg) is effective.

The situation in dogs and cats is quite different from that in ruminants, and treatment for tapeworm infections is necessary for several reasons. Heavy infection with cestodes can cause digestive disturbances or pruritus ani when segments are passed, but the aesthetic requirements of the owner are usually a more pressing reason for treatment. Several species of *Taenia* infect the dog as the definitive host. In some species, the sheep is the intermediate host, where the effects can include acute coenurosis ('gid') or tissue damage with carcase condemnation, which may cause substantial economic loss. The dog is the definitive host for *Echinococcus granulosus* and effective treatment is important because the parasite causes hydatidosis in the intermediate hosts which include humans, the horse and meat animals (particularly sheep). In human infections, the massive hydatid cysts which develop (usually in the lungs) probably reflect the slow growth of the cyst and the fact that infection usually occurs in childhood. Rupture of a cyst can generate secondary cysts, however. Radiological and/or immunological confirmation of hydatid disease is usually followed by the surgical removal of the cysts. In Australia, for example, the prevalence of the disease in humans corresponds roughly to the number of sheep in the area.

Anticestodal drugs

Arecoline

This parasympathomimetic used to be indicated for treating cestode infections in dogs, but it has now been replaced by equally effective and much safer drugs. An arecoline purge (5–15 mg) is still sometimes used as the only effective means of diagnosing *Echinococcus granulosus* infection in dogs, since the eggs are indistinguishable from those of *Taenia* species and the adult tapeworm must be identified. This is not possible with other anthelmintics because the worms are killed and subsequently digested.

Broad-spectrum drugs

Nitroscanate and the benzimidazoles, fenbendazole and mebendazole, were described in the previous section as drugs used in nematode infections. They are also effective against some tapeworm species (see Table 22.6), and fenbendazole and mebendazole are also licensed in the UK for use in cats.

Narrow-spectrum drugs

Three drugs are currently used specifically for their efficacy against cestodes in dogs and cats and occasionally in other species when treatment is considered necessary (Table 22.6).

Praziquantel
Praziquantel (Fig. 22.1) is generally acknowledged to have unsurpassed activity against tapeworms in dogs and cats, particularly when *Echinococcus granulosus* is present. It is also effective against *Moniezia* species in ruminants, but these worms rarely cause a clinical problem, and should be effectively controlled if oxfendazole, fenbendazole or albendazole is used to treat concurrent nematode infections.

The drug is formulated for oral or parenteral administration and is effective against mature and immature forms of tapeworms. Injection may be subcutaneous or intramuscular, but the latter is preferred when *E. granulosus* is suspected. It acts by impairing the normal tegument function of the parasite which makes it permeable to excessive glucose loss and susceptible to the host's proteolytic enzymes. Thus, whole tapeworms or even recognizable segments are rarely voided.

Praziquantel has a good safety margin and can be administered to pregnant and young animals without dietary restriction.

Dose

dog and cat	5 mg/kg p.o.; 3.5–7.5 mg/kg s.c. or i.m.
horse	10 mg/kg p.o.

Bunamidine
Bunamidine (Fig. 22.1) is administered orally to dogs and cats and is effective against all the common tapeworm species, but repeated dosing is necessary in *E. granulosus* infections. Bunamidine is highly effective against adult *E. granulosus*, but less so against immature forms. Since the prepatent period for this parasite is about 47 days, a 6-weekly dosing schedule is necessary in intensive control programmes. Overdosage commonly causes severe vomiting and diarrhoea. Deaths have occasionally been reported from cardiac failure,

which may have been due to bunamidine sensitization of the heart to catecholamines, leading to ventricular fibrillation.

Dose

dog, cat   20–40 mg/kg p.o.

Niclosamide

Niclosamide (Fig. 22.1) is effective against cestodes in horses and sheep, but as mentioned previously, specific treatment is rarely necessary in sheep. It is marketed for oral administration to dogs and cats for treating infestations by *Taenia* and *Dipylidium* species. Activity against *E. granulosus* is poor and the manufacturers recommend using four times the normal dose in such infections; praziquantel would be more appropriate.

Niclosamide acts by blocking exogenous respiration and glucose uptake by inhibiting the anaerobic incorporation of phosphate into ATP. The worms then become susceptible to the host's proteolytic enzymes and are partially digested.

The drug has a good safety margin and can be used in pregnant and young animals.

Dose

dog, cat   125 mg/kg p.o.

Helminth control programmes in dogs

Toxocara and *Ascaris* can be assumed to be present in virtually every litter of pups. Control protects the pups from the deleterious effects of severe infestation and it is important to minimize the public health risk of visceral larva migrans (see p. 496).

The ultimate source of infection for adults and pups is the embryonated egg. Pups can also be infected by larvae *in utero* and also from the dam's milk. Furthermore, the drugs which have been described, when used at the normal dose rate, are only effective against ascarids in the gut; they do not kill somatic larvae in the tissues, so repeated dosing is necessary.

Ideally, dosing of pups should begin at about 2 weeks of age (when the first prenatally transmitted worms are susceptible) and should continue at fortnightly intervals until about 3 months of age. Further treatment at 6 months of age and then at yearly intervals will deal with the small number of adult worms which sometimes affect older dogs.

A more recent control technique—using fenbendazole at high daily dosage —overcomes the obstacle of conventional anthelmintic dosing, namely its ineffectiveness against somatic larvae, which are the most important source of infection for pups *in utero*. Fenbendazole, at high daily dosage (see p. 504), substantially reduces the worm burden in pups by killing somatic larvae in the bitch. Such programmes do not obviate the need for good hygiene to reduce the risk of reinfection from embryonated eggs.

Cestode infections can be treated in dogs with the effective drugs which are now available, but control also requires that the life cycle of the parasite is broken to minimize infection. For instance, the life cycle of *Dipylidium* involves the flea (occasionally the louse) as the intermediate host. In this infection, anthelmintic therapy in dogs and cats must be accompanied by effective control of the associated ectoparasites.

The control of *Echinococcus granulosus* infection is important because of its public health significance. Hydatid disease in humans (one of the intermediate hosts) is mainly confined to areas where there is contact between dogs (definitive host) and extensively grazed sheep (important intermediate hosts). National control schemes are in operation in various parts of the world and are usually based on the following general principles:

1. Collection of data to define local epidemiological patterns.
2. Registration of all working, hunting and pet dogs in the district.
3. Routine (3-monthly) treatment of all dogs with an appropriate anthelmintic.
4. An intensive education programme emphasizing that all sheep carcasses must be buried and that untreated offal is not fed to dogs.

There is little public health risk associated with *Taenia* species. Control is based on the use of effective anthelmintics in dogs and prevention of reinfection by strict dietary control as the metacestode forms are all found in meat animals.

CHAPTER 23

ECTOPARASITICIDES

The ectoparasiticides are products used to treat skin diseases caused by arthropod parasites, chiefly arachnids (ticks and mites) or insects (flies, lice and fleas). The term pesticide is often used synonymously with ecto-parasiticide, as is insecticide, although by strict definition, the insecticides are only active against flies, lice and fleas.

The control of ectoparasites of domesticated animals is important. In addition to the discomfort and sometimes allergic responses they cause, heavy infestation leads to losses in production due to unthriftiness and damage to fleece and hides. Some ectoparasites are vectors for transmission of other diseases. For example, ticks transmit the virus causing louping-ill in sheep and the protozoan parasite causing babesiasis in cattle; fleas are intermediate hosts for the tapeworm *Dipylidium*, which infests dogs. Control of ectoparasites of animals is also necessary to prevent transmission of diseases to in-contact humans. Common examples are skin lesions caused by mites (*Sarcoptes* and *Cheyletiella*) and fleas from small animals.

Selective toxicity to ectoparasites is due to the more rapid absorption of the pesticide through the chitinous cuticle of the parasite than the skin of the host. Furthermore, many pesticides act on nervous tissue, which in ectoparasites is located near the cuticle. Another factor accounting for selective toxicity is that mammals are better endowed than the parasites with enzymes that rapidly metabolize some pesticides, such as the organophosphates.

Nevertheless, pesticides are potentially toxic to mammals and, in turn, to humans. It is important to observe the manufacturer's directions with reference to factors such as method of use, disposal of waste dips and empty containers, possible toxic reactions if used with other products, the use of protective clothing by the operator and withdrawal periods when used on food animals.

The extensive use of pesticides in agriculture (including horticulture) causes public concern. They can poison wildlife (bees and fish are particularly susceptible) or can be passed along the food chain to the human consumer. This has led to government bans on the use of certain organochlorine pesticides in many countries.

Populations of ectoparasites develop resistance to pesticides in a similar manner to bacteria, which become resistant to antibiotics as a result of selection pressure. Some individuals, by spontaneous mutation, possess genes which confer resistance so that this resistance is heritable. When exposed to the pesticide, the resistant organisms multiply while the susceptible ones are destroyed. Again, analogous to antibiotic resistance in bacteria, there is often cross-resistance; for example, ectoparasites resistant to one organophosphorus compound are usually resistant to other organophosphates. A pesticide with a different mode of action should then be used. When the selection pressure of the pesticide is removed, the population usually slowly reverts to sensitivity.

In some cases, resistance to pesticides can be overcome by incorporating compounds which inhibit the parasite's ability to destroy the pesticide. Piperonyl butoxide, itself a weak insecticide, acts in this way with the insecticidal pyrethrins, resulting in a clinically useful synergism. Theoretically, this same synergism could be used with other pesticides, such as the organophosphates, which are also hydroxylated by the same mixed function oxidase system as the pyrethrins. In practice, this is not feasible because the toxic effects of the organophosphates on the mammal are also likely to be enhanced.

Classification

The number of products for controlling ectoparasite infestations is large because, in many cases, the same active compound is marketed in different formulations, such as aerosol spray and wash. In this account, representative examples of each class or chemical group of compounds will be described, with an indication of the formulations available. Manufacturers' data sheets should be consulted for details of methods of use and withdrawal periods.

The main classes of pesticides are benzyl benzoate, naturally occurring compounds, amitraz, organochlorine compounds, organophosphorus compounds and carbamates.

Benzyl benzoate

This was commonly used as an emulsion or tincture for treating mange (except demodectic mange) in horses, dogs and pigs, but has been superseded by more effective treatments. It is contraindicated in cats.

Benzyl benzoate is still used occasionally as one choice of insect repellant in treating 'sweet itch' in ponies, a distressing hypersensitivity reaction to the bites of *Culicoides* midges. The emulsion is diluted with liquid paraffin and applied to affected areas of the mane and tail. Systemic corticosteroids are also used in acutely affected animals. Affected and known susceptible animals should be stabled during the period of dusk from April to October (in the northern hemisphere) when midges are active, and a fly repellant used in the stable. Some clinicians simply maintain a film of Liquid Paraffin B.P. on the skin and hair of the mane and tail. This prevents midges from coming in contact with the skin and appears to be as effective as a pesticide dressing.

Naturally occurring compounds

Derris

Derris consists of the dried roots and rhizomes of exotic leguminous plants (*Derris* spp.) and contains several pesticide residues, of which the main active ingredient is rotenone. Rotenone inhibits the oxidation of pyruvate and glutamate. Selective toxicity is due to selective uptake through the cuticle and by ingestion. It is poorly absorbed through mammalian skin (and gut if skin dressings are ingested) but should not be used in cats. It is used in sheep dips in Australia. Rotenone is toxic to bees and fish (it was originally used in South East Asia as a fish poison) and care is necessary in disposing of waste skin washes.

Before the development of organophosphorus pesticides, derris was used to treat warble infestation in cattle. It is used as a wash or bath against fleas and lice in dogs (not cats) and large animals, but probably less commonly than the newer products described below. However, it is still one of the few effective treatments for demodectic mange in dogs.

Demodectic mange presents as a localized (squamous) or generalized (pustular) form. The parasite is found in the skin (hair follicles) of most healthy dogs and is transmitted from the bitch early in the neonatal period. Pustular demodicosis is apparently associated with T-cell lymphocyte suppression. This is currently considered to originate as a specific, hereditary T-cell defect, thus allowing the parasite to multiply and to induce a humoral agent which causes generalized T-cell suppression. It is commonly recommended that carrier bitches should not be used for breeding.

Although now discontinued in the UK, 3 per cent alcoholic solution (for effective skin penetration) of rotenone diluted and used according to the manufacturer's instructions, is a very effective treatment, even for generalized demodicosis. This form is often associated with secondary bacterial deep pyoderma and sensitivity testing is necessary to select an appropriate systemic antibiotic for concurrent use (see p. 430). Treatment should be continued for about 3 weeks and is effective in more than 90 per cent of cases.

Generalized demodicosis associated with secondary pyoderma is severely pruritic but the use of corticosteroids is contraindicated. Corticosteroids are likely to enhance the immunosuppression already present, thus favouring multiplication of mites and bacteria. Corticosteroids are also contraindicated in localized demodicosis because they can predispose to the development of the generalized form.

Pyrethrum

The exotic pyrethrum plant (*Chrysanthemum cinerariaefolium*) contains several insecticidal esters called pyrethrins. These are effective against flies, lice and fleas, but not mites. Pyrethrins are very rapid in action, being well absorbed through the chitinous cuticle (and in common with most pesticides through the gills of fish) to poison the nervous system by affecting the fluxes of Na^+ and K^+ associated with action potentials. Pyrethrins are commonly formulated as insecticidal aerosol sprays for domestic use and their rapid 'knock down' action is very obvious.

The selective toxicity of pyrethrins is very favourable. They are among the least toxic of all pesticides to mammals and birds because any pyrethrin which is absorbed is rapidly metabolized by mixed function oxidases. These enzymes are not normally very active in insects but their activity can increase after exposure to pyrethrins, with the consequent development of resistance. Pyrethrins are therefore often formulated with a synergist.

Pyrethrins have been largely replaced for therapeutic purposes by synthetic pyrethroids, but synergised preparations of pyrethrins are available for the control of fleas, lice and ticks on dogs and flies on horses and cattle.

Synthetic pyrethroids were developed to overcome the disadvantage of the natural pyrethrins, namely their instability when exposed to light. While this makes pyrethrins safe pesticides, it also follows that they have no persistent effect and frequent applications are impracticable in large flocks or herds. In contrast the synthetic pyrethroids are stable in the atmosphere and on the animal so that a useful, persistent effect is achieved. Selective toxicity is good, but manufacturers' directions must be observed, particularly when products such as aerosols are dispensed. For example, cats may occasionally show hyperaesthesia following the enthusiastic use of permethrin aerosols by owners. There is no specific antidote, but undisturbed confinement in a darkened receptacle has proved effective in cases reported to date.

The following pyrethroids are currently available in the UK:

Permethrin

Permethrin (Fig. 23.1) is marketed in several formulations. A concentrated water-miscible oil preparation, diluted as instructed, is sprayed onto cattle to control fly infestation. The same formulation is used topically on horses as an alternative to benzyl benzoate in the treatment of sweet itch.

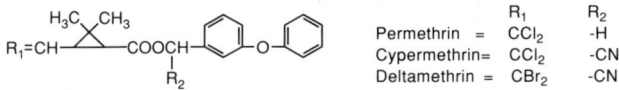

		R_1	R_2
Permethrin	=	CCl_2	-H
Cypermethrin	=	CCl_2	-CN
Deltamethrin	=	CBr_2	-CN

Figure 23.1 Structures of insecticidal pyrethroids.

Permethrin is also available as a ready-to-use solution, applied as a measured dose along the mid-line of the neck and back to control flies and lice on cattle. One application protects for several weeks. This product and other 'pour-on' and 'spot-on' preparations are formulated in such a way that the active principle spreads over the skin surface of the animal.

A novel formulation of permethrin is flexible PVC ear tags, which are impregnated with insecticide and can be used to control flies on cattle for up to 4 months. The permethrin rubs off the surface of the tag onto the skin and is spread by normal body movements.

Permethrin is also formulated as dusting powder, shampoo and aerosol sprays for the control of flea infestation in dogs and cats, giving protection against infestation for up to 2 weeks.

Flea infestation is considered to be the most important cause of parasitic skin disease of cats in the UK and the cat flea is the most common variety found on dogs. In addition to the damage caused by self-trauma or hypersensitivity reactions, the parasites produce papular urticarial reactions in humans. Effective eradication is therefore important. Corticosteroids or (in cats) megestrol acetate (2.5–5.0 mg twice weekly) are sometimes used to reduce pruritus, but not as a substitute for parasiticidal therapy.

For effective flea control, all animals in the household must be treated and attention given to their environment. Fleas are facultative parasites and spend much of their life cycle in carpets, furnishings and the animals' bedding. The environment should be vacuum cleaned and a suitable parasiticide applied. A combination of permethrin and methoprene is available as an aerosol which both kills adult fleas and stops the development of hatching eggs. Alternatives are organophosphates (e.g. iodofenphos and dichlorvos, either alone or in combination). These preparations are for application to carpets, etc. and not directly onto the animals.

Cypermethrin

Cypermethrin (Fig. 23.1) is similar to permethrin in formulations, indications and residual action. Sprays of diluted concentrate are used to control flies on cattle and horses, lice on cattle and red mite on poultry. Impregnated PVC ear tags are available to provide control of flies on cattle for up to 5 months. A ready-to-use solution is applied along the neck and back to control flies, lice and ticks on sheep and lice on goats.

Tetramethrin and phenothrin

Tetramethrin and phenothrin are other examples of synthetic pyrethroids. They are formulated together in an aerosol spray for the control of fleas on dogs and cats to provide a rapid action and sufficient persistence to protect against reinfestation for up to 2 weeks.

Deltamethrin

Deltamethrin (Fig. 23.1) is formulated in an oil base for use in cattle, sheep and pigs as a 'spot on' application of a measured dose to the mid-line of the back. The product gives protection for several weeks against lice and flies on cattle, lice on pigs, and flies, lice, ticks and keds on sheep. For effective use on sheep, the fleece should be parted and the dose applied to the skin. As with similar spot-on and pour-on formulations, the drug spreads over the skin surface.

Ivermectin

The avermectins are a group of lactones produced by the actinomycete *Streptomyces avermitilis*, and dihydroavermectin B_1 (ivermectin) has a remarkably broad spectrum of chemotherapeutic activity. Ivermectin is potent and is effective at a dose of 0.2 mg/kg (0.3 mg/kg in pigs) against a range of endoparasites and ectoparasites. It is currently licensed in the UK for oral administration in horses, sheep and goats and subcutaneous injections in pigs, beef cattle and non-lactating dairy cattle. There are recent and promising reports of the large-scale use of ivermectin to treat river blindness (onchocerciasis) in humans.

The action of ivermectin is probably due to its ability to block transmission in the nervous system of susceptible parasites. Gamma-amino butyric acid (GABA) is an inhibitory transmitter in nervous tissue and there is evidence that ivermectin acts by indirectly stimulating GABA receptors. Selective toxicity is good; for example, up to 30 times the therapeutic dose does not cause toxic effects in cattle.

Ivermectin is contraindicated in cattle producing milk for human consumption. As with all medicinal products, the manufacturers' data sheets should be consulted for current recommendations on withdrawal periods and special precautions in handling the product and disposal of containers.

Clinical applications

In addition to its use as an effective anthelmintic against gastrointestinal and lungworms (see Chapter 22), the indications for ivermectin include the control of various ectoparasites.

In horses, ivermectin is effective against the gastric stages of *Gasterophilus* species (bot flies). Stomach bots are of little clinical significance, but dosing in November–January (in the northern hemisphere) removes them and breaks the life cycle of these nuisance flies. Ivermectin can be used to control warbles, sucking lice and mange mites (*Psoroptes* and *Sarcoptes*) in cattle. The drug is less effective against chorioptic mange and biting lice. Lice and mange mites which infest pigs can be eradicated with ivermectin, as can the larval stages of the nasal fly, *Oestrus ovis*, in sheep. Although the data sheets only indicate the use of ivermectin as an anthelmintic in goats, there are recent reports that the drug is most effective in the treatment of sarcoptic mange. The incidence of this condition in the UK appears to be increasing and it is considered to be the most difficult to treat of the mange infestations in goats.

At the time of writing, ivermectin is not licensed in the UK for use in small animals, such as dogs and cats, but there are good reports of its efficacy in treating mange. Adverse reactions have been reported in dogs, particularly in the Collie breeds. Ivermectin is used in Australia for heartworm disease prophylaxis in dogs and eliminates the tissue stage of the larva (*Dirofilaria immitis*) for up to 30 days after infection.

Ivomec injection (formulation for cattle) has been used in cats (0.1 ml s.c.) with excellent results in killing ear mites after one administration. A second injection was sometimes necessary after 3 weeks. This dose regimen has proved very effective in controlling ear mites, other mange mites, fleas, lice and worms, with no adverse reactions in the animals.

Amitraz

Amitraz is one of a group of compounds known as triazapentadienes (Fig. 23.2) and is used in certain parts of the world, including some states of Australia (NSW and Queensland) and the UK, as a dip formulation for effective control of ticks in sheep, goats and deer. The mode of action of the drug is not known.

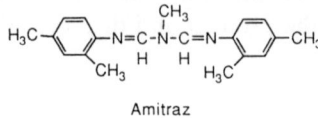

Amitraz

Figure 23.2 Structure of amitraz.

In the UK it is licensed for use in dogs for treating demodectic mange. The formulation (5 per cent) is diluted and used as a wash at weekly intervals for at least 3 weeks after signs have subsided or until live mites cannot be identified in skin scrapings. Treatment is effective but there are reports of resistance, and the recovery rate appears to be comparable with treatment involving derris as described above. Some animals with generalized demodectic mange will require repeated treatment because, as described earlier, this condition is associated with an immunological deficiency.

Amitraz is safe if used as directed, but is contraindicated in cats and in chihuahuas, where severe idiosyncratic reactions may occur. It is also available as a concentrate (12.5 per cent) for preparing dips and sprays for use on pigs, cattle and sheep (the spray can be used to disinfect buildings and in a pour on (2 per cent) solution. Amitraz is used to control mange and lice on pigs and cattle, and to control ticks, lice and keds on sheep. Tick collars impregnated with amitraz are available in Australia.

Organochlorine compounds

The chlorinated hydrocarbons were formerly very widely used to control a variety of insect pests both on crops and on animals. They are stable and thus had a persistent action; for example, when used as sheep dips their effectiveness lasted for many weeks. The compounds are also fat-soluble, which led to accumulating tissue residues in animals and thence in humans. Effects on the food chain, particularly fish and birds (the latter eating treated grain and crops), were quite disastrous, especially in raptors. Consequently, the use of these compounds is strictly controlled in many parts of the world. In the UK, gamma-benzene hexachloride (lindane, gamma-BHC) and bromocyclen are the only organochlorine compounds permitted for use on animals. The use of lindane is restricted in Australia, New Zealand and the USA because of the problems of residues in food animals.

Gamma-BHC (lindane)

Lindane has a broad spectrum of activity against mites (not *Demodex*), including sheep scab, and is a constituent of various UK government-approved sheep scab dips. It is effective against fleas, lice and ticks and is a versatile, economical pesticide, but resistance does develop fairly readily and has been reported most commonly in lice.

The mode of action is believed to be similar to that of DDT (dicophane). It is absorbed through the cuticle and affects the nervous system, disrupting action potentials to cause paralysis and death.

Acute toxicity in mammals is also manifested by effects on nervous tissue with muscle tremors, convulsions and sometimes respiratory paralysis as the main signs. Cats are particularly susceptible and care must be taken to observe the manufacturers' directions when using shampoos or wettable powders for baths. Affected animals should be treated with intravenous calcium borogluconate and barbiturates.

Lindane is formulated in a variety of ways. It is incorporated into several brands of ear drops to eliminate *Otodectes* mites, usually with antibacterials. Dusting powders, shampoos and wettable powders for baths are commonly used against other mange mites (except *Demodex*) and these are also effective against fleas and lice. When used in sheep dips, lindane is sometimes formulated with an organophosphate. Lindane is also incorporated with proflavine in a cream which will prevent fly attack of open wounds for up to 7 days.

Bromocyclen (Alugan)

Bromocyclen has a broad spectrum of pesticidal activity similar to that of lindane. It is therefore a versatile and economical drug, but as with lindane, resistant ectoparasites can be a problem. Bromocyclen is effective against fleas, lice, sheep keds and most types of mange mites except *Demodex*. In the U.K. it is licensed for use in all domesticated species except poultry because of the danger of residues in eggs.

Bromocyclen is formulated as a dusting powder (used directly on animals and their bedding), aerosol spray and concentrate powder for preparing washes, dips or sprays. Cats are particularly susceptible, as with lindane, to the toxic effects of bromocyclen. The aerosol or dusting powder, rather than the bathing formulation, should normally be used in this species.

Organophosphorus compounds

These compounds are typically esters or amides or phosphoric or thiophosphoric acids. Some of the original organophosphates were developed as nerve gases for use in chemical warfare, but not all organophosphates are equally toxic and many are now used as pesticides against a wide range of parasites in farm and companion animals.

The organophosphates are anticholinesterases. Thus, following rapid absorption through the cuticle of the parasite, they form stable complexes with the cholinesterase in the nervous system which inhibits the metabolism of acetylcholine and kills the parasite. Some compounds have direct anticholinesterase action. Others, mainly phosphorothionates, have no anticholinesterase activity *per se*, and are activated in the body by metabolism to organophosphates.

Resistance of various ectoparasites to organophosphorus compounds is increasing and several mechanisms of resistance have been described.

Organophosphates can also form stable complexes with mammalian cholinesterases, but selectivity arises because mammals are better endowed than parasites with enzymes that metabolize organophosphates. Metabolism is mainly by liver microsomal enzymes, which inactivate the compounds by hydrolysis or dealkylation; other enzymes in the kidney and plasma assist the process.

However, the cholinesterase-organophosphate complex is stable, and recovery seems to depend more on the synthesis of new cholinesterase than on the dissociation of the complex, which is variable, depending on the particular organophosphate. Thus, organophosphate which is absorbed and is not rapidly inactivated by metabolism, reduces cholinesterase levels, in some cases sufficiently to cause signs of toxicity.

It is interesting to note that the phosphorothionates are among the safest of this group of compounds. They are precursors of active metabolites and are commonly used in formulations for systemic absorption (see below). A proportion of the inactive precursor is metabolized directly to inactive metabolites and if this process is less efficient in the parasites, it may also contribute to selectivity.

Toxic effects due to organophosphorus pesticides are uncommon when the products are used as directed. Organophosphates are lipid-soluble and are so rapidly absorbed through mucous membranes that care is necessary, particularly when using aerosols, to ensure that none is inhaled. These agents are also absorbed through the skin and manufacturers' directions concerning protective clothing should be observed.

If cholinesterase levels are sufficiently lowered, signs of cholinergic poisoning, manifested as the muscarinic and nicotinic effects of acetylcholine, become apparent. These are variable combinations of salivation, diarrhoea, muscle tremor, convulsions and respiratory failure. In such cases, any residues on the skin should be washed off with soap and water. The muscarinic effects of the excess acetylcholine, which are responsible for many of the toxic signs, are readily antagonized by atropine. The initial dose may be given intravenously at a rate of 1–2 mg/kg or to effect mydriasis. Subsequent doses are administered subcutaneously at about hourly intervals as necessary.

Oximes such as pralidoxime are specific antidotes (up to 10 mg/kg i.v.), acting by splitting the cholinesterase-organophosphorus complex, but unfortunately they are only effective within a few hours of exposure to the pesticide.

Clinical uses

Many organophosphorus products are currently licensed for various uses in all domesticated animals. Only representative examples will therefore be mentioned to illustrate the different formulations and uses. Data sheets should be consulted for details of dosage or application and precautions in use.

Two or more formulations of an organophosphorus compound (e.g. an impregnated collar and aerosol spray, or an organophosphate anthelmintic and a pesticide) should not be used concurrently because of the increased risk of toxicity. Similarly, organophosphates should not be used concurrently with other anticholinesterases (e.g. carbamates) or with other drugs which stimulate acetylcholine receptors (e.g. levamisole; see Chapter 22), or which are inactivated by cholinesterases (e.g. the muscle relaxant, suxamethonium).

Aerosol sprays containing dichlorvos and fenitrothion are widely used to control fleas, lice, ticks and mange mites on cats and dogs. They are clean and easy to use, but when dispensed, the client must be warned against over-enthusiastic application.

Insecticidal collars impregnated with dichlorvos or diazinon are available for cats and dogs. They are claimed to provide protection against fleas for several months, but their efficacy is questionable, particularly in hypersensitized animals. The fleas have to feed (which induces the allergic response) before being killed by ingesting the pesticide.

Aqueous suspensions of coumaphos, diazinon, chlorofenvinphos or mixtures of these are used as washes, dips or sprays in horses, cattle, sheep, pigs and goats against flies, lice, ticks and mange mites.

Oil-based solutions of fenthion and phosmet are formulated for pour-on use in cattle to treat warbles, lice and mange. A proportion of the active principle is absorbed through the skin into the circulation to affect all stages of warble fly larvae. Treatment for warbles must not be undertaken during December to mid-March (in the northern hemisphere) when the larvae are migrating through the epidural fat. Killing the larvae in this site may cause a local reaction and damage the spinal cord.

Cythioate is a phosphorothionate formulated for oral administration as tablets. It is licensed for use in cats to control fleas and in dogs to control fleas, ticks and demodectic mange. The drug is well absorbed from the gut, widely distributed in the tissues and the maximum effect persists for up to 8 hours, after which is it rapidly eliminated. Ectoparasites are killed when they ingest body fluids. The margin of safety between recommended repeated oral dose and toxicity is stated to be 10-fold in the dog and 20-fold in the cat.

Dose

cythioate

cat   1.5 mg/kg as a single weekly dose for 4 weeks, then every second week to control reinfestation

dog   3 mg/kg as a single dose twice weekly. To control fleas and ticks, the dosage is continued for 4 weeks, then every second week to control reinfestation. To treat demodectic mange, 3 mg/kg as a single dose twice weekly for at least 6 weeks and for a maximum of 6 months if necessary.

Carbamates

The carbamates, like the organophosphorus compounds, are anticholinesterases. They combine with the enzyme more rapidly than the organophosphates, but are potentially less toxic to mammals because the enzyme-carbamate complex dissociates within about 3 hours. Toxic effects (similar to organophosphorus poisoning), which are apparently uncommon, are thus readily controlled with atropine. Formulations of propoxur and carbaryl licensed for use in dogs and cats are classified as GSL products in the UK (*see* Appendix 1), which indicates their relative safety.

Propoxur is used to control fleas. It is incorporated in insecticidal collars for dogs and an aerosol for use on dogs and cats. Carbaryl is formulated as a shampoo to control fleas in dogs and cats.

Selection of pesticides

The simplified summary shown in Table 23.1, based on the manufacturers' recommendations for the representative products included in the text, is intended for initial reference in drug selection. The text and data sheets should then be consulted for details of contraindications in particular species and efficacy against, for example, various types of mites.

Table 23.1 Selection of pesticides

	Flies	Lice	Fleas	Ticks	Mites (not *Demodex*)	*Demodex*
Derris		\	\			\
Pyrethrins		\	\	\		
Permethrin	\	\	\			
Cypermethrin	\	\		\	\	
Tetramethrin and Phenothrin			\			
Deltamethrin	\	\		\		
Ivermectin	\	\			\	
Amitraz		\		\	\	\
Lindane		\	\	\	\	
Bromocyclen		\	\		\	
Dichlorvos and Fenitrothion		\	\	\	\	
Dimpylate	\	\		\	\	
Crotoxyphos	\	\		\	\	
Coumaphos	\	\		\	\	
Fenthion	\	\			\	
Phosmet	\	\			\	
Cythioate			\	\		\
Propoxur			\			
Carbaryl			\			

CHEMOTHERAPY AND IMMUNOTHERAPY OF NEOPLASIA

Surgery (including cryosurgery), radiation therapy, chemotherapy and immuno-therapy are all employed in the treatment of neoplasia. Laser microsurgery, hyperthermia and photoradiation therapy are currently being investigated as alternative measures for cancer management. Of the more conventional treatments, consideration of only chemotherapy and immunotherapy is appro-priate here. However, it should be appreciated that combination therapy is common and hence reference should be made to texts on surgery, radiation and oncology to obtain fuller information.

The main objectives of chemotherapy are to palliate the disease and allow the patient a good quality of life. Complete cures are only rarely effected. Careful selection of patients for chemotherapy considerably increases the chances of achieving useful and meaningful results. Before the institution of a chemotherapy regime, the veterinarian must:

1. Conduct a full and detailed clinical and radiological examination of the patient. The tumour should be clinically staged and a full laboratory examination should be performed.
2. Conduct a histological examination of the tumour to enable a prognosis to be made.
3. Carefully explain and discuss the prognosis and treatment with the owner. It is also necessary to describe the incidence and nature of the side-effects of the proposed medication.
4. Assess the available information regarding the disease process and the pharmacology of the chemotherapeutic agents under consideration.

Drugs used in the chemotherapy of cancer exert their anti-neoplastic action in a variety of different ways, but the underlying mechanism involves interference with cell growth and division. Mitosis, the period during which the division of cells takes place, usually takes about 30 to 60 minutes and can be regarded as the start of the cell cycle. The cell then either enters a resting phase (gap$_0$ or G$_0$), which is of variable duration, or proceeds directly to G$_1$, the period during which synthesis of the cellular components required for DNA replication occurs. The duration of G$_1$ varies and may be between 10 and 72 hours. The next 10 to 20 hours, when DNA is synthesized, is referred to as the synthesis (S) phase and this is followed by another gap (G$_2$) phase which lasts for 1–3 hours. In this final phase before the next cell division, RNA and proteins are synthesized and the mitotic spindle apparatus is formed.

Tumours consist of a heterogeneous population of cells. The cells may differ in a number of ways, including their capacity to metastasize, their rate of growth and division and their susceptibility to chemotherapeutic agents. The growth fraction of a tumour is a measure of the proportion of cells within the tumour which are dividing. The action of chemotherapeutic agents depends on interference with cell growth and division, and thus the extent to which such drugs will be effective in treatment of tumours depends, to a considerable extent, on the growth fraction of the tumour. The prime aim of chemotherapy is to destroy as many tumour cells as possible, whilst minimizing the toxicity to normal tissue cells. These cells are only spared from toxic effects because, although their rate of growth may be faster than that of malignant tissue, their growth fraction is much smaller. Some normal cells, such as bone marrow progenitor cells and intestinal epithelial cells, divide at a greater rate and have a high growth fraction. This is reflected in the low therapeutic index of most drugs used in cancer chemotherapy and the most commonly observed toxic effects of myelosuppression and gastrointestinal disorders.

The growth fraction of tumours is also related to tumour size. In the early stages of growth, when the tumour is small, the growth fraction is high. As the size of the tumour increases, the proportion of cells in the resting phase increases and the growth fraction is reduced. This pattern of growth, known as Gompertzian growth, has an important bearing on the response of tumours to chemotherapeutic agents. These drugs are most effective in rapidly dividing cells and are thus more effective against tumours in the early stages of growth, when the growth fraction is highest.

Anti-cancer drugs which exert their action at a particular phase of the cell cycle are referred to as 'cell cycle phase specific agents'. For example, drugs which inhibit the formation of DNA in the synthesis phase of the cell cycle, or which inhibit mitosis, are included in this classification. These drugs are most effective when used in the treatment of tumours with a high growth fraction. Cell cycle phase non-specific drugs act independently of the cell cycle phase and are more effective against cells with a low growth fraction.

In general, the number of cancer cells killed by any drug is proportional to the dose of drug used. Thus, the use of higher doses is associated with an increase in the number of cancer cells killed. A further factor to be considered is that a constant proportion of cells is killed by each dose of drug. The clinical implications of these kinetics are of major importance. For example, a tumour containing 10^{12} cells may weigh 1 kg. If the tumour was treated with a drug which killed 99.99 per cent of these cells, its size would be reduced to approximately 100 mg and the patient would be considered to be in clinical remission. However, there would still be 10^8 malignant cells present and any one of these could initiate further growth and eventual relapse. In order to achieve total cell kill, the use of combinations of drugs is common in cancer chemotherapy.

It follows from the above that, wherever possible, maximal doses of anti-cancer drugs should be used. Since underdosage reduces the efficacy of the drugs and increases the likelihood of tumour recurrence, and since overdosage increases the likelihood of toxicity, accurate dosing with chemotherapeutic drugs is essential. Thus the more accurate system of dosing according to body surface area rather than body weight is preferred. This index is proportional to metabolic mass and takes into account the higher metabolic rate of smaller animals.

Chemotherapeutic agents

The drugs which are used for chemotherapy of tumours can be divided into a number of categories, depending on their mode of action and the different stages in the cell growth cycle at which they work.

1. Alkylating agents—these cause cross-linking and breaking of DNA molecules, interfering with DNA replication and transcription.
2. Antimetabolites—these mimic normal substrates needed for nucleic acid synthesis. They inhibit cellular enzymes or lead to the production of non-functional molecules.
3. Plant alkaloids.
4. Anti-tumour antibiotics—these bind to DNA and inhibit DNA and RNA synthesis.
5. Hormones—these include sex hormones, which are effective in malignancies associated with reproductive organs, and glucocorticoids, which are cytolytic for lymphoid tissues and are therefore useful in the treatment of haemolymphatic malignancies. The mechanism of their anti-tumour action is not clear.
6. Miscellaneous agents—agents with a variety of modes of action.

Alkylating agents

These are drugs which replace a hydrogen atom in a molecule of DNA with an alkyl group. Alkylation of the N7 position in the guanine residue in the DNA molecule is one of the crucial reactions. The resulting alteration to the guanine structure prevents replication of the DNA. Many alkylating agents are powerful mutagens, teratogens and carcinogens.

Cyclophosphamide

Cyclophosphamide (Fig. 24.1) is the most widely used and one of the most potent alkylating agents in veterinary medicine. It can be used alone or in combination therapy (which is often preferable) for treatment of lymphosarcoma and other sarcomas, mastocytomas, transmissible venereal tumours and bladder carcinomas. It is activated by hepatic microsomal enzymes and should not be used in animals with compromised liver function. The activation of cyclophosphamide is inhibited by prednisolone and other corticosteroids that inhibit microsomal enzyme activity. Concurrent administration of these agents may thereby reduce the efficacy of cyclophosphamide. The main toxic effects are bone marrow depression and haemorrhagic cystitis in dogs. In cats the main toxic effects are in the gastrointestinal tract and include anorexia, nausea and vomiting. Toxicity may be reduced by administration of the drug in alternate weeks.

Ipophosphamide is structurally related to cyclophosphamide and there is little difference in their efficacy or toxicity.

Dose

dog, cat   50 mg/m^2 p.o. every second day or 100–200 mg/m^2 i.v. every 3 weeks (maximum recommended dose for dogs 250 mg/m^2).

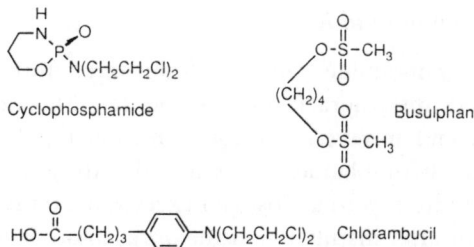

Figure 24.1 Alkylating agents used in cancer chemotherapy.

Chlorambucil

Chlorambucil (Fig. 24.1) is used in lymphosarcoma and leukaemia. Myelo-suppression and vomiting are seen in some dogs. It can be used as a substitute for cyclophosphamide if cystitis develops. Mild leucopenia and thrombocytopenia are the most likely toxic effects.

Dose

dog, cat   2 mg/m^2 p.o. every 24–48 h or 20 mg/m^2 every 2 weeks.

Busulphan

Busulphan (Fig. 24.1) may be useful in the treatment of granulocytic leukaemia. It has also been advocated for human patients with polycythaemia vera and it may be of use in this condition in dogs.

Dose

dog, cat   initial dose 3–6 mg/m^2 p.o. daily until white cell count approaches normal values. Maintenance dose 2 mg/m^2 daily.

Melphalan

This agent has been suggested for the treatment of lymphoreticular neoplasms, osteosarcomas, and mammary and lung tumours.

Dose

Multiple myeloma
dog, cat

1.5 mg/m^2 p.o. daily for 7–14 days, followed by no therapy for 2–3 weeks. The cycle is then repeated.

Lymphoproliferative disorders   up to 5 mg/m^2 p.o. every second day.

Triethylene thiophosphoramide

Triethylene thiophosphoramide can be administered intravenously, but is usually administered intrathoracically for pleural effusion resulting from thoracic metastases and intravesically for transitional cell carcinoma of the bladder. In animals with bladder tumours, the drug is administered by catheter into the bladder at a total dose not exceeding 30 mg/m^2. The bladder is catheterized 1 hour after instillation of the drug, in order to reduce toxicity. It has also been injected locally into mastocytomas, but further evaluation of the success of this treatment is required.

Antimetabolites

Antimetabolites are structural analogues of normal metabolites required for the synthesis of purines and pyrimidines. They are S phase-specific, i.e. active only against those cells in the synthesis phase of the cycle, during which DNA is being produced. Thus, increasing the efficacy of antimetabolites is best achieved by utilization of a dose schedule which maximizes the exposure of as many cells in the S phase as possible. Toxic effects include leucopenia, thrombocytopenia and anaemia. Nausea and vomiting may also occur.

Methotrexate

Methotrexate (Fig. 24.2) is the N10 methyl derivative of aminopterin and structurally it is similar to dihydrofolate. It inhibits the enzyme dihydrofolate reductase, which normally catalyses the conversion of dihydrofolate to tetrahydrofolate, an essential cofactor in the synthesis of DNA, RNA and protein. Toxic effects include myelosuppression, destruction of intestinal epithelium and hepatic necrosis. Leucoverin, a reduced folate, will mitigate these effects. Methotrexate has been used successfully in combination with vincristine and cyclophosphamide for treatment of transmissible venereal tumours. Synergistic effects have been observed with methotrexate and cytosine arabinoside used concurrently, but there have also been reports of antagonism, so the clinical outcome with this combination is uncertain.

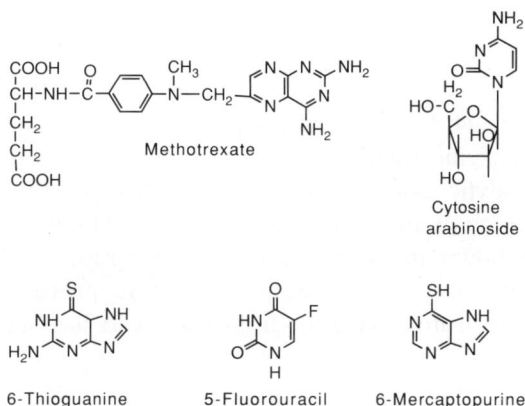

Figure 24.2 Structures of antimetabolites.

Dose

dog, cat   2.5 mg/m^2 p.o. or i.v. daily (dose frequency is adjusted according to toxicity).

6-Mercaptopurine

This (Fig. 24.2) acts by suppression of purine biosynthesis and inhibition of interconversion reactions among the intermediate compounds in purine metabolism. It is only of limited value in the treatment of leukaemia and lymphosarcoma due to its haematological toxicity.

Dose

50 mg/m^2 p.o. daily, until response or toxicity, then 50 mg/m^2 every second day or as necessary.

6-Thioguanine

6-Thioguanine (Fig. 24.2) inhibits the growth of tumours, apparently by its substitution for guanine in the synthesis of nucleic acid. It is fairly well tolerated by cats. The main toxic effect is on the bone marrow but it can produce myocarditis and interstitial nephritis. It has been used in the treatment of lymphosarcoma in the dog, but bone marrow depression was a very common and prolonged side-effect.

Dose

dog, cat   25 mg/m^2 p.o. daily (up to 40 mg/m^2 p.o. daily) for a maximum of 5 days. Repeat at 20–30-day intervals.

5-Fluorouracil

5-Fluorouracil (Fig. 24.2) is a pyrimidine analogue. Its major action is the inhibition of the enzyme thymidylate synthetase, which is required for the synthesis of thymidylic acid, a precursor of DNA. Further evaluation of the drug, either alone or in combination, for the therapy of mammary and gastrointestinal tumours in dogs and cats is required. Toxic reactions to 5-fluorouracil can be severe. In addition to myelosuppression and intestinal epithelial damage, neurotoxicity in both dogs and cats has been described.

Dose

dog   50–200 mg/m^2 i.v., once weekly

Cytosine arabinoside (cytarabine)

This drug (Fig. 24.2) is a pyrimidine nucleoside; it has been used in combination with other drugs in the treatment of lymphosarcoma and mastocytoma. It is one of the few chemotherapeutic agents able to cross the blood–brain barrier. It inhibits DNA polymerase by competitive inhibition of deoxycytidine triphosphate. The drug is inactivated by cytidine deaminase and thus the cytotoxic effect on cell metabolism is of short duration (half-life less than 20 minutes). Since the S phase of the cell cycle lasts for 10–20 hours, continuous infusion of the drug increases the number of susceptible cells exposed and administration by intravenous infusion is common.

Dose

dog, cat   100 mg/m² s.c. or by i.v. infusion for 4 days in dogs and 2 days in cats.
20 mg/m² by intrathecal injection every 1–5 days.

Plant alkaloids

Vincristine

Vincristine (Fig. 24.3) was isolated from the periwinkle plant (*Vinca rosea*). It is a cell cycle phase specific agent. The drug exerts its action by binding to dimeric tubulin, a protein which polymerizes to form the microtubules comprising the mitotic spindle, thereby impairing the formation of normal mitotic spindles. Thus cell division is arrested in metaphase. In immune-mediated thrombocytopenia, the accumulation of vincristine in thrombocytes results in targeted drug delivery to the mononuclear cells responsible for platelet phagocytosis. It is also of value in the treatment of lymphosarcoma and mastocytoma, especially when it is used in combination with other chemotherapeutic agents (as above). Myelosuppression is not as serious as with many of the other cytotoxic agents. Intestinal stasis, leading to constipation can occur. Neurotoxicity in both dogs and cats may occur. Great care should be taken to avoid extravascular leakage as the drug is very irritant.

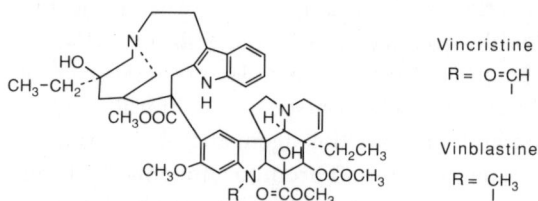

Figure 24.3 Structures of the *Vinca* alkaloids.

Dose

dog, cat   0.5–0.7 mg/m^2 i.v. weekly or 2-weekly.

Combination therapy:
Initially

vincristine sulphate	0.5 mg/m^2 i.v. once weekly
cytosine arabinoside	100 mg/m^2 i.v. or s.c. daily, for 4 days
cyclophosphamide	50 mg/m^2 p.o. every alternate day
prednisolone	20 mg/m^2 p.o. twice daily for one week then half dose daily.

Maintenance

vincristine sulphate	0.5 mg/m^2 every second day
cyclophosphamide	50 mg/m^2 every second day
prednisolone	20 mg/m^2 every second day

Vinblastine

Vinblastine (Fig. 24.3) is a *Vinca* alkaloid closely related to vincristine. Its mechanism of action is the same as that of vincristine. It is used in the therapy of lymphoma and mast cell tumours. Bone marrow suppression, nausea and vomiting are likely side-effects.

Dose

dog, cat   2.0–2.5 mg/m^2 i.v. weekly or 2-weekly

Antibiotics

This group of drugs is derived from soil microorganisms of the *Streptomyces* genus. Many of these drugs exert their anti-cancer action by the formation of a stable complex with DNA and thereby inhibit DNA and/or RNA synthesis, cause DNA strand scission and interfere with cell replication.

Actinomycin D

Actinomycin D (dactinomycin) intercalates between adjacent guanine cytosine base pairs of double-stranded DNA and inhibits DNA-dependent RNA synthesis. Like the other drugs with similar mechanisms of action, the effect of actinomycin D is cell cycle non-specific. Clinical experience is relatively limited in the dog and cat, but this agent may be of value in the treatment of bone and soft tissue sarcomas. Thrombocytopenia, leukaemia and vomiting may occur. It has been suggested that toxicity may limit the use of actinomycin D in dogs and cats.

Dose

dog, cat   0.5–1.5 mg/m^2 i.v. every 2–3 weeks, or up to once weekly.

Doxorubicin hydrochloride

Doxorubicin (Fig. 24.4) belongs to the anthracycline group of antibiotic anti-cancer agents; it is the most widely used of these in veterinary medicine. A closely related drug, daunorubicin (Fig. 24.4), is more commonly used in humans. The actions of these drugs include inhibition of DNA and RNA synthesis and DNA strand scission by intercalation with DNA bases, alteration of membrane fluidity and ion transport, and generation of the semiquinine free radical and oxygen radicals. The free radicals interact with DNA in the same way as the alkylating agents and are responsible for cell membrane damage and DNA cleavage. Doxorubicin has been used effectively in a variety of soft tissue solid tumours and in combination with other drugs in the treatment of osteosarcoma in dogs following amputation. Bone marrow suppression and gastrointestinal side-effects are common but these are likely to be reversed after cessation of dosing. The generation of free radicals is thought to be responsible for the cardiac toxicity of doxorubicin, which may be irreversible and which restricts the clinical use of the drug. In cats, renal toxicity and alopecia have been reported; the latter occurs with high doses of doxorubicin.

Dose

doxorubicin
> dog   30 mg/m^2 i.v. every third week
>   do not exceed 240 mg/m^2 total dose
> cat   25–30 mg/m^2 i.v. every third week

daunorubicin
> cat   15–30 mg/m^2 i.v., repeated at 3-weekly intervals.

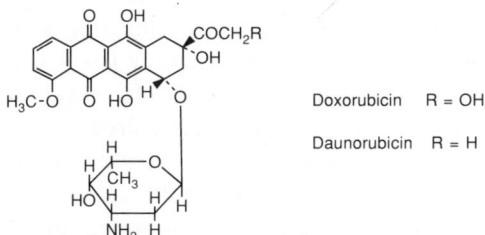

Doxorubicin R = OH

Daunorubicin R = H

Figure 24.4 Structure of the anthracycline antibiotic anti-cancer drugs.

Bleomycin

Bleomycin consists of a mixture of different glycopeptides. Like the other antibiotic anti-cancer drugs, the actions of bleomycin depend on initial binding to DNA. Single- and double-strand breaking of DNA, inhibition of DNA synthesis and free radical generation are all likely to contribute to the final response. Unlike the previously described antibiotics, the action of bleomycin is cell cycle specific and its administration leads to the accumulation of cells in the G_2 phase, which normally lasts for 1–3 hours. During this period RNA and proteins are synthesized and the mitotic spindle apparatus is formed. Bleomycin has been used in dogs and cats for the treatment of squamous cell carcinoma. Some tumour regression has been observed but serious pulmonary side-effects, in particular interstitial pneumonia or pulmonary scarring, can occur. Bleomycin is the only drug used in cancer chemotherapy that does not cause bone marrow suppression.

Dose

dog, cat   10–15 units/m² i.v. weekly (to a maximum of 250 units/m²).

Hormones

Steroid hormones, including glucocorticoids and sex hormones, are used in human and veterinary medicine in the treatment of a number of tumour types. Cancers which originate in mammary and prostate glands may retain some of the properties of cells in those glands, and therefore may be stimulated or inhibited by changes in hormonal balance. Alteration of hormone balance has been shown to be effective in inhibiting the growth of some of these tumours. The effect may depend on the presence of hormone-specific receptor proteins in the cytoplasm of the cancer cells. Hormone–receptor complexes formed in the cytoplasm translocate to the nucleus, where the subsequent synthesis of proteins is affected. In general, a tumour which contains, for example, oestrogen receptors, may regress in the absence of endogenous oestrogens or after administration of oestrogen receptor antagonists or androgens.

It is well recognized that early ovariectomy has a sparing influence on the incidence of canine mammary carcinoma. However, although cytoplasmic receptors for oestrogens, progestogens and androgens have been demonstrated in these tumours, there is no real evidence that ovariectomy is beneficial once tumours have appeared. Hormone receptors have not yet been demonstrated in feline tumours. Canine adenocarcinomas appear to have a higher incidence of oestrogen receptors than mixed mammary tumours, and these receptors are the target of some of the therapeutic agents currently under development.

In human medicine, mammary tumours which can be shown to contain oestrogen receptors generally respond well to removal of hormone-secreting glands or to agents which act as antagonists at oestrogen receptors. The anti-oestrogen, tamoxifen, produces regression in some human breast carcinomas but some of the comparative studies with this drug have been disappointing. Tamoxifen may produce pyometra in the bitch.

Oestrogens

Oestrogens can be used to block the growth-stimulating effects of androgens in cells with androgen receptors. The effect may be due to an inhibition of the release of luteinizing hormone from the pituitary and subsequent reduction of testicular androgen production. Oestrogens have been used as palliative therapy in hyperplasia of the prostate and anal adenoma in dogs. The most commonly used drugs are diethylstilboestrol, ethinyloestradiol and stilboestrol diphosphate. Toxic effects of these include feminization, fluid retention, alopecia and myelodepression. Since long-term oestrogen therapy in dogs may cause life-threatening, irreversible bone marrow failure, prostatic hyperplasia may also be treated by castration and anal tumours by surgery and/or radiotherapy.

Dose

ethinyloestradiol   5–10 mg s.c. weekly for 4 weeks,
                       then once per month.

Androgens

Dromostanalone propionate and testosterone propionate have been used somewhat empirically in canine mammary carcinomas. Surgery remains the treatment of choice in most canine and feline mammary tumours and further studies are necessary to properly define the appropriate use of hormone therapy.

Corticosteroids

Corticosteroids, including prednisolone, prednisone, dexamethasone and beta-methasone, are lympholytic and antimitotic on lymphoid tissue. The mechanism of action of these hormones is not clearly defined and may involve plasma membrane receptors and/or cytosolic receptors. They are used frequently in combination therapy for lymphosarcoma and mastocytoma. Large doses of hydrocortisone (up to 200 mg) can be administered intravenously in an attempt to avoid tracheostomy in cases of lymphosarcoma with respiratory obstruction and dyspnoea due to enlarged submandibular lymph nodes or tonsils. The reduction in volume of the malignant tissue is usually rapid and routine combination therapy is then instituted.

Dogs with lymphosarcoma on corticosteroid therapy often become more active and somewhat rejuvenated, although polydipsia and polyuria are common. A variety of toxic effects, such as loss of skin collagen, muscle weakness, 'pot belly' and diabetes (Cushingoid syndrome), are often seen after prolonged administration. The immunosuppressive activity of the corticosteroids may cause problems in cancer patients receiving other immunodepressant drugs.

Dose

dog, cat prednisolone from 10 mg/m^2 p.o. every 48 hours to 60 mg/m^2 p.o. daily.

Miscellaneous

L-Asparaginase

L-Asparaginase is an enzyme isolated from bacterial sources for therapeutic use. It catalyses the breakdown of extracellular asparagine. Normal cells are unaffected by the drug because they synthesize their own asparagine but lymphoma cells are unable to perform this synthesis. The subsequent inhibition of protein synthesis results in cell death. Resistant tumour cells can develop during treatment. L-Asparaginase can produce regressions in canine lymphosarcoma and lymphatic leukaemia. It may be used alone or in combination with vincristine, cytosine arabinoside, cyclophosphamide and prednisolone. Because L-asparaginase is a foreign protein, anaphylactic reaction may occur after repeated administration. Although intraperitoneal injection has been recommended, the intramuscular route appears to be more convenient and satisfactory. It is an expensive drug, which, after reconstitution has a short shelf-life.

Dose

dog, cat 10 000–30 000 units/m^2 s.c. or i.m. every 1–4 weeks

Hydroxyurea

Hydroxyurea inhibits the enzyme ribonucleotide reductase and thereby inhibits DNA synthesis. The effect is thus specific for the S-phase of the cell cycle.

Hydroxyurea has been used in the therapy of leukaemia and mastocytoma. The main toxic effect is on the bone marrow, but recovery soon occurs after therapy is discontinued.

Dose

dog, cat   50 mg/kg p.o. daily or 80 mg/kg p.o. every 3 days.

Mitotane

Mitotane is of value in the treatment of Cushing's syndrome, which arises as a result of adrenocortical hyperplasia or adenoma. Cells of both the zona fasciculata and zona reticulosa are selectively destroyed while the effect on the zona glomerulosa is slight.

Dose

dog   up to 50 mg/kg p.o. (in divided doses, administered with food) daily for 10 days and then once per week.

Nitrosoureas

This group includes carmustine, lomustine, semustine and streptozocin. A number of these compounds have been advocated for use in humans, but information on their use in domestic animals is sparse. Streptozocin has been used in the treatment of islet cell carcinoma, but it produces severe nephrotoxicity. Carmustine has been used in malignant melanoma and plasma cell myeloma and for tumours of the central nervous system.

Cisplatin

The mechanism of action of cisplatin (Fig. 24.5) is similar to that of the alkylating agents. The heavy metal platinum is bound to chlorine atoms, which are ionized intracellularly. This causes inter- and intrastrand cross-linking of DNA, which inactivates the DNA as a template for RNA synthesis. In dogs the drug is most frequently used in the treatment of transitional cell carcinoma. It is also effective in the treatment of osteosarcoma and lymphoma and in some carcinomas of nasal, salivary and squamous origins. Its use is contraindicated in cats, where it has been reported to cause idiosyncratic, often fatal vasculitis within the pulmonary system.

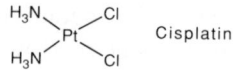

Figure 24.5 Cisplatin.

Dose

dog   50–70 mg/m² i.v. infusion (saline diuresis before and after treatment and appropriate collection of urine for safe disposal are required).

Combination therapy

Drugs chosen for use in combination must have a proven cytostatic or cytotoxic effect when used singly, or should be capable of arresting the neoplastic cell at a particular stage of the cycle when it is susceptible to other drugs. When two drugs are used in combination, the fraction of tumour cells killed by one drug is independent of the fraction killed by the other drug. While the true academic approach is to select drugs that kill cells in different ways biochemically, this has proved quite difficult in practice and many drug combinations have been developed somewhat empirically. Experimentally, it has been shown that the emergence of populations resistant to individual drugs can be delayed if a combination of several drugs is used. If there is little overlap of toxicity, then it is possible to use almost maximum doses of each individual agent without greatly increasing the overall toxicity. A good example of this is provided by vincristine, which has a less toxic effect on bone marrow than most of the potent anti-cancer drugs and has been used successfully in many combination regimes.

Treatment of drug toxicity

The main problem with most of the cytotoxic drugs used in veterinary practice is bone marrow depression. A severe lymphopenia, granulopenia and thrombocytopenia can lead to toxic signs such as pyrexia, infection, haemorrhages and, in some instances, death. A particularly dangerous sign is a total white blood cell count below 10 per cent of normal values. If this occurs, then cytotoxic therapy should be stopped and broad-spectrum antibiotics administered.

Renal toxicity is observed in older cats and dogs when alkylating agents and some other cytotoxic drugs are given. Fluid therapy should be instituted, the causative drugs should be discontinued and the regime changed.

Cyclophosphamide is a useful drug in veterinary practice but it can produce cystitis, particularly after prolonged usage. This toxicity can be reduced by feeding additional salt, maintaining a high water intake, administering the drug in the morning and ensuring that the patient urinates before going to sleep at night. Concurrent corticosteroid therapy promotes renal perfusion and increases urine production, thus reducing the risk of cystitis. Following the diagnosis of cystitis, administration of cyclophosphamide should be stopped, sensitivity tests conducted and antibiotic therapy initiated. Severe cases of haemorrhagic cystitis have responded favourably to infusion of the bladder with 1 per cent formalin.

Cardiac toxicity is a serious problem with doxorubicin and extreme care must be taken with dosage. Bleomycin therapy should be discontinued immediately if clinical signs of impaired lung function are observed or if pulmonary changes are detected on X-ray.

A number of cytotoxic drugs are teratogens and they are contraindicated in pregnant or breeding animals. The carcinogenic effect of the drugs is of little import in cases of clinical neoplasia but extreme care should be exercised by the veterinary surgeon or the person handling the agents. Skin contamination, ingestion or inhalation of the drugs should be avoided at all times. This applies particularly to such agents as actinomycin D, which is a powerful mutagen, even in small quantities. Attention should be paid to the appropriate disposal of cytotoxic waste.

Immunotherapy

Anti-tumour immune responses may be mediated by macrophages, T-cells, B-cells and natural killer cells. Activation of these cells by tumour-associated antigens, interferon or lymphokines stimulates the release of lymphokines and cytokines, such as interleukins and interferon, which regulate the immune response. Tumour necrosis factor and lysosomal enzymes released from activated macrophages are also important in mediating cytotoxic effects. The combined functioning of these cells is believed to be important in immunosurveillance and anti-tumour activity. Immunotherapy (or biologic therapy) depends on modulation of cytotoxic effector functions and enhancement of natural defences against tumour-associated antigens.

Non-specific immunomodulators currently under investigation include levamisole, bacille Calmette–Guérin (BCG) and *Propionibacterium acnes* (formerly *Corynebacterium parvum*). Results from trials using the anthelmintic, levamisole, in humans have been inconsistent. This drug has also proved disappointing in the treatment of both canine and feline mammary tumours and canine lymphosarcoma. The methanol-extractable residue of BCG (MER-BCG) has been evaluated in both human and animal cancer patients. While some benefit in humans has been shown, there is little evidence of efficacy in animals to date. Results from experiments with muramyl dipeptide (MDP), an active component of the BCG cell wall, and muramyl tripeptide (MTP) indicate these substances may be effective in immunotherapy of malignancies. *P. acne* has been shown to retard disease in dogs with malignant melanoma and, as with MDP and MTP, further investigations are warranted.

The endogenous agents which are normally involved in the immune response may prove useful as therapeutic agents in cancer. Among those which are currently being investigated are interferons, interleukins and tumour necrosis factor. An alternative approach involves the administration of anti-tumour antibodies to cancer patients. Such monoclonal antibodies can be administered alone or can be coupled to chemotherapeutic or radioactive agents. This facilitates specific targeting of the drugs and doses can be reduced accordingly. Toxicity and side-effects may be significantly reduced.

Immunotherapy is still under investigation. There have been some promising results from *in vitro* studies and studies in human and animal patients. Further data from veterinary clinical trials are required to establish its future place in the treatment of cancer in animals.

CHAPTER 25

ANTISEPTICS AND DISINFECTANTS

Pathogenic microorganisms from an infected animal may leave the animal in a number of ways, including in droplets of moisture which are breathed, coughed or sneezed out, in cells from skin or hair and in excretions including urine, faeces and milk. The pathogens are usually able to survive in the environment outside the animal, sometimes for years (e.g. *Bacillus anthracis*), and thereby infect other susceptible animals. A disinfectant is any agent that destroys pathogenic microorganisms on inanimate objects. These agents are usually toxic to host cells as well and are not suitable for systemic administration. They may also be too toxic for topical application. Those disinfectants which can be topically applied are referred to as antiseptics.

Disinfection is one of the measures which may be employed to break the cycle of infectious diseases in animals. To be effective, it must be used in combination with careful attention to husbandry techniques and the maintenance of a clean environment for the animals. Physical or chemical methods can be used for disinfection. Physical methods include ultraviolet light, osmotic pressure and heat, with moist heat being more effective than dry heat. The processes of disinfection can be applied to aspects other than the animal and its environment, including the disinfection of animal feed, water and waste as well as disinfection of animal products, including meat, eggs and milk. These topics are beyond the scope of this book and only chemical disinfectants for use in the immediate environment of the animals, and antiseptics (i.e. compounds applied to skin or living tissue) are described in this chapter.

A variety of disinfectants is available and each possesses, to a greater or lesser extent, the properties of an ideal agent (Table 25.1). In practice, a number of factors influence the effectiveness of disinfectants. The presence of organic matter is one of the most important environmental factors which influences disinfectant activity. Animal-derived matter, such as blood, pus or

Table 25.1 Properties of an ideal disinfectant

Broad spectrum of activity
Rapid action
Unaffected by environmental factors (pH, temperature, humidity)
Low toxicity for animals, non-irritant
Non-corrosive, non-staining, odourless
Water-soluble with detergent action
Not inactivated by protein
Chemically stable
Economical, simple to use

faeces, and environmental matter, such as soil or food residues, are thought to react with the preparation, thus reducing the amount available for disinfection. Effective cleaning prior to disinfection, especially the removal of dried films of organic matter, greatly increases the chances of successful disinfection. For example, changes in pH may alter the activity of the disinfectant chemical, the nature of the cell surface to which it is applied, and the partitioning of active constituent(s) within the vehicle and the microbial cell. Any of these changes may affect the antimicrobial activity of the preparation.

Phenols

Phenolic disinfectants (including phenol itself, cresols and xylenols) are often obtained from coal tar. The chemical structures of some of the agents in this group are shown in Fig. 25.1. These compounds alter cell wall permeability and denature proteins, thereby inactivating enzymes. Antibacterial activity increases with halogen substitution and nitration. The group has bactericidal activity for both Gram-positive and Gram-negative organisms and is effective against yeasts and fungi. Viruses vary in their susceptibility to phenols and

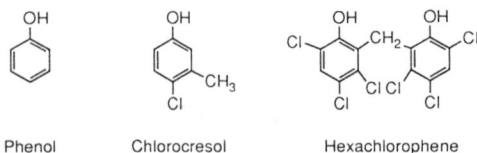

Figure 25.1 Phenolic disinfectants.

bacterial spores are resistant. Cresol is a mixture of cresols and phenols which results from distillation of coal tar. Lysol, a solution of cresol with soap, is more soluble in water and is widely used as a disinfectant. One major advantage of lysol is that its antimicrobial activity is relatively unaffected by the presence of organic matter. Hexachlorophene is one of the halogenated phenols which is used in soaps for surgical scrubs. Single applications are probably no more effective than ordinary soap but with repeated use a deposit of hexachlorophene on the skin exerts a prolonged bacteriostatic effect.

Phenols need to be handled with caution since they are rapidly absorbed through the skin and can cause severe burns. Swallowing agents of this type can be fatal. Dogs and cats are particularly sensitive to the toxic effects of these disinfectants and care is required to avoid poisoning through skin absorption or accidental ingestion.

Acids and alkalis

Bacteria are inhibited at high or low pH. Fungal infections of the skin may be treated by formulations of salicylic, benzoic or undecanoic acids, and citric acid is effective against foot-and-mouth virus. Skin and hides which have been contaminated by anthrax spores can be disinfected with 2.5 per cent hydrochloric acid.

Caustic soda (sodium hydroxide) is normally used as a disinfectant as a 2 per cent solution in hot or boiling water. At this concentration, it is effective against many common bacteria and at higher concentrations (>5 per cent) it is lethal to anthrax spores. Calcium hydroxide (hydrated lime), as a 20 per cent suspension, and sodium carbonate (4 per cent w/v) are also used for disinfection).

Acids are corrosive and alkalis cause severe burns, and thus care to avoid contact with skin and eyes is essential. Swallowing either strong acids or strong alkalis can be fatal.

Detergents

Detergents are agents which reduce surface and interfacial tensions and have cleansing effects. Cationic surfactants, in which the hydrophilic, polar portion of a surface-active molecule has a positive charge, are weak detergents, but have strong bactericidal properties. In contrast, anionic surfactants generally have weak antimicrobial effects and are strong detergents. In all cases, the activity of the compounds is limited to bacteria and is markedly reduced in the presence of organic matter. Cationic detergents antagonize the actions of anionic detergents and vice versa.

Cationic bactericides

These are usually quaternary ammonium compounds and include the mono-quaternary compounds, cetrimide and benzalkonium chloride (Fig. 25.2), and bisquaternary compounds, such as hedaquinium and dequalinium, which all react with phospholipids in the cell membrane and may also denature bacterial protein. The group is effective against both Gram-positive and Gram-negative bacteria but spores, fungi and some viruses (especially non-enveloped) are resistant to their effects. Acid pH reduces their efficacy as does the presence of any residual soap (anionic detergent).

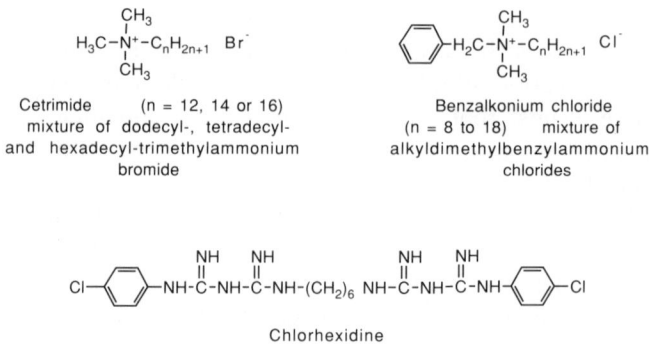

Cetrimide (n = 12, 14 or 16)
mixture of dodecyl-, tetradecyl-
and hexadecyl-trimethylammonium
bromide

Benzalkonium chloride
(n = 8 to 18)   mixture of
alkyldimethylbenzylammonium
chlorides

Chlorhexidine

Figure 25.2 Cationic bactericides.

Cetrimide and benzalkonium chloride are most commonly used. Toxicity is not usually a problem if the preparation is used in accordance with directions. In general, toxic effects of the quaternary ammonium compounds may include central nervous system depression and hypotension. Convulsions and coma may also occur.

Anionic surfactants

This group includes soaps and sodium lauryl sulphate. Anionic surfactants are usually the sodium or potassium salts of fatty acids and when dissolved in water are strongly alkaline. The effectiveness of these preparations is associated with the removal of grease and dirt as well as surface secretions and desquamated epithelium with the bacteria contained therein. They also have some limited activity against Gram-positive bacteria. Antibacterial activity is markedly increased at pH <3.0.

Aldehydes

Glutaraldehyde and formaldehyde are the most important of the aldehydes, although others have antimicrobial activity. The activity of these agents is due to a reaction with amino and sulphydryl groups in microbial protein and with imino groups in nucleic acid. Glutaraldehyde is active in its monomeric form but can also exist as a dimer, trimer or a polymer. It is more active at alkaline pH, but is also liable to lose activity due to polymer formation. Thus it is usually purchased as an acid solution and the pH is adjusted just prior to use. Unlike many other disinfectants, the presence of organic matter does not appear to reduce the effectiveness of glutaraldehyde. Bacteria and their spores, mycelial and spore forms of fungi and some viruses are sensitive to glutaraldehyde.

Formaldehyde is also lethal to bacteria, bacterial spores, fungi and some viruses, but its sporicidal action is slower than that of glutaraldehyde. It is one of the approved agents (in the UK) for use in foot-and-mouth and swine vesicular diseases.

Both glutaraldehyde and formaldehyde are potentially toxic to humans and animals. Ingestion may cause depression of the central nervous system and cardiovascular collapse. Formaldehyde vapour is intensely irritant to mucous membranes.

Alcohols

Both Gram-negative and non-sporing Gram-positive bacteria are sensitive to alcohols, which precipitate protein and denature lipids. Ethanol has been widely used as a skin disinfectant but is less satisfactory for the sterilization of instruments because it has no effect on spores. Since some water is required for a disinfectant effect, 60–75 per cent solutions of ethanol are most effective. Absolute ethanol is a poor disinfectant.

Oxidizing compounds

Hydrogen peroxide

The release of a hydroxyl free radical by hydrogen peroxide and the subsequent DNA strand breakage is responsible for the bactericidal, sporicidal and virucidal actions of this agent. In addition, it reacts with sulphydryl and amino groups in enzymes, thereby inactivating them. When hydrogen peroxide is applied to tissues, the action of the enzyme catalase results in the rapid release of O_2. The bubbles aid the disinfection process by adding a mechanical cleaning action.

Other oxidizing agents

These include sodium perborate and benzoyl peroxide, which both cause the release of oxygen, and potassium permanganate, which is a strong oxidizing agent although it does not release gaseous oxygen.

Chlorine and chlorine-releasing disinfectants

Chlorine is a strong oxidizing agent and chlorine-releasing compounds are effective disinfectants. The activity of these compounds depends on the formation of hypochlorous acid. Enzymes and protoplasmic components are oxidized and the permeability of bacterial cell walls is altered. Sodium hypochlorite and calcium hypochlorite (chlorinated lime) are widely used. Although these agents have a wide spectrum of antibacterial activity, their antimicrobial activity is reduced as the pH increases and also in the presence of organic matter. Other chlorine-releasing compounds include chloramine-T, dichloramine-T and di- and tri-chloroisocyanuric acids. Chlorine-releasing disinfectants may corrode metals or bleach materials with which they come into contact. These agents are also extremely toxic and ingestion or inhalation may be fatal.

Iodine compounds

Iodine is less reactive than chlorine. As with chlorine, the activity of iodine is reduced in the presence of organic matter and at alkaline pH. The major disadvantages of iodine include irritation and a delay in wound healing. It may also produce skin sensitization. So, although iodine has rapid lethal effects against bacteria and their spores, moulds, yeasts and viruses, it should not be used, especially on open wounds.

Iodophores (e.g. povidone-iodine) are compounds in which iodine is solubilized with surface-active agents. These compounds retain the germicidal effects of iodine, which are associated with the presence of free iodine, but not the unwanted actions. At pH <4, even in the presence of organic matter, iodophores remain effective disinfectants. They are widely used as disinfectants and antiseptics, especially for skin preparation prior to surgery.

Dyes

Acridines, quinones and triphenylmethane dyes all have antimicrobial activity. They are more effective at alkaline pH, exerting (relatively slow) activity against both Gram-positive and Gram-negative organisms. Acridine derivatives, including acriflavine, proflavine and aminacrine hydrochloride, are used as topical antiseptics for skin and wound dressing.

Miscellaneous

Chlorhexidine (Fig. 25.2) is a biguanide which disrupts the bacterial cell wall by reacting with negatively charged groups on proteins or lipopolysaccharides and acidic phospholipids. It is effective against both Gram-positive and Gram-negative bacteria and also against some fungi. Organic matter and acid pH reduce its activity.

Vapour-phase disinfectants

Ethylene oxide (C_2H_4O) is effective against bacteria and their spores, fungi, yeasts and viruses. The gas reacts with carboxyl, amino, sulphydryl and hydroxyl groups in protein and also with DNA and RNA. It is able to penetrate paper and cellophane and is widely used as a sterilizing agent. The gas can be irritant and may cause nausea, vomiting and skin rashes.

Sulphur dioxide, produced by burning sulphur, is also effective as a gaseous disinfectant. Its action depends on the gas dissolving in water on the surfaces to be disinfected, with the consequent formation of sulphurous acid, which is bactericidal. It should be noted, however, that the acid may also affect fabric and metal.

Other vapour-phase disinfectants are available, but they are less effective and/or more toxic than ethylene oxide and are therefore less commonly used. These include formaldehyde, methyl bromide and propylene oxide.

CHAPTER 26

DRUG INTERACTIONS

Drug interactions are said to occur when the action of a particular drug is modified by the presence of one or more other drugs. In these cases, the patient demonstrates an uncharacteristic response to one or more of the drugs involved. The modified reaction can involve a variation in the therapeutic or toxic effects of the drug, or an effect not observed when the drug is administered alone.

It is widely accepted that drug interactions do occur and that these can be dangerous or even life threatening: a number of deaths, in both man and animals, due to drug interactions are recorded in the literature. However, there are marked differences of opinion about the frequency of clinically significant drug interactions, and it is important to maintain a clinical perspective or the importance of drug interactions may be overestimated. It is also important to attempt to assess the clinical significance in veterinary medicine of those interactions which are of theoretical importance or have only been reported in the medical literature.

Not all drug interactions are dramatic or dangerous. Drugs may be deliberately combined to achieve a synergistic effect or to limit the occurrence of side-effects. These interactions form part of normal veterinary practice, such as the administration of neostigmine preceded by an antimuscarinic agent, to reverse the action of non-depolarizing muscle relaxants in anaesthesia while avoiding excessive muscarinic activity. Drug interactions may also be useful in situations where the toxic effects of one drug are decreased by the administration of another, as in the case of atropine administration to treat poisoning with an organophosphorus compound, or the use of orally administered charcoal in the management of ingested poisons. The therapeutic use of these drug interactions depends on knowledge of the pharmacology of the drugs involved. The vast majority of undesirable interactions are unpredicted and experience precedes an understanding of the mechanism.

It is only occasionally that interactions and their mechanisms are predicted. A good example of this is the inhibition of suxamethonium metabolism by ecothiopate eye drops, which was anticipated before the first human clinical cases were reported.

A classification of drug interactions on the basis of their mechanisms may aid in their prediction and thereby prevent the undesirable consequences and may also suggest therapeutically useful interactions. Such a classification also provides a framework for continual awareness of potential interactions and should contribute to the rational management of drug interactions when they occur. The following is an attempt to provide such a classification, but it must be appreciated that the suggested mechanisms are often tentative and that future pharmacokinetic or pharmacodynamic studies may provide alternative explanations for the observed interactions.

Two broad categories can be used for initial classification of drug interactions: *in vitro* incompatibilities and *in vivo* mechanisms.

In vitro incompatibilities include those interactions in which mixing of two drugs before administration, or the addition of a drug to infusion fluids, reduces the therapeutic potency of the drug or drugs. Because of the possibility of this type of drug interaction, it is generally considered poor practice to mix products or vehicles in the same syringe. Chemical reactions (hydrolysis, oxidation, reduction or complex formation) may not produce a visible change in the appearance of the drug, despite the fact that chemical alteration of the active ingredients has occurred. These changes may only be detectable by analysis. In contrast, changes in colour and/or turbidity are more likely to occur when physically incompatible compounds are mixed. In these cases, the altered appearance of the solution is a useful warning to avoid using the mixture. A selected group of *in vitro* incompatibilities, which are of relevance to veterinary practice, is shown in Table 26.1. Two examples

Table 26.1 Incompatibilities of parenteral drugs

Drug	Incompatible with:
Acetylpromazine maleate	Phenylbutazone sodium
Ampicillin sodium (and other semisynthetic penicillins)	Many incompatibilities*
Atropine sulphate	Barbiturates, diazepam
Barbiturates	Many incompatibilities*
Benzylpenicillin sodium	Many incompatibilities*
Calcium gluconate	Carbonates, phosphates, sulphates, promethazine hydrochloride, tetracyclines
Chloramphenicol sodium succinate	Erythromycin, hydrocortisone sodium succinate, gentamicin, penicillins, tetracyclines, chlorpromazine hydrochloride, vitamins B and C

Table 26.1 (continued)

Drug	Incompatible with:
Chlorpromazine hydrochloride	Chloramphenicol sodium succinate, atropine sulphate, hydrocortisone sodium succinate, tetracyclines, sulphonamides, vitamins B and C, phenylbutazone sodium
Diazepam	Many incompatibilities*
Droperidol	Barbiturates
Fentanyl	Barbiturates
Heparin sodium	Aminoglycosides, benzylpenicillin sodium, hydrocortisone sodium succinate, tetracyclines, pethidine hydrochloride, atropine sulphate, promethazine hydrochloride, tylosin
Gentamicin sulphate	Carbenicillin (and other penicillins), heparin sodium, sulphonamides, chloramphenicol sodium succinate, cephalosporins
Hydrocortisone sodium succinate	Chloramphenicol sodium succinate, heparin sodium, aminoglycosides, tetracyclines, barbiturates, promethazine hydrochloride, chlorpromazine hydrochloride, tylosin
Ketamine hydrochloride	Barbiturates
Lincomycin	Penicillins
Methylprednisone sodium succinate	Calcium gluconate, benzylpenicillin, tetracyclines, pethidine hydrochloride, thiopentone sodium, sulphonamides, vitamins B and C
Pethidine hydrochloride	Barbiturates, heparin sodium, methylprednisolone sodium succinate, sodium bicarbonate
Phenylbutazone sodium	Acetylpromazine hydrochloride, chlorpromazine hydrochloride
Potassium chloride	Adrenaline, sulphadiazine sodium
Prednisolone sodium phosphate	Calcium gluconate, promethazine hydrochloride
Promethazine hydrochloride	Many incompatibilities*
Streptomycin sulphate	Calcium gluconate, sodium bicarbonate, heparin sodium, tylosin
Sulphonamides	Many incompatibilities*
Suxamethonium chloride	Thiopentone and other alkaline solutions
Tetracyclines	Preparations with a high concentration of sodium or calcium salts, penicillins, cephalosporins, heparin sodium, barbiturates, chloramphenicol sodium succinate, hydrocortisone sodium succinate, sodium bicarbonate, tylosin
Tylosin	Heparin sodium, hydrocortisone sodium succinate, streptomycin, tetracyclines
Vitamin B complex	Many incompatibilities*

*Do not mix with other drugs.

Note: Adapted from P. E. B. Reilly and J. P. Isaacs, *Veterinary Record*, **112**, 29–33, 1983.

of particular interest are the precipitation which occurs following the mixing of thiopentone and suxamethonium and the precipitation which can follow the addition of calcium salts to sodium bicarbonate solution.

Reports of the interactions between drugs and intravenous infusion fluids are often inconsistent and difficult to summarize. This is due to a variety of factors, which include differences in the amount of drug and its degree of dilution, failure to take into account differences in the pH of the diluting solution and the difficulty in the detection of slow losses of drug potency. The only general rule is that loss of potency of a drug prepared in an infusion increases with time and decreases with refrigeration.

When drugs are to be administered by intravenous infusion, the common recommendation is that normal saline, with a pH of around 4, be used as the diluent. The pH of 5 per cent dextrose solution can vary between 3.5 and 6.5 and thus it is less suitable as a vehicle for intravenous drugs. Sodium bicarbonate and Hartmann's solution should not be used as diluents without careful compatibility checks. In the case of Hartmann's solution, not only is the pH high, but Ca^{2+} may contribute to drug interactions. Drugs known to be incompatible with Hartmann's solution include tetracyclines, nitrofurantoin and ascorbic acid. Examples of other important *in vitro* incompatibilities of drugs and parenteral solutions are shown in Table 26.2, with suggested compatible fluids. Only mixtures which are likely to be encountered in a veterinary clinical situation have been included.

Table 26.2 Compatibility of drugs with intravenous fluids

Drug	Incompatible i.v. fluids	Compatible i.v. fluids*
Ampicillin sodium	Dextrose solutions, dextran	Normal saline, Compound Sodium Lactate
Adrenaline	Sodium bicarbonate and other solutions with pH >5.5	Normal saline
Benzylpenicillin	Dextrose solutions	Normal saline
Cloxacillin sodium	Dextrose solutions >5%	Normal saline, Ringer's solution, dextrose saline
Diazepam	Addition to i.v. fluids not recommended, insoluble in most solutions	
Gentamicin sulphate	Any solution where the concentration of gentamicin >1 g/l	Normal saline, dextrose, dextrose saline
Heparin sodium	Dextrose solutions	Compatible with most
Magnesium sulphate	Sodium bicarbonate	Normal saline, dextrose, dextrose saline

Table 26.2 (continued)

Drug	Incompatible i.v. fluids	Compatible i.v. fluids*
Methylprednisolone sodium succinate	Compound Sodium Lactate (depends on drug concentration)	Normal saline, dextrose, dextrose saline (depends on drug concentration)
Noradrenaline bitartrate	Normal saline, sodium bicarbonate	Dextrose, dextrose saline
Oxytetracycline hydrochloride	Solutions containing Ca^{2+} or Mg^{2+}, dextrose	Normal saline
Oxytocin	Dextran 12%	Dextrose 5%, normal saline
Sodium bicarbonate	Compound Sodium Lactate, Ringer's solution, Ca^{2+}-containing solutions	Normal saline, dextrose, dextrose saline
Vitamin B complex with vitamin C	Sodium bicarbonate	Normal saline, dextrose, dextrose saline, Compound Sodium Lactate

*Potency of drug solutions may decrease with time.
Note: Adapted from P. E. B. Reilly and J. P. Isaacs, *Veterinary Record*, **112**, 29–33, 1983.

Adverse drug interactions which occur *in vivo* can be classified into those which interfere with drug disposition and those which are due to interaction at the receptor site. The former group can be further subdivided into those which involve alterations of the absorption, protein-binding, metabolism and/or excretion of the drug.

Drug interactions causing altered absorption

The absorption of orally administered drugs through the gastrointestinal tract can be affected by several mechanisms. It is also possible to alter the uptake of drugs administered by the intramuscular or subcutaneous routes and those given by inhalation.

In many instances, preparations containing the same active ingredient have been shown to differ in respect of the rate and extent of release of the drug and its absorption, i.e. the bioavailability of different formulations may vary considerably (see Chapter 1). Variations in the rate of dissolution of a drug in the alimentary tract can be due to differences in the physical properties of the drug or due to interactions between the drug and formulation adjustments. Differences in bioavailability occur most commonly with drugs which are only sparingly soluble. The most commonly prescribed drugs in which variations in bioavailability may cause problems include digoxin, some steroids and antibiotics such as tetracyclines and chloramphenicol. Sulphonamides and phenylbutazone also have low solubility and consequently variable bioavailability. It should be noted here that bioavailability refers to both rate and extent of absorption and that during continuous dosage therapy, variations in the extent of drug absorption of a drug are more important than variations in the rate of its absorption.

A large number of drug preparations are available for oral administration to animals and thus interactions between drugs in the alimentary tract may be considered to be of some importance. However, the actual modification of the rate or extent of absorption of one drug by another in the alimentary tract is relatively uncommon. Although the possibility of such interactions can be predicted from a prior knowledge of the chemical, physical and pharmacological properties of the drug, it is well established that many of the predicted reactions have not been shown to be of clinical significance.

Absorption of drugs from the gastrointestinal tract may be reduced by the presence of adsorbents, such as kaolin and charcoal. In these cases, the active drug is absorbed onto the kaolin or charcoal and a marked reduction in drug absorption may result.

Some drugs are known to undergo chemical reactions within the alimentary tract and these may alter absorption. The classic example is the oral administration of some of the tetracycline antibiotics and the concurrent ingestion of food (especially milk products), antacids or laxatives containing divalent or trivalent cations. The interaction is probably due to the formation of relatively insoluble chelates which cannot be absorbed. Chelation of Fe^{2+} and Fe^{3+} ions in oral iron preparations, when these are administered with tetracyclines, reduces the absorption of iron. Since chelation is most marked under conditions of raised pH, such iron preparations should not be administered by the oral route to patients receiving antacids containing sodium bicarbonate.

Gastrointestinal pH is likely to have a profound effect on the absorption of orally administered drugs. As described in Chapter 1, the non-ionized (fat-soluble) form of a drug diffuses most readily through membranes and thus any change in pH which shifts the equilibrium towards the formation of the non-ionized form would increase absorption. Thus an increase in gastrointestinal pH would be expected to slow the absorption of weak acids and increase that of weak bases. The reverse would occur if pH decreased. A decreased absorption in the presence of antacids has been demonstrated in the case of some acidic drugs, including barbiturates, penicillin and phenylbutazone.

This predicted effect may also be associated with an alteration of the rate of dissolution and solubility of the drugs by the antacid. Furthermore, changes in the rate of gastric emptying (see below) induced by the antacid may contribute to the observed alteration of the absorption of drugs administered concurrently.

Acidic drugs with a low pK_a are absorbed rapidly through the stomach wall, and neutralization of such drugs is likely to increase their dissociation and thereby decrease their absorption. Hence administration of alkalis with acetylsalicylic acid or ascorbic acid reduces the absorption of these compounds.

In general, absorption of orally administered drugs from the small intestine is more rapid than from the stomach. Thus, drugs which delay gastric emptying usually decrease the rate of absorption of other drugs administered concurrently and increase the time to peak effect. Decreased gastric emptying will also decrease the availability of drugs which are metabolized or degraded in the stomach. Such alterations in gastric emptying may be important in the case of most of the penicillins, which are degraded by gastric acid. Drugs which are known to inhibit gastric emptying, and hence the rate and sometimes the extent of absorption of another drug, include atropine, morphine and aspirin. Many of the drugs involved have anticholinergic properties and these drugs will also reduce the secretion of gastric acid. This latter effect is unpredictable since the secretion of hydrochloric acid is largely under hormonal rather than vagal control. The main and predictable effect of anticholinergic drugs is to reduce gastrointestinal tract motility. In cases where the drug is absorbed from the stomach, prolonged contact with the mucosa may increase the total amount of drug absorbed. Metoclopramide is a drug used to increase the rate of gastric emptying (Chapter 14) and as such will reduce the time to peak effect of many other drugs administered concurrently.

The presence of food in the stomach reduces the rate of gastric emptying and thus often slows the absorption of drugs. A reduction in the rate of absorption is generally of minor significance in continuous dosing schedules, providing the total amount of drug absorbed is not altered. However, in some cases bioavailability is reduced when drugs are administered with food (e.g. penicillin and tetracycline; see above). Such drugs should be given either at least half an hour before or two hours after a meal. In contrast, the absorption of griseofulvin is enhanced by a fatty meal, possibly as a result of stimulation of bile secretion which can enhance the absorption of a highly lipid-soluble drug.

Absorption from the gastrointestinal tract can also be altered by changes in gut flora and enzymes. For example, the usual form of folic acid in the diet is folate polyglutamate, but this is not absorbed and the enzyme folate conjugase in the intestinal mucosa is required to convert the substrate to folic acid. Phenytoin has been shown to inhibit the activity of folate conjugase and thereby induce a folic acid deficiency in some species. Alteration of gut flora may lead to drug interactions which are independent of altered absorption. For instance, there are reports in the literature that some antibiotics inhibit the gut flora that synthesize vitamin K and thereby potentiate the action of oral anticoagulants.

Most drugs are absorbed by a passive, non-saturable process and it is unlikely in these cases that interactions will occur in the absorption process. Although some drugs, including phenytoin, ethanol and neomycin, have been shown to inhibit absorption of both drugs and nutrients in ingested food, there is very little information available on this subject in domestic animals.

When drugs are administered by intramuscular or subcutaneous injection, a delay in absorption may be produced by the addition of adrenaline to the formulation. Other methods to delay absorption include the combination of insulin with protamine, and of penicillin with procaine. In contrast, addition of hyaluronidase to drug formulations results in more rapid absorption.

In the case of administration of drugs by inhalation, the second gas effect may be considered as a drug interaction. The alveolar concentration of one gas or vapour, such as halothane, increases due to the administration of another gas, such as nitrous oxide. The alveolar concentration of a drug can also be increased by an agent which increases alveolar ventilation and the most commonly used one is carbon dioxide. Conversely, alveolar concentration is decreased when the alveolar ventilation is reduced by respiratory depressant drugs such as opioids.

Drug interactions and protein-binding

Binding of drugs to plasma proteins is easily demonstrated and is well documented in the literature. The amount of drug bound to plasma proteins can sometimes account for the major portion of the total drug present in the body. In these circumstances, the therapeutic (and toxic) effects of the drug are mediated by the very small portion of free drug. When a second drug, which displaces the first from its protein-binding sites, is administered the displaced drug markedly increases the levels of free drug available to exert both therapeutic and toxic effects and a clinically significant drug interaction may occur. These are most likely if the displaced drug has a low therapeutic index, is strongly bound to plasma proteins, is present in low concentrations and is slowly eliminated. Low albumin concentration, such as occurs in liver disease, also increases the risk of significant drug interactions.

The displacement of drugs from protein-binding sites is the mechanism of drug interaction responsible for many instances of warfarin toxicity. This anticoagulant is used in the treatment of navicular disease (see page 205) and widely used in human medicine. At equilibrium, about 98 per cent of warfarin is bound to plasma proteins. Thus it is a difficult drug to use and attention to detail of dose adjustment and awareness of potential drug interactions are necessary to avoid life-threatening haemorrhage. Poisoning of animals with warfarin is still a relatively common occurrence. Animals on any medication which may reduce the plasma protein-binding of warfarin, such as non-steroidal anti-inflammatory drugs, may be expected to be more severely affected.

One of the major roles of serum albumin is the transport of endogenous compounds, including fatty acids, bilirubin and corticosteroids. Such substances may be displaced by drugs which bind to the carrier sites. For example, acidic anti-rheumatic drugs such as indomethacin, oxyphenbutazone and salicylates can displace corticosteroids from binding sites on the globulin transcortin. It has been suggested that this interaction may account for some of their anti-rheumatic activity.

Drug interactions in drug metabolism

Although lipid-solubility of drugs is important in their ability to be absorbed and reach their sites of action, very lipid-soluble substances undergo almost 100 per cent reabsorption in the renal tubules and thereby resist elimination. In general, elimination of drugs follows their metabolism to more hydrophilic compounds which undergo less reabsorption in the kidney. The metabolism is catalysed by a variety of enzymes, many of which are not substrate-specific but also metabolize a number of endogenous compounds. The lack of substrate specificity is important in that the metabolism of a number of drugs may be altered by any agent which either increases the synthesis of an enzyme or reduces its activity.

Some drugs are able to stimulate the production of drug-metabolizing enzymes. Drug interactions, usually involving a loss of therapeutic activity, may result from the consequent increase in the rate of metabolism. These are particularly important when the drugs are involved in the maintenance of vital physiological functions, such as the control of blood sugar levels or blood clotting. The extent of enzyme induction varies widely with species and the extent of exposure to other, similar agents. Thus it is often difficult to predict the extent of drug interactions arising from enzyme induction. Since the process of enzyme induction requires the synthesis of new proteins, it can take a number of days for the full induction potential of a drug to be realized.

Several hundred drugs are known to induce drug-metabolizing enzymes. The list includes hypnotics, sedatives, hypoglycaemic drugs, muscle relaxants, analgesics, antihistamines, steroid and thyroid hormones and many polycyclic aromatic hydrocarbons. These agents represent a diverse group of compounds with different chemical and pharmacological properties. The only common factor appears to be their high lipid-solubility.

Phenobarbitone is one of the most well-known enzyme-inducing drugs. Clinically significant interaction can occur when it is used in combination with phenytoin in the treatment of epilepsy. Adjustment of phenytoin dosage in these circumstances may be required to avoid therapeutic failure. Phenobarbitone has also been shown to reduce the therapeutic efficacy of concurrently administered chloramphenicol, griseofulvin and cortisol. Similarly, the efficacy of systemic corticosteroid therapy may be reduced by concurrent administration of phenylbutazone or phenytoin.

Metabolism of a drug may also be inhibited by other drugs. This would result in prolongation of the biological half-life of the drug and an increase in therapeutic efficacy. Of course, potentiation of toxicity is also possible. The drugs which are most likely to be involved in clinically important interactions of this type are those with a low therapeutic index, where inhibition of metabolism is likely to cause toxic effects. The inhibition is usually competitive and it may require several days of drug administration before the concentration of the inhibitor reaches a level at which inhibition of metabolism of the other drug results in a clinically significant effect. In most cases, the enzymes involved in drug metabolism are not saturated by the dose of drug, and the functional reserve of catalytic capacity prevents the development of observable and clinically significant interaction.

The irreversible inactivation by chloramphenicol of a major group of metabolic enzymes does have important consequences in animal medicine. Chloramphenicol is a substrate for cytochrome P_{450}-dependent monooxygenases of liver endoplasmic reticulum. It is rapidly metabolized to a reactive product, which covalently binds to the enzyme and irreversibly inactivates it. Thus other drugs administered concurrently show marked increases in potency. For example, the duration of pentobarbitone-induced anaesthesia in cats and dogs is greatly prolonged following chloramphenicol therapy. The potentiating effect can still be seen 3 weeks after cessation of chloramphenicol administration in dogs. This delay in return to normal function may be associated with the time required for membrane protein turnover and replacement of inactive enzyme by newly synthesized protein.

Drug interactions and drug excretion

There are a number of different drug interaction mechanisms which involve renal excretion. Drugs which alter renal blood flow modify the renal clearance of other drugs. Also, since only free drug is filtered at the glomerulus, drugs which displace others from protein-binding sites may increase the rate of renal excretion of the displaced drug. Furthermore, carriers for active tubular transport have a limited capacity, and competition for these tubular secretion mechanisms will also alter the excretion of competing drugs and can lead to drug interactions. Clinically significant interactions of this type usually involve competing anions.

Drugs which alter urinary pH can alter the extent of tubular reabsorption of ionizable drugs. Alkalinization of the urine with, for example, sodium bicarbonate, increases the degree of ionization of weak acids in the tubular lumen. Uptake of the ionized form into the blood is thereby reduced and the excretion of the drug is enhanced. This effect may be of use in therapy with sulphonamides where crystalluria, due to precipitation of poorly soluble unionized sulphonamide in tubular urine with a low pH, can occur. Urinary alkalinization increases the excretion of the sulphonamides and prevents the development of crystalluria. Conversely, drugs which acidify the urine, such as ascorbic acid or ammonium chloride, are contraindicated during sulphonamide therapy.

Alterations in urine flow may also be important in drug interactions. For example, water or osmotic diuresis increases drug excretion rates. In some situations, diuretics compete with other drugs for tubular transport carriers and this may decrease the renal excretion of the drug.

Interactions at drug receptor sites

Drugs may interact at receptor sites in a competitive manner, e.g. morphine–naloxone, or by interference with some part of the pathway leading to the receptor site. Some of the most commonly recognized interactions (both therapeutically useful and potentially dangerous) come into this group. In many of these cases, the exact mechanism of the interaction is not clear and the discussion below is arranged according to the therapeutic application of the drugs.

Neuromuscular blocking agents, antibiotics and general anaesthetics

Aminoglycoside antibiotics (streptomycin, dihydrostreptomycin, neomycin, gentamicin and kanamycin) have been shown to produce skeletal neuro-muscular blockade. The mechanism of this effect involves competition with acetylcholine for its receptors at the skeletal neuromuscular junction, similar to that which occurs with tubocurarine, gallamine and pancuronium. Thus combinations of aminoglycoside antibiotics and non-depolarizing neuromuscular blockers can lead to excessive muscle relaxation. Other chemotherapeutic agents, including lincomycin, clindamycin and the polymyxins, also exert a neuromuscular blocking effect and the use of non-depolarizing neuromuscular blocking agents in patients being treated with these is not recommended.

The effects of non-depolarizing neuromuscular blocking agents are potentiated by some general anaesthetics, including ether, halothane, methoxyflurane and enflurane. Thus in patients anaesthetized with these agents, reduced doses of neuromuscular blockers should be used. Furthermore, the combined neuromuscular relaxant effects of parenterally administered aminoglycoside antibiotics and the general anaesthetics above may lead to respiratory failure.

The acetylcholinesterase inhibitor neostigmine is commonly used to reverse the neuromuscular block produced by the non-depolarizing agents (see below). Neostigmine, however, should not be used for this purpose in patients treated with the depolarizing agent suxamethonium as potentiation of the initial depolarization may prolong the effect of suxamethonium. Furthermore, since the metabolism of suxamethonium by plasma pseudocholinesterase can be inhibited by some anticholinesterases, these will also prolong the duration of action of concurrently administered suxamethonium. Other drugs, including promethazine, diphenhydramine and chlorpromazine, also inhibit the enzyme and can thereby potentiate suxamethonium-induced neuromuscular blockade. The use of suxamethonium should be avoided in animals being treated with these drugs.

Halothane, one of the most widely used inhalation anaesthetics, causes cardiovascular depression, which results in reduced heart rate and blood pressure. Methoxyflurane also has a depressor effect. Use of adrenaline and noradrenaline to reverse the hypotension should be avoided because their arrhythmogenic activity is increased in the presence of these general anaesthetics (and many others). Similarly, the use of sympathomimetic amines for the treatment of cardiac arrest occurring during the use of these anaesthetics should be avoided.

Acetylcholinesterase inhibitors

With the exception of edrophonium and neostigmine, acetylcholinesterase inhibitors are most widely used in veterinary practice as anthelmintics and pesticides. They are potentially toxic to humans and animals and many instances of poisoning, accidental or deliberate, have been recorded. Toxicity is characterized by excessive cholinergic stimulation, which leads to vomiting and salivation as early signs. In these cases, vomiting should not be controlled by the use of neuroleptic drugs such as phenothiazine derivatives, nor by metoclopramide. Manufacturers of anthelmintic preparations containing dichlorvos or levamisole recommend that concomitant use of phenothiazine tranquillizers should be avoided.

Many of the acetylcholinesterase inhibitors also inhibit plasma pseudo-cholinesterase, and their potential for interactions with suxamethonium is described above. Although some of the anticholinesterases (like malathion) do not have this effect, it may be best to avoid the use of suxamethonium in all cases.

Analgesics

The effects of narcotic analgesics can be antagonized by naloxone, a pure opioid antagonist. Nalorphine is a partial agonist and therefore cannot be used to antagonize the effects of drugs such as pentazocine, which is also a partial agonist.

Anticholinesterases increase the analgesic effects of morphine. It is possible that this interaction is associated with an increased level of acetylcholine in the brain, since potentiation occurs only with those anticholinesterases which cross the blood–brain barrier.

Fentanyl and droperidol have synergistic effects which have been observed under clinical conditions. Doses which do not produce analgesia when administered alone, will do so when administered in combination. This effect is of clinical importance in the technique of neuroleptanalgesia. However, it should also be noted that doses of the two drugs which do not produce respiratory depression when administered alone, do so when administered in combination.

Antibiotics and other antimicrobials

Alterations in urinary pH may reduce the effectiveness of a number of antibiotics and antimicrobials used for the treatment of urinary tract infections. For example, under acidic conditions, the antibacterial actions of erythromycin, cephaloridine and aminoglycoside antibiotics are reduced. In contrast, the efficacy of the tetracyclines, nitrofurantoin and the urinary antiseptics nalidixic acid, hexamine and mandelic acid is enhanced under acidic conditions. Urinary pH may also alter the solubility of substances excreted via the kidneys, such as sulphonamides and their metabolites. These are more soluble at alkaline pH and therefore urinary acidifiers should not be administered to patients taking sulphonamides.

Cardiac glycosides

Cardiac glycosides act by inhibiting the enzyme which regulates the transport of Na^+ and K^+ across the myocardial cell membrane (see page 211).

The result is a decrease in the concentration of intracellular K^+. This effect can be exacerbated by the concurrent administration of diuretics which increase K^+ excretion. This interaction is likely to be responsible, at least in part, for the increased toxic effects of glycosides in patients also receiving diuretics. It is generally recommended that potassium supplements should be considered for all patients being treated with cardiac glycosides where K^+ depletion by concurrently administered diuretics may increase glycoside toxicity.

It is clear that drug interactions are of considerable importance in the practice of veterinary medicine. The likelihood of such interactions is increasing with the increased tendency to employ multiple drug therapy. Some of the interactions are dangerous, to the point of being life-threatening, others may be deliberately employed to improve treatment. A sound understanding of the pharmacodynamics and pharmacokinetics of the drugs involved is necessary to anticipate the former and most effectively employ the latter.

DRUGS AND THE LAW

In all developed countries the manufacture, importation and distribution of medicinal products are controlled by law. In the UK, controls are effected under the provisions of the Medicines Act (1968) and the Misuse of Drugs Act (1971). The Orders and Regulations of these Acts allow for modifications to be made without the need for new Acts to be introduced. In this way, subsidiary legislation can be readily passed when, for example, new products are developed. Details of the legislation are available in a booklet, *Legislation Affecting the Veterinary Profession in the United Kingdom*, which is published and updated annually by the Royal College of Veterinary Surgeons. The overall aim of the legislation is to control matters associated with the safety, quality and efficacy of medicines, for human and animal use.

In order to maintain high standards of safety and practice in the prescription and retailing of veterinary medicines, the British Veterinary Association has formulated a Code of Practice for the Sale or Supply of Animal Medicines by Veterinary Surgeons (*Veterinary Record*, September 1990) and a Code of Practice for Prescribing Medicinal Products by Veterinary Surgeons (*Veterinary Record*, September 1991). These codes are recommended by the British Veterinary Association, Royal College of Veterinary Surgeons and Ministry of Agriculture, Fisheries and Food (MAFF) and incorporate many of the changes associated with the control of prescribing, dispensing and selling animal medicines by European law which became effective at the start of 1992.

The Medicines Act (1968)

The Medicines Act is essentially a licensing system which is administered by the Secretaries of State for Health and Agriculture, who are advised by the Medicines Commission and a number of expert committees. The expert committee most concerned with veterinary medicine is the Veterinary Products Committee, which reports to the Minister of Agriculture. The work of the Committee also includes the promotion of efforts to collect and investigate information relating to adverse reactions to veterinary medicines. These effects include those observed in animals receiving the drugs and also those in any persons who handle the drug during its administration to animals. Reports of adverse reactions may be made by veterinarians on forms which are available from the Veterinary Medicines Directorate, Freepost, Woodham Lane, New Haw, Addlestone, Surrey KT15 3NB.

Before a new drug can be tested in the field, an Animal Test Certificate, issued by the Veterinary Products Committee, is required. The projected trial procedure must be justified in terms of the pharmacological activity and pharmacokinetics of the drug and the dosage and formulation to be used. The manufacture, sale and supply of the product for the purposes of the test can then proceed.

The control of importation, manufacture and distribution of medicines is controlled by the issue of three types of licences: product licences, manufacturer's licences and wholesale dealer's licences. Product licences are held by 'the person responsible for the composition' of the product or by the importer, and allow the sale, supply, import or export of the product concerned.

Since 1971, a system has been in place which requires a new drug to be approved for veterinary use by the Veterinary Products Committee before marketing. A much larger volume of data which relates to the synthesis, purity, stability, pharmacological activity, pharmacokinetics, therapeutic efficacy and adverse effects must be submitted by the manufacturers. This is carefully scrutinized by the Committee in relation to the projected use of the drug and the alternative therapy available. If the application is successful, a Full Product Licence is granted to the manufacturer or importer. Preparations on the market before 1971 were granted Product Licences of Right but this is an interim provision and these products will have to be withdrawn if they do not meet the requirements for new drugs. Drugs which are adopted from human medicine have undergone a similar examination by the relevant authorities before their approval for human use.

Where there has been a breach of the licensing conditions for a product it may be necessary to alter the product licence or to amend the product literature accordingly.

Where the professional judgement of a veterinarian dictates that a particular medicinal product is indicated for the treatment of an animal or herd under his/her care, exemption from the licensing restrictions is usually granted under the Act. Thus, the veterinarian is able to prepare or procure the manufacture of the product without a licence. On the issue of a prescription for a medicinal product by the veterinarian, this exemption is extended to the pharmacist. These exemptions may not apply to certain immunological products, such as poultry vaccines. Other vaccines may be prepared without a licence only if they are autogenous. Plasma and serum for passive immunization may be prepared without a licence only if it is intended for use within the same herd as the source animal.

Data sheets

A data sheet must be supplied by the manufacturer for each product which is promoted. The information which must be included in the data sheets is laid down in the Medicines (Data Sheet) Regulations (1972) and is required to be updated every 15 months.

The data sheet forms a standard reference for the veterinarian and includes basic information on indications, dosage and precautions for the product. If a product is used for purposes other than those indicated on the data sheet, the veterinarian does so at his/her own risk and without recourse to the licence holder. Further information about a product may be available on request from the licence holder. The National Office of Animal Health Ltd. publishes a Compendium of Data Sheets for Veterinary Products every 15 months which serves as a useful reference source.

Classification of medicinal products

The Medicines Act (1968) classifies medicinal products into five main legal categories:

1. GSL—A preparation which comes within the General Sales List. These do not require a prescription and can be sold by anyone.
2. P—A pharmacy medicine, which can be sold by a retail pharmacy. Very few veterinary medicinal products fall into this category.
3. PML—The Pharmacy and Merchant's List, which contains preparations that come within Schedule 1 to The Medicines (Exemptions from Restrictions on the Retail Sale or Supply of Veterinary Drugs) Order (1984), as amended, and can thus be sold by a retail pharmacy or a registered agricultural merchant.
4. POM—A Prescription Only Medicine. Products in this category can only be supplied by a veterinarian or by a pharmacist according to the prescription of a veterinarian. Prescriptions for POMs must fulfil strict requirements (see Appendix 2).
5. CD—Controlled drugs, which are divided into five schedules, according to the Misuse of Drugs Regulations 1985 (see below).

Veterinarians are bound by the Act, apart from ethical considerations, to supply or prescribe P, PML or POM drugs only for animals or herds which are under their care.

In addition to the categories described above, the non-general sales list of veterinary products is permitted by The Medicines (Exemptions from Restriction on the Retail Sale or Supply of Veterinary Drugs) Order 1985 (with later amendments). Preparations in the list are detailed in Schedules 1 to 4 of the Order and may be sold by pharmacists, agricultural merchants and certain other persons:

Schedule 1

This comprises the Merchant's List or Farmer's List of PML products which includes anthelmintics, vaccines, certain growth promoters and sheep dips. The Code of Practice for Merchants Selling or Supplying Veterinary Drugs states the rules relating to the sale of products in Schedule 1. These products can only be sold to a farmer or a person who maintains animals for business purposes. No prescription or pharmacist's supervision is required for their sale.

Schedules 2 and 3

These are concerned with medicated feedstuffs. Where medicinal products are to be incorporated into animal fodder it must be in accordance with the Product Licence, Animal Test Certificate or the veterinarian's written direction (VWD). Where a PML product is intended for incorporation at a specified concentration for a particular species, a VWD is not mandatory for the incorporation or subsequent supply of the final feed. If the product is to be added in any way not in accord with the product licence, a VWD is required. The incorporation of POMs into feedstuffs and their supply requires detailed, unambiguous instructions from the veterinarian. It is illegal to authorize the incorporation of a medicine which is not licensed for in-feed use. Forms and advisory notes are available from the British Veterinary Association. If there is any doubt that the form complies with the statutory requirements, the VWD will not be accepted by the compounder.

Schedule 4

This contains a limited range of horse wormers which saddlers, registered merchants and pharmacists are permitted to sell.

An important aspect of the safety of medicines used in veterinary practice relates to the residues of drugs in the carcasses of animals intended for human consumption. The monitoring of such agents in animal products in the UK is the responsibility of the Ministry of Agriculture, Fisheries and Food (MAFF). In recent years EC legislation to prohibit or control the use of some substances in food animals has been enacted. The MAFF, with the co-operation of a number of interested organizations, was also responsible for the development of the Code of Practice for the Safe Use of Veterinary Medicines on Farms. The Code stresses the importance of recording the use of medicines and observation of withdrawal periods.

Labelling requirements

Medicinal products

There are precise requirements for the labelling of containers and packages of medicinal products produced by the pharmaceutical companies which are detailed in the Regulations of the Medicines Act 1968. When these medicines (GSL, PML, P or POM) are supplied or sold by a veterinarian (or by a pharmacist under the veterinarian's instructions) for administration to animals under his/her care they are defined as 'dispensed medicines' and, as such, are exempt from detailed labelling requirements. The labels of 'dispensed medicines' must, however, always clearly, legibly and indelibly indicate:

1. The name of the person who has possession or control of the animal or herd and the address of the premises where the animal or herd is kept, or the address of one such site.
2. The name and address of the veterinarian.
3. The date of dispensing.
4. The words 'for animal treatment only', unless the container or package is too small for this to be reasonably included.
5. The words 'keep out of the reach of children', or words to that effect.
6. If the preparation is an embrocation, liniment, lotion, liquid antiseptic or other liquid preparation or gel for external use only, the words 'for external use only'.
7. If the product contains hexachlorophene and is for oral administration for the prevention or treatment of fluke disease in sheep or cattle, a warning that protective clothing must be worn by the operator when the product is being administered. If the product is for use in cattle, a warning that it must not be used in lactating cows.
   Note: Particulars relating to items 6 and 7 must be enclosed in a rectangle. If any of the required information appears on the supplier's label, it need not be repeated by the dispenser.

The provision of information relating to the name of the product, directions for use and precautions relating to the use of the product is not mandatory, and may be added at the discretion of the dispensing veterinarian. Where the product is being dispensed by a pharmacist according to the prescription of a veterinarian, instructions to include this additional information may be given (see page 577).

The relevant withdrawal period should always be stated on medicinal products for food animals.

Dispensed medicinal products to be incorporated into animal feedstuff and medicated animal feedstuff.

If the drug or preparation concerned has been granted a product licence, the container and the package must bear the manufacturer's labelling particulars when dispensed. Furthermore, items 1–7 (above) must appear on both the container and the package when dispensed medicinal products are to be incorporated into animal feedstuff.

Dispensing requirements

Although there is no legal requirement to dispense capsules or tablets in child-resistant containers, this is good practice unless there is a clear reason for doing otherwise. Paper envelopes and plastic bags are unacceptable as the sole container for medicinal products. Liquid products which are intended for external use (apart from eye or ear drops, which may be dispensed in the original pack), should be dispensed in fluted bottles unless the volume exceeds 1.14 l. Liquids intended to be consumed should be dispensed in plain glass bottles.

Record keeping

Although, at the time of writing, there are no formal requirements for the maintenance of records other than those for Schedule 2 drugs listed below, it is likely that EC legislation relating to record keeping will soon apply to other drugs. Products which are likely to be included in the legislation include those for use in food-producing animals which are POMs and any P, PML or GSL products where a withdrawal period must be observed. The records should contain the following information relating to each incoming or outgoing transaction: date, identity of the product, manufacturer's batch number, quantity received, quantity supplied, name and address of recipient, name and address of prescribing veterinarian (where applicable). These records should be kept available for inspection for three years.

The Misuse of Drugs Act (1971)

The Misuse of Drugs Act (1971) places more stringent controls on drugs which are considered to be 'dangerous or otherwise harmful' and restricts their supply, purchase and possession to authorized persons. Veterinarians who use drugs which fall under the provisions of this Act for legitimate professional purposes are considered to be authorized persons provided that all transactions are carried out in accordance with the restrictions defined in the Act and Regulations. The Misuse of Drugs Regulations (1985) classifies controlled drugs into five schedules, as shown in Table A1.1.

The Misuse of Drugs Regulations (1985) lay down special requirements relating to the writing of prescriptions for products coming within Schedules 2 and 3 (see Appendix 2). Drugs listed in Schedules 2 and 3 may only be obtained by a veterinarian by submitting a signed requisition which includes the name and address of the veterinarian, the purpose for which the drug is required and the total quantity required.

Table A1.1 Drug Schedules under the Misuse of Drugs Act (1971)

Schedule 1:	Includes cannabis and hallucinogens such as lysergic acid diethylamide (LSD). No recognized therapeutic uses. Veterinarians have no general authority to possess or use these drugs.
Schedule 2:	Includes drugs with a high abuse potential, e.g. narcotic analgesics (etorphine, morphine, pethidine, etc.), quinalbarbitone and amphetamine. Special prescription/requisition requirements and entry in controlled drugs register. Must be stored in a locked container.
Schedule 3:	Includes diethylpropion, pentazocine and some barbiturates (e.g. pentobarbitone). Special prescription/requisition requirements but no entry in the controlled drugs register. Locked storage only for diethylpropion.
Schedule 4:	Devoted to the benzodiazepines. Exempted from restrictions as controlled drugs when used in veterinary practice.
Schedule 5:	Includes some preparations containing codeine, morphine, cocaine and pholcodine. Exempted from restrictions as controlled drugs when used in veterinary practice.

Records of controlled drugs

The requirements for the maintenance of records relating to the purchase, administration and supply of controlled substances by the veterinarian concerns only drugs which are listed in Schedule 2. Entries must be made in a bound book which constitutes the register of controlled drugs, which must be kept on all premises where stocks of scheduled drugs are held. The register, which is used only for the purpose of maintaining records of transactions in scheduled drugs, may be purchased in a printed form or prepared as shown in Fig. A1.1. In either case, a separate register must be kept for each class of drug (where a class of drugs is any drug and its salts, stereoisomers and any preparation in which it is contained). Each record in the register is essentially a balance sheet for the drug concerned and relates the amount in stock to the amounts supplied on requisition and prescription. For the purposes of veterinary practice, the administration of a controlled drug to an animal is regarded as the supply of the drug to the owner of the animal. Details of the prescribed supply of a Schedule 2 drug by a pharmacist need not be included in the records of the prescribing veterinarian; these will be kept by the pharmacist concerned. Information relating to the receipt, administration or dispensing of a drug in Schedule 2 must be recorded, in chronological order, in the register within 24 hours of the transaction. No entry may be cancelled, obliterated or altered. Corrections must be made by marginal note or footnote, giving the date on which the correction was made. Registers must be retained for 2 years from the date of the last entry. Unrequired stocks of controlled drugs may be destroyed but entries of transactions of this nature must be witnessed by an authorized person (Drug Squad Officer or Home Office Inspector).

Police officers are empowered by the Act to enter the premises of a veterinarian and inspect the register and stocks of controlled drugs. Failure to keep adequate

Figure A1.1

Registers of controlled drugs obtained and supplied by a veterinary surgeon

IMMOBILON			
Date on which supply received	**Name and address of person or firm**	**Amount obtained**	**Form in which obtained**
13 January 1992	A. Mann Ltd., 2 Walsall Rd., Farnfield, Essex	2 × 21 ml	Small Animal Immobilon

PETHIDINE				
Date on which the transaction was effected	**Name and address of person or firm supplied**	**Particulars as to licence or authority of person or firm supplied to be in possession**	**Amount supplied**	**Form in which supplied**
20 January 1992	C. Sawyer, 12 Ross Way Farnfield	Dispensed	6 × 50 mg	Pethidine tablets
10 February 1992	J. Smith 10 The Avenue	Direct administration	25 mg	Pethidine injection 1 ml

Figure A1.1 Registers of controlled drugs obtained and supplied by a veterinary surgeon.

records, or the irresponsible supply of controlled drugs, may be dealt with by the Home Secretary, who has the power to prohibit the veterinarian from prescribing, administering or supplying controlled drugs. The law also provides for imprisonment of a veterinarian who is convicted of illegal supply of controlled drugs. Furthermore, the Royal College of Veterinary Surgeons Disciplinary Committee has the authority to remove from the Register the name of any veterinarian who is convicted of an offence under the Act.

Storage of controlled drugs

Schedule 2 drugs must be kept in a locked receptacle which can be opened only by the veterinarian or someone authorized by him/her. Each member of a practice should hold only one key. A locked car is not considered a locked receptacle within the meaning of the Misuse of Drugs (Safe Custody) Regulations (1973). Only the minimum quantity of controlled drugs which are consistent with the routine need and emergencies of the practice should be stored.

Of the drugs in Schedule 3, only the appetite suppressant diethylpropion must be stored in a locked receptacle. No special storage restrictions apply to drugs in Schedules 4 and 5 but it is clearly good practice to prevent the access to drugs of any kind by unauthorized persons.

Medicated feeds

There is an understandable public concern about what goes into food animals and then possibly into the human food chain. For example, premixes and additives (now called intermediate feeds) containing antibacterials, anthelmintics or coccidiostats are commonly incorporated into pig and poultry feeds for convenient mass therapy. Specified antibacterials (currently: avoparin, avilomycin, bacitracin zinc, bambera-mycin, monensin sodium, salmomycin, spiramycin, tylosin and virginiamycin) are licensed for in-feed use for growth promotion. It must be ensured that medicating feeds does not result in drug residues in meat and eggs.

UK legislation controlling medicated animal feeds was recently consolidated and extended by the Medicines (Medicated Animal Feeding Stuffs) Regulations 1989 (S.I. 1989, No: 2320) which also implement relevant EC directives. The legislation is designed principally to protect the public against medication residues from food animals.

The regulations apply to anyone who incorporates a medicinal product of any description in animal feedstuff, including liquid feed such as whey or skimmed milk, 'in the course of a business carried on by him': i.e. 'home-mixers' (e.g. farmers, keepers of zoo animals and keepers of dogs for business purposes) are affected, as well as commercial feed compounders. However, the legislation does not affect the owner of a companion animal administering a medicinal product by mixing it in the feed, since no business is involved, nor does it affect a farmer or similar person 'top-dressing' feed or medicating via the drinking water.

Registered feed compounders

The 1989 Regulations require all feed compounders—commercial and home mixers—who add medicines to feeds to register with the Royal Pharmaceutical Society of Great Britain (or the Department of Agriculture in Northern Ireland), who enforce the legislation and associated Codes of Practice.

Part A of the Register relates to feed compounders proposing to incorporate medicinal products at a dilution rate of less than 2 kg/tonne, i.e. where products more potent than those relevant to Part B are being incorporated; hence, the registration requirements are aimed primarily at commercial feed compounders.

Persons registered in Part A have to comply with the requirements of a stringent Category A Code of Practice, which covers premises, equipment, personnel and training, documentation and quality assurance. Failure to observe any of the provisions of the Code may lead to removal from the Register.

Part B of the Register relates to compounders and home mixers incorporating medicinal products at a dilution rate of 2 kg/tonne or more. They have to comply with the requirements of a Category B Code of Practice, which are generally less stringent than those for Category A; they are designed to ensure that the minimum EC and UK standards are satisfied. Again, failure to comply with the requirements of the Code may lead to refusal to register or removal from the Register.

The Regulations exempt fish farmers from the requirement to be on the Register.

Authority to medicate feedstuffs

A medicinal product, whether PML or POM, may only be incorporated in an animal feedstuff by an appropriately registered person (see above) in accordance with either (i) a relevant product licence or animal test certificate containing provisions—e.g. inclusion rates, species limitations—concerning incorporation of the product; or (ii) the Veterinary Written Direction (VWD) issued by veterinarians for the treatment of animals under their care.

PML products (e.g. coccidiostats, growth promoters) are primarily intended for incorporation at specified concentrations for particular species, and a VWD is not mandatory for incorporation or subsequent supply of the final feed. However, if they are to be incorporated at higher levels, or in any way not in accordance with the advice on the label of the product, a VWD is required. A VWD is generally mandatory for incorporation of a POM product, and certainly before such medicated feed is supplied to a farmer.

Veterinary Written Direction (VWD)

Medicinal products to be included in feed must, by law, be licensed for in-feed use, although the veterinarian may authorize use for species or conditions other than those specified in the product licence.

Prepared VWD pads are available from the BVA and advice on the completion of the VWD, and particularly on recommending withdrawal periods, has been provided in a composite statement by MAFF, RCVS and BVA. The statement emphasizes that the choice of medicinal product for inclusion in feed must be restricted to licensed products. They should, wherever possible, be used in accordance with the data sheet instructions as regards inclusion rates, target species and withdrawal periods.

When a licensed product is used for an unlicensed indication (e.g. non-target species), the following standard withdrawal periods should be used:

Eggs (all species)	7 days
Milk (all species)	7 days
Meat from poultry and mammals	28 days
Meat from fish	500 degree days*

*Cumulative total of the mean daily water temperature in degrees Celsius on each day following the last treatment.

These standard withdrawal periods represent a minimum and veterinarians should always consider whether a longer period is more appropriate. The standard withdrawal periods are kept under review and may be changed in the light of new scientific evidence.

Section III of the VWD need only be completed in two emergency situations:

1. If incorporation of a product is required at less than 2 kg/tonne and the compounder or farmer is not on Part A of the Register.
2. If the compounder is not on Part A or Part B of the Register.

In either case, the person incorporating the medicinal product must send a copy of the VWD to the Royal Pharmaceutical Society of Great Britain or Department of Agriculture of Northern Ireland (DANI) within 28 days of incorporation.

PRESCRIPTION WRITING

In order for drugs to be dispensed by a pharmacist for animal use, a prescription written by the veterinarian is required. A number of criteria must be satisfied before a prescription is deemed to be acceptable and the information which must be included and the conventions of prescription writing are outlined below and summarized in Table A2.1.

Table A2.1 Legal requirements for prescriptions

Prescription only medicines	Schedule 2 and 3 drugs
Written in ink (or otherwise indelible)	Written in ink (or otherwise) indelible)
Prescriber's address	Prescriber's address
Name and address of person to whom drug is to be delivered*	Name and address of person to whom drug is to be delivered*
Date of writing*	Date of writing*
	Total quantity (in words and figures), form and strength of preparation (where appropriate)†*
	The dose*
	The words 'For Animal Treatment Only'
Declaration that the drug is for an animal or herd under the care of the prescriber	Declaration that the drug is for an animal or herd under the care of the prescriber
Prescriber's signature*	Prescriber's signature*
Indication that the prescriber is a veterinary surgeon or practitioner	Indication that the prescriber is a veterinary surgeon or practitioner

*The information must be handwritten.
†Does not apply to prescriptions for phenobarbitone or phenobarbitone sodium.

In the UK the precise format of a drug prescription depends on the classification of that drug under the Medicines Act 1968 (see Appendix 1). The formal requirements for the prescription of POMs (prescription only medicines) and drugs controlled under Schedules 2 and 3 of the Misuse of Drugs Regulations 1985 are clearly defined and preparations containing these drugs may not be dispensed unless all the requirements have been fulfilled. Prescriptions for PML products (pharmacy and merchant's list), pharmacy (P) medicines and General Sale List (GSL) preparations have no corresponding formal requirements, but if a standard prescription format is adopted there is less chance of ambiguity and error.

An example of a prescription is shown in Fig. A2.1. The drug to be dispensed, pethidine, is listed in Schedule 2 of the Misuse of Drugs Regulations 1985, and strict requirements are operative. Prescriptions are now most commonly written in English, but the use of Latin terms and abbreviations persists and remains acceptable. Some of the more commonly used Latin terms and their meanings are given in Table A2.2.

A. N. Other & A. Signature M'sRCVS
20 Long Lane, Seaford. RP2 3YZ
April 15, 1993

For Mrs. B. Client's dog
65 Vale Road
Seaford

R

Tablets Pethidine 50mg

Send 10 (ten)

Label give one tablet every 12 hours

For Animal Treatment Only

This prescription is issued in respect of an animal under my care

A. Signature MRCVS

Figure A2.1 A sample prescription. Prescriptions for Schedule 2 and 3 controlled drugs must be indelible. To minimize the possibility of forgery, the particulars shown underlined must be handwritten by the veterinary surgeon (except in the case of phenobarbitone and phenobarbitone sodium).

A prescription consists of the following components:

The Heading

The address of the prescribing veterinarian (which is usually printed).
The name and address of the client.
The date of the prescription.
The species of the patient may be included (to allow the pharmacist to check the dose).

The Superscription

The symbol ℞—an abbreviation of the word 'recipe' (this is now traditional rather than obligatory).

Table A2.2 Latin abbreviations used in prescriptions

Abbreviation	Latin	English
aa	ana	of each
a.c.	ante cibum	before food
ad	ad	up to
ad lib.	ad libitum	no limit (on amount to be used)
aeq.	aequalis	equal
agit.	agita	shake
altern.d.	alterno die	on alternate days
ante	ante	before
aq.	aqua	water
b.i.d.	bis in die	twice daily
b.d.s.	bis in die sumenda	to be taken twice a day
c.	cum	with
circa	circa	around
div.	divide	divide
dos.	dosis	dose
et	et	and
ext., extemp.	extemplo	immediately
ft.	fiat	let it be made
gtt.	gutta(e)	drops(s)
h.	hora	hour
id.	idem	the same
m.	misce	mix
m.d.u.	more dictu utendus	use as directed
mist.	mistura	mixture
mitt.	mitte	send
mor. dict.	more dicto	as directed
n.r., non rep.	non repetatur	do not repeat
non	non	not
o.m.	omne mane	every morning
o.n.	omne nocte	every evening
p.c., post cib.	post cibum	after food
p.r.n.	pro re nata	when needed

Table A2.2 (continued)

Abbreviation	Latin	English
parv.	parvus	small
pulv.	pulvis	powder
q.h.	quaque hora	every hour
q.q.h.	quaque quattuor horas	every four hours
Q.R.	quantum rectum	the correct quantity
q.s.	quantum sufficiat	sufficient
℞	recipe	recipe
r., rep., repet.(n)	repetatur	repeat (n times)
s	sine	without
s.o.s., si. op. sit.	si opus sit	if necessary
ss	semis	one half
sig.	signetur	write (on label)
solv.	solve	dissolve
stat.	statim	immediately
suff.	sufficiens	sufficient
t.d.s.	ter in die sumendus	to be given three times daily
t.i.d.	ter in die	three times daily
ut dict.	ut dictum	as directed
ut supr.	ut supra	as above

The Inscription

The name of the drug and the form and strength of the preparation to be dispensed. This is now most commonly the name (generic or brand) of a manufactured product but, occasionally, the pharmacist may be required to follow a recipe to prepare the medicine.
Note:
This is a formal requirement for drugs in Schedules 2 and 3 (MDA), but it is good prescribing practice to include this information on all prescriptions.

The prescriber may choose to specify a particular proprietary brand, in which case it will be dispensed. If the drug is prescribed by an approved (generic) name, the pharmacist may dispense any proprietary brand of that drug or preparation.

The Subscription

The prescriber instructs the pharmacist as to the nature of the final product (mixture, ointment, etc.) if a recipe, rather than a commercial preparation, is involved. The quantity to be dispensed is specified and the term 'send' is also used here.

The Signature

This is not (as might be expected) the signature of the prescriber, but is a set of instructions to be written on the label of the dispensed product. The words 'For Animal Treatment Only' must appear on all prescriptions for Schedule 2 and 3 drugs, and may be printed on the prescription form.

Note:
Although dosage information and special precautions related to the use of the medicine are mandatory only for Schedule 2 and 3 drugs, instructions for the inclusion of this information on all prescriptions are strongly recommended.

Declaration for POMs/controlled drugs

Prescriptions for these drugs must contain the statement 'This prescription is issued in respect of an animal under my care' (or some similar declaration). This may be printed on the prescription form.

If the prescriber wishes a repeat to be dispensed, the instructions are included at this point.

Prescriber's signature

The prescriber's signature and qualifications are written at the end of the prescription. This is optional for drugs which are not listed as POMs or controlled drugs.

Validity

Prescriptions for POMs are valid for 6 months from the date of issue and those for Schedule 2 and 3 drugs for 13 weeks. Where repeats are specified, they may be dispensed after the expiry of the original prescription. Prescriptions are only valid if the prescriber's address is in the UK.

INDEX

Where applicable, main entries are indicated by bold type.